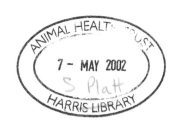

D1514841

CLINICAL PEDIATRIC NEUROLOGY

FOURTH EDITION

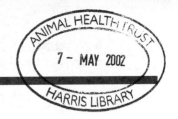

CLINICAL PEDIATRIC NEUROLOGY

A Signs and Symptoms Approach

Gerald M. Fenichel, MD

Professor and Chairman
Department of Neurology
Vanderbilt University School of Medicine
Nashville, Tennessee

W.B. SAUNDERS COMPANY
A Harcourt Health Sciences Company
Philadelphia London St. Louis Sydney Toronto

W.B. SAUNDERS COMPANY
A Harcourt Health Sciences Company

The Curtis Center
Independence Square West
Philadelphia, Pennsylvania 19106

Library of Congress Cataloging-in-Publication Data

Fenichel, Gerald M.
   Clinical pediatric neurology : a sign and symptoms approach / Gerald M. Fenichel.—
4th ed.

     p. ; cm.
   Includes bibliographical references and index.

   ISBN 0–7216–9234–6

   1. Pediatric neurology.   2. Nervous system—Diseases—Diagnosis.   I. Title.
   [DNLM: 1. Nervous System Diseases—Child.   2. Nervous System Diseases—Infant.   3.
Nervous System Diseases—diagnosis. WS 340 F333c 2001]

   RJ486.F46 2001

   618.92′8—dc21   00–061239

CLINICAL PEDIATRIC NEUROLOGY   ISBN 0–7216–9234–6

Printed in the United States of America

Last digit is the print number: 9   8   7   6   5   4   3   2   1

Preface

MUCH HAS HAPPENED in the 4 years since the third edition was published. The rapidity with which new information is emerging in genetics is astounding. It is not possible to stay current using print-based resources. I recommend two Web-based resources that I have used extensively: *Online Medelian Inheritance in Man* (http://www.ncbi.nih.gov/omim) and *GeneClinics* (http://www.geneclinics.org). The future of textbook publishing may be somewhat in doubt, but I suspect that the need to hold a book may last for another generation.

The main intent of this book is to provide an approach to the common presenting problems of children with disorders of the nervous system. I have maintained the general organization of the third edition, but the reader will find considerable change in the content of the fourth edition. The text remains a manual of practical information, much of it derived from my own experience. I have felt free to indicate my own biases concerning patient management in situations where a single standard of practice is not established.

I am grateful to the following colleagues who provided counsel: Patrick J.M. Lavin (Neuro-ophthalmology), Thomas L. Davis (Movement Disorders), and Neil Green (Orthopedic Surgery); and to Jeffrey Creasy, who provided new MRI images, and to Mrs. Lester Tilley, who keeps my office running so that I have the opportunity to write.

Gerald M. Fenichel, MD

Contents

Chapter 1
Paroxysmal Disorders

PAROXYSMAL DISORDERS ARE characterized by the sudden onset of neurological dysfunction. In children, such events often clear
completely and are caused by disturbance of ion
channels (*channelopathies*). Examples of channelopathies are genetic epilepsies, migraine, periodic paralysis, and paroxysmal movement disorders.

Approach to
Paroxysmal Disorders

The diagnosing physician almost never wit-
nesses the paroxysmal event. The nature of the
event must be surmised by listening to the eyewitness description offered by a family member
or, even worse, to the secondhand description
that the parent heard from the teacher. Most
"spells" are not seizures, and epilepsy is not a
diagnosis of exclusion. "Spells" seldom remain
unexplained after being viewed. Because observation of the spell is critical to diagnosis, the
event in question should be recorded on videotape. Most families either own or can borrow
a video camera; even if the camera must be pur-
chased, *it is more cost effective than brain imaging studies, and at least the family has something useful to show for the expenditure.*

Two questions must be asked. Has this ever
happened before? Does anyone else in the family
have similar episodes? It is remarkable how often this important information is not offered
unless requested. Episodic symptoms that last
only seconds and cause no abnormal signs are
rarely explained and usually do not warrant laboratory investigation. The differential diagnosis
of paroxysmal disorders is somewhat different

in the neonate, infant, child, and adolescent, and
is best presented by age groups.

Paroxysmal Disorders
of Newborns

Seizures are the main paroxysmal disorder of
the newborn. The challenge for the clinician is
to differentiate seizure activity from normal neonatal movements and from pathological movements caused by other mechanisms (Table 1-1).

Approach to Diagnosis

Seizure Patterns

Seizures in newborns, especially those who are
premature, are poorly organized and difficult
to distinguish from normal activity. Newborns
with hydranencephaly or atelencephaly are capable of generating the full variety of neonatal
seizure patterns. This supports the notion that
seizures may arise from the brainstem as well
as the hemispheres. Seizures arising in the brainstem may be confined there by the absence of
myelinated pathways for propagation. For the
same reason, seizures originating in one hemi-

Table 1-1
**Movements That Resemble
Neonatal Seizures**

Benign nocturnal myoclonus
Jitteriness
Nonconvulsive apnea
Normal movement
Opisthotonos
Pathological myoclonus

---

sphere are unlikely to spread beyond the contiguous cortex or to produce secondary bilateral synchrony.

Table 1-2 lists clinical patterns that have been associated with epileptiform discharges in newborns. This classification is useful but does not do justice to the rich variety of patterns actually observed or take into account that 50% of prolonged epileptiform discharges on the electroencephalogram (EEG) are not associated with visible clinical changes. Generalized tonic-clonic seizures do not occur. Many newborns suspected of having generalized tonic-clonic seizures are actually *jittery* (see Jitteriness, discussed later in this chapter). Newborns paralyzed with pancuronium to assist mechanical ventilation pose a special problem in seizure identification. In this circumstance physicians may be alerted to the possibility of seizures by the presence of rhythmic increases in systolic arterial blood pressure, heart rate, and oxygenation.

The term *subtle seizures* encompasses several different patterns in which tonic or clonic movements of the limbs are lacking. EEG monitoring has consistently failed to show that such movements are associated with epileptiform activity. One exception is tonic deviation of the eyes, which is almost always a seizure manifestation.

The definitive diagnosis of neonatal seizures often requires EEG monitoring. This is best accomplished with split-screen 16-channel video-EEG, but an ambulatory EEG cassette capable of marking the time of events can also be used. Epileptiform activity in the newborn is usually widespread and can be detected even when the newborn is clinically asymptomatic.

Focal Clonic Seizures

CLINICAL FEATURES. Repeated, irregular jerking movements affecting one limb or both limbs on one side are characteristic of focal clonic sei-

---

Table 1-2
Seizure Patterns in Newborns

Apnea with tonic stiffening of body
Focal clonic movements of one limb or both limbs on one side
Multifocal clonic limb movements
Myoclonic jerking
Paroxysmal laughing
Tonic deviation of the eyes upward or to one side
Tonic stiffening of the body

---

zures. The movements are rarely sustained for long periods, and they do not "march" as though spreading along the motor cortex. *In an otherwise alert and responsive full-term newborn, focal clonic seizures always indicate a cerebral infarction or hemorrhage.* In newborns with states of decreased consciousness, focal clonic seizures may indicate a focal infarction superimposed on a generalized encephalopathy.

DIAGNOSIS. During the seizure, the EEG may show a unilateral focus of high-amplitude sharp waves adjacent to the rolandic fissure. The discharge can spread to involve contiguous areas in the same hemisphere and can be associated with unilateral seizures of the limbs and adversive movements of the head and eyes. The interictal EEG usually shows focal slowing or amplitude attenuation.

Newborns with focal clonic seizures should be evaluated immediately using noncontrast-enhanced computed tomography (CT) or ultrasound to look for intracerebral hemorrhage. If the CT is normal, contrast-enhanced CT or magnetic resonance imaging (MRI) should be done 3 days later to look for cerebral infarction. Ultrasound is not useful in detecting small cerebral infarctions.

Multifocal Clonic Seizures

CLINICAL FEATURES. In multifocal clonic seizures, migratory jerking movements are noted in first one limb and then another; facial muscles may be involved as well. The migration appears random and does not follow expected patterns of epileptic spread. Movements in one limb are sometimes prolonged, suggesting a focal rather than a multifocal seizure. The multifocal nature is detected later, when nursing notes are found to be contradictory concerning the side or the limb affected. Multifocal clonic seizures are a neonatal equivalent of generalized tonic-clonic seizures. They are ordinarily associated with severe, generalized cerebral disturbances such as hypoxic-ischemic encephalopathy.

DIAGNOSIS. Multifocal epileptiform activity can usually be detected on a standard EEG. If epileptiform activity is not seen, a 24-hour monitor is recommended.

Myoclonic Seizures

CLINICAL FEATURES. Brief, repeated extension and flexion movements of the arms, the legs, or all limbs characterize myoclonic seizures. They constitute an uncommon seizure pattern in the newborn, but their presence suggests severe, diffuse brain damage.

DIAGNOSIS. No specific EEG pattern is associated with myoclonic seizures in the newborn. Myoclonic jerks are often seen in babies born to drug-addicted mothers. Whether these movements are seizures, jitteriness, or myoclonus (discussed later) is uncertain.

Tonic Seizures

CLINICAL FEATURES. Tonic seizures are characterized by extension and stiffening of the body, usually associated with apnea and upward deviation of the eyes. Tonic posturing without the other features is rarely a seizure manifestation. Tonic seizures are more common in premature than in full-term newborns and usually indicate structural brain damage rather than a metabolic disturbance.

DIAGNOSIS. Tonic seizures in premature newborns are often a symptom of intraventricular hemorrhage and are an indication for ultrasound study. Tonic posturing also occurs in newborns with forebrain damage, not as a seizure manifestation but as a disinhibition of brainstem reflexes. Prolonged disinhibition results in *decerebrate posturing,* an extension of the body and limbs associated with internal rotation of the arms, dilation of the pupils, and downward deviation of the eyes. Decerebrate posturing is often encountered as a terminal sign in premature infants with intraventricular hemorrhage caused by pressure on the upper brainstem (see Chapter 4).

Tonic seizures and decerebrate posturing must also be distinguished from *opisthotonos,* a prolonged arching of the back not necessarily associated with eye movements. Opisthotonos is probably caused by meningeal irritation and is seen in kernicterus, infantile Gaucher disease, and some aminoacidurias.

Apnea

CLINICAL FEATURES. An irregular respiratory pattern with intermittent pauses of 3 to 6 seconds, often followed by 10 to 15 seconds of hyperpnea, is regularly seen in premature infants. The pauses are not associated with significant alterations in heart rate, blood pressure, body temperature, or skin color. This respiratory pattern, termed *periodic breathing,* is caused by immaturity of the brainstem respiratory centers. The incidence of periodic breathing correlates directly with the degree of prematu-

rity. Apneic spells are more common during active than quiet sleep.

Apneic spells of 10 to 15 seconds are detectable at some time in almost all premature and some full-term newborns. Apneic spells of 10 to 20 seconds are usually associated with a 20% reduction in heart rate. Longer episodes of apnea are almost invariably associated with a 40% or greater reduction in heart rate. The frequency of these apneic spells correlates with brainstem myelination. Even at 40 weeks conceptional age, premature newborns continue to have a higher incidence of apnea than do full-term newborns. The incidence of apnea sharply decreases in all infants at 52 weeks conceptional age.

DIAGNOSIS. Apneic spells in an otherwise normal-appearing newborn should be considered a sign of brainstem immaturity and not a pathological condition. The sudden onset of apnea and states of decreased consciousness, especially in premature newborns, suggests an intracranial hemorrhage with brainstem compression. Immediate ultrasound examination is indicated.

Apneic spells are almost never a seizure manifestation unless they are associated with tonic deviation of the eyes, tonic stiffening of the body, or characteristic limb movements. The absence of bradycardia in association with prolonged apnea suggests the possibility of seizures.

MANAGEMENT. Short episodes of apnea do not require intervention.

Benign Nocturnal Myoclonus

CLINICAL FEATURES. Sudden jerking movements of the limbs during sleep occur in normal people of all ages (see Chapter 14). They appear primarily during the early stages of sleep as repeated flexion movements of the fingers, wrists, and elbows. The jerks are never consistently localized, are not stopped by gentle restraint, but end abruptly with arousal. When prolonged, they may be misdiagnosed as focal clonic or myoclonic seizures.

DIAGNOSIS. Nocturnal myoclonus can be distinguished from seizures and jitteriness because it occurs solely during sleep, it is not activated by a stimulus, and the EEG is normal.

MANAGEMENT. Treatment is not required. Anticonvulsant drugs may increase the frequency of myoclonus by causing sedation.

Jitteriness

CLINICAL FEATURES. Jitteriness or tremulousness is an excessive response to stimulation. A low-frequency, high-amplitude shaking of the limbs and jaw is provoked by touch, noise, or motion. Jitteriness is commonly associated with a low threshold for the Moro reflex, but it can occur in the absence of any apparent stimulation and be confused with myoclonic seizures.

DIAGNOSIS. Jitteriness usually occurs in newborns with perinatal asphyxia that may have seizures as well. It can be distinguished from seizures by EEG monitoring, by the absence of eye movements or alteration in respiratory pattern, and by the presence of stimulus activation. Jitteriness is also encountered in newborns of addicted mothers and in newborns with metabolic disorders.

MANAGEMENT. Reduced stimulation decreases jitteriness. However, newborns of addicted mothers require sedation to facilitate feeding and to decrease energy expenditure.

Differential Diagnosis of Seizures

Seizures are a feature of almost all brain disorders in the newborn. The time of onset of the first seizure is very helpful in determining the cause (Table 1-3). Seizures occurring during the first 24 hours, and especially in the first 12 hours, are usually due to hypoxic-ischemic encephalopathy. Sepsis, meningitis, and subarachnoid hemorrhage are next in frequency, followed by intrauterine infection and trauma. Direct drug effects, intraventricular hemorrhage at term, and pyridoxine dependency are relatively rare causes of seizures.

During the period from 24 to 72 hours after birth, seizures are most commonly caused by intraventricular hemorrhage in premature newborns, by subarachnoid hemorrhage and cerebral contusion in large full-term newborns, and by sepsis and meningitis at all gestational ages. Focal clonic seizures in full-term newborns are usually caused by cerebral infarction, intracerebral hemorrhage, or venous thrombosis. Cerebral dysgenesis causes seizures at this time and remains an important cause of seizures throughout infancy. All other conditions are relatively rare. Newborns with metabolic disorders are usually lethargic and feed poorly before the onset of seizures.

After 72 hours, inborn errors of metabolism, especially aminoacidurias, become a more important consideration because protein and glucose feedings have been initiated. A battery of screening tests for metabolic disorders is outlined in Table 1-4. Herpes simplex infection is transmitted during delivery and does not be-

---

Table 1-3
Differential Diagnosis of Neonatal Seizures by Peak Time of Onset

24 Hours
Bacterial meningitis and sepsis (see Chapter 4)
Direct drug effect
Hypoxic-ischemic encephalopathy
Intrauterine infection (see Chapter 5)
Intraventricular hemorrhage at term (see Chapter 4)
Laceration of tentorium or falx
Pyridoxine dependency
Subarachnoid hemorrhage

24 to 72 Hours
Bacterial meningitis and sepsis (see Chapter 4)
Cerebral contusion with subdural hemorrhage
Cerebral dysgenesis (see Chapter 18)
Cerebral infarction (see Chapter 11)
Drug withdrawal
Glycine encephalopathy
Glycogen synthase deficiency
Hypoparathyroidism-hypocalcemia
Idiopathic cerebral venous thrombosis
Incontinentia pigmenti
Intracerebral hemorrhage (see Chapter 11)
Intraventricular hemorrhage in premature newborns (see Chapter 4)
Pyridoxine dependency
Subarachnoid hemorrhage
Tuberous sclerosis
Urea cycle disturbances

72 Hours to 1 Week
Familial neonatal seizures
Cerebral dysgenesis (see Chapter 18)
Cerebral infarction (see Chapter 11)
Hypoparathyroidism
Idiopathic cerebral venous thrombosis
Intracerebral hemorrhage (see Chapter 11)
Kernicterus
Methylmalonic acidemia
Nutritional hypocalcemia
Propionic acidemia
Tuberous sclerosis
Urea cycle disturbances

1 Week to 4 Weeks
Adrenoleukodystrophy, neonatal (see Chapter 6)
Cerebral dysgenesis (see Chapter 18)
Fructose dysmetabolism
Gaucher disease type 2 (see Chapter 5)
GM_1 gangliosidosis type 1 (see Chapter 5)
Herpes simplex encephalitis
Idiopathic cerebral venous thrombosis
Ketotic hyperglycinemias
Maple syrup urine disease, neonatal
Tuberous sclerosis
Urea cycle disturbances

---

come symptomatic until the second half of the first week. Among the conditions that cause early seizures and can also cause late seizures are cerebral dysgenesis, cerebral infarction, intracerebral hemorrhage, and familial neonatal seizures.

Table 1-4
Screening for Inborn Errors of Metabolism That Cause Neonatal Seizures

Blood Glucose Low
Fructose 1,6,-diphosphatase deficiency
Glycogen storage disease, type 1
Maple syrup urine disease

Blood Calcium Low
Hypoparathyroidism
Maternal hyperparathyroidism

Blood Ammonia High
Argininosuccinic acidemia
Carbamylphosphate synthetase deficiency
Citrullinemia
Methylmalonic acidemia (may be normal)
Multiple carboxylase deficiency
Ornithine transcarbamylase deficiency
Propionic acidemia (may be normal)

Blood Lactate High
Fructose 1,6,-diphosphatase deficiency
Glycogen storage disease, type 1
Mitochondrial disorders
Multiple carboxylase deficiency

Metabolic Acidosis
Fructose 1,6,-diphosphatase deficiency
Glycogen storage disease, type 1
Maple syrup urine disease
Methylmalonic acidemia
Multiple carboxylase deficiency
Propionic acidemia

Hypoxic-Ischemic Encephalopathy

Asphyxia at term is almost always an intrauterine event, and hypoxia and ischemia occur together; the result is hypoxic-ischemic encephalopathy (HIE). Acute total asphyxia often leads to death from circulatory collapse. Survivors are born comatose, have evidence of lower cranial nerve dysfunction, and always have severe neurological handicaps (Roland et al, 1998).

The usual mechanism of HIE in surviving full-term newborns is partial, prolonged asphyxia. The fetal circulation accommodates to reductions in arterial oxygen by maximizing blood flow to the brain, and to a lesser extent the heart, at the expense of other organs.

Clinical experience indicates that the fetus may be subjected to considerable hypoxia without the development of brain damage. The incidence of cerebral palsy among full-term newborns with a 5-minute Apgar score of 0 to 3 is only 1% if the 10-minute score is 4 or higher. Any episode of hypoxia sufficiently severe to cause brain damage also causes derangements in other organs. Newborns with mild HIE always have a history of irregular heart rate and usually pass meconium. Those with severe HIE may have lactic acidosis, elevated serum concentrations of hepatic enzymes, enterocolitis, renal failure, and fatal myocardial damage.

CLINICAL FEATURES. Mild HIE is relatively common. The newborn is lethargic but not unconscious immediately after birth. Other characteristic features are jitteriness and sympathetic overactivity (tachycardia, dilatation of pupils, and decreased bronchial and salivary secretions). Muscle tone is normal at rest, tendon reflexes are normoreactive or hyperactive, and ankle clonus is usually elicited. The Moro reflex is complete, and repetitive extension and flexion movements are generated by a single stimulus. Seizures are not an expected feature, and their occurrence suggests concurrent hypoglycemia or the presence of a second condition.

Symptoms diminish and disappear during the first few days, although some degree of overresponsiveness may persist. Newborns with mild HIE are believed to recover normal brain function completely. They are not at greater risk for later epilepsy or learning disabilities.

Newborns with severe HIE are stuporous or comatose immediately after birth, and respiratory effort is usually periodic and insufficient to sustain life. Seizures begin within the first 12 hours. Hypotonia is severe, and tendon reflexes, the Moro reflex, and the tonic neck reflex are absent as well. Sucking and swallowing are depressed or absent, but the pupillary and oculovestibular reflexes are present. Most of these newborns have frequent seizures, which may be appreciated only on EEG, that progress to status epilepticus. The response to anticonvulsant drugs is usually incomplete. Generalized increased intracranial pressure characterized by coma, bulging of the fontanelles, loss of pupillary and oculovestibular reflexes, and respiratory arrest develops between 24 and 72 hours of age.

The newborn may die at this time or may remain stuporous for several weeks. The encephalopathy begins to subside after the third day, and seizures decrease in frequency and eventually stop. Jitteriness is common as the child becomes arousable. Tone increases in the limbs during the succeeding weeks. Neurological sequelae are expected in newborns with severe HIE who remain comatose for more than a week.

DIAGNOSIS. EEG and CT are helpful in determining the severity and prognosis of HIE. In mild HIE the EEG background rhythms are normal or lacking in variability. In severe HIE the background is always abnormal and shows suppression of background amplitude. The degree of suppression correlates well with the severity of HIE. The worst case is a flat EEG or one with a burst-suppression pattern. A bad outcome is invariable if the amplitude remains suppressed for 2 weeks or a burst-suppression pattern is present at any time. Epileptiform activity may also be present but is less predictive of the outcome than is background suppression.

Two to 4 days after severe prolonged partial asphyxia, CT shows the cerebral edema as decreased tissue attenuation of the hemispheres. Repeat CT or MRI after 1 month shows the full extent of injury. Survivors of near-total asphyxia have decreased tissue attenuation in the basal ganglia and thalamus.

MANAGEMENT. The management of HIE in newborns requires immediate attention to derangements in several organs and correction of acidosis. Clinical experience indicates that control of seizures, maintenance of adequate ventilation and perfusion, and prevention of fluid overload increase the chance of a favorable outcome. Intracranial pressure may be lessened by the simple procedure of elevating the head to 30 degrees and reducing fluids by 10%.

The use of phenobarbital to treat seizures in newborns is detailed in a separate section. If high dosages of phenobarbital prove ineffective, other drugs are unlikely to be successful. Seizures usually cease spontaneously during the second week, and anticonvulsants should be stopped after a further 2 weeks of control. The incidence of later epilepsy among infants who had neonatal seizures caused by HIE is 30% to 40%. Continuing anticonvulsant therapy after the initial seizures have stopped does not influence the outcome (Hellström-Westas et al, 1995).

Trauma and Intracranial Hemorrhage

Neonatal head trauma occurs most often in large term newborns of primiparous mothers. Usually labor was prolonged and extraction was difficult because of fetal malposition or a precipitous delivery before the maternal cervix was sufficiently dilated. Intracranial hemorrhage may be subarachnoid, subdural, or intraventricular. Intraventricular hemorrhage is discussed in Chapter 4.

Idiopathic Cerebral Venous Thrombosis

Cerebral venous thrombosis in newborns may be caused by coagulopathies, polycythemia, sepsis, and asphyxia. Cerebral venous thrombosis, especially that involving the superior sagittal sinus, also occurs without known predisposing factors.

CLINICAL FEATURES. The initial symptom is focal seizures or lethargy beginning anytime during the first month. Intracranial pressure remains normal, lethargy slowly resolves, and seizures respond to phenobarbital. The long-term outcome is uncertain and probably depends upon the extent of hemorrhagic infarction of the hemisphere.

DIAGNOSIS. CT is satisfactory for diagnosis, but MRI provides a more comprehensive assessment of the involved vessels and the extent of brain damage.

MANAGEMENT. Anticoagulation does not influence the outcome and is not recommended.

Primary Subarachnoid Hemorrhage

CLINICAL FEATURES. Blood in the subarachnoid space probably originates from tearing of the superficial veins by shearing forces during a prolonged delivery with the head engaged. Mild HIE is often associated with subarachnoid hemorrhage, but the newborn is usually well when an unexpected seizure occurs on the first or second day of life. Lumbar puncture is performed because of suspected sepsis, and blood is found in the cerebrospinal fluid. Most newborns with subarachnoid hemorrhages will be neurologically normal later.

DIAGNOSIS. CT is useful to document the extent of hemorrhage. Blood is present in the interhemispheric fissure and the supratentorial and infratentorial recesses. Routine ultrasound does not reliably show blood in the subarachnoid space. Epileptiform activity may be seen on the EEG, but the background is not suppressed. This indicates that seizures are not caused by HIE and that the prognosis is more favorable. Clotting studies should be performed to exclude the possibility of a coagulopathy.

MANAGEMENT. Seizures usually respond to phenobarbital. Specific therapy is not available for the hemorrhage, and posthemorrhagic hydrocephalus is uncommon.

Subdural Hemorrhage

CLINICAL FEATURES. Subdural hemorrhage is usually the consequence of a tear in the tentorium near its junction with the falx. The tear is caused by excessive vertical molding of the head in vertex presentation, anteroposterior elongation of the head in face and brow presentations, or prolonged delivery of the aftercoming head in breech presentation. Blood collects in the posterior fossa and may produce brainstem compression. The initial features are those of mild to moderate HIE. Clinical evidence of brainstem compression is delayed for 12 hours or longer and is characterized by irregular respiration, an abnormal cry, declining consciousness, hypotonia, seizures, and a tense fontanelle. Intracerebellar hemorrhage is sometimes present. Mortality is high, and neurological impairment among survivors is common.

DIAGNOSIS. CT or ultrasound can be used to visualize subdural hemorrhages.

MANAGEMENT. Small hemorrhages do not require treatment, but large collections should be evacuated surgically to relieve brainstem compression.

Hypoglycemia

A transitory, asymptomatic hypoglycemia can be detected in 11% of newborns during the first hours after delivery and before oral feeding is initiated. Hypoglycemia is not associated with neurological impairment later in life. Symptomatic hypoglycemia may result from cerebral stress or inborn errors of metabolism (Table 1-5).

Table 1-5
Causes of Neonatal Hypoglycemia

Primary Transitional Hypoglycemia
Complicated labor and delivery
Intrauterine malnutrition
Maternal diabetes
Prematurity

Secondary Transitional Hypoglycemia
Asphyxia
Central nervous system disorders
Cold injuries
Sepsis

Persistent Hypoglycemia
Aminoacidurias
    Maple syrup urine disease
    Methylmalonic acidemia
    Propionic acidemia
    Tyrosinosis
Congenital hypopituitarism
Defects in carbohydrate metabolism
    Fructose 1–6, diphosphatase deficiency
    Fructose+ intolerance
    Galactosemia
    Glycogen storage disease, type 1
    Glycogen synthase deficiency
Hyperinsulinism
Organic acidurias
    Glutaric aciduria type 2
    3-Methyl glutaryl-CoA lyase deficiency

CLINICAL FEATURES. The time of onset of symptoms depends upon the underlying disorder. Early onset is generally associated with perinatal asphyxia or intracranial hemorrhage and late onset with inborn errors of metabolism. Hypoglycemia is rare and mild among newborns with classic maple syrup urine disease, ethylmalonic aciduria, and isovaleric acidemia and is invariably severe in those with 3-methylglutaconic aciduria, glutaric aciduria type 2, and disorders of fructose metabolism.

The syndrome includes any of the following symptoms: apnea, cyanosis, tachypnea, jitteriness, high-pitched cry, poor feeding, vomiting, apathy, hypotonia, seizures, and coma. Symptomatic hypoglycemia is often associated with later neurological impairment.

DIAGNOSIS. Neonatal hypoglycemia is defined as a whole blood glucose concentration of less than 20 mg/dl (1 mmol/L) in premature and low-birth-weight newborns, less than 30 mg/dl (1.5 mmol/L) in term newborns during the first 72 hours, and less than 40 mg/dl (2 mmol/L) in full-term newborns after 72 hours.

MANAGEMENT. Normal blood glucose concentrations can be restored by intravenous administration of glucose, but the underlying cause must be determined before definitive treatment can be provided.

Hypocalcemia

Hypocalcemia is defined as a blood calcium concentration less than 7 mg/dl (1.75 mmol/L). The onset of hypocalcemia in the first 72 hours after delivery is associated with low birth weight, asphyxia, maternal diabetes, transient neonatal hypoparathyroidism, maternal hyperparathyroidism, and the DiGeorge syndrome. Later-onset hypocalcemia is seen in children fed evaporated cow's milk and other improper formulas, in maternal hyperparathyroidism, and in the DiGeorge syndrome.

Hypoparathyroidism in the newborn may result from maternal hyperparathyroidism or may be a transitory phenomenon of unknown cause. Hypocalcemia occurs in less than 10% of stressed newborns and enhances their vulnerability to seizures, but it is rarely the primary cause.

DiGeorge Syndrome

The DiGeorge syndrome is associated with microdeletions of chromosome 22q11. The phenotype can be explained by disturbance of cervical neural crest migration into the derivatives of the pharyngeal arches and pouches. Organs derived from the third and fourth pharyngeal pouches (thymus, parathyroid gland, and great vessels) are hypoplastic.

CLINICAL FEATURES. The acronym CATCH is used to describe the phenotype of cardiac abnormality, T-cell deficit, clefting (multiple minor facial anomalies), and hypocalcemia (Burn, 1999). The symptoms may be due to congenital heart disease, hypocalcemia, or both. Jitteriness and tetany usually begin in the first 48 hours after delivery. The peak onset of seizures is on the third day but may be delayed for 2 weeks. Many affected newborns die of cardiac causes during the first month; survivors fail to thrive and have frequent infections because of the failure of cell-mediated immunity.

DIAGNOSIS. In newborns who come to medical attention because of heart disease, hypocalcemia may be suspected when a prolonged Q-T interval is detected on the electrocardiogram (ECG). All newborns with symptoms of hypocalcemia should be examined for cardiac defects.

MANAGEMENT. Hypocalcemia generally responds to parathyroid hormone or to oral calcium and vitamin D.

Aminoacidopathies

Maple Syrup Urine Disease

The neonatal form of maple syrup urine disease (MSUD) is caused by an almost complete absence (less than 2% of normal) of branched-chain ketoacid dehydrogenase (BCKD). BCKD is composed of six subunits, but the main abnormality in MSUD is deficiency of the E1 subunit on chromosome 19q13.1–q13.2. Leucine, isoleucine, and valine cannot be decarboxylated, and they accumulate in blood, urine, and tissues (Figure 1-1). Later-onset forms are described in Chapters 5 and 10. The defect is transmitted by autosomal recessive inheritance.

CLINICAL FEATURES. Affected newborns appear healthy at birth, but lethargy, feeding difficulty, and hypotonia develop after ingestion of protein. Seizures begin in the second week and are associated with the development of cerebral edema. Once seizures begin, they continue with increasing frequency and severity. Without therapy, cerebral edema becomes progressively worse and results in coma and death within 1 month.

DIAGNOSIS. Rapid screening of urine for MSUD can be accomplished by the addition of ferric chloride, which colors urine deep blue, or with 2,4-dinitrophenylhydrazine, which causes a cloudy yellow precipitate. The diagnosis is established by showing increased plasma concentrations of the three branch-chained amino acids or enzyme deficiency in peripheral leukocytes. Heterozygotes have diminished levels of enzyme activity.

MANAGEMENT. Hemodialysis may be necessary to correct the life-threatening metabolic acidosis. A trial of thiamine (10–20 mg/kg/day) is given because a thiamine-responsive MSUD variant exists. All natural protein intake must be stopped, and dehydration, electrolyte imbalance, and metabolic acidosis corrected. A special diet, low in branched-chain amino acids, may prevent further encephalopathy and should be started immediately by nasogastric tube. Newborns diagnosed in the first 2 weeks and treated rigorously have the best prognosis.

Glycine Encephalopathy

Glycine encephalopathy (nonketotic hyperglycinemia) is caused by a defect in the glycine cleaving system. It is inherited as an autosomal recessive trait.

CLINICAL FEATURES. Affected newborns are normal at birth but become irritable and refuse feeding anytime from 6 hours to 8 days after delivery. The onset of symptoms is usually within 48 hours but may be delayed by a few weeks in milder allelic forms. Hiccupping is an early and continuous feature; some mothers relate that the child hiccupped in utero. Progressive lethargy, hypotonia, respiratory disturbances, and myoclonic seizures follow. Some newborns survive the acute illness, but their subsequent course is characterized by mental retardation, epilepsy, and spasticity.

DIAGNOSIS. During the acute encephalopathy the EEG demonstrates a burst-suppression pattern, which later evolves into hypsarrhythmia during infancy. MRI shows partial agenesis of the corpus callosum. The diagnosis is established by showing hyperglycinemia, and especially elevated concentrations of glycine in the cerebrospinal fluid, in the absence of hyperammonemia or organic acidemia.

MANAGEMENT. No therapy has proven to be effective. Hemodialysis provides only temporary relief of the encephalopathy, and diet therapy has not proved successful in modifying the course. Diazepam, a competitor for glycine receptors, in combination with choline, folic acid, and sodium benzoate, may stop the seizures. Benzoate doses as high as 750 mg/kg are toler-

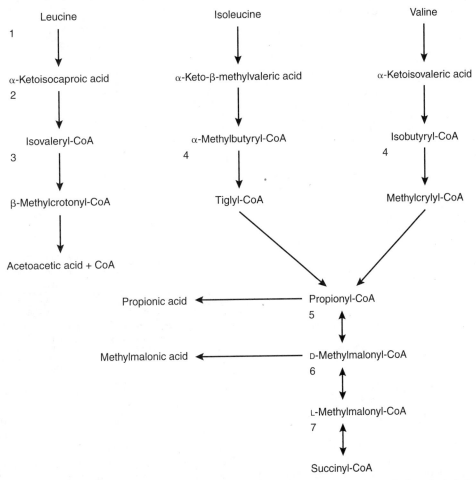

Figure 1-1. Branched-chain amino acid metabolism. 1. Transaminase system; 2. Branched-chain α-ketoacid dehydrogenase; 3. Isovaleryl-CoA dehydrogenase; 4. α-Methyl branched-chain acyl-CoA dehydrogenase; 5. Propionyl-CoA carboxylase (biotin cofactor); 6. Methylmalonyl-CoA racemase; 7. Methylmalonyl-CoA mutase (adenosylcobalamin cofactor).

ated and should be tried. Carnitine deficiency may be associated, and treatment with L-carnitine, 100 mg/kg/day, may increase the glycine conjugation with benzoate (Hamosh et al, 1998).

Urea Cycle Disturbances

Carbamyl phosphate synthetase (CPS) deficiency, ornithine transcarbamylase (OTC) deficiency, citrullinemia, argininosuccinic acidemia, and argininemia (arginase deficiency) are the disorders caused by defects in the enzyme systems responsible for urea synthesis (Figure 1-2). Arginase deficiency does not cause symptoms in the newborn. OTC deficiency is an X-linked trait; all others are transmitted by autosomal recessive inheritance. The prevalence of urea cy-

cle enzyme deficiencies is estimated to be 1 : 30,000 live births.

CLINICAL FEATURES. The clinical features of urea cycle disorders are due to ammonia intoxication (Table 1-6). Progressive lethargy, vomiting, and hypotonia may develop on the first day after delivery, even before the initiation of protein feeding, and are followed by progressive loss of consciousness and seizures on subsequent days. Vomiting and lethargy correlate well with plasma ammonia concentrations greater than 200 μg/dl (120 μmol/L); coma with concentrations greater than 300 μg/dl (180 μmol/L); and seizures with those greater than 500 μg/dl (300 μmol/L). Death follows quickly in untreated newborns. Newborns with partial deficiency of CPS and female carriers of OTC deficiency may become symptomatic after ingesting a large protein load.

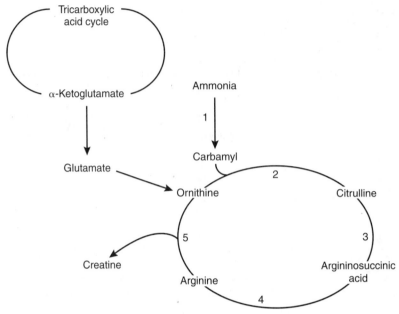

Figure 1-2. Ammonia metabolism. 1. Carbamyl phosphate synthetase (CPS); 2. Ornithine transcarbamylase (OTC); 3. Argininosuccinate synthetase (AS); 4. Argininosuccinate lyase (AL); 5. Arginase.

DIAGNOSIS. The diagnosis of a urea cycle disturbance should be suspected in every newborn with a compatible clinical syndrome and hyperammonemia without organic acidemia. Hyperammonemia can be life-threatening, and diagnosis within 24 hours is essential. The blood ammonia concentration should be analyzed immediately and the plasma studied for acid-base status and concentrations of quantitative amino acids, creatinine, sodium, potassium, chloride, calcium, glucose, free and total carnitine, and lactate. A spot urine sample should be analyzed for quantitative amino acids, orotic acid, organic acids, and carnitine concentrations.

The diagnosis is established by identification of the specific enzyme defect in hepatic tissue or peripheral leukocytes.

MANAGEMENT. Treatment cannot await specific diagnosis in newborns with symptomatic hyperammonemia due to inborn errors of urea synthesis. Nitrogen intake is limited to 1.2 to 2.0 g/kg/day, and a large percentage of the protein content should be essential amino acids. Arginine concentrations are low in all inborn errors of urea synthesis except for arginase deficiency and must be supplemented. Alternative pathways for nitrogen excretion must be provided. In addition to removal of ammonia by peritoneal dialysis or hemodialysis, waste nitrogen excretion through pathways other than urea synthesis can be promoted by sodium benzoate and phenylacetic acid (Maestri et al, 1995). Nitrogen can be removed by peritoneal dialysis when blood ammonia concentrations become dangerously high.

Long-term management of disorders of urea synthesis requires a protein-restricted diet and arginine supplementation. Sodium benzoate and sodium phenylacetate should be continued as well. Even with optimal supervision, episodes of hyperammonemia may occur and may lead to coma and death. In such cases, intravenous

---

Table 1-6
Causes of Neonatal Hyperammonemia

Liver Failure

Primary Enzyme Defects in Urea Synthesis
Argininosuccinic acidemia
Carbamyl phosphate synthetase deficiency
Citrullinemia
Ornithine transcarbamylase deficiency

Other Disorders of Amino Acid Metabolism
Glycine encephalopathy
Isovaleric acidemia
Methylmalonic acidemia
Multiple carboxylase deficiency
Propionic acidemia

Transitory Hyperammonemia of Prematurity

---

administration of sodium benzoate, sodium phenylacetate, and arginine, coupled with nitrogen-free alimentation, is indicated. Peritoneal dialysis or hemodialysis is indicated if the patient does not respond to drug therapy.

Organic Acid Disorders

Organic acid disorders are characterized by the accumulation of compounds, usually ketones or lactic acid, that cause acidosis in biological fluids. More than 50 organic acid disorders have been described. They can be caused by abnormalities in vitamin metabolism, lipid metabolism, glycolysis, the citric acid cycle, oxidative metabolism, glutathione metabolism, and 4-aminobutyric acid metabolism. The clinical presentations vary considerably and are described in several chapters. Defects in the further metabolism of branched-chain amino acids are the organic acid disorders that most often cause neonatal seizures.

Isovaleric Acidemia

Isovaleric acid is a fatty acid derived from leucine. Its conversion to propionyl-coenzyme A (CoA) is metabolized by the enzyme isovaleryl-CoA dehydrogenase (see Figure 1-1). Isovaleric acidemia is transmitted by autosomal recessive inheritance, and the heterozygote state can be detected in cultured fibroblasts.

CLINICAL FEATURES. Two phenotypes are associated with the same enzyme defect. One is an acute, overwhelming disorder of the newborn; the other is a chronic infantile form. Newborns are normal at birth but within a few days become lethargic, refuse to feed, and vomit. The clinical syndrome is similar to MSUD except that the urine is described as smelling like "sweaty feet" instead of maple syrup. Sixty percent of affected newborns die within 3 weeks. The survivors have a clinical syndrome identical to the chronic infantile phenotype.

DIAGNOSIS. Isovaleric acidosis is detected by the excretion of isovaleryl-lysine in the urine. Isovaleryl-CoA dehydrogenase activity can be assayed in cultured fibroblasts. The clinical phenotype correlates not with the percentage of residual enzyme activity, but with the ability to detoxify isovaleryl-CoA with glycine.

MANAGEMENT. Dietary restriction of protein, especially leucine, decreases the occurrence of later psychomotor retardation. L-Carnitine, 50 mg/kg/day, is a beneficial supplement to the diet of some children with isovaleric acidemia.

In acutely ill newborns, oral glycine, 250 to 500 mg/day, in addition to protein restriction and carnitine, lowers mortality.

Propionic Acidemia

Propionyl-CoA is formed as a catabolite of methionine, threonine, and the branched-chain amino acids. Its further carboxylation to D-methylmalonyl-CoA requires the enzyme propionyl-CoA carboxylase and the coenzyme biotin (see Figure 1-1). Isolated deficiency of propionyl-CoA carboxylase causes propionic acidemia (Hamilton et al, 1995). The defect is transmitted as an autosomal recessive trait.

CLINICAL FEATURES. Most affected children appear normal at birth; symptoms may begin as early as the first day after delivery but can be delayed for months or years. In newborns, the symptoms are nonspecific: feeding difficulty, lethargy, hypotonia, and dehydration. The subsequent course is characterized by recurrent attacks of profound metabolic acidosis often associated with hyperammonemia, which respond poorly to buffering. Untreated newborns rapidly become dehydrated, have generalized or myoclonic seizures, and become comatose.

Hepatomegaly caused by a fatty infiltration occurs in 28% of patients. Neutropenia, thrombocytopenia, and occasionally pancytopenia may be present. A bleeding diathesis accounts for massive intracranial hemorrhage in some newborns. Children who survive beyond infancy develop infarctions in the basal ganglia.

DIAGNOSIS. Propionic acidemia should be considered in any newborn with ketoacidosis but must also be considered in newborns with hyperammonemia without ketoacidosis, since an erroneous diagnosis of carbamyl phosphate synthesis deficiency may be suggested. Propionic acidemia is the probable diagnosis when the plasma concentrations of glycine and propionate and the urinary concentrations of glycine, methylcitrate, and beta-hydroxypropionate are increased. While the urinary concentration of propionate may be normal, the plasma concentration is always elevated, without a concurrent increase in the concentration of methylmalonate.

The definitive diagnosis of propionic acidemia is established by showing a deficiency of enzyme activity in peripheral blood leukocytes or in skin fibroblasts. Prenatal diagnosis is accomplished by detecting methylcitrate, a unique metabolite of propionate, in the amniotic fluid and by showing deficient enzyme activity in amniotic fluid cells.

MANAGEMENT. The newborn in ketoacidosis requires dialysis to remove toxic metabolites, parenteral fluids to prevent dehydration, and protein-free nutrition. Restricting protein intake to 0.5 to l.5 g/kg/day decreases the frequency and severity of subsequent attacks. Oral administration of L-carnitine reduces the ketogenic response to fasting and may be useful as a daily supplement. Biotin supplementation is often used, although its benefit has not been established.

Methylmalonic Acidemia

D-Methylmalonyl-CoA is racemized to L-methylmalonyl-CoA by the enzyme D-methylmalonyl racemase and then isomerized to succinyl-CoA, which enters the tricarboxylic cycle. The enzyme D-methylmalonyl-CoA mutase catalyzes the isomerization. The cobalamin (vitamin B_{12}) coenzyme adenosylcobalamin is a required cofactor. Several defects in this pathway are known; all are transmitted by autosomal recessive inheritance. Mutase deficiency is the most common abnormality. Propionyl-CoA, propionic acid, and methylmalonic acid accumulate and cause hyperglycinemia and hyperammonemia. Each of the enzyme defects responsible for methylmalonic acidemia is believed to be transmitted as an autosomal recessive trait.

CLINICAL FEATURES. Affected children appear normal at birth. In 80% of those with complete mutase deficiency, the symptoms appear during the first week after delivery; those with defects in the synthesis of adenosylcobalamin generally show symptoms after 1 month. Symptoms include lethargy, failure to thrive, recurrent vomiting, dehydration, respiratory distress, and hypotonia after the initiation of protein feeding. Leukopenia, thrombocytopenia, and anemia are present in more than one half of patients. Intracranial hemorrhage may result from a bleeding diathesis. The outcome for newborns with complete mutase deficiency is usually poor. Most die within 2 months of diagnosis; survivors have recurrent acidosis, growth retardation, and mental retardation.

DIAGNOSIS. The diagnosis should be suspected in any newborn with metabolic acidoses, especially if associated with ketosis, hyperammonemia, and hyperglycinemia. The diagnosis is confirmed by the demonstration of an increased concentration of methylmalonate in the plasma and urine. The specific enzyme defect can be determined in fibroblasts. Techniques for prenatal detection are available.

MANAGEMENT. Affected newborns can be divided into those who are cobalamin responsive and those who are not (Nicolaides et al, 1998). Those with mutase deficiency are managed like those in propionic acidemia. The long-term results are poor. Vitamin B_{12} supplementation is useful in some defects of adenosylcobalamin synthesis, and hydroxocobalamin, 1 mg, should be administered while the definitive diagnosis is awaited. Treatment is then maintained with protein restriction (0.5 to l.5 g/kg/day) and hydroxocobalamin, 1 mg, weekly. As in propionic acidemia, oral supplementation of L-carnitine reduces ketogenesis in response to fasting.

Herpes Simplex Encephalitis

Herpes genitalis (herpes simplex virus type 2, HSV-2) accounts for the majority of herpetic infections of the newborn. The newborn is most commonly infected during the second stage of labor by contact with maternal genital herpes, which is asymptomatic or unrecognized in 60% to 80% of women. Symptomatic infections occur in 8% of newborns whose mothers have a history of recurrent genital HSV infection. The risk of contamination at birth is greatest when the mother has primary genital herpes involving the cervix at delivery and the newborn is premature and delivered with instrumentation, including scalp electrodes.

CLINICAL FEATURES. The clinical spectrum of perinatal HSV infection is considerable. Among symptomatic newborns, two thirds have disseminated disease and one third have localized involvement of the brain, eyes, skin, or mouth. Whether disseminated or localized, approximately half of infections involve the central nervous system. The overall mortality rate is 62%, and 50% of survivors have permanent neurological impairment.

The onset of symptoms may be as early as the fifth day but is usually in the second week. A vesicular rash is present in 30%, usually on the scalp after vertex presentation and on the buttocks after breech presentation. Conjunctivitis, jaundice, and a bleeding diathesis may be present. The first symptoms of encephalitis are irritability and seizures. Seizures may be focal or generalized and are frequently refractory to therapy. Neurological deterioration is progressive and characterized by coma and quadriparesis.

DIAGNOSIS. The EEG is always abnormal and shows a periodic pattern of slow waves or spike discharges. The cerebrospinal fluid examination shows a lymphocytic leukocytosis, red blood cells, and an elevated protein concentration. Diagnosis is established by culturing the virus or by viral identification in the cerebrospinal fluid using the polymerase chain reaction (Whitley and Lakeman, 1995).

MANAGEMENT. The best treatment is prevention. Recurrent genital herpes in adults can be suppressed by administration of acyclovir, 800 mg, as a single oral dose. All women with genital herpes at term whose membranes are intact or have been ruptured for less than 4 hours should be delivered by cesarean section. Acyclovir, 10 mg/kg every 8 hours for 10 to 14 days, is recommended for therapy in the newborn, but 10% of those with disseminated disease will relapse within 2 weeks after completion of the course. Mortality remains 50% or greater in newborns with disseminated disease.

Drug Withdrawal

Marijuana, alcohol, narcotic-analgesics, and hypnotic-sedatives are the drugs most commonly used during pregnancy. Marijuana and alcohol do not cause drug dependence in the fetus and are not associated with withdrawal symptoms. Hypnotic-sedatives, such as barbiturates, do not ordinarily produce withdrawal symptoms unless very large doses are ingested. Phenobarbital has a sufficiently long half-life in newborns that sudden withdrawal does not occur.

The prototype of narcotic withdrawal in the newborn is with heroin or methadone, but a similar syndrome occurs with codeine and propoxyphene.

CLINICAL FEATURES. Symptoms of opiate withdrawal are more severe and tend to occur earlier in full-term (first 24 hours) than in premature (24 to 48 hours) newborns. The initial feature is a coarse tremor, present only during the waking state, which can shake an entire limb. This is followed by irritability, a shrill, high-pitched cry, and hyperactivity. The newborn seems hungry but has difficulty feeding and vomits afterward. Diarrhea and other symptoms of autonomic instability are common.

Myoclonic jerking is present in 10% to 25% of newborns undergoing withdrawal. Whether these movements are seizures or jitteriness is not clear. Definite seizures occur in fewer than 5%.

Maternal use of cocaine during pregnancy is associated with premature delivery, growth retardation, and microcephaly. Newborns exposed to cocaine in utero or after delivery through the breast milk often show features of cocaine intoxication including tachycardia, tachypnea, hypertension, irritability, and tremulousness.

DIAGNOSIS. Drug withdrawal should be suspected and anticipated in every newborn whose mother has a history of substance abuse. Even when such a history is not available, the combination of irritability, hyperactivity, and autonomic instability should provide a clue to the diagnosis. Careful questioning of the mother concerning her use of prescription and nonprescription drugs is imperative. Specific drug identification is accomplished by blood and urine analyses.

MANAGEMENT. Symptoms remit spontaneously in 3 to 5 days, but appreciable mortality occurs among untreated newborns. Phenobarbital, 8 mg/kg/day, or chlorpromazine, 3 mg/kg/day, relieves symptoms and reduces mortality. Morphine, meperidine, opium, and methadone are not sufficiently secreted in breast milk to cause or relieve addiction in the newborn.

The occurrence of seizures does not in itself indicate a poor prognosis. The long-term outcome is closely related to the other risk factors associated with substance abuse in the mother.

Bilirubin Encephalopathy

Unconjugated bilirubin is bound to albumin in the blood. *Kernicterus,* a yellow discoloration of the brain that is especially severe in the basal ganglia and hippocampus, occurs when the serum unbound or free fraction becomes excessive. An excessive level of the free fraction in an otherwise healthy newborn is approximately 20 mg/dl (340 μmol/L). Kernicterus was an important complication of hemolytic disease from maternal-fetal blood group incompatibility, but this condition is now uncommon. Other causes of hyperbilirubinemia in full-term newborns are generally managed without difficulty. Critically ill premature infants with respiratory distress syndrome, acidosis, and sepsis are the group at greatest risk. In such newborns an unbound serum concentration of 10 mg/dl (170 μmol/L) may be sufficient to cause bilirubin encephalopathy, and even the albumin-bound fraction may pass the blood-brain barrier.

CLINICAL FEATURES. Three distinct clinical phases of bilirubin encephalopathy occur in full-term newborns with untreated hemolytic disease. Hypotonia, lethargy, and a poor sucking reflex are noted within 24 hours of delivery. Bilirubin staining of the brain is already evident in newborns who die during this first clinical phase. On the second or third day, the newborn becomes febrile and shows increasing tone and opisthotonic posturing. Seizures are not a constant feature but may occur at this time. The third phase is characterized by apparent improvement with normalization of tone. This may cause second thoughts about the accuracy of the diagnosis, but the improvement is short-lived. Evidence of neurological dysfunction begins to appear toward the end of the second month, and the symptoms become progressively worse throughout infancy.

In premature newborns, the clinical features are subtle and may lack the phases of increased tone and opisthotonos. The majority of affected premature infants are believed to die in the newborn period.

The typical clinical syndrome after the first year includes extrapyramidal dysfunction, usually athetosis, which occurs in virtually every case (see Chapter 14); disturbances of vertical gaze, upward more often than downward, in 90%; high-frequency hearing loss in 60%; and mental retardation in 25%.

DIAGNOSIS. In newborns with hemolytic disease, a clinical diagnosis can be presumed on the basis of significant hyperbilirubinemia and a compatible evolution of symptoms. However, the diagnosis is difficult to establish in critically ill premature newborns, whose brain damage is more often caused by asphyxia and its consequences than by kernicterus.

The brainstem auditory evoked response (BAER) may be useful in assessing the severity of bilirubin encephalopathy and its response to treatment. The auditory nerve and pathways are especially susceptible to bilirubin encephalopathy. The generators of wave I and wave V of the BAER are the auditory nerve and the inferior colliculus, respectively. The latency of both waves increases in proportion to the concentration of free albumin and decreases after exchange transfusion.

MANAGEMENT. Maintaining serum bilirubin concentrations below the toxic range, either by phototherapy or exchange transfusion, prevents kernicterus. Once kernicterus has occurred, further damage can be limited, but not reversed, by lowering serum bilirubin concentrations.

Pyridoxine Dependency

Pyridoxine dependency is a rare disorder transmitted as an autosomal recessive trait. It is caused by impaired glutamic decarboxylase activity. The gene locus is 2q31. Neurotoxic concentrations of glutamate are measured in the cerebrospinal fluid.

CLINICAL FEATURES. Multifocal clonic seizures begin almost immediately after birth and progress rapidly to status epilepticus. However, a later onset, even after the first year, does not exclude the diagnosis. The seizures are refractory to standard anticonvulsants and respond only to pyridoxine. If pyridoxine supplementation is discontinued, seizures return within 3 weeks.

DIAGNOSIS. In most cases the diagnosis is suspected because a sibling was affected by the same syndrome and died. In the absence of a family history of the disorder, the diagnosis need be considered only in newborns with continuous seizures. The infantile-onset variety may be characterized by intermittent myoclonic seizures, focal clonic seizures, or generalized tonic-clonic seizures. The EEG is continuously abnormal because of generalized or multifocal spike discharges. An intravenous injection of pyridoxine, 100 mg, stops the clinical seizure activity and often converts the EEG to normal in less than 10 minutes.

Pyridoxine-responsive seizures also occur in newborns of mothers treated with isoniazid. The onset of seizures is in the third week after delivery.

MANAGEMENT. A lifelong dietary supplement of pyridoxine, which varies from 10 to 30 mg/kg/day, prevents further seizures. The higher dose is used during infancy and the smaller dose in childhood. Subsequent psychomotor development is best when treatment is initiated early, but this does not ensure a normal outcome. The dose needed to prevent mental retardation may be higher than that needed to stop seizures.

Incontinentia Pigmenti (Bloch-Sulzberger Syndrome)

Incontinentia pigmenti is a rare neurocutaneous syndrome involving the skin, teeth, eyes, and central nervous system. It is transmitted as an X-linked trait (Xq28) that is lethal in the hemizygous male (Francis and Sybert, 1997).

CLINICAL FEATURES. The female-to-male ratio is 20:1. An erythematous and vesicular rash resembling epidermolysis bullosa is present on the flexor surfaces of the limbs and lateral aspect of the trunk at birth or soon thereafter. Neurological disturbances occur in fewer than half of the cases. In newborns, the prominent feature is the onset of seizures on the second or third day, often confined to one side of the body. The rash persists for the first few months and is replaced by a verrucous eruption that lasts for weeks or months. Between 6 and 12 months of age, pigment is deposited in the previous area of rash in bizarre polymorphic arrangements. The pigmentation later regresses and may disappear. Residual neurological handicaps may include mental retardation, epilepsy, hemiparesis, and hydrocephalus.

DIAGNOSIS. Clinical diagnosis is based on the character of the rash. Biopsy of the rash during the vesicular stage provides histological confirmation.

MANAGEMENT. Neonatal seizures caused by incontinentia pigmenti usually respond to standard anticonvulsant drugs.

Benign Familial Neonatal Seizures

In some families, several members have seizures in the first weeks of life but do not have epilepsy or other neurological abnormalities later on. The trait is transmitted by autosomal dominant inheritance, and the abnormal gene locus is on chromosome 20.

CLINICAL FEATURES. Brief multifocal clonic seizures develop during the first week, sometimes associated with apnea. The onset may be delayed as long as 4 weeks. With or without treatment, the seizures usually stop spontaneously within 6 weeks. Febrile seizures occur in up to one third of children; some have febrile seizures without neonatal seizures. Epilepsy develops later in life in 10% to 15% of affected newborns.

DIAGNOSIS. The syndrome should be suspected when seizures develop without apparent cause in a healthy newborn. Laboratory tests, including the interictal EEG, show no abnormalities. During a seizure, the initial apnea and tonic activity are associated with flattening of the EEG; generalized spike-wave discharges occur during the clonic activity. A family history of neonatal seizures is critical to diagnosis but may not be discovered until the grandparents are interviewed; parents are frequently unaware that they had neonatal seizures.

MANAGEMENT. Phenobarbital is usually effective to stop seizures. After 4 weeks of complete seizure control the drug can be tapered and discontinued. If seizures return, a longer trial should be initiated.

Treatment of Neonatal Seizures

Animal studies suggest that continuous seizure activity, even in the normoxemic brain, may cause brain damage by inhibiting protein synthesis and breaking down polyribosomes. In premature newborns, an additional concern is that the increased cerebral blood flow associated with seizures will increase the risk of intraventricular hemorrhage. Protein binding of anticonvulsant drugs may be impaired in premature newborns and the free fraction concentration may be toxic, whereas the measured protein-bound fraction appears therapeutic.

The initial steps in managing newborns with seizures are to maintain vital function, identify and correct the underlying cause (i.e., hypocalcemia) when possible, and rapidly provide a therapeutic blood concentration of an anticonvulsant drug when needed.

Phenobarbital

Intravenous phenobarbital is the treatment of choice for newborns with seizures. A unitary relationship usually exists between the intravenous dose of phenobarbital in milligrams per kilogram of body weight and the blood concentration in micrograms per milliliter measured 24 hours after the load. A blood concentration of 20 μg/ml can be safely achieved with a single intravenous loading dose of 20 mg/kg injected at a rate of 5 mg/min. The usual maintenance dose is 4 mg/kg/day, but those who do not respond to the initial load should be given additional boluses of 10 mg/kg to a total of 40 mg/kg. Phenobarbital monotherapy is effective in 70% to 85% of newborns with seizures when blood levels of 40 μg/ml are achieved. In term newborns with intractable seizures from hypoxic-ischemic encephalopathy, additional boluses of phenobarbital can be used to achieve a blood concentration of 70 μg/ml, because such newborns are always being ventilated. If such concentrations of phenobarbital are ineffective, the addition of other drugs is unlikely to be helpful.

The half-life of phenobarbital in newborns varies from 50 to 200 hours, and additional doses should be administered only on the basis of current blood concentration information.

After the 10th day the half-life shortens as the result of enzyme induction, and a steady state is easier to achieve.

Phenytoin

Parenteral phenytoin is safely administered intravenously as fosphenytoin sodium. Oral doses of phenytoin are poorly absorbed in newborns. A therapeutic blood concentration of 15 to 20 μg/ml (40 to 80 μmol/L) can be safely achieved by a single intravenous injection of 20 mg/kg at a rate of 0.5 mg/kg/min. The half-life is long during the first week, and further administration should be based on current knowledge of the blood concentration. Most newborns require a maintenance dosage of 5 to 10 mg/kg/day.

Duration of Therapy

Seizures caused by an acute, self-limited encephalopathy, such as hypoxic-ischemic encephalopathy, do not ordinarily require prolonged maintenance therapy. In most newborns seizures stop when the acute encephalopathy is over. Therefore therapy should be discontinued after 2 weeks of complete seizure control. If seizures recur, anticonvulsant therapy can be reinitiated.

In contrast to newborns with seizures caused by acute encephalopathy, those with seizures caused by cerebral dysgenesis should be treated continuously. Eighty percent will be epileptic in childhood.

Paroxysmal Disorders in Children Less Than 2 Years Old

The pathophysiology of paroxysmal disorders is more varied in infants than in newborns (Table 1-7). Seizures, especially febrile seizures, are the main cause of paroxysmal disorders, but apnea and syncope (breath-holding spells) are relatively common as well. Infants with paroxysmal disorders are frequently referred for neurological consultation because of the suspicion of seizures. The determination of which "spells" are seizures is often difficult and relies more on obtaining a complete description of the spell than on laboratory test results. The parents should be asked to provide a sequential history. If more than one spell occurred, they should first describe the one that was best observed or most recent. The following questions should be in-

Table 1-7
Paroxysmal Disorders in Children Younger Than 2 years

Apnea and Breath-holding
Cyanotic
Pallid

Dystonia
Glutaric aciduria (see Chapter 14)
Transient paroxysmal dystonia of infancy

Migraine
Benign paroxysmal vertigo (see Chapter 10)
Cyclic vomiting
Paroxysmal torticollis (see Chapter 14)

Seizures
Febrile seizures
    Epilepsy triggered by fever
    Infection of the nervous system
    Simple febrile seizure
Nonfebrile seizures
    Generalized tonic-clonic seizures
    Partial seizures
        Benign familial infantile seizures
        Ictal laughter
Myoclonic seizures
    Infantile spasms
    Benign myoclonic epilepsy
    Severe myoclonic epilepsy
    Myoclonic status
    Lennox-Gastaut syndrome

Stereotypies (see Chapter 14)

cluded: What was the child doing before the spell? Did anything provoke the spell? Did the child's color change? If so, when and to what color? Did the eyes move in any direction? Was one part of the body affected more than another?

In addition to obtaining a home video of the spell, ambulatory, prolonged split-screen video-EEG monitoring is the only way to identify the nature of unusual spells. Seizures characterized by decreased motor activity with indeterminate changes in the level of consciousness arise from the temporal, temporoparietal, or parieto-occipital regions, while seizures with motor activity usually arise from the frontal, central, or frontoparietal areas (Acharya et al, 1997).

Apnea and Syncope

Infant apnea is defined as cessation of breathing for 15 seconds or longer, or for less than 15 seconds if accompanied by bradycardia. Premature newborns with respiratory distress syndrome may continue to have apneic spells as infants, especially if they are neurologically abnormal. Persistent apnea is often thought to be a seizure manifestation, but EEG monitoring in children with this condition rarely shows epileptiform activity in association with apneic spells or episodic tonic posturing.

Breath-holding spells with loss of consciousness occur in almost 5% of infants. They are caused by a disturbance in central autonomic regulation probably transmitted by autosomal dominant inheritance with incomplete penetrance. Approximately 20% to 30% of parents of affected children have a history of the condition. The term *breath-holding* is a misnomer because breathing always stops in expiration. Cyanotic and pallid varieties have been described; cyanotic spells are three times more common than pallid spells. Most children experience only one or the other, but 20% have both.

The spells are involuntary responses to adverse stimuli. In approximately 80% of affected children the spells begin before 18 months of age, and in all cases they start before 3 years of age. The last episode usually occurs by age 4 and no later than age 8.

Cyanotic Syncope

CLINICAL FEATURES. Cyanotic spells are usually provoked by anger, frustration, or fear. If the infant's sibling takes away a toy, the child cries and then stops breathing in expiration. Cyanosis develops rapidly, followed quickly by limpness and loss of consciousness. Crying may not precede cyanotic episodes that are provoked by pain.

If the attack lasts for only a few seconds, the infant may resume crying on awakening. Most spells, especially the ones referred for neurological evaluation, are longer and are associated with tonic posturing of the body and trembling movements of the hands or arms. The eyes may roll upward. These movements are regarded as seizures by even experienced observers, but they are probably a brainstem release phenomenon. Concurrent EEG shows flattening of the record, not epileptiform activity.

After a short spell, the child rapidly recovers and seems normal immediately; after a prolonged spell, the child first arouses and then goes to sleep. Once an infant begins having breath-holding spells, the frequency increases for several months and then declines, and finally the spells cease.

DIAGNOSIS. The typical sequence of cyanosis, apnea, and loss of consciousness is critical for diagnosis. Cyanotic syncope is often misdiag-

nosed as epilepsy because of lack of attention to the precipitating event. It is not sufficient to ask, "Did the child hold his breath?" The question conjures up the image of breath-holding during inspiration. Instead, questioning should be focused on precipitating events, absence of breathing, facial color, and family history. The family often has a history of breath-holding spells.

Between attacks the EEG is normal. During an episode the EEG first shows diffuse slowing and then rhythmic slowing during the tonic-clonic activity.

MANAGEMENT. Piracetam, 40 mg/kg/day, showed a 92% reduction in spells compared to 30% for placebo (Donma, 1998). The drug is not available in the United States, but levetiracetam is very similar and may be useful. However, I believe that picking up the child, which is the natural act of the mother or other observer, prolongs the spell. People who have lost consciousness because of decreased cerebral perfusion should not be placed in an upright position. I always caution parents to hold the child with the head in a dependent position.

Most important is to identify the nature of the spell and explain that it is harmless. Children do not die during breath-holding spells, and the episodes always cease spontaneously. Does anyone know an adult who has breath-holding spells?

Pallid Syncope

CLINICAL FEATURES. Pallid syncope is usually provoked by a sudden, unexpected, painful event such as a bump on the head. The child rarely cries but instead becomes white and limp and loses consciousness. These episodes are truly terrifying to behold. Parents invariably believe the child is dead and begin mouth-to-mouth resuscitation. After the initial limpness the body may stiffen, and clonic movements of the arms may occur. As in cyanotic syncope, these movements represent a brainstem release phenomenon, not seizure activity. The duration of the spell is difficult to determine because the observer is so frightened that seconds seem like hours. Afterward the child often falls asleep and is normal on awakening.

DIAGNOSIS. Pallid syncope is the result of reflex asystole. An attack sometimes can be provoked by pressure on the eyeballs to initiate a vagal reflex. I do not recommend provoking an attack as an office procedure. The diagnosis can be made by the history alone.

MANAGEMENT. As with cyanotic spells, the major goal is to reassure the family that the child will not die during an attack. The physician must be very convincing.

Febrile Seizures

An infant's first seizure often occurs at the time of fever. Three explanations are possible: (1) an infection of the nervous system; (2) an underlying seizure disorder in which the initial seizure is triggered by the stress of fever, although subsequent seizures may be afebrile; or (3) a *simple febrile seizure,* a genetic age-limited epilepsy in which seizures occur only with fever. Infections of the nervous system are discussed in Chapters 2 and 4. *Children who have seizures from encephalitis or meningitis do not wake up afterward; they are usually comatose.* The distinction between epilepsy and simple febrile seizures is sometimes difficult and may require time rather than laboratory tests.

CLINICAL FEATURES. Febrile seizures not caused by infection or another definable cause occur in approximately 4% of children. Only 2% of children whose first seizure is associated with fever will have nonfebrile seizures (epilepsy) by age 7. The most important predictor of subsequent epilepsy is an abnormal neurological or developmental state. Complex seizures—defined as prolonged, focal, or multiple—and a family history of epilepsy slightly increase the probability of subsequent epilepsy (Berg and Shinnar, 1996).

A single, brief, generalized seizure occurring in association with fever is likely to be a simple febrile seizure. The seizure need not occur during the time when fever is rising. "Brief" and "fever" are difficult to define. Parents do not use stopwatches, and when a child is having a seizure, seconds seem like minutes. A prolonged seizure is one that is still in progress after the family has contacted the doctor or has left the house for the emergency room. Postictal sleep should not be counted as seizure time. Similarly, body temperature is not measured during a seizure and may be considerably different 30 minutes later.

Simple febrile seizures are familial and probably transmitted by autosomal dominant inheritance with incomplete penetrance. One third of infants who have a first simple febrile seizure will have a second one at the time of a subsequent febrile illness, and half of these will have a third febrile seizure. The risk of recurrence is increased if the first febrile seizure occurs before 18 months of age or at a body temperature less than 40°C (Berg et al, 1997). More than three episodes of simple febrile seizures are unusual and suggest that the child may later have nonfebrile seizures.

DIAGNOSIS. Any child who is thought to have an infection of the nervous system should undergo a lumbar puncture for examination of the cerebrospinal fluid. Approximately one quarter of children with bacterial or viral meningitis have seizures. Ninety percent are obtunded after the seizure, and the other 10% have nuchal rigidity or complex seizures that suggest meningitis.

In contrast, infants who have simple febrile seizures usually look normal after the seizure. Lumbar puncture is not needed following a brief, generalized seizure from which the child recovers rapidly and completely, especially if the fever subsides spontaneously or is otherwise explained.

Blood cell counts, measurements of glucose, calcium, electrolytes, urinalysis, and EEG on a routine basis are not cost effective and should not be performed. The decision for laboratory testing can be individualized to the circumstances of the case. EEG should be performed on every infant who is not neurologically normal or who has a family history of epilepsy. MRI is indicated in infants with prolonged focal febrile seizures. Many will show a preexisting hippocampal abnormality (VanLandingham et al, 1998).

MANAGEMENT. Because only one third of children with an initial febrile seizure have a second seizure, treating every affected child is unreasonable. The low-risk group with a single, brief, generalized seizure should not be treated. No evidence has shown that a second or third simple febrile seizure, even if prolonged, causes epilepsy or brain damage (Verity et al, 1998).

As a rule, I recommend anticonvulsant prophylaxis only if I believe the child has a condition other than simple febrile seizures, and I follow these guidelines:

1. Infants with an abnormal neurological examination or developmental delay should be considered candidates for prophylactic anticonvulsant therapy.

2. When the initial febrile seizure is complex (multiple, prolonged, or focal) but the child recovers rapidly and completely, treatment is not indicated unless the family has a history of nonfebrile seizures.

3. A family history of simple febrile seizures or other known genetic epilepsies is a relative contraindication to therapy.

4. Children who have frequent and prolonged febrile seizures should be treated. The alternatives are prophylactic phenobarbital or oral administration of diazepam, 0.33 mg/kg, every 8 hours during a febrile illness. The side effects of diazepam—ataxia, lethargy, and irritability—are transitory.

Nonfebrile Seizures

Disorders that produce nonfebrile tonic-clonic or partial seizures in infancy are not substantially different from those that cause nonfebrile seizures in childhood (see the following section). Major risk factors for the development of epilepsy in infancy and childhood are congenital malformations, neonatal seizures, and a family history of epilepsy.

A complex partial seizure syndrome that has its onset during infancy, sometimes in the newborn period, is *ictal laughter* associated with hypothalamic hamartoma. The attacks are brief, occur several times each day, and may be characterized by pleasant laughter or giggling. At first the laughter is thought to be normal, but then facial flushing and pupillary dilatation are noted. With time the child begins to have drop attacks and generalized seizures and undergoes personality change. Precocious puberty may be an associated condition.

A first partial motor seizure before the age of 2 is associated with a recurrence rate of 87%, whereas with a first seizure at a later age the rate is 51%. The recurrence rate after a first nonfebrile, asymptomatic, generalized seizure is 60% to 70% at all ages. The younger the age at onset of a nonfebrile seizure of any type, the more likely that the seizure is symptomatic rather than idiopathic.

Approximately 25% of children who have recurrent seizures during the first year, excluding neonatal seizures and infantile spasms, are developmentally or neurologically abnormal at the time of the first seizure. The initial EEG has prognostic significance; normal EEG results are associated with a favorable neurological outcome.

Intractable seizures in children less than 2 years of age are often associated with later mental retardation. The seizure types with the greatest probability of mental retardation in descending order are myoclonic, tonic-clonic, complex partial, and simple partial.

Benign familial infantile epilepsy is transmitted by autosomal dominant inheritance and has its onset as early as 3 months. The gene locus, on chromosome 19, is different from the locus for benign familial neonatal seizures. Motion arrest, decreased responsiveness, staring or blank eyes, and mild convulsive movements of the limbs characterize the seizures. They are easily controlled with anticonvulsant drugs and stop spontaneously within 2 to 4 years.

Myoclonus and Myoclonic Seizures

Infantile Spasms

Infantile spasms are age-dependent myoclonic seizures that occur with an incidence of 25 per 100,000 live births in the United States and Western Europe. An underlying cause can be determined in approximately 75% of patients; congenital malformations and perinatal asphyxia are common causes, and tuberous sclerosis accounts for 20% of cases in some series (Table 1-8). Despite considerable concern in the past, pertussis immunization is not a cause of infantile spasms.

The combination of infantile spasms, agenesis of the corpus callosum (as well as other midline cerebral malformations), and retinal malformations is referred to as *Aicardi syndrome*. All affected children are females, and the disorder is believed to be transmitted as an X-linked dominant trait with hemizygous lethality in males.

CLINICAL FEATURES. The peak age at onset is between 4 and 7 months, and onset always occurs before 1 year of age. The spasm can be a flexor or an extensor movement; some children have both. Spasms generally occur in clusters, shortly after the infant awakens from sleep, and are not activated by stimulation. A rapid flexor spasm involving the neck, trunk, and limbs is followed by a tonic contraction sustained for 2 to 10 seconds. Less severe flexor spasms are characterized only by dropping of the head and abduction of the arms or by flexion at the waist resembling colic. Extensor spasms resemble the second component of the Moro reflex: the head moves backward and the arms are suddenly spread. Whether flexor or extensor, the movement is almost always symmetric and brief.

When the cause of spasms is identifiable (symptomatic spasms), the infant is usually abnormal neurologically or developmentally when the spasms begin. Microcephaly is common in this group. Prognosis depends on the cause, but as a rule the symptomatic group does poorly.

Table 1-8
Neurocutaneous Disorders Causing Seizures in Infancy

Incontinentia Pigmenti
Seizure type
    Neonatal seizures
    Generalized tonic-clonic
Cutaneous manifestations
    Erythematous bullae (newborn)
    Pigmentary whorls (infancy)
    Depigmented areas (childhood)

Linear Nevus Sebaceous Syndrome
Seizure type
    Infantile spasms
    Lennox-Gastaut syndrome
    Generalized tonic-clonic
Cutaneous manifestation
    Linear facial sebaceous nevus

Neurofibromatosis
Seizure type
    Generalized tonic-clonic
    Partial complex
    Partial simple motor
Cutaneous manifestations
    Café au lait spots
    Axillary freckles
    Neural tumors

Sturge-Weber Syndrome
Seizure type
    Epilepsia partialis continuans
    Partial simple motor
    Status epilepticus
Cutaneous manifestation
    Hemifacial hemangioma

Tuberous Sclerosis
Seizure type
    Neonatal seizures
    Infantile spasms
    Lennox-Gastaut syndrome
    Generalized tonic-clonic
    Partial simple motor
    Partial complex
Cutaneous manifestations
    Abnormal hair pigmentation
    Adenoma sebaceum
    Café au lait spots
    Depigmented areas
    Shagren patch

Idiopathic spasms characteristically occur in children who had been developing normally at the onset of spasms and have no history of prenatal or perinatal disorders. Neurological findings, including head circumference, are normal. Approximately 40% of children with idiopathic spasms are neurologically normal or only mildly retarded subsequently.

DIAGNOSIS. The delay from spasm onset to diagnosis is often considerable. Infantile spasms are so unlike the usual perception of seizures that even experienced pediatricians may be slow to realize the significance of the movements. Colic is often considered and treated for several weeks before seizures are suspected.

Infantile spasms must be differentiated from benign myoclonus of early infancy, benign myoclonic epilepsy of infants, severe myoclonic epilepsy of infancy, and the Lennox-Gastaut syndrome (Table 1-9). However, there is some reason to believe that infantile spasms, severe myoclonic epilepsy, and the Lennox-Gastaut syndrome are a continuum of epileptic encephalopathies.

The EEG is the single most important test for diagnosis. However, EEG findings vary with the duration of recording, sleep state, and underlying disorder. Hypsarrhythmia is the usual pattern recorded during the early stages of infantile spasms. A chaotic and continuously abnormal background of very high voltage and random slow waves and spike discharges are characteristic. The spikes vary in location from moment to moment and at times become generalized, but they are never repetitive. Typical hypsarrhythmia is most often recorded during wakefulness or active sleep. During quiet sleep, greater interhemispheric synchrony occurs and the background may have a burst-suppression appearance.

The EEG may transiently become normal immediately upon arousal, but when spasms occur, either an abrupt attenuation of the background or high-voltage slow waves appear. Within a few weeks the original chaotic pattern of hypsarrhythmia is replaced by greater interhemispheric synchrony. The distribution of epileptiform discharges changes from multifocal to generalized,

Table 1-9
Electroencephalographic (EEG) Appearance in Myoclonic Seizures of Infancy

Seizure Type	EEG Appearance
Infantile spasms	Hypsarrhythmia
	Slow spike and wave
	Burst-suppression
Benign myoclonus	Normal
Benign myoclonic epilepsy	Spike and wave (3 cps)
	Polyspike and wave (3 cps)
Severe myoclonic epilepsy	Polyspike and wave (>3 cps)
Lennox-Gastaut syndrome	Spike and wave (2–2.5 cps)
	Polyspike and wave (2–2.5 cps)

and the generalized discharges are followed by attenuation of the record.

MANAGEMENT. Hormonal therapy with adrenocorticotropic hormone (ACTH) or corticosteroids is effective in stopping infantile spasms, but it need not be used in every case. Hormonal therapy does not affect the outcome in infants whose spasms are due to prenatal or perinatal brain abnormalities. Clonazepam, nitrazepam, or vigabatrin (Vigevano and Cillo, 1997) should be tried first and often proves effective, at least temporarily. Vigabatrin is especially useful when the spasms are caused by tuberous sclerosis (Hancock and Osborne, 1999). Unfortunately it is not available in the United States because of safety concerns; it causes visual field defects.

Levetiracetem may also be useful. Valproate monotherapy controls spasms in 70% of infants when doses of 100 to 300 mg/kg are used, but it is not a drug of first choice because of an unacceptable rate of fatal hepatotoxicity in this age group. However, since fatal hepatotoxicity occurs mainly in infants with certain inborn errors of metabolism, I use it when infantile spasms are known to be secondary to hypoxic-ischemic encephalopathy or tuberous sclerosis.

If pharmacological therapy fails, hormonal therapy should be initiated. However, clonazepam should be continued in neurologically abnormal infants; ACTH or prednisone usually provides only temporary respite from seizures, and long-term anticonvulsant therapy is needed. ACTH may be more beneficial than prednisone (Baram et al, 1996). The ideal dose and duration of ACTH or prednisone have not been established. ACTH gel is usually given twice daily as an intramuscular injection of 75 U/m² for 2 to 6 weeks and then tapered to zero during a 1-week period. Prednisone, 2 mg/kg/day, is administered orally for 2 weeks and then tapered over 2 weeks.

The response to hormonal therapy is never graded; control is either complete or not at all. Even when the response is favorable, one third of patients have relapses during or after the course of treatment. Failure to respond and relapses occur more often in symptomatic than idiopathic cases. A second course of treatment is effective in 75% of cases in which the first course was successful, albeit at the price of increased adverse reactions.

High-dose pyridoxine should be considered in the treatment of infantile spasms when ACTH fails initially or relapses occur. Some cases of infantile spasms or other seizures of infancy may be atypical presentations of pyridoxine-dependent seizures. However, in most cases the anticonvulsant properties of pyridoxine and ACTH are unrelated to their physiological functions. The recommended dosage of pyridoxine is 30 to 40 mg/kg/day.

Some children with idiopathic infantile spasms who are refractory to medical therapy have an area of cortical abnormality demonstrable by some combination of positron emission tomography (PET), closed-circuit television EEG, and MRI. Surgical removal of the area, which usually proves to contain dysplastic tissue, often provides seizure control.

Benign Myoclonus of Infancy

CLINICAL FEATURES. Many series of patients with infantile spasms include a small number with normal EEG results. Such infants cannot be distinguished from others with infantile spasms by clinical features because the age at onset and the appearance of the movements are the same. The spasms occur in clusters, frequently at mealtime. Clusters increase in intensity and severity over a period of weeks or months and then abate spontaneously. After 3 months the spasms usually stop altogether, and although they may recur occasionally, no spasms occur after 2 years of age. Affected infants are normal neurologically and developmentally and remain so afterward. The term *benign myoclonus* is used because the spasms are believed to be an involuntary movement and not a seizure.

DIAGNOSIS. A normal EEG result distinguishes this group from other types of myoclonus in infancy. The MRI findings are also normal.

MANAGEMENT. Infants who are neurologically normal and have normal EEGs should not be treated.

Benign Myoclonic Epilepsy

CLINICAL FEATURES. Benign myoclonic epilepsy is a rare disorder of uncertain cause. A genetic basis is presumed because one third of patients have family members with epilepsy. Onset is between 4 months and 2 years of age. Affected infants are neurologically normal at the onset of seizures and remain so afterward. The seizures are characterized by brief myoclonic attacks, which may be restricted to head nodding or may be so severe as to throw the child to the floor. The head drops to the chest, eyes roll upward, arms are thrown upward and outward, and legs flex. Myoclonic seizures may be single or repetitive, but consciousness is not lost. No other seizure types are observed in infancy, but generalized tonic-clonic seizures may occur in adolescence.

DIAGNOSIS. During a seizure the EEG shows generalized 3 cycles/sec (cps) spike-wave or polyspike-wave discharges. Sensory stimuli do not activate seizures. The pattern is consistent with primary, generalized epilepsy.

MANAGEMENT. Valproate produces complete seizure control. If left untreated, seizures may persist for years. The use of valproate is potentially dangerous in infants because of hepatotoxicity. Levetiracetem may be useful.

Early-Onset Progressive Encephalopathy with Migrant, Continuous Myoclonus

This syndrome may be the same as severe myoclonic epilepsy, described in the following section. Continuous, multifocal, myoclonic jerks begin during early infancy and later progress to generalized tonic-clonic seizures (Gaggero et al, 1996). The initial neurological examination and EEG are normal. However, the infant eventually develops hypotonia and ataxia, the EEG shows epileptiform activity that may be generalized or focal, and neuroimaging shows cortical atrophy.

Severe Myoclonic Epilepsy

Severe myoclonic epilepsy is an important but poorly understood syndrome. A seemingly healthy infant has a seizure and then undergoes progressive neurological deterioration that ends in a chronic brain damage syndrome. Because its cause is unknown, the disorder is blamed on any and all preceding events. It is often, but improperly, blamed on immunization.

CLINICAL FEATURES. A family history of epilepsy is present in 25% of cases. The first seizures are frequently febrile, are usually prolonged, and can be generalized or focal clonic in type. Febrile and nonfebrile seizures recur, sometimes as status epilepticus. Generalized myoclonic seizures appear after 1 year of age. At first mild and difficult to recognize as a seizure manifestation, they later become frequent and repetitive and disturb function. Partial complex seizures with secondary generalization may also occur. Coincident with the onset of myoclonic seizures are the slowing of development and the gradual appearance of ataxia and hyperreflexia.

DIAGNOSIS. The initial differential diagnosis is febrile seizures. Because the febrile seizures are usually prolonged and sometimes focal, epilepsy

should be suspected. A specific diagnosis is not possible until the appearance of myoclonic seizures in the second year.

Interictal EEG findings are normal at first. Paroxysmal abnormalities appear in the second year and are characterized by generalized spike-wave and polyspike-wave complexes with a frequency greater than 3 cps. Discharges are activated by photic stimulation, drowsiness, and quiet sleep.

MANAGEMENT. The seizures are resistant to therapy with anticonvulsant drugs. Valproate and benzodiazepines should be tried first, then levetiracetem or zonisamide Carbamazepine may increase seizure frequency.

Biotinidase Deficiency

This relatively rare disorder is transmitted as an autosomal recessive trait. It is caused by defective biotin absorption or transport and was previously called *late-onset multiple (holo) carboxylase deficiency.*

CLINICAL FEATURES. Age at onset is usually around 3 months (Suormala et al, 1997). Seizures and hypotonia are the initial features. The seizures may be generalized tonic-clonic, myoclonic, or infantile spasms. Other features that may be seen initially or develop later are ataxia, respiratory disturbances, dermatitis, and alopecia.

DIAGNOSIS. Ketoacidosis, hyperammonemia, and organic aciduria are present, as in holocarboxylase deficiency. Biotinidase deficiency should be suspected when the onset of symptoms is after the newborn period. The diagnosis is established by showing biotinidase deficiency in serum.

MANAGEMENT. Treatment with biotin, 5 to 20 mg/day, successfully reverses most of the symptoms if started during early infancy, and may prevent mental retardation.

Lennox-Gastaut Syndrome

The triad of seizures (atypical absence, atonic, and myoclonic), 1.5–2 Hz spike-wave complexes on EEG, and mental retardation characterize the Lennox-Gastaut syndrome. In most children the seizures are secondary to underlying brain damage, but some are primary epilepsies. The term *myoclonic-astatic epilepsy* is sometimes reserved for the Lennox-Gastaut syndrome when it occurs as a primary epilepsy (Wheless and Constantinou, 1997).

CLINICAL FEATURES. The peak age at onset is 3 to 5 years; less than half of the cases begin before age 2. An underlying cause can be identified in approximately 60%; neurocutaneous disorders such as tuberous sclerosis, perinatal disturbances, and postnatal brain injuries are most common. Twenty percent of children with the Lennox-Gastaut syndrome have a history of infantile spasms, sometimes with a seizure-free interval before development of the syndrome.

Although the syndrome can begin in a normal child, most children are identified as neurologically abnormal before its onset. The first seizures may be generalized tonic-clonic or focal clonic but are usually tonic. Stiffening of the body, upward deviation of the eyes, dilatation of the pupils, and alteration in the respiratory pattern are the characteristic features of tonic seizures. The seizures frequently occur during sleep, and enuresis may be an associated condition.

Atypical absence seizures occur in almost every patient. In addition to the stare, trembling of the eyelids and mouth occurs, followed by loss of facial tone so that the head leans forward and the mouth hangs open. Atonic seizures are characterized by sudden dropping of the head or body, at times throwing the child to the ground. More than 90% of patients are mentally retarded by 5 years of age.

DIAGNOSIS. An EEG is essential for diagnosis. The characteristic feature during atypical absence or atonic seizures is a generalized burst of 2- to 2.5-cps spike-wave complexes. Tonic seizures are associated with 1-cps slow waves followed by generalized rapid discharges without postictal depression.

In addition to EEG, a thorough evaluation is needed to look for an underlying cause. Special attention should be given to skin manifestations suggesting a neurocutaneous syndrome (see Table 1-8). MRI is useful for the diagnosis of congenital malformations, postnatal disorders, and neurocutaneous syndromes.

MANAGEMENT. Seizures are difficult to control with drugs, and the ketogenic diet should be considered when drugs fail. Valproate and clonazepam are usually the most effective drugs. Lamotrigine, felbamate, and topiramate have shown promise as add-on drugs. Vigabatrin, not available in the United States, may be the most effective (Delanty and French, 1998).

Migraine

CLINICAL FEATURES. Migraine attacks are uncommon in infancy, but when they occur, the clinical features are often paroxysmal and suggest the possibility of seizures. Cyclic vomiting is probably the most common manifestation. Attacks of vertigo (see Chapter 10) or torticollis (see Chapter 14) may be especially perplexing, and some infants have attacks in which they rock back and forth and appear uncomfortable.

DIAGNOSIS. Benign paroxysmal vertigo is sufficiently stereotyped in presentation to be recognizable as a migraine variant. Other syndromes often remain undiagnosed until the episodes evolve into a typical migraine pattern. A history of migraine in one parent, usually the mother, is essential for diagnosis.

MANAGEMENT. Antimigraine drugs are generally not used for infants.

Paroxysmal Disorders of Childhood

Like infants, children with paroxysmal disorders are generally thought to have seizures until proven otherwise. Seizures are the most common paroxysmal disorder requiring medical consultation. Syncope, especially presyncope, is considerably more common but is generally diagnosed and managed at home unless associated symptoms suggest a seizure.

Migraine is probably the most common causes of paroxysmal neurological disorders in childhood; its incidence is 10 times greater than that of epilepsy. Migraine syndromes that may suggest epilepsy are described in Chapters 2, 3, 10, 11, 14, and 15.

Sleep disorders often have a paroxysmal quality and may be confused with complex partial seizures. Adding to the confusion is the fact that complex partial seizures are often activated by sleep.

Syndromes Simulating Seizures

Paroxysmal Dyskinesia

Paroxysmal dyskinesia occurs in four different syndromes: paroxysmal kinesigenic dyskinesia (PKD); paroxysmal nonkinesigenic dyskinesia (PNKD), also known as *familial paroxysmal choreoathetosis*; supplementary sensorimotor seizures; and paroxysmal nocturnal dystonia (Lüders, 1996). The first two are not seizure disorders. They are mainly distinguished by whether or not the dyskinesia is provoked by movement. The second two are epilepsies and are discussed elsewhere in this chapter. PNKD is transmitted as an autosomal dominant trait that has been linked to chromosome 2q.

CLINICAL FEATURES. PKD usually begins in childhood. Most cases are sporadic. The paroxysms are precipitated by sudden movement or startle and usually last less than a minute. Several attacks occur each day. Each attack may include dystonia, choreoathetosis, or ballismus (see Chapter 14). One or both sides of the body can be affected. Some patients have an "aura" described as tightness or tingling of the face or limbs.

PNKD begins in childhood or early adult life (Fink et al, 1997). Only a few attacks occur each year, but they last for several hours or days. Although most attacks occur spontaneously, they are also precipitated by caffeine and alcohol. Consciousness is always preserved during attacks of paroxysmal dyskinesia, and life expectancy is not shortened.

DIAGNOSIS. Ictal and interictal EEGs are normal. Children with EEG evidence of epileptiform activity should be considered to have a seizure disorder and not a paroxysmal dyskinesia.

MANAGEMENT. Phenytoin in ordinary anticonvulsant dosages is effective in PKD but not in PNKD. PNKD is difficult to treat, but clonazepam taken daily or at the first sign of an attack may reduce the frequency or severity of attacks. Gabapentin is effective in some children (Chudnow et al, 1997).

Hyperventilation Syndrome

Hyperventilation induces alkalosis by altering the proportion of blood gases. This is more readily accomplished in children than in adults.

CLINICAL FEATURES. During times of emotional upset, the respiratory rate and depth may increase insidiously, first appearing like sighing and then as obvious hyperventilation. The occurrence of tingling of the fingers disturbs the patient further and may induce greater hyperventilation. Headache is an associated symptom. If hyperventilation is allowed to continue, the patient may lose consciousness.

DIAGNOSIS. The observation of hyperventilation as a precipitating factor of syncope is essential to diagnosis. Often patients are unaware that they were hyperventilating, and probing questions are needed to elicit the history in the absence of a witness.

MANAGEMENT. An attack in progress can be aborted by having the patient breathe into a paper bag.

Narcolepsy-Cataplexy

Narcolepsy-cataplexy is a sleep disorder characterized by an abnormally short latency from sleep onset to rapid eye movement (REM) sleep. REM sleep is attained in less than 20 minutes instead of the usual 90 minutes. Normal REM sleep is characterized by dreaming and severe hypotonia. In narcolepsy-cataplexy these phenomena occur during wakefulness.

CLINICAL FEATURES. Onset may occur at any time from early childhood to middle adulthood, usually in the second or third decade and rarely before age 5 (Aldrich, 1998). The syndrome has four components:

1. *Narcolepsy* refers to short sleep attacks. Three or four attacks occur each day, most often during monotonous activity, and are difficult to resist. Half of the patients are easy to arouse from a sleep attack, and 60% feel refreshed afterward. Narcolepsy is usually a lifelong condition.

2. *Cataplexy* is a sudden loss of muscle tone induced by laughter, excitement, or startle. Almost all patients who have narcolepsy have cataplexy as well. The patient may collapse to the floor and then arise immediately. Partial paralysis, affecting just the face or hands, is more common than total paralysis. Two to four attacks occur daily, usually in the afternoon. They are embarrassing but do not cause physical harm.

3. *Sleep paralysis* occurs in the transition between sleep and wakefulness. The patient has generalized hypotonia and, although mentally awake, is unable to move any body part. Partial paralysis is less common. The attack may end spontaneously or when the patient is touched. Two thirds of patients with narcolepsy-cataplexy also experience sleep paralysis once or twice each week. Occasional episodes of sleep paralysis may occur in people who do not have narcolepsy-cataplexy.

4. *Hypnagogic hallucinations* are vivid, usually frightening, visual and auditory perceptions occurring at the transition between sleep and wakefulness: a sensation of dreaming while awake. They are reported as an associated event by half of the patients with narcolepsy-cataplexy. Episodes occur less than once a week.

DIAGNOSIS. The syndrome should be recognizable by the history. However, the symptoms are embarrassing or sound "crazy" to the patient, and considerable prompting is often needed to elicit a full history.

Narcolepsy can be difficult to distinguish from other causes of excessive daytime sleepiness. The multiple sleep latency test is the standard for diagnosis. Patients with narcolepsy enter REM sleep within a few minutes of falling asleep.

MANAGEMENT. Symptoms of narcolepsy-cataplexy are distressing and often associated with emotional disturbances. The realization that narcolepsy is not a mental disorder is comforting.

Methylphenidate or pemoline is usually prescribed for narcolepsy but should be given with some caution because of potential abuse. Small doses should be used on schooldays or workdays and no medicine, if possible, on weekends and holidays. When not taking medicine, patients should be encouraged to schedule short naps.

Modafinil, a new wake-promoting agent distinct from stimulants, has been tested in a placebo-controlled trial in adults (US Modafinil in Narcolepsy Multicenter Study Group, 1998). Once daily treatment with 200 or 400 mg decreased daytime sleepiness with minimal side effects.

Selegiline, a monoamine oxidase inhibitor, is useful in reducing the frequency of sleep attacks and cataplexy. Cataplexy also can be treated with fluoxetine, 20 mg/day; trihexyphenidyl, 2 mg three times a day; or imipramine, 50 mg three times a day.

Night Terrors

Night terrors are a partial arousal from non-rapid eye movement (non-REM) sleep.

CLINICAL FEATURES. The onset usually occurs by 4 years of age and almost always by age 6. Two hours after falling asleep the child awakens in a terrified state, does not recognize people, and is inconsolable. An episode usually lasts for 5 to 15 minutes but can last for an hour. During this time the child screams incoherently, may run if not restrained, and then goes back to sleep. Afterward, the child has no memory of the event.

Most children with night terrors experience an average of one or more episodes each week. Night terrors stop by 8 years of age in one half of affected children but continue into adolescence in one third.

DIAGNOSIS. Half of the children with night terrors are also sleepwalkers, and many have a family history of either sleepwalking or night terrors. The diagnosis should be based on the history alone. A sleep laboratory evaluation may be helpful in unusual circumstances when the possibility of seizures cannot be excluded.

MANAGEMENT. Treatment is not needed, and regular bedtime sedation should be avoided except when spells are very frequent and intolerable to the family. Clonidine, starting at 0.1 mg at bedtime and slowly increased, may be useful to treat night terrors and sleepwalking.

Startle Disease

Startle disease, also called *hyperekplexia*, is a rare disorder transmitted as an autosomal dominant trait (Tijssen et al, 1997). The abnormal gene is a subunit of the glycine receptor on chromosome 5q33-35.

CLINICAL FEATURES. The onset is at birth or during infancy. When the onset is at birth, the newborn may appear hypotonic during sleep and develop generalized stiffening on awakening. Apnea and an exaggerated startle response may be associated signs. Hypertonia in the newborn is unusual. Rigidity diminishes but does not disappear during sleep. Tendon reflexes are brisk, and the response spreads to other muscles.

The stiffness resolves spontaneously during infancy, and by 3 years of age the children are normal; however, episodes of stiffness may recur during adolescence or early adult life in response to startle, cold exposure, or pregnancy. Throughout life, affected individuals show a pathologically exaggerated startle response to visual, auditory, or tactile stimuli that would not startle normal individuals. In some, the startle is associated with a transitory, generalized stiffness of the body that causes falling without protective reflexes, often leading to injury. The stiffening response is often confused with the stiffman syndrome (see Chapter 8).

DIAGNOSIS. A family history of startle disease is critical to the diagnosis but may be difficult to elicit because of partial expression or embarrassment. Startle disease can be differentiated from startle-provoked epileptic seizures because in startle disease the EEG is always normal.

MANAGEMENT. Valproate or clonazepam is useful in abolishing the falling attacks and reducing the startle. The natural history of the disease is variable; some patients improve spontaneously, but others get worse.

Syncope

Syncope is loss of consciousness because of a transitory decline in cerebral blood flow. This may be caused by an irregular cardiac rate or rhythm or by alterations of blood volume or distribution.

CLINICAL FEATURES. Syncope is a common event in otherwise healthy children, especially in the second decade. The mechanism is a vasovagal reflex by which an emotional experience produces peripheral pooling of blood. The reflex may also be stimulated by overextension or sudden decompression of viscera, by the Valsalva maneuver, and by stretching with the neck hyperextended. Fainting in a hot, crowded church when the worshiper rises to stand after prolonged kneeling is especially common. Healthy children do not faint while lying down and rarely while seated. Fainting from anything but standing or arising suggests a cardiac arrhythmia and requires further investigation.

The child may first feel faint (described as "faint," "dizzy," or "light-headed") or may lose consciousness without warning. The face is drained of color, and the skin is cold and clammy. With loss of consciousness the child falls to the floor. Consciousness may be regained rapidly, or stiffening of the body and trembling movements of the arms may occur. The latter is not a seizure. The stiffening and trembling are more common when the reduction of cerebral blood flow is exaggerated and prolonged because the child is prevented from falling. A short period of confusion may follow, but recovery is complete within minutes.

DIAGNOSIS. The criteria for differentiating syncope from seizures are the precipitating factors and the child's appearance. Seizures do not produce pallor and cold, clammy skin. *Always inquire about the child's color in all children having an initial evaluation for seizures.* Laboratory investigations are not cost effective when syncope occurs in expected circumstances and the results of the clinical examination are normal. Recurrent orthostatic syncope requires investigation of autonomic function, and any suspicion of cardiac abnormality deserves ECG monitoring. Always ask the child if irregular heart rate or beats are noted at the time of syncope or at other times.

MANAGEMENT. Infrequent syncopal episodes of obvious cause do not require treatment.

Migraine and Epilepsy

Migraine and epilepsy are thought to be linked because (1) they are both familial, paroxysmal, and associated with transitory neurological disturbances, (2) the incidence of epilepsy is increased in migraine sufferers, and the incidence of migraine is increased in epileptics, (3) headache can be a seizure manifestation, and (4) abnormal EEGs are common in both disorders.

CLINICAL FEATURES. In children who have epilepsy and migraine, both disorders may have a common aura and one may provoke the other. Basilar migraine (see Chapter 10) and benign occipital epilepsy best exemplify the fine line between epilepsy and migraine. Both are characterized by seizures, headache, and epileptiform activity.

DIAGNOSIS. The diagnosis is based on the clinical features. Asymptomatic central spikes are observed in 9% of children with migraine compared with 1.9% of healthy children.

MANAGEMENT. Children who have both epilepsy and migraine must be treated for each condition separately.

Staring Spells

Daydreaming is a pleasant escape for people of all ages. Children feel the need for escape most acutely when in school and may stare vacantly out the window to the place where they would rather be. Daydreams can be hard to break, and a child may not respond to verbal commands. Neurologists, who often recommend EEG, see many dreamers. Sometimes the EEG shows sleep-activated central spikes or another abnormality not related to staring, which may lead the physician to prescribe inappropriate anticonvulsant drug therapy.

Absence and complex partial seizures are both characterized by staring. They are usually distinguishable because absence is brief (5 to 15 seconds) and the child feels normal immediately afterward, while complex partial seizures usually last for more than 1 minute and are followed by fatigue. The associated EEG patterns and the response to treatment are quite different, and precise diagnosis is needed before treatment is initiated.

Absence seizures occur in four epileptic syndromes: childhood absence epilepsy, juvenile absence epilepsy, juvenile myoclonic epilepsy, and epilepsy with grand mal on awakening (Janz, 1997). All four syndromes are genetic disorders transmitted as an autosomal dominant trait. The phenotypes have considerable overlap. The most significant difference is the age at onset.

Childhood and Juvenile Absence Epilepsy

Childhood absence epilepsy begins between ages 6 and 8 years and juvenile absence epilepsy between ages 10 and 16 years. One may be a continuum of the other. As a rule, adolescent onset is associated with a higher frequency of generalized tonic-clonic seizures and is more likely to persist into adult life. Development of generalized tonic-clonic seizures or myoclonic seizures during treatment of absence predicts lack of remission and progression to juvenile myoclonic epilepsy (Wirrell et al, 1996).

CLINICAL FEATURES. The reported incidence of epilepsy in families of children with absence varies from 15% to 40%. Concurrence in monozygotic twins is 75% for seizures and 85% for the characteristic EEG abnormality.

Affected children are otherwise healthy. Typical attacks last for 5 to 10 seconds and occur up to 100 times each day. The child stops ongoing activity, stares vacantly, sometimes with rhythmic movements of the eyelids, and then resumes activity. Aura and postictal confusion never occur. Longer seizures may last for up to 1 minute and are indistinguishable by observation alone from complex partial seizures. Associated features may include myoclonus, increased or decreased postural tone, picking at clothes, turning of the head, and conjugate movements of the eyes. Occasional children and adults are brought to emergency departments in a confusional state caused by absence status (see Chapter 2).

Approximately 50% of children with absence have at least one generalized tonic-clonic seizure. Many are first brought for medical care because of a tonic-clonic seizure, even though absence attacks have occurred undiagnosed for months or years. The occurrence of a generalized tonic-clonic seizure in an untreated child does not change the diagnosis, prognosis, or treatment plan.

DIAGNOSIS. The EEG is pathognomonic. Bilaterally synchronous and symmetric paroxysms of 3-cps spike-wave complexes appear concurrently with the clinical seizure (Figure 1-3). The amplitude of discharge is greatest in the frontocentral regions. Although the discharge begins with a frequency of 3 cps, it may slow to 2 cps as it ends. Hyperventilation almost always activates the discharge. The interictal EEG is usually normal. When it is abnormal, the typical features are focal or multifocal spike discharges or diffuse slowing. Children with interictal abnormalities are more likely to have mental retardation or developmental delay.

Although the EEG pattern of discharge is stereotyped, variations on the theme in the form of multiple spike and wave discharges are also acceptable. During sleep, the discharges often lose their stereotypy and become polymorphic in form and frequency but remain generalized.

Once a correlation between clinical and EEG findings is made, looking for an underlying disease is unnecessary. Absence epilepsy is distinguished from juvenile myoclonic epilepsy (see later discussion on Myoclonic Seizures) by the absence of myoclonic seizures.

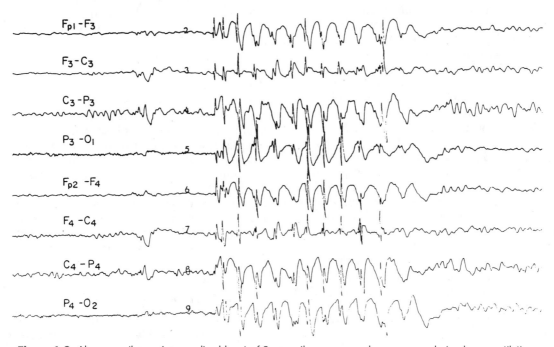

Figure 1-3. Absence epilepsy. A generalized burst of 3-cps spike-wave complexes appears during hyperventilation.

MANAGEMENT. Ethosuximide and valproate are equally effective in the treatment of absence, with each providing complete relief of seizures in 80% of children. Ethosuximide is preferred because of its lower incidence of serious side effects. If neither drug alone provides seizure control, they can be used in combination at reduced dosages or lamotrigine can be substituted for one or both drugs (see Lamotrigine, later on, for precautions concerning the combination of valproate and lamotrigine). The EEG becomes normal if treatment is successful, and repeating the EEG is useful to confirm the seizure-free state.

Children with only a 3-cps spike-wave on EEG should first be treated with ethosuximide alone, even if a tonic-clonic seizure occurred before initiation of therapy. If tonic-clonic seizures recur after therapy is initiated, valproate should be substituted for ethosuximide. Clonazepam is sometimes useful in the treatment of refractory absence. Carbamazepine may accentuate the seizures and cause absence status.

Complex Partial Seizures

Complex partial seizures arise in the cortex, most often the temporal lobe, but can originate from the frontal or parietal lobes as well. Complex partial seizures (discussed more fully in a later section) may be symptomatic of an underlying focal disorder.

CLINICAL FEATURES. Complex partial seizures occur spontaneously or may be activated by sleep. Most last 1 to 2 minutes and rarely less than 30 seconds. An aura is reported in fewer than 30% of children. It is usually a nondescript unpleasant feeling, but may also be a stereotyped auditory hallucination or abdominal discomfort. The first feature of the seizure can be staring, automatic behavior, tonic extension of one or both arms, or loss of body tone. Staring is associated with a change in facial expression and is followed by automatic behavior. Automatisms vary from facial grimacing and fumbling movements of the fingers to walking, running, and resisting restraint. Automatic behavior in a given patient tends to be similar from seizure to seizure.

The seizure usually terminates with a period of postictal confusion, disorientation, or lethargy. Transitory aphasia is sometimes present. Secondary generalization is likely if the child is not treated or if treatment is abruptly withdrawn.

Partial complex status epilepticus is a rare event characterized by impaired consciousness, staring alternating with wandering eye movements, and automatisms of the face and hands. Such children may arrive at the emergency department in a confused or delirious state (see Chapter 2).

DIAGNOSIS. The etiology of complex partial seizures is heterogeneous, and a cause is often not determined. Contrast-enhanced MRI should be done in all cases. It may reveal a low-grade glioma or dysplastic tissue, especially migrational defects.

An EEG should be recorded in both the waking and sleeping states. Hyperventilation and photic stimulation are not useful as provocative measures. Results of a single EEG may be normal in the interictal period, but repeated EEGs usually reveal either a spike or slow-wave focus in the frontal or temporal lobe or multifocal abnormalities. During the seizure, repetitive focal spike discharges occur in the involved area of cortex, which change to spike-slow wave complexes and then slow waves with amplitude attenuation as the seizure ends.

MANAGEMENT. Carbamazepine, phenytoin, primidone, and valproate are effective for seizure control, and the choice should be based on cost, side effects, and dosage schedule. Topiramate and lamotrigine are useful as add-on therapy in children whose seizures are hard to control.

Temporal lobectomy should be considered when seizures are refractory to anticonvulsant drugs (see section on Surgical Approaches to Childhood Epilepsy).

Myoclonic Seizures

Myoclonus is a brief, involuntary muscle contraction (jerk) that may represent (1) a seizure manifestation, as in infantile spasms, (2) a physiological response to startle or to falling asleep, or (3) an involuntary movement either alone or in combination with tonic-clonic seizures (see Table 14-8). Myoclonic seizures are often difficult to distinguish from myoclonus (the movement disorder) on clinical grounds alone. Essential myoclonus and other disorders in which myoclonus is not a seizure are discussed in Chapter 14.

Juvenile Myoclonic Epilepsy

Juvenile myoclonic epilepsy (JME) is a hereditary disorder, probably inherited as an autosomal dominant trait. The responsible gene has been mapped to the short arm of chromosome 6 (Serratosa et al, 1996).

CLINICAL FEATURES. Males and females are affected equally. Seizures in affected children and their affected relatives may be tonic-clonic, myoclonic, or absence. The usual age at onset of absence seizures is 7 to 13 years; of myoclonic jerks, 12 to 18 years; and of generalized tonic-clonic seizures, 13 to 20 years.

The myoclonic seizures are brief, bilateral but not always symmetric, flexor jerks of the arms, which may be repetitive. The jerk sometimes affects the legs, causing the patient to fall. The highest frequency of myoclonic jerks is in the morning. Consciousness is usually retained so that the patient is aware of the jerking movement. Seizures are precipitated by sleep deprivation, alcohol ingestion, and awakening from nocturnal or daytime sleep.

Most patients also have generalized tonic-clonic seizures, and one third experience absence but are otherwise normal neurologically. The potential for seizures of one type or another continues throughout adult life.

DIAGNOSIS. Diagnosis is often delayed until a generalized tonic-clonic seizure brings the child to medical attention. The interictal EEG in JME consists of bilateral, symmetrical spike and polyspike-and-wave discharges of 3.5–6 Hz, usually maximal in the frontocentral regions (Figure 1-4). Photic stimulation often provokes

a discharge. Focal EEG abnormalities may occur.

MANAGEMENT. Valproate is the treatment of choice and provides complete relief of seizures in 75% of cases. Lamotrigine, levetiracetam, topiramate, or zonisamide can be used in patients who do not tolerate valproate. Treatment is lifelong.

Progressive Myoclonus Epilepsies

The term *progressive myoclonus epilepsies* is used to cover several progressive disorders of the nervous system characterized by (1) myoclonus; (2) seizures that may be tonic-clonic, tonic, or myoclonic; (3) progressive mental deterioration; and (4) cerebellar ataxia, involuntary movements, or both. Some of these disorders are due to specific lysosomal enzyme deficiencies, whereas others are probably mitochondrial disorders (Table 1-10).

Lafora Disease

Lafora disease is a rare hereditary disease probably transmitted by autosomal recessive inheritance.

CLINICAL FEATURES. Onset is between 11 and 18 years of age, with the mean at age 14. Tonic-clonic or myoclonic seizures are the initial feature in 80% of cases. Myoclonus becomes progressively worse, may be segmental or massive,

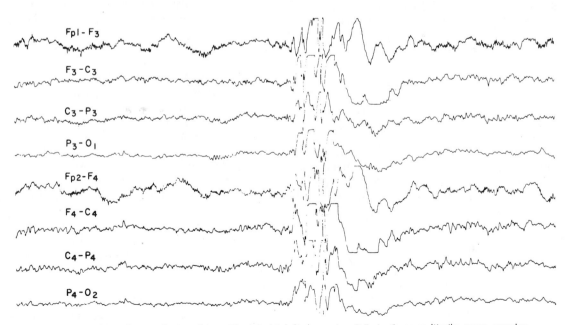

Figure 1-4. Juvenile myoclonic epilepsy. The interictal discharge is a 3.5- to 6-cps multispike-wave complex.

Table **1-10**
Progressive Myoclonus Epilepsies

Ceroid lipofuscinosis, juvenile form (see Chapter 5)
Glucosylceramide lipidosis (Gaucher type 3) (see Chapter 5)
Lafora disease
Myoclonus epilepsy and ragged-red fibers (see Chapter 5)
Ramsay-Hunt syndrome (see Chapter 10)
Sialidoses (see Chapter 5)
Unverricht-Lundborg syndrome

and is increased by movement. Mental retardation begins early and is relentlessly progressive. Ataxia, spasticity, and involuntary movements occur late in the course. Death occurs 5 to 6 years after the onset of symptoms.

DIAGNOSIS. The EEG is normal at first and later develops nonspecific generalized polyspike discharges that are not activated by sleep. The background becomes progressively disorganized and epileptiform activity more constant. Photosensitive discharges are a regular feature late in the course.

Antemortem diagnosis is sometimes accomplished by showing periodic acid-Schiff (PAS)–positive inclusion bodies consisting of aggregates of filaments composed of polyglucasans in biopsy specimens of liver or sweat gland, but these may be absent even in late stages of the disease.

MANAGEMENT. The seizures become refractory to most anticonvulsant drugs, but the combination of valproate, clonazepam, and phenobarbital should be tried. Treatment of the underlying disease is not available.

Unverricht-Lundborg Syndrome

Unverricht-Lundborg syndrome is clinically similar to Lafora disease, except that inclusion bodies are not present. It is transmitted by autosomal recessive inheritance. The syndrome is most often reported in Finland and other Baltic countries but has a worldwide distribution. A combination of valproate, clonazepam, and phenobarbital is effective for seizure control.

Reading Epilepsy

Reading epilepsy may be a variant of juvenile myoclonic epilepsy; many children with reading epilepsy experience myoclonic jerks of the limbs shortly after arising in the morning (Radhakrishnan et al, 1995).

CLINICAL FEATURES. Age at onset is usually in the second decade. Myoclonic jerks involving orofacial and jaw muscles develop while reading. Reading time before seizure onset is variable. The initial seizure is almost always in the jaw and is described as "jaws locking or clicking." Other initial features are quivering of the lips, choking in the throat, or difficulty speaking. Myoclonic jerks of the limbs may follow, and some children experience a generalized tonic-clonic seizure if they continue reading. Generalized tonic-clonic seizures may also occur at other times.

DIAGNOSIS. The history of myoclonic jerks during reading and during other processes requiring higher cognitive function is critical to the diagnosis. The interictal EEG usually shows generalized discharges, and brief spike-wave complexes can be provoked by reading that are simultaneous with jaw jerks.

MANAGEMENT. Some patients can control their seizures without the use of anticonvulsant drugs by quitting reading at the first sign of orofacial or jaw jerks. Most require anticonvulsant therapy. Phenytoin or carbamazepine is effective.

Partial Seizures

This section discusses several different seizure types of focal cortical origin other than complex partial seizures. Such seizures may be purely motor or purely sensory or may affect higher cortical function. The benign childhood partial epilepsies are the most common cause of partial seizures in children. Benign centrotemporal (rolandic) epilepsy and benign occipital epilepsy are the most common forms. The various benign partial epilepsy syndromes begin and cease at similar ages, have a similar course, and occur in the members of the same family. It seems likely that they are different phenotypic expressions of the same genetic defect.

Partial seizures are also secondary to underlying diseases, which can be focal, multifocal, or generalized. Intractable partial seizures are often caused by neuronal migrational disorders and gliomas. Cerebral cysticercosis is an important cause in Mexico and Central America (Carpio et al, 1998). MRI is recommended for all children with intractable focal seizures. Many may be candidates for surgical therapy.

Any seizure that originates in the cortex may discharge into the brainstem, causing a generalized tonic-clonic seizure (secondary generalization). If the discharge remains localized for a few seconds, the patient experiences a focal seizure or an aura before losing consciousness. Often the secondary generalization occurs so rapidly that a tonic-clonic seizure is the initial symptom. In such cases, cortical origin of the seizure may be detectable on EEG. However, normal EEG findings are common during a simple partial seizure and do not exclude the diagnosis.

Acquired Epileptiform Aphasia

Acquired aphasia associated with epileptiform activity on EEG in children is called the *Landau-Kleffner syndrome*. The syndrome appears to be a disorder of auditory processing. The cause is unknown except for occasional cases associated with temporal lobe tumors.

CLINICAL FEATURES. Age at onset ranges from 2 to 11 years, with 75% beginning between 3 and 10 years. The first symptom may be aphasia or epilepsy. Aphasia is initially characterized by auditory verbal agnosia. The child has difficulty understanding what is said, spontaneous speech is reduced, and deafness or autism develops. Seizures, which may be partial or generalized, occur in 80% of children. Atypical absence is sometimes the initial feature and may be associated with continuous spike and slow waves during slow-wave sleep. Hyperactivity and personality change are noted in one half of affected children and may be caused by aphasia. Intelligence is not affected, and the neurological examination is otherwise normal.

Recovery of language is more likely to occur if the syndrome begins before 7 years of age. Seizures cease generally by age 10 and always by age 15.

DIAGNOSIS. Acquired epileptiform aphasia, as the name implies, can be differentiated from autism and hearing loss because the diagnosis requires that the child have normal language and cognitive development prior to onset of symptoms and normal hearing. The EEG shows multifocal cortical spike discharges with a predilection for the temporal and parietal lobes. Involvement is bilateral in 88% of cases. An intravenous injection of diazepam may normalize the EEG and improve speech transiently, but this should not suggest that aphasia is caused by epileptiform activity. Instead, both features reflect an underlying cerebral disorder.

MRI is needed in every case to exclude the rare possibility of a temporal lobe tumor.

MANAGEMENT. Standard anticonvulsant drugs such as carbamazepine and phenytoin usually control the seizures but do not improve speech. Corticosteroid therapy, especially early in the course, may normalize the EEG and provide long-lasting remission of aphasia and seizures.

Recovery of speech in 11 of 14 children was reported from one medical center after subpial intracortical transection of the epileptic focus in the speech area (Morrell et al, 1995).

Acquired Epileptiform Opercula Syndrome

This syndrome and *autosomal dominant rolandic epilepsy and speech apraxia* are probably the same entity (Scheffer et al, 1995). They are probably different from acquired epileptiform aphasia but may represent a spectrum of the same underlying disease process.

CLINICAL FEATURES. Onset is before age 10 years. Brief nocturnal seizures occur that mainly affect the face and mouth but may become secondarily generalized. Oral dysphasia, inability to initiate complex facial movements (blowing out a candle), speech dysphasia, and drooling develop concurrently with seizure onset. Cognitive dysfunction is associated. Familial cases are transmitted by autosomal dominant inheritance with anticipation.

DIAGNOSIS. The EEG shows centrotemporal discharges or status epilepticus during slow wave sleep.

MANAGEMENT. The dysphasia does not respond to anticonvulsant drugs.

Autosomal Dominant Nocturnal Frontal Lobe Epilepsy

This epilepsy syndrome is characterized by bizarre behavior and motor features during sleep, which are often misdiagnosed as a sleep or psychiatric disorder (Hayman et al, 1997). The abnormal gene is located on chromosome 20q and may be allelic with one of the genes for benign neonatal familial epilepsy. It is transmitted as an autosomal dominant trait with a penetrance rate of approximately 70%.

CLINICAL FEATURES. Seizures begin in childhood and usually persist into adult life. Most attacks occur when dozing or first falling off to sleep. Clusters of 4 to 11 seizures, each lasting less than a minute, occur in one night. A vocalization, usually a gasp or grunt that awakens the individual, is common. Other auras include special sensory sensations, psychic phenomena (fear, malaise, etc.), shivering, and difficulty breathing. This is followed by thrashing or tonic stiffening with superimposed clonic jerks. The eyes are open, and the individual is aware of what is happening; many sit up and try to grab on to a bed part.

DIAGNOSIS. The family history is important to the diagnosis, but many family members may not realize that their own attacks are seizures or want others to know that they experience such bizarre symptoms. The interictal EEG is usually normal, and concurrent video-EEG is often required to capture the event. During a seizure the discharge is generalized and distributed diffusely. The initial ictal EEG is often obscured by movement artifact.

Children who have seizures when awake and no family history of epilepsy may have supplementary sensorimotor seizures (see later section on Supplementary Sensorimotor Seizures).

MANAGEMENT. Carbamazepine is usually effective in preventing seizures.

Benign Occipital Epilepsy of Childhood

Benign occipital epilepsy of childhood is probably transmitted by autosomal dominant inheritance. It may be a phenotypic variation of benign rolandic epilepsy. Both epilepsies are commonly associated with migraine (Andermann and Zifkin, 1998).

CLINICAL FEATURES. Age at onset is usually between 4 and 8 years. One third of patients have a family history of epilepsy, frequently benign rolandic epilepsy. The initial seizure manifestation can consist of (1) visual hallucinations, usually flashing lights or spots; (2) blindness, hemianopia, or complete amaurosis; (3) visual illusions, such as micropsia, macropsia, or metamorphasia; or (4) loss of consciousness lasting for up to 12 hours. More than one feature may occur simultaneously. The visual aura may be followed by unilateral clonic seizures, complex partial seizures, or generalized tonic-clonic seizures. Afterward, the child may have migraine-like headaches and nausea. Attacks occur when the child is awake or asleep, but the greatest frequency is at the transition from wakefulness to sleep. Seizures may be induced by photic stimulation or by playing video games.

DIAGNOSIS. Results of the neurological examination, CT, and MRI are normal. The interictal EEG shows unilateral or bilateral high-amplitude, occipital spike-wave discharges with a frequency of 1.5 to 2.5 cps. The discharges are inhibited by eye opening and enhanced by light sleep. A similar interictal pattern is seen in some children with absence epilepsy, suggesting a common genetic disorder among different benign genetic epilepsies. During a seizure, rapid firing of spike discharges occurs in one or both occipital lobes.

Epilepsy associated with ictal vomiting is a variant of benign occipital epilepsy (Panayiotopoulos et al, 1999). Seizures occur during sleep and are characterized by vomiting, eye deviation, speech arrest, or hemiconvulsions.

MANAGEMENT. Complete seizure control is usually accomplished with standard anticonvulsant drugs. Typical seizures never persist beyond 12 years of age. However, not all children with occipital discharges have a benign epilepsy. Persistent or hard-to-control seizures raise the question of a structural abnormality in the occipital lobe, and MRI is indicated.

Benign Rolandic Epilepsy of Childhood

Benign rolandic epilepsy of childhood is a genetic disorder transmitted as an autosomal dominant trait. Forty percent of close relatives have a history of febrile seizures or epilepsy (Wirrell, 1998).

CLINICAL FEATURES. The age at onset is between 3 and 13 years, with a peak at 7 to 8 years. Seizures almost always stop spontaneously by age 14. Even without drug therapy, 10% of patients have only one seizure, 70% have infrequent seizures, and only 20% have frequent seizures. With drug therapy, 20% have isolated seizures and 6% have frequent seizures. Seventy percent of children have seizures only while asleep, 15% only when awake, and 15% both awake and asleep.

The typical seizure wakes the child from sleep. Paresthesias occur on one side of the mouth, followed by ipsilateral twitching of the face, mouth, and pharynx, resulting in speech arrest and drooling. Consciousness is preserved. The seizure lasts for 1 or 2 minutes. Daytime seizures do not generalize, but nocturnal seizures in children younger than 5 years old often spread to the arm or evolve into a generalized tonic-clonic seizure.

DIAGNOSIS. Results of neurological examination and brain imaging studies are normal. Interictal EEG shows unilateral or bilateral spike discharges in the central or centrotemporal region. The spikes are typically of high voltage and are activated by drowsiness and sleep. The frequency of spike discharge does not correlate with the subsequent course. Children with typical clinical seizures and EEG abnormalities do not require neuroimaging. However, MRI is warranted in those with atypical features or hard-to-control seizures and may show a low-grade glioma.

MANAGEMENT. Treatment is not needed if seizures are infrequent and only nocturnal. A single bedtime dose of phenobarbital is usually satisfactory for seizure control. After 2 years of treatment, medication can be withdrawn and 80% of patients remain seizure free. Those who resume having seizures should be treated until age 14. All children eventually stop having seizures whether they are treated or not.

Epilepsia Partialis Continuans

Focal motor seizures that do not stop spontaneously are termed *epilepsia partialis continuans*. This is an ominous symptom and almost always indicates an underlying cerebral disorder. Possible causes include infarction, hemorrhage, tumor, and inflammation. Every effort should be made to stop the seizures with intravenous anticonvulsant drugs (see later section on Treatment of Status Epilepticus). The response to anticonvulsant drugs and the outcome depend on the underlying cause.

Hemiconvulsions-Hemiplegia Syndrome (Rasmussen Syndrome)

Rasmussen syndrome is a poorly understood disorder that was originally described as focal viral encephalitis. However, an infectious etiology has never been established.

CLINICAL FEATURES. Focal jerking frequently begins in one body part, usually one side of the face or one hand, and then spreads to contiguous parts. Trunk muscles are rarely affected. The rate and intensity of the seizures vary at first, but then become more regular and persist during sleep. The seizures defy treatment and progress to affect first both limbs on one side of the body and then the limbs on the other side. Progressive hemiplegia develops and remains after seizures have stopped.

DIAGNOSIS. EEG shows continuous spike discharges originating in one portion of the cortex, with spread to contiguous areas of the cortex and to a mirror focus on the other side. Secondary generalization may occur. MRI should be performed in every case. The initial imaging studies are usually normal, but repeat studies

after 6 months show atrophy of the hemisphere with dilation of the ipsilateral ventricle. PET shows widespread hypometabolism of the affected hemisphere at a time when the spike discharges are still localized. The cerebrospinal fluid is usually normal, although a few monocytes may be present.

MANAGEMENT. The treatment of Rasmussen syndrome is especially difficult. Standard anticonvulsant therapy is not effective in stopping seizures, and progressive hemiplegia is the rule. The use of immunosuppressive therapy is recommended by some and antiviral therapy by others. These medical approaches are rarely successful. Early hemispherectomy is the treatment of choice.

Temporal Lobe Epilepsy

Temporal lobe epilepsy in children may be primary or secondary (Harvey et al, 1997). Primary temporal lobe epilepsy is inherited as an autosomal dominant trait. Among children with secondary temporal lobe epilepsy, a history of an antecedent illness or event is obtained in 29% of children, and MRI shows a structural abnormality in 38%.

CLINICAL FEATURES. Seizure onset in primary temporal lobe epilepsy occurs in adolescence or later. The seizures consist of simple psychic (déjà vu, cognitive disturbances, illusions and hallucinations) or autonomic (nausea, tachycardia, sweating) symptoms. Secondary generalization is unusual. Seizure onset in secondary temporal lobe epilepsy is during the first decade and often occurs during an acute illness. The seizures are usually complex partial in type, and secondary generalization is more common.

DIAGNOSIS. A single EEG in children with primary temporal lobe epilepsy is likely to be normal. The frequency of interictal temporal lobe spikes is low, and prolonged video-EEG studies are often needed for diagnosis. The incidence of focal interictal temporal lobe spikes is 78% in children with secondary temporal lobe epilepsy, but detection may require several EEG studies.

MANAGEMENT. Monotherapy with phenytoin or carbamazepine is usually satisfactory for seizure control in both types.

Generalized Tonic-Clonic Seizures

Generalized tonic-clonic seizures are the most common seizures of childhood. They are dramatic and frightening events that invariably demand medical attention. Seizures that are prolonged or repeated without recovery are termed *status epilepticus*. Many children with generalized tonic-clonic seizures have a history of febrile seizures during infancy (Scheffer and Berkovic, 1997). Some of these represent a distinct autosomal dominant disorder. The diagnostic considerations in a child who has had a generalized tonic-clonic seizure are summarized in Table 1-11.

CLINICAL FEATURES. The onset may occur anytime after the neonatal period, but the onset of primary generalized epilepsy without absence is usually during the second decade. With absence, age at onset shifts to the first decade.

The initial feature is sudden loss of consciousness. The child falls to the floor, and the body stiffens (tonic phase). Repetitive jerking movements of the limbs follow (clonic phase); these movements at first are rapid and rhythmic and then become slower and more irregular as the seizure ends. The eyes roll backward in the orbits; breathing is rapid and deep, causing saliva to froth at the lips; and urinary and fecal incontinence may occur. Seizures are followed by a postictal sleep from which arousal is difficult. Afterward, the child appears normal but may have sore limb muscles and a painful tongue, bitten during the seizure.

DIAGNOSIS. A first generalized tonic-clonic seizure requires laboratory evaluation. The extent of evaluation must be individualized. Important determining factors include neurological findings, family history, and known precipitating factors. An eyewitness report of focal features at the onset of the seizure, or the recollection of an aura, indicates a partial seizure with secondary generalization.

During the seizure the EEG shows generalized repetitive spikes in the tonic phase and then periodic bursts of spikes in the clonic phase. The clonic portion is usually obscured by movement artifact. As the seizure ends, the background rhythms are slow and the amplitude is attenuated.

Table 1-11

Diagnostic Considerations for a First Nonfebrile Tonic-Clonic Seizure after 2 Years of Age

Acute encephalopathy or encephalitis (see Chapter 2)
Isolated unexplained seizure
Partial seizure of any cause with secondary generalization
Primary generalized epilepsy
Progressive disorder of the nervous system (see Chapter 5)

Between seizures, brief generalized spike or spike-wave discharges that are polymorphic in appearance may occur. Discharge frequency is sometimes increased by drowsiness and light sleep. The presence of focal discharges indicates that the tonic-clonic seizure was secondarily generalized.

The cerebrospinal fluid is normal following a brief tonic-clonic seizure due to primary epilepsy. However, prolonged or repeated seizures may cause leukocytosis (up to 80 cells/mm^3 with a polymorphonuclear predominance). The protein concentration can be mildly elevated, but the glucose concentration is normal.

MANAGEMENT. I do not start prophylactic anticonvulsant therapy in an otherwise normal child who has had a single unexplained seizure. The recurrence rate is probably less than 50% after 1 year. Phenobarbital, phenytoin, and carbamazepine are equally effective in children with recurrent seizures that require treatment. Status epilepticus must be treated with intravenous drugs (see later section on Treatment of Status Epilepticus).

Epilepsy with Generalized Tonic-Clonic Seizures on Awakening

Epilepsy with generalized tonic-clonic seizures on awakening is not linked to the JME gene locus on chromosome 6 (Greenberg et al, 1995). The mode of inheritance is unknown.

CLINICAL FEATURES. Onset occurs in the second decade, and 90% of seizures occur on awakening, regardless of the time of day. Seizures also occur with relaxation in the evening. Absence and myoclonic seizures may occur.

DIAGNOSIS. The EEG shows a pattern of idiopathic generalized epilepsies.

MANAGEMENT. Treatment is similar to that of JME.

Pseudoseizures

"Hysterical" seizures are an effective method of seeking attention and secondary gain. They occur more often in adolescence than childhood and more often in females than males (3 : 1). A history of sexual abuse is common in women who experience pseudoseizures. People with pseudoseizures may also have true seizures; the pseudoseizures begin when true seizures come under control, and the secondary gain of epilepsy is lost.

CLINICAL FEATURES. Pseudoseizures rarely simulate true seizures but sometimes may be difficult to distinguish by observation alone. The clinical features include a rich variety of motor and behavioral phenomena, but three broad patterns are often observed:

1. Unilateral or bilateral motor activity characterized by tonic posturing and tremulousness in which the patient's movements are thrashing or jerking rather than tonic-clonic; different movements may occur simultaneously.

2. Behavioral or emotional changes in which distress or discomfort is expressed, followed by semipurposeless, but not stereotyped, behaviors such as fumbling with objects or walking.

3. Periods of unresponsiveness.

Attacks may be precipitated and ended by suggestion. Patients usually do not hurt themselves and are not incontinent.

DIAGNOSIS. Pseudoseizures usually occur at home and are believed to be real. If the child has epilepsy, the seizures are reported by telephone to the physician and drug schedules are needlessly revised, often to the patient's detriment. The possibility of pseudoseizures must be considered when frequent seizures develop in children whose epilepsy has recently come under control. Children who do not have epilepsy and in whom pseudoseizures develop are frequently brought to an emergency department and may be given anticonvulsant drugs before any investigation is initiated. It is then difficult to stop the medications and obtain a baseline EEG. Most pseudoseizures are diagnosed by observation alone. When doubt remains, video-EEG monitoring is the best method of diagnosis.

MANAGEMENT. The diagnosis of pseudoseizures should be presented in a positive and supportive manner. The diagnosis does not mean that the person is crazy or faking. The spells can be stopped, but not with anticonvulsant drugs. Psychiatric referral is not always necessary, but psychological counseling is often needed. Determining the secondary gain provided by seizures and offering alternative methods of satisfaction is the best approach to treatment. Most children with pseudoseizures stop having attacks once the diagnosis is established.

Video Game-Induced Seizures

Children who experience seizures while playing video games usually have a photosensitive seizure disorder that is demonstrable on EEG during intermittent photic stimulation. Two thirds

have primary generalized epilepsy (generalized tonic-clonic, absence, and juvenile myoclonic epilepsy), and the rest have partial epilepsies, usually benign occipital epilepsy.

Anticonvulsant Drug Therapy

The goal of anticonvulsant therapy is to achieve the maximum normal function by balancing seizure control against drug toxicity (Greenwood and Tennison, 1999).

Indications for Starting Therapy

Prophylactic therapy should be initiated whenever there is a reasonable expectation that seizures will recur. Juvenile myoclonic epilepsy and absence epilepsy should always be treated, not only because more seizures are expected, but also because uncontrolled absence impairs education. After a first unexplained and untreated seizure, less than half of otherwise normal children will have a second seizure. The risk of recurrence after a second untreated generalized tonic-clonic seizure is 90%, but the recurrence rate in children with partial seizures is considerably lower because of the benign cortical epilepsies of childhood. Further, the chance of ultimately providing seizure control is not influenced by delaying therapy and allowing more seizures to occur (Musicco et al, 1997). *In an otherwise normal child who is not driving a car, it is reasonable to withhold therapy after a first unexplained seizure until a second seizure occurs.*

Discontinuing Therapy

Children who have seizures during an acute encephalopathy (e.g., anoxia, head trauma, encephalitis) should be treated with anticonvulsant drugs. When the acute encephalopathy is over and seizures have stopped, anticonvulsant therapy should be discontinued. Only a minority of children will have epilepsy later on, and they can be treated when seizures recur. It is not established that later epilepsy can be prevented by the continuous use of anticonvulsant drugs after an acute encephalopathy.

Pooled data on epilepsy in children suggest that anticonvulsant therapy can be successfully discontinued in children whose seizures have been controlled for 2 years. *I suspect that many otherwise normal children who were started on anticonvulsant medication after a first seizure and then remain seizure free for 2 years should not have received medication in the first place.* The decision to stop therapy, like the decision to start therapy, should be individualized to the child and the cause of the epilepsy. Children who are neurologically abnormal (remote symptomatic epilepsy) and those with specific epileptic syndromes that are known to persist into adult life are likely to have recurrences, while those with benign epilepsies of childhood are likely to remain seizure free. Three fourths of relapses occur during the withdrawal phase and in the 2 years thereafter. Contrary to popular belief, seizures are not caused by the rapid withdrawal of anticonvulsant drugs in a person who does not need them. Seizures occur in people with epilepsy when the blood concentration is no longer therapeutic, without regard to the rate of decline. As a general rule, I try to stop anticonvulsant therapy 1 year before driving age in children who are seizure free and neurologically normal.

Principles of Therapy

Therapy should be started with a single drug. Most children with epilepsy achieve complete seizure control with monotherapy. Even patients whose seizures are never controlled are likely to do better on the smallest number of drugs. Polytherapy poses several problems: (1) drugs compete with each other for protein binding sites, (2) one drug can increase the rate and pathway of catabolism of a second drug, (3) drugs have cumulative toxicity, and (4) compliance is more difficult.

When more than one drug is needed, drugs that have different spectrums of activity or mechanisms of action should be chosen. Only one drug should be changed at a time. If several changes are made simultaneously, it is impossible to determine which drug is responsible for a beneficial or an adverse effect.

Anticonvulsant drugs should not be administered more often than three times each day. With many drugs an acceptable steady state can be attained using a twice-a-day regimen, and some can be administered once a day. Compliance falls when drugs are taken more than twice each day. *It is difficult to remember to take medicine when you are not in pain to prevent something from happening.*

Blood Concentrations

The development of techniques to measure blood concentrations of anticonvulsant drugs was an important advance in the treatment of epilepsy. Measuring total drug concentrations, protein-bound and free fractions, is customary even though the free fraction is responsible for efficacy and toxicity. While the ratio of free to bound fractions is relatively constant, some drugs have a greater affinity for binding protein than other drugs and will displace them when used together. The free fraction of the displaced drug is then increased and causes toxicity even though the measured total drug concentration is "therapeutic."

Reference values of drug concentrations are guidelines. Some patients are seizure free with concentrations that are below the reference value, and others are unaffected by apparently toxic concentrations.

Most anticonvulsants follow first-order kinetics; that is, blood levels increase proportionately with increases in the oral dose. The main exception is phenytoin, whose metabolism changes from first-order to zero-order kinetics when the enzyme system responsible for its catabolism is saturated. Then a small increment in oral dose produces large increments in blood concentration.

The half-lives of the anticonvulsants listed in Table 1-12 are at steady state. Half-lives are generally longer when a patient is first exposed to a drug. Steady state is usually achieved after five half-lives. Similarly, five half-lives are required to eliminate a drug after administration has been discontinued. Drug half-lives vary from individual to individual and may be shortened or increased by the concurrent use of other anticonvulsants, antibiotics, and antipyretics. This is one reason that children with epilepsy may have a toxic response to a drug or increased seizures at the time of a febrile illness.

Some anticonvulsants are metabolized to active metabolites that have anticonvulsant and toxic properties. With the exception of phenobarbital derived from primidone, these metabolites are not usually measured. Active metabolites may provide seizure control or have toxic effects when the blood concentration of the parent compound is low.

Adverse Reactions

Many anticonvulsant drugs irritate the gastric mucosa and cause nausea and vomiting. When this occurs, symptoms may be relieved by taking smaller doses at more frequent intervals, using enteric-coated preparations, and administering the drug after meals.

Table **1-12**
Anticonvulsant Drugs for Children

Drug	Initial Dosage	Maintenance Dosage	Blood Concentration (μg/ml)	Half-Life (hours)
Carbamazepine	5 mg/kg/day	10–35 mg/kg/day	4–12	14–27
Clonazepam	0.025 mg/day	1–3 mg/day	*	20–40
Clorazepate	3.75 mg/bid	15–60 mg/day	*	20–60
Ethosuximide	10–15 mg/kg/day	15–40 mg/kg/day	*	30–40
Felbamate	15 mg/kg/day	15–45 mg/kg/day	40–80	20–23
Gabapentin	10 mg/kg/day	30–60 mg/kg/day	***	5–7
Lamotrigine	0.6 mg/kg/day**	5–15 mg/kg/day	***	25 (monotherapy) 12 (polytherapy)
Levetiracetam	15 mg/kg/day	45 mg/kg	***	5
Oxcarbazepine	10 mg/kg/day	20–40 mg/kg/day	***	9
Phenobarbital	3–5 mg/kg/day	5–10 mg/kg/day	15–40	35–73
Phenytoin	5–10 mg/kg/day	5–10 mg/kg/day	10–25	24
Primidone	5 mg/kg/day	10–25 mg/kg/day	8–12	8–22
Tiagabine	4 mg/day	4–32 mg/day	***	16
Topiramate	1 mg/kg/day	1–9 mg/kg/day	***	18–30
Valproate	20 mg/kg/day	30–60 mg/kg/day	50–100	6–15
Vigabatrin	40–60 mg/kg/day	60–80 mg/kg/day	***	Days
Zonisamide	1.5 mg/kg/day	6 mg/kg/day	***	24

* Not clinically useful.
** Dosage depends on concomitant therapy with other drugs (see text).
*** Not established.

Toxic adverse reactions are dose related. All anticonvulsant drugs cause sedation when blood concentrations are excessive. Subtle cognitive and behavioral disturbances, which are recognized only by the patient or family, often occur at low blood concentrations. The patient's observation of a toxic effect should not be discounted because the blood concentration is within the therapeutic range. As doses are increased, attention span, memory, and interpersonal relations may become seriously impaired. This is especially common with barbiturates but can occur with any drug.

Idiosyncratic reactions are not entirely dose related. They may occur on the basis of hypersensitivity (usually manifest as rash, fever, and lymphadenopathy) but may also be caused by the production of toxic metabolites. Idiosyncratic reactions are not always predictable, and the patient's observation should be respected, even when the reaction was not previously reported.

Notwithstanding package inserts and threats of litigation, routine laboratory studies of blood counts and organ function in a healthy child are neither cost effective nor helpful. I prefer to do studies based on clinical features.

Selection of an Anticonvulsant Drug

The use of generic drugs is difficult to avoid in managed care health programs. Unfortunately, several different manufacturers provide generic versions of each drug; the bioavailability and half-life of these products vary considerably, and maintaining a predictable blood concentration may be difficult. Common reasons for loss of seizure control in children who were previously seizure free are noncompliance and changing from the brand name to a generic drug or from one generic to another. Patients should ask their pharmacist to tell them when their source of generic drug is going to change.

The drugs most often selected for the treatment of generalized tonic-clonic and partial seizures are carbamazepine, oxcarbazepine, phenobarbital, and phenytoin. Clonazepam, felbamate, levetiracetam, topiramate, valproate, and zonisamide are used in refractory cases. Levetiracetam, topiramate, valproate, and zonisamide are effective against many different seizure types. However, all are more expensive than several older drugs and need not be chosen first when other drugs are equally effective.

The initial drugs used to treat absence seizures are either ethosuximide or valproate. Those used initially to treat myoclonic seizures are valproate, lamotrigine, levetiracetam, and benzodiazepines (clonazepam, clorazepate, and nitrazepam). The ketogenic diet is an alternative to drug therapy. ACTH, prednisone, and pyridoxine provide transitory relief of intractable seizures in infants (see Infantile Spasms), but they are not ordinarily used in older children.

Carbamazepine (Tegretol, Tegretol-XR, Novartis; Carbitrol, Shire Richmond)

INDICATIONS. Partial seizures, primary or secondary generalized tonic-clonic seizures. Contraindicated in the treatment of absence and myoclonic seizures.

ADMINISTRATION. Approximately 85% of the drug is protein bound. Carbamazepine induces its own metabolism, and the initial dose should be 25% of the maintenance dose to prevent toxicity. The usual maintenance dosage is 15 to 20 mg/kg/day to provide a blood concentration of 4 to 12 μg/ml. However, 30 mg/kg/day is often required in infants. The half-life at steady state is 5 to 27 hours, and children usually require doses three times a day. Two long-acting preparations are available.

Concurrent use of cimetidine, erythromycin, fluoxetine, and propoxyphene interferes with carbamazepine metabolism and causes toxicity.

ADVERSE EFFECTS. A depression of peripheral leukocytes is expected but is rarely sufficient (absolute neutrophil count less than 1,000) to warrant discontinuation of therapy. It is reasonable to measure the white blood cell count 6 weeks after therapy is started. Repeated white blood cell counts each time the patient returns for a routine follow-up visit are not cost effective and do not allow the prediction of life-threatening events. The most informative time to repeat the white blood cell count is concurrently with a febrile illness.

Cognitive disturbances occur within the therapeutic range. Sedation, ataxia, and nystagmus occur at toxic blood concentrations. Nonepileptic myoclonus is an allergic reaction.

Clonazepam (Klonopin, Roche)

INDICATIONS. Clonazepam is used to treat infantile spasms, myoclonic seizures, absence, and partial seizures.

ADMINISTRATION. The initial dosage is 0.025 mg/kg/day in two divided doses. Increments of 0.025 mg/kg are recommended every 3 to 5 days as needed and tolerated. The usual maintenance dosage is 0.1 mg/kg/day in three divided doses. Most children cannot tolerate dosages of more than 0.15 mg/kg/day. Therapeutic blood concentrations are 0.02 to 0.07 μg/ml; 47% of the drug is protein bound, and the half-life is 20 to 40 hours. The rectal route may be used for maintenance.

ADVERSE EFFECTS. Toxic effects with dosages within the therapeutic range include sedation, cognitive impairment, hyperactivity, and excessive salivation. Idiosyncratic reactions are unusual.

Clorazepate (Tranxene, Abbott)

INDICATIONS. Adjunct therapy for refractory myoclonic and partial seizures. Clorazepate should not be used as a primary anticonvulsant.

ADMINISTRATION. The smallest dosage, a 3.75-mg capsule, is given once each day and increased by one capsule every 3 days as needed and tolerated. Maintenance dosage is 1 to 3 mg/kg/day in three divided doses. The total dosage is limited by toxicity, and blood concentration measurements are not useful.

ADVERSE EFFECTS. Sedation occurs within the therapeutic range and limits usefulness. Higher doses cause ataxia, diplopia, and impairment of cognitive function.

Ethosuximide (Zarontin, Parke-Davis)

INDICATIONS. Treatment of absence; also useful for myoclonic absence.

ADMINISTRATION. The drug is absorbed rapidly, and peak blood concentrations appear within 4 hours. The half-life is 30 hours in children and up to 60 hours in adults. The initial dosage is 10–15 mg/kg/day in three divided doses after meals to avoid gastric irritation. Increments of 10 mg/kg/day are administered as needed and tolerated to provide seizure control without adverse effects. The total dosage is limited by toxicity, and blood concentration measurements are not useful.

ADVERSE EFFECTS. The common adverse reactions are nausea and abdominal pain. These symptoms occur within the therapeutic range and limit the drug's usefulness.

Felbamate (Felbatol, Wallace Laboratories)

INDICATIONS. Felbamate has a wide spectrum of anticonvulsant activity. It is useful in refractory partial and generalized seizures, the Lennox-Gastaut syndrome, atypical absence, and atonic seizures.

ADMINISTRATION. Felbamate is rapidly absorbed after oral intake and is not affected by food or antacids. Maximal plasma concentrations occur in 2 to 6 hours. The initial dosage is 15 mg/kg/day in three divided doses. Nighttime doses should be avoided if the drug causes insomnia. Increments of 15 mg/kg are made weekly if needed to a total dose of approximately 45 mg/kg/day. The total dosage is limited by toxicity, and blood concentration measurements are not useful.

ADVERSE EFFECTS. Initially, adverse effects of felbamate were thought to be mild and dose related (nausea, anorexia, insomnia, weight loss) except when used in combination with other anticonvulsants. The addition of felbamate increases the plasma concentrations of phenytoin and valproate as much as 30%. The carbamazepine serum concentration falls, but the concentration of its active epoxide metabolite increases almost 50%.

Postmarketing experience showed that felbamate causes fatal liver damage and aplastic anemia. Regular monitoring of blood counts and liver function is required. However, this is a valuable drug and should be used with informed consent.

Gabapentin (Neurontin, Parke-Davis)

INDICATIONS. This drug is used more often for pain and dystonia than for seizures, the only approved indication. It is not a primary anticonvulsant but is used mainly as add-on therapy for refractory partial-onset seizures.

ADMINISTRATION. Gabapentin is rapidly absorbed, not protein bound, does not induce hepatic enzymes, does not interact with other drugs, and is excreted unchanged in the urine. The dosage is 30–60 mg/kg/day, and a therapeutic blood level has not been established.

ADVERSE EFFECTS. These are usually mild and mainly consist of somnolence, dizziness, and ataxia. However, behavioral side effects of tantrums and aggressive behavior may occur in children.

Lamotrigine (Lamictal, Glaxo Wellcome)

INDICATIONS. Lamotrigine is useful in absence epilepsy, atonic seizures, juvenile myoclonic epilepsy, the Lennox-Gastaut syndrome, and par-

tial seizures. The spectrum of activity is similar to that of valproate.

ADMINISTRATION. The initial dosage is 0.5 mg/kg/day. The dosage is then slowly increased to achieve a maintenance dosage of 5–15 mg/kg/day. This is a slow process, and the main disadvantage of using lamotrigine as a primary drug is the long interval required to achieve seizure control. A therapeutic plasma concentration has not been established. The concomitant use of lamotrigine and other anticonvulsants shortens the half-life of lamotrigine but does not lower the blood concentration of the other drugs. In contrast, the concomitant use of valproate markedly extends the half-life of lamotrigine. The initial dose and the incremental doses of lamotrigine must be reduced by 50% when administered to children who are taking valproate.

ADVERSE EFFECTS. The main allergic reaction is rash, which is more likely to occur if the drug dosage is increased rapidly. Other adverse effects consist mainly of dizziness, ataxia, diplopia, and headache.

Levetiracetam (Keppra, UCB Pharma)

INDICATIONS. Levetiracetam has a broad spectrum of activity and can be used for many of the same seizure types that respond to valproate.

ADMINISTRATION. Levetiracetam is only available in tablet form but the tablets easily dissolve in water. Although the half-life is short, the duration of efficacy is longer, and twice daily dosing is recommended. The dosages in children are not established and the suggestions in Table 1-12 are approximate.

ADVERSE EFFECTS. Levetiracetam is not metabolized by the liver. It is metabolized in the blood and excreted in the urine. The main adverse effect is drowsiness.

Oxcarbazepine (Trileptal, Novartis)

INDICATIONS. Oxcarbazepine is the active breakdown product of carbamazepine. It has the same therapeutic profile as carbamazepine.

ADMINISTRATION. Oxcarbazepine can be substituted for carbamazepine on a mg per mg basis.

ADVERSE EFFECTS. The main adverse effect is drowsiness, but this is not as severe as with carbamazepine.

Phenobarbital

INDICATIONS. Tonic-clonic and simple partial seizures.

ADMINISTRATION. Oral absorption is slow, and daily doses are better given with the evening meal than at bedtime if seizures are hypnagogic. Since intramuscular absorption requires 1 to 2 hours, the intramuscular route should not be used for rapid loading (see Treatment of Status Epilepticus); 50% of the drug is protein bound, and 50% is free.

Initial and maintenance dosages are 3 to 5 mg/kg/day. The half-life is 50 to 140 hours in adults, 35 to 70 hours in children, and 50 to 200 hours in term newborns. Because of the very long half-life at all ages, once-a-day doses are usually satisfactory, and steady-state blood concentrations should be measured after 2 weeks of therapy. Therapeutic blood concentrations are 15 to 40 μg/ml.

ADVERSE EFFECTS. Hyperactivity is the most common and limiting side effect in children. Adverse behavioral changes occur in one half of children between ages 2 and 10. Parents should be warned of this possibility at the onset of therapy. Behavioral changes are dose related, and other barbiturates that are converted to phenobarbital produce the same adverse effects at equivalent phenobarbital blood concentrations.

Phenobarbital has no life-threatening side effects. Drowsiness and cognitive dysfunction, rather than hyperactivity, are the usual adverse effects after 10 years of age. Infants tolerate phenobarbital well, and it remains the drug of choice for oral use in newborns and infants. Rash is the main idiosyncratic reaction.

Phenytoin (Dilantin, Parke-Davis)

INDICATIONS. Tonic-clonic seizures, partial seizures, status epilepticus.

ADMINISTRATION. Oral absorption is slow and unpredictable in newborns, erratic in infants, and probably not reliable until 3 to 5 years of age. Even in adults there is considerable individual variability. Once absorbed, phenytoin is 70% to 95% protein bound. A typical maintenance dosage is 7 mg/kg/day in newborns and 5 mg/kg/day in children. The half-life is up to 60 hours in term newborns, up to 140 hours in premature infants, 5 to 14 hours in children, and 10 to 34 hours in adults. Capsules are usually taken in two divided doses, but tablets are more rapidly absorbed and may require three divided doses a day. Rapid oral loading of phenytoin can be achieved by giving three times the maintenance dosage. Parenteral phenytoin has been replaced by fosphenytoin sodium (see discussion of Status Epilepticus). The usual thera-peutic range is 10 to 20 μg/ml, and once within that range, dosage increments must be small.

ADVERSE EFFECTS. The major adverse reactions are hypersensitivity, gum hypertrophy, and hirsutism. Hypersensitivity reactions usually occur within 6 weeks of the initiation of therapy and are characterized by rash, fever, and lymphadenopathy. Once such a reaction has occurred, the drug should be discontinued. Concurrent use of antihistamines is not appropriate management. Continued use of the drug may produce a Stevens-Johnson syndrome or a lupus-like disorder.

Gum hypertrophy is caused by a combination of phenytoin metabolites and plaque on the teeth. Persons with good oral hygiene are unlikely to have gum hypertrophy. The importance of good oral hygiene should be discussed at the onset of therapy. Hirsutism is rarely a problem, and then only for girls. When it occurs, the drug can be discontinued without permanent harm. Memory impairment, decreased attention span, and personality change may occur at therapeutic concentrations, but they occur less often and are less severe than with phenobarbital.

Primidone (Mysoline, Ayerst)

INDICATIONS. Tonic-clonic and partial seizures.

ADMINISTRATION. Primidone is metabolized to at least two active metabolites, phenobarbital and phenyl-ethyl-malonamide (PEMA). The half-life of primidone is 6 to 12 hours, and that of PEMA is 20 hours. The usual maintenance dosage is 10 to 25 mg/kg/day, but the initial dosage should be 25% of the maintenance dosage or intolerable sedation occurs. A therapeutic blood concentration of primidone is 8 to 12 μg/ml. The blood concentration of phenobarbital derived from primidone is generally four times greater, but this ratio is altered when other anticonvulsant drugs are administered concurrently.

ADVERSE EFFECTS. The adverse effects are the same as for phenobarbital, except that the risk of intolerable sedation from the first tablet is great.

Tiagabine (Gabitral, Abbott)

INDICATIONS. Adjunctive therapy for partial-onset and generalized seizures.

ADMINISTRATION. The initial single-day dose is 0.2 mg/kg/day. This is increased every 2 weeks by 0.2 mg/kg until optimal benefit is achieved or adverse reactions occur. Most children tolerate doses of 4.0 to 6.0 mg/day.

ADVERSE EFFECTS. The most common adverse effects are somnolence and difficulty concentrating.

Topiramate (Topamax, Ortho)

INDICATIONS. Used mainly as adjunctive therapy for partial-onset seizures and the Lennox-Gastaut syndrome.
ADMINISTRATION. The initial dose is 1–2 mg/kg/day, increased incrementally to up to 9 mg/kg/day bid.
ADVERSE EFFECTS. Fatigue and altered mental status occur at toxic dosages.

Valproate (Depakene, Abbott)

INDICATIONS. Valproate is used mainly for generalized seizures and is especially useful for mixed seizure disorders. Included are myoclonic seizures, simple absence, myoclonic absence, myoclonus, and tonic-clonic seizures.
ADMINISTRATION. Oral absorption is rapid, and the half-life is 6 to 15 hours. Doses three times a day are needed to achieve constant blood concentrations. An enteric-coated capsule (Depakote) slows absorption and allows twice-a-day doses in many children.

The initial dosage is 20 mg/kg/day. Increments of 10 mg/kg/day are administered to provide a blood concentration of 50 to 100 μg/ml. Blood concentrations of 80 to 120 μg/ml are often required to achieve seizure control. Protein binding is 95% at blood concentrations of 50 μg/ml and 80% at 100 μg/ml. Therefore doubling the blood concentration increases the free fraction eightfold. Valproate has a strong affinity for plasma proteins and displaces other anticonvulsant drugs.

Valproate is absorbed when given rectally and can be administered by this route when oral administration is not possible. A peak concentration is attained 3 hours after rectal administration, and the serum concentration is approximately 75% of the oral dose.
ADVERSE EFFECTS. Valproate has dose-related and idiosyncratic hepatotoxicity. Dose-related hepatotoxicity is harmless and is characterized by increased serum concentrations of transaminases. Important dose-related effects are a reduction in the platelet count, pancreatitis, and hyperammonemia. Thrombocytopenia may result in serious bleeding after trivial injury, while pancreatitis and hepatitis are both associated with nausea and vomiting. Hyperammonemia, caused by interference with the urea cycle, causes cognitive disturbances and nausea. These adverse reactions are reversible when the daily dose is reduced. Plasma carnitine concentrations are reduced in children taking valproate, and some believe that carnitine supplementation helps relieve cognitive impairment.

The major idiosyncratic reaction is fatal liver necrosis attributed to the production of an aberrant and toxic metabolite. The major risk (1 : 800) is in children younger than 2 years of age who are receiving polytherapy. Many such cases may not be caused by valproate, or valproate alone, but by an underlying inborn error of metabolism. Fatal hepatotoxicity has not been reported in children over 10 years of age treated with valproate alone.

The clinical manifestations of idiosyncratic hepatotoxicity are similar to those of Reye syndrome (see Chapter 2). They may begin after 1 day of therapy or may not appear for 6 months. No reliable way exists to monitor patients for idiosyncratic hepatotoxicity or to predict its occurrence.

Vigabatrin

INDICATIONS. Unfortunately, vigabatrin is not approved for use in the United States. It is an excellent drug for the treatment of infantile spasms and partial seizures.
ADMINISTRATION. Vigabatrin is a very-long-acting drug and needs only single-day dosing, but twice-daily dosing is preferable to reduce adverse effects. The initial dose is 10 mg/kg/day. The dose is increased incrementally, as needed and tolerated, up to 100 mg/kg/day.
ADVERSE EFFECTS. Visual field defects are the adverse reaction that prevented approval for the use of this drug in the United States. The defect is rare and consists of circumferential field constriction with nasal sparing. Behavioral problems, fatigue, confusion, and gastrointestinal upset are usually mild and dose related.

Zonisamide (Zonegran, Elan pharmaceuticals)

INDICATIONS. Like levetiracetam, zonisamide has a broad spectrum of activity and can be used both for primary generalized epilepsy and partial onset epilepsy.
ADMINISTRATION. Zonisamide is a very-long-acting drug and can be administered once or twice daily. The dose in children is not fully established and the dose suggested in Table 1-12 is approximate.

ADVERSE EFFECTS. The most common adverse effects are drowsiness and anorexia.

Treatment of Status Epilepticus

Status epilepticus is defined as a prolonged single seizure (longer than 20 minutes) or repeated seizures without interictal recovery. Generalized tonic-clonic status is life-threatening and is the most common emergency in pediatric neurology. Status may be caused by a new acute illness such as encephalitis, a progressive neurological disease, loss of seizure control in a known epileptic, or a febrile seizure in an otherwise normal child. The outcome is mainly determined by the cause. Recurrence of status epilepticus is most likely in children who are neurologically abnormal and is rare in children with febrile seizures.

Absence status and complex partial status are often difficult to identify as status epilepticus. The child may appear to be in a confusional state.

Immediate Management

Prolonged seizures or clusters of seizures in children with known epilepsy can sometimes be managed at home with rectal diazepam to prevent or abort status epilepticus. A rectal diazepam gel is commercially available, or the intravenous preparation can be given rectally (0.4 mg/kg) through a lubricated syringe. Pharmacists can make up suppositories for home use. If the rectal dose fails to stop the seizures, the child should be brought to an emergency service.

Status epilepticus is a medical emergency requiring prompt attention. Initial assessment should be rapid and includes cardiorespiratory function, a history leading up to the seizure, and a neurological examination. A controlled airway must be established immediately and mechanical ventilation made available. Venous access is established next. Blood is withdrawn for measurement of glucose, electrolytes, and anticonvulsant concentrations when applicable. Other tests (i.e., a toxic screen) are performed as indicated. After blood is withdrawn, an intravenous infusion of saline solution is started for the administration of anticonvulsant drugs. An intravenous bolus of a 50% glucose solution, 1 mg/kg, is then administered.

Drug Treatment

The ideal drug for treating status epilepticus is one that acts rapidly, has a long duration of action, and does not produce sedation. Benzodiazepines (diazepam and lorazepam) are used widely for this purpose, but they are inadequate by themselves because their duration of action is brief. In addition, children who are given intravenous benzodiazepines after a prior load of barbiturate often have respiratory depression. If diazepam is chosen as a first drug, the dose is 0.2 mg/kg, not to exceed 10 mg at a rate of 1 mg/min. Lorazepam may be preferable to diazepam because of its longer duration of action. The usual dosage in children 12 years of age or younger is 0.1 mg/kg. After age 12 it is 0.07 mg/kg.

My preference is intravenous fosphenytoin because it has a long duration of action, does not produce respiratory depression, and does not impair consciousness. The initial dose is 20 mg/kg (calculated as phenytoin equivalents). It can be administered intravenously or intramuscularly, but the intravenous route is preferred. Unlike phenytoin, which had to be injected at a rate not to exceed 0.5 mg/kg/min to avoid cardiac toxicity, fosphenytoin can be injected more rapidly and prior benzodiazepine therapy is not needed. Infants generally require 30 mg/kg.

Fosphenytoin is usually effective unless status epilepticus is caused by a severe, acute encephalopathy. EEG should be done in children who fail to wake up at an expected time after the clinical signs of status have stopped to be certain that electrical status is terminated.

When fosphenytoin fails, several alternatives are available; my preference is pentobarbital coma. The patient should have been transferred from the emergency department to an intensive care unit, intubated, and mechanically ventilated. After an arterial line is placed, the patient's blood pressure, cardiac rhythm, body temperature, and blood oxygen saturation are monitored.

With an EEG monitor recording continuously, 10 mg/kg boluses of pentobarbital are infused until a burst-suppression pattern appears on the EEG (Figure 1-5); a minimum of 30 mg/kg is generally required. Hypotension is the most serious complication and requires treatment with vasopressors. It is generally not observed until 40 to 60 mg/kg is administered. Barbiturates tend to accumulate, and the usual dosage needed to maintain pentobarbital coma is 3 mg/kg/h. The coma can be maintained safely for several days. The EEG should be checked several times each day for the burst-suppression pattern. The coma can be lifted every 24 to 48 hours to see whether the seizures have stopped.

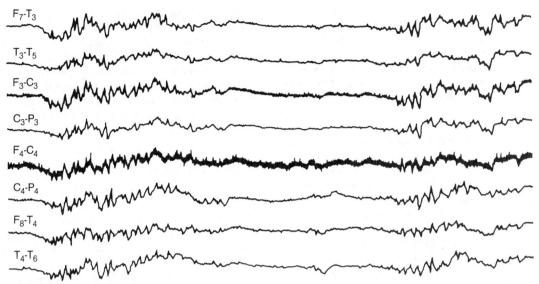

Figure 1-5. Burst-suppression pattern in pentobarbital coma. Long intervals of amplitude suppression are interrupted by bursts of mixed frequencies.

The Ketogenic Diet

Fasting as a treatment for epilepsy was recorded in antiquity. During the 1920s, when barbiturates and bromides were the only available anticonvulsant drugs, diet-induced ketosis was introduced to mimic fasting. This method became less popular with the introduction of effective pharmacotherapy, but it is being used again to treat children whose seizures are refractory to anticonvulsant drugs at nontoxic levels (Freeman et al, 1998). The diet is most effective in infants and young children whose diet is more easily supervised. A diet that consists of 60% medium-chain triglycerides, 11% long-chain saturated fat, 10% protein, and 19% carbohydrate is commonly used. The main side effects are abdominal pain and diarrhea.

The ketogenic diet causes a prompt elevation in plasma ketone bodies that are used by the brain as an energy source. The mechanism of action is not established. The ketogenic diet is most effective for control of myoclonic seizures, infantile spasms, atonic/akinetic seizures, and mixed seizures of the Lennox-Gastaut syndrome.

Vagal Nerve Stimulation

Vagal nerve stimulation (VNS) is a treatment for refractory seizures that uses a programmed stimulus from a chest-implanted generator via coiled electrodes tunneled to the left cervical vagus nerve (Morris et al, 1999). Voice changes or hoarseness are the main adverse effects. A 50% reduction in seizure frequency is achieved in approximately 40% of people with epilepsy. VNS has been used extensively in adults and children.

Surgical Approaches to Childhood Epilepsy

Surgery is sometimes recommended for children with epilepsy that is intractable to optimal anticonvulsant therapy. Surgery is never a substitute for good medical therapy, and anticonvulsant drugs are often needed after surgery is performed. Three procedures are used: hemispherectomy, interhemispheric commissurotomy, and temporal lobectomy. None of these procedures is new, and all have gone through phases of greater or lesser popularity since being introduced.

Hemispherectomy

Hemispherectomy, or more correctly hemidecortication, has been used exclusively for children with intractable epilepsy and hemiplegia. The original procedure consisted of removing the cortex of one hemisphere along with a variable portion of the underlying basal ganglia. The extent of surgery depended partly upon the underlying disease. The resulting cavity communicated with the third ventricle and became lined with a subdural membrane. The immediate results were good. Seizures were relieved in about 80% of children, and behavior and spasticity were improved without deterioration of intellectual function or motor function in the hemiparetic limbs.

However, late complications of hemorrhage, hydrocephalus, and hemosiderosis occurred in up to 35% of children and were sometimes fatal. It is believed that the subdural membrane repeatedly tears, bleeding into the ventricular system and staining the ependymal lining and the pia arachnoid with iron.

Because of these complications, less radical alternatives are generally preferred. These alternatives are the Montreal-type hemispherectomy and interhemispheric commissurotomy. The Montreal-type hemispherectomy is a modified procedure in which most of the damaged hemisphere is removed but portions of the frontal and occipital lobes are left in place, disconnected from the other hemisphere and brainstem. The best results are obtained when presurgical evaluation with single photon emission computed tomography (SPECT) or PET shows that only one hemisphere is abnormal and the source of seizures.

Interhemispheric Commissurotomy

Disconnecting the hemispheres from each other and from the brainstem is an alternative to hemispherectomy in children with intractable epilepsy and hemiplegia. This operation is also used to decrease the occurrence of secondary generalized tonic-clonic seizures from partial or minor generalized seizures. The efficacy of commissurotomy and hemispherectomy in children with infantile hemiplegia is probably comparable, but the efficacy of commissurotomy in other forms of epilepsy has not been established.

Complete and partial commissurotomies have been recommended. Complete commissurotomy entails division of the entire corpus callosum, anterior commissure, one fornix, and the hippocampal commissure. Complete commissurotomies may be performed in one stage or two. Partial commissurotomies vary from division of the corpus callosum and hippocampal commissure to division of only the anterior portion of the corpus callosum.

Two immediate, but transitory, postoperative complications may follow interhemispheric commissurotomy: (1) a syndrome of mutism, left arm and leg apraxia, and urinary incontinence and (2) hemiparesis. They are both more common after one-stage, complete commissurotomy than after two-stage procedures or partial commissurotomy and are probably caused by prolonged retraction of one hemisphere during surgery. Long-term complications may include stuttering and poorly coordinated movements of the hands.

Temporal Lobectomy

The results of temporal lobectomy depend upon the selection criteria and the skill of the epileptology team. Complete seizure relief should be attainable in more than half of children with intractable partial complex seizures of temporal lobe origin (Gilliam et al, 1997). Only children who have a unilateral temporal focus are candidates for surgery. PET is proving valuable for identifying the epileptic focus. The surgical procedure is a subpial resection of the superior temporal gyrus, hippocampus, and amygdala. Intraoperative EEG determines the extent of resection. Benign tumors, gliomas, and ganglioneuromas are found in 12% of the specimens. The most common complication is superior quadrantanopsia (40%) and the most serious complication is aphasia (10%), which is usually transitory.

References

Acharya JN, Wyllie E, Lüders HO, et al. Seizure symptomatology in infants with localization-related epilepsy. *Neurology* 1997;48:189–196.

Aldrich MS. Diagnostic aspects of narcolepsy. *Neurology* 1998;50(suppl 1):S2–S7.

Andermann F, Zifkin B. The benign occipital epilepsies of childhood: An overview of the idiopathic syndrome and of the relationship to migraine. *Epilepsia* 1998;4:S9–S23.

Baram TZ, Mitchell WG, Tournay A, et al. High-dose corticotropin (ACTH) versus prednisone for infantile spasms: A prospective, randomized, blinded study. *Pediatrics* 1996;97:375–379.

Berg AT, Shinnar S. Unprovoked seizures in children with febrile seizures: Short-term outcomes. *Neurology* 1996; 47:562–568.

Berg AT, Shinnar S, Darefsky AS, et al. Predictors of recurrent febrile seizures. A prospective cohort study. *Arch Pediatr Adolesc Med* 1997;151:371–378.

Burn J. Closing time for CATCH22. *J Med Genet* 1999; 36:737–738.

Carpio A, Escobar A, Hauser WA. Cysticercosis and epilepsy: A critical review. *Epilepsia* 1998;39:1025–1040.

Chudnow RS, Mimbela RA, Owen DB, et al. Gabapentin for familial paroxysmal dystonic choreoathetosis. *Neurology* 1997;49:1441–1442.

Connolly MB, Langill L, Wong PKH, et al. Seizures involving the supplementary sensorimotor area in children: A video-EEG analysis. *Epilepsia* 1995;36:1025–1032.

Delanty N, French J. Treatment of Lennox-Gastaut syndrome: Current recommendations. *CNS Drugs* 1998; 10:181–188.

Donma MM. Clinical efficacy of piracetum in treatment of breath-holding spells. *Pediatr Neurol* 1998;18:41–45.

Fink JK, Hedera P, Mathay JG, et al. Paroxysmal dystonic choreoathetosis linked to chromosome 2q: Clinical analysis and proposed pathophysiology. *Neurology* 1997; 49:177–183.

Francis JS, Sybert VP. Incontinentia pigmenti. *Semin Cut Med Surg* 1997;16:54–60.

Freeman JM, Vining EPG, Pillas DJ, et al. The efficacy of the ketogenic diet—1998: A prospective evaluation of intervention in 150 children. *Pediatrics* 1998;102:1358–1363.

Gaggero R, Baglietto MP, Curia R, et al. Early-onset progressive encephalopathy with migrant, continuous myoclonus. *Child Nerv Syst* 1996;12:254–261.

Gilliam F, Wyllie EW, Kashden J, et al. Epilepsy surgery outcome: Comprehensive assessment in children. *Neurology* 1997;48:1368–1374.

Greenberg DA, Durner M, Resor S, et al. The genetics of idiopathic generalized epilepsies of adolescent onset: Differences between juvenile myoclonic epilepsy and epilepsy with random grand mal and with awakening grand mal. *Neurology* 1995;45:942–946.

Greenwood RS, Tennison MB. When to start and stop anticonvulsant therapy in children. *Arch Neurol* 1999; 56:1073–1077.

Hamilton RL, Haas RH, Nyhan WL, et al. Neuropathology of propionic acidemia: A report of two patients with basal ganglia lesions. *J Child Neurol* 1995;10:25–30.

Hamosh A, Maher JF, Bellus GA, et al. Long term use of high-dose benzoate and dextromethorphan for the treatment of nonketotic hyperglycinemia. *J Pediatr* 1998; 132:709–713.

Hancock E, Osborne JP. Vigabatrin in the treatment of infantile spasms in tuberous sclerosis: Literature review. *J Child Neurol* 1999:1471–1474.

Harvey AS, Berkovic SF, Wrennall JA, et al. Temporal lobe epilepsy in childhood: Clinical, EEG, and neuroimaging findings and syndrome classification in a cohort with new-onset seizures. *Neurology* 1997;49:960–968.

Hayman M, Scheffer LE, Chinvarun Y, et al. Autosomal dominant nocturnal frontal lobe epilepsy: Demonstration of frontal focal onset and intrafamilial variation. *Neurology* 1997;49:969–975.

Hellström-Westas L, Blennow G, Lindroth M, et al. Low risk of seizure recurrence after early withdrawal of antiepileptic treatment in the neonatal period. *Arch Dis Child* 1995;72:F97–F101.

Janz D. The idiopathic generalized epilepsies of adolescence childhood and juvenile age of onset. *Epilepsia* 1997; 38:4–11.

Lüders HO. Paroxysmal choreoathetosis. *Eur Neurol* 1996;36(suppl 1):20–23.

Maestri NE, Clissold DB, Brusilow SW. Long-term survival of patients with argininosuccinate synthetase deficiency. *Pediatrics* 1995;127:929–935.

Morrell F, Whisler WW, Smith MC, et al. Landau Kleffner syndrome: Treatment with subpial intracortical transection. *Brain* 1995;118:1529–1546.

Morris GL III, Mueller WM. The Vagal Nerve Stimulation Group. Long-term treatment with vagus nerve stimulation in patients with refractory epilepsy. *Neurology* 1999;53:1731–1735.

Musicco M, Beghi E, Solari A, et al. Treatment of first tonic-clonic seizures does not improve the prognosis of epilepsy. *Neurology* 1997;49:991–998.

Nicolaides P, Leonard J, Surtees R. Neurological complications of methylmalonic acidaemia. *Arch Dis Child* 1998;78:508–512.

Panayiotpoulos CP. Extraoccipital benign childhood partial seizures with ictal vomiting and excellent prognosis. *J Neurol Neurosurg Psychiatry* 1999;66:82–85.

Radhakrishnan K, Silbert PL, Klass DW. Reading epilepsy: An appraisal of 20 patients diagnosed at the Mayo Clinic, Rochester, Minnesota, between 1949 and 1989, and delineation of the syndrome. *Brain* 1995;118:75–89.

Roland EH, Poskitt K, Rodriguez E, et al. Perinatal hypoxic-ischemic thalamic injury: Clinical features and neuroimaging. *Ann Neurol* 1998;44:161–166.

Scheffer IE, Berkovic SF. Generalized epilepsy with febrile seizures plus a genetic disorder with heterogeneous clinical phenotypes. *Brain* 1997;120:479–490.

Scheffer IE, Jones L, Pozzebon M, et al. Autosomal dominant Rolandic epilepsy and speech dyspraxia: A new syndrome with anticipation. *Ann Neurol* 1995;38:633–642.

Serratosa JM, Delgado-Escueta AV, Medina MT, et al. Clinical and genetic analysis of a large pedigree with juvenile myoclonic epilepsy. *Ann Neurol* 1996;39:187–195.

Suormala T, Fowler B, Duran M, et al. Five patients with a biotin-responsive defect in holocarboxylase formation: Evaluation of responsiveness to biotin therapy in vivo and comparative biochemical studies in vitro. *Pediatr Res* 1997;41:666–673.

Tijssen MAJ, Padberg GW, van Dijk JG. The startle pattern in the minor form of hyperekplexia. *Arch Neurol* 1997;54:388–393.

US Modafinil in Narcolepsy Multicenter Study Group. Randomized trial of modafinil for the treatment of pathological somnolence in narcolepsy. *Ann Neurol* 1998;43:88–97.

Van Hove JLK, Kishnani P, Muenzer J, et al. Benzoate therapy and carnitine deficiency in non-ketotic hyperglycinemia. *Am J Med Genet* 1995;59:444–453.

VanLandingham KE, Heinz ER, Cavazos JE, et al. Magnetic resonance imaging evidence of hippocampal injury after prolonged focal febrile convulsions. *Ann Neurol* 1998;43:413–426.

Verity C, Greenwood R, Golding J. Long-term intellectual and behavioral outcomes of children with febrile convulsions. *N Engl J Med* 1998;338:1723–1728.

Vigevano F, Cilio MR. Vigabatrin versus ACTH as first-line treatment for infantile spasms: A randomized, prospective study. *Epilepsia* 1997;38:1270–1274.

Wheless JW, Constantinou JEC. Lennox-Gastaut syndrome. *Pediatr Neurol* 1997;17:203–211.

Whitley R, Lakeman F. Herpes simplex virus infections of the nervous system: Therapeutic and diagnostic considerations. *Clin Infect Dis* 1995;20:414–420.

Wirrell EC. Benign epilepsy of childhood with centrotemporal spikes. *Epilepsia* 1998;39(suppl):S32–S34.

Wirrell EC, Camfield CS, Camfield PR, et al. Long-term prognosis of typical childhood absence epilepsy: Remission or progression to juvenile myoclonic epilepsy. *Neurology* 1996;47:912–918.

Chapter 2
Altered States of Consciousness

THE TERMS USED in this textbook to describe states of decreased consciousness are provided in Table 2-1. With the exception of *coma,* these definitions are not standard. However, they are more precise and therefore more useful than such terms as *semicomatose* and *semistuporous.* The term *encephalopathy* is used to describe a diffuse disorder of the brain in which at least two of the following symptoms are present: (1) altered states of consciousness, (2) altered cognition or personality, and (3) seizures. *Encephalitis* is an encephalopathy accompanied by cerebrospinal fluid pleocytosis.

Lack of responsiveness is not always caused by lack of consciousness. For example, infants with botulism (see Chapter 6) may have such severe hypotonia and ptosis that they cannot move their limbs or eyelids in response to stimulation. They appear to be in a coma or stupor but are actually alert. The locked-in syndrome (a brainstem disorder in which the individual can process information but cannot respond) and catatonia are other examples of diminished responsiveness in the alert state.

Progression from consciousness to coma may be characterized by increased or decreased neuronal excitability. Patients with increased neuronal excitability (the *high road*) become restless and then confused; next, tremor, hallucinations, and delirium (an agitated confusional state) develop. Myoclonic jerks may occur. Seizures herald the end of delirium and are followed by stupor or coma. Table 2-2 summarizes the differential diagnosis of the high road to coma. Tumors and other mass lesions are not expected causes. Instead, the diagnosis is weighted in favor of metabolic, toxic, and inflammatory disorders.

Decreased neuronal excitability (the *low road*) lacks an agitated stage. Instead, awareness

Table 2-1
States of Decreased Consciousness

Term	Definition
Lethargy	Difficult to maintain the aroused state
Obtundation	Responsive to stimulation other than pain*
Stupor	Responsive only to pain*
Coma	Unresponsive to pain

* Responsive indicates cerebral alerting, not just reflex withdrawal.

progressively deteriorates from lethargy to obtundation, to stupor, and to coma. The differential diagnosis is considerably larger than that with the high road and includes mass lesions and other causes of increased intracranial pressure (Table 2-3). Conditions that cause recurrent encephalopathies are listed in Table 2-4. A comparison of Tables 2-2 and 2-3 shows a considerable overlap between conditions whose initial features are agitation and confusion and those that begin with lethargy and coma; therefore the disorders responsible for each are described together to prevent repetition.

Diagnostic Approach to Delirium

Any child with the acute behavioral changes of delirium (agitation, confusion, delusions, or hallucinations) should be assumed to have an organic encephalopathy until proven otherwise. Delirium is usually caused by a toxic or metabolic disorder diffusely affecting both cerebral hemispheres. Schizophrenia should not be a con-

Table 2-2
Causes of Agitation and Confusion

Epileptic
Absence status (see Chapter 1)
Complex partial seizure (see Chapter 1)

Infectious Disorders
Bacterial infections
    Cat scratch disease
    Meningitis (see Chapter 4)
Rickettsial infections
    Lyme disease
    Rocky Mountain spotted fever
Viral infections
    Aseptic meningitis
    Arboviruses
    Herpes simplex encephalitis
    Measles encephalitis
    Postinfectious encephalomyelitis
    Reye syndrome

Metabolic and Systemic Disorders
Disorders of osmolality
    Hypoglycemia
    Hyponatremia
Endocrine disorders
    Adrenal insufficiency
    Hypoparathyroidism
    Thyroid disorders
Hepatic encephalopathy
Inborn errors of metabolism
    Disorders of pyruvate metabolism (see Chapter 5)
    Medium-chain acyl-CoA dehydrogenase (MCAD) deficiency
    Respiratory chain disorders (see Chapters 5, 6, 8, 10)
    Urea cycle disorder, heterozygote (see Chapter 1)
Renal disease
    Hypertensive encephalopathy
    Uremic encephalopathy

Migraine
Acute confusional
Aphasic
Transient global amnesia

Psychological
Panic disorder
Schizophrenia

Toxic
Immunosuppressive drugs
Prescription drugs
Substance abuse
Toxins

Vascular
Congestive heart failure
Embolism
Hypertensive encephalopathy
Lupus erythematosus
Subarachnoid hemorrhage
Vasculitis

sideration in a prepubertal child with acute delirium. *Delusions* are fixed beliefs that cannot be altered by reason. The paranoid delusions of schizophrenia are logical to the patient and frequently part of an elaborate system of irrational thinking in which the patient feels menaced. Delusions associated with organic encephalopathy are less logical, are not systematized, and tend to be stereotyped.

A *hallucination* is the perception of sensory stimuli that are not present. Visual hallucinations are almost always caused by organic encephalopathy, and auditory hallucinations, especially if accusatory, usually indicate psychiatric illness. Stereotyped auditory hallucinations that represent a recurring memory are an exception and suggest temporal lobe seizures;

History and Physical Examination

Delirious children, even with stable vital function, must be assessed rapidly because the potential for deterioration to a state of diminished consciousness is always present. A careful history must be obtained of (1) the events leading to the behavioral change, (2) drug or toxic exposure (prescription drugs are more often at fault than substances of abuse, and a medicine cabinet inspection should be ordered in every home the child has visited), (3) a personal or family history of migraine or epilepsy, (4) recent or concurrent fever, infectious disease, or systemic illness, and (5) a previous personal or family history of encephalopathy.

Examination of the eyes, in addition to determining the presence or absence of papilledema, provides other etiological clues. Small or large pupils that respond poorly to light, nystagmus, or impaired eye movements suggest a drug or toxic exposure. Fixed deviation of the eyes in one lateral direction may indicate that (1) the encephalopathy has focal features, (2) seizures are a cause of the confusional state, or (3) seizures are part of the encephalopathy. The general and neurological examinations should specifically include a search for evidence of trauma, needle marks on the limbs, meningismus, and cardiac disease.

Laboratory Investigations

Laboratory evaluation should be individualized; not every test is essential for each clinical situation. The first step is to obtain blood and urine tests. Studies of potential interest include culture, complete blood count; sedimentation rate;

Table 2-3
Causes of Lethargy and Coma

Epilepsy
Postictal state (see Chapter 1)
Status epilepticus (see Chapter 1)

Hypoxia-Ischemia
Cardiac arrest
Cardiac arrhythmia
Congestive heart failure
Hypotension
    Autonomic dysfunction
    Dehydration
    Hemorrhage
    Pulmonary embolism
Near-drowning
Neonatal (see Chapter 1)

Increased Intracranial Pressure
Cerebral abscess (see Chapter 4)
Cerebral edema (see Chapter 4)
Cerebral tumor (see Chapters 4 and 10)
Herniation syndromes (see Chapter 4)
Hydrocephalus (see Chapters 4 and 18)
Intracranial hemorrhage
    Spontaneous (see Chapter 4)
    Traumatic

Infectious Disorders
Bacterial infections
    Cat scratch disease
    Gram-negative sepsis
    Hemorrhagic shock and encephalopathy syndrome
    Meningitis (see Chapter 4)
    Toxic shock syndrome
Rickettsial infections
    Lyme disease
    Rocky Mountain spotted fever
Viral infections
    Aseptic meningitis
    Arboviruses
    Herpes simplex encephalitis
    Measles encephalitis
    Postinfectious encephalomyelitis
    Reye syndrome
Postimmunization encephalopathy

Metabolic and Systemic Disorders
Disorders of osmolality
    Diabetic ketoacidosis (hyperglycemia)
    Hypoglycemia

Hypernatremia
Hyponatremia
Endocrine disorders
    Adrenal insufficiency
    Hypoparathyroidism
    Thyroid disorders
Hepatic encephalopathy
Inborn errors of metabolism
    Disorders of pyruvate metabolism (see Chapter 5)
    Glycogen storage disorders (see Chapter 1)
    Medium-chain acyl-CoA dehydrogenase (MCAD) deficiency
    Respiratory chain disorders (see Chapter 5, 6, 8, 10)
    Urea cycle disorder, heterozygote (see Chapter 1).
Renal disorders
    Acute uremic encephalopathy
    Chronic uremic encephalopathy
    Dialysis encephalopathy
    Hypertensive encephalopathy
Other metabolic disorders
    Burn encephalopathy
    Hypomagnesemia
    Parenteral hyperalimentation
    Vitamin B complex deficiency

Migraine Coma
Toxic
Immunosuppressive drugs
Prescription drugs
Substance abuse
Toxins

Trauma
Concussion
Contusion
Intracranial hemorrhage
    Epidural hematoma
    Subdural hematoma
    Intracerebral hemorrhage
Neonatal (see Chapter 1)

Vascular
Hypertensive encephalopathy
Intracranial hemorrhage, nontraumatic (see Chapter 4)
Lupus erythematosus (see Chapter 11)
Neonatal idiopathic cerebral venous thrombosis (see Chapter 1)
Vasculitis (see Chapter 11)

---

toxicity screen; blood concentrations of glucose, electrolytes, calcium and phosphorus, urea nitrogen, ammonia, and thyroid-stimulating hormone; and liver function tests. If possible, computed tomography (CT) of the head should be performed while the results of these tests are pending. If sedation is required to perform the study, a short-acting benzodiazepine is preferred. Nondiagnostic blood studies and normal CT results are an indication for lumbar puncture to look for infection or increased intracranial

pressure. A manometer should always be available to measure cerebrospinal fluid pressure.

An electroencephalogram (EEG) can be useful in the evaluation of delirious patients and should be obtained at an opportune time. Findings are almost always abnormal in acute organic encephalopathies and normal in psychiatric illnesses. The minimal EEG finding in encephalopathy is slowing of the posterior rhythm. Diffuse theta and delta activity, absence of faster frequencies, and intermittent rhythmic

Table 2-4
Causes of Recurrent Encephalopathy

Burn encephalopathy
Epilepsy
Hashimoto thyroiditis
Hypoglycemia
Increased intracranial pressure (recurrent)
Medium-chain acyl-CoA dehydrogenase (MCAD) deficiency
Mental disorders
Migraine
Mitochondrial disorders
Pyruvate metabolism disorders
Substance abuse
Urea cycle disorder

delta activity are characteristic of severe enceph-alopathies. Specific abnormalities may include epileptiform activity consistent with absence or complex partial status; triphasic waves indicat-ing hepatic or uremic encephalopathy; and peri-odic lateralizing epileptiform discharges in one temporal lobe, suggesting herpes encephalitis.

Diagnostic Approach to Lethargy and Coma

The diagnostic approach to states of diminished consciousness in children is similar to that sug-gested for delirium, except for greater urgency. Progressive decline in the state of consciousness can be caused by diffuse or multifocal distur-bances of the cerebral hemispheres or by focal injury to the brainstem. The anatomic site of abnormality can often be determined by physi-cal examination.

History and Physical Examination

The historical data to be obtained are the same as for delirium, except that mass lesions are an important consideration. Further inquiry must be made concerning trauma or preceding symp-toms of increasing intracranial pressure.

Physical examination is directed at determin-ing both the anatomical site of disturbed cere-bral function and its cause. The important vari-ables in locating the site of abnormality are state of consciousness, pattern of breathing, pupillary size and reactivity, eye movements, and motor responses. Lethargy and obtundation are gener-ally caused by mild depression of hemispheric function. Stupor and coma are characteristic of much more extensive disturbance of hemi-spheric function or involvement of the dienceph-alon and upper brainstem. Derangements of the dominant hemisphere may have a greater effect on consciousness than derangements of the non-dominant hemisphere.

Cheyne-Stokes respiration, in which periods of hyperpnea alternate with periods of apnea, is usually caused by bilateral hemispheric or di-encephalic injuries, but can result from bilateral damage anywhere along the descending path-way between the forebrain and upper pons. Alertness, pupillary size, and heart rhythm may vary during Cheyne-Stokes respiration. Alert-ness is greater during the waxing portion of breathing. Lesions just ventral to the aqueduct or fourth ventricle cause a sustained, rapid, deep hyperventilation (central neurogenic hyperven-tilation). Abnormalities within the medulla and pons affect the respiratory centers and cause three different patterns of respiratory control: (1) *apneustic breathing,* a pause at full inspira-tion; (2) *ataxic breathing,* haphazard breaths and pauses without a predictable pattern; and (3) *Ondine's curse,* failure of automatic breath-ing when asleep.

The pupillary light reflex is usually retained in metabolic disturbances, and its absence in a comatose patient indicates a structural abnor-mality. The major exception is drugs: fixed dila-tion of the pupils in an alert patient is caused by topical administration of mydriatics. In co-matose patients, hypothalamic damage causes unilateral pupillary constriction and a Horner's syndrome; midbrain lesions cause midposition fixed pupils; pontine lesions cause small but re-active pupils; and lateral medullary lesions cause a Horner's syndrome.

Tonic lateral deviation of both eyes indicates a seizure originating in the hemisphere opposite to the direction of gaze or a destructive lesion in the hemisphere in the direction of gaze. Ocular motility can be assessed in comatose patients by instilling ice water sequentially 15 minutes apart in each ear to chill the tympanic membrane. Ice water in the right ear causes both eyes to deviate rapidly to the right and then slowly return to the midline. The rapid movement to the right is a brainstem reflex, and its presence indicates that much of the brainstem is intact. Abduction of the right eye with failure of left eye adduction indicates a lesion in the medial longitudinal fas-ciculus (see Chapter 15). The slow movement that returns the eyes to the left requires a cortico-pontine pathway originating in the right hemi-sphere and terminating in the left pontine lateral gaze center. Its presence indicates unilateral hemispheric function. Skew deviation, the deviation of one eye above the other (hypertropia), usually indicates a lesion of the brainstem or cerebellum) (Leigh and Zee, 1999).

Trunk and limb position at rest, spontaneous movements, and response to noxious stimuli must be carefully observed. Spontaneous movement of all limbs generally indicates a mild depression of hemispheric function without structural disturbance. Monoplegia or hemiplegia, except when in the postictal state, suggests a structural disturbance of the contralateral hemisphere. An extensor response of the trunk and limbs to a noxious stimulus is termed *decerebrate rigidity*. The most severe form is called *opisthotonos*: the neck is hyperextended and the teeth are clenched; the arms are adducted, hyperextended, and hyperpronated; and the legs are extended with the feet plantar flexed. Decerebrate rigidity indicates brainstem compression and should be considered an ominous sign whether present at rest or in response to noxious stimuli. Flexion of the arms and extension of the legs is termed *decorticate rigidity*. It is uncommon in children except following head injury and indicates hemispheric dysfunction with brainstem integrity.

Laboratory Investigations

Laboratory investigations are similar to those described for the evaluation of delirium. Head CT with contrast enhancement should be performed promptly in order to exclude the possibility of a mass lesion and herniation. It is a great error to send a child whose condition is uncertain for CT without someone in attendance who knows how to monitor deterioration and intervene appropriately.

Hypoxia and Ischemia

Hypoxia and ischemia usually occur together. Prolonged hypoxia causes personality change first and then loss of consciousness; acute anoxia results in immediate loss of consciousness.

Prolonged Hypoxia

CLINICAL FEATURES. Prolonged hypoxia can result from severe anemia (oxygen-carrying capacity reduced by at least half), congestive heart failure, chronic lung disease, and neuromuscular disorders.

The best-studied model of prolonged, mild hypoxia involves ascent to high altitudes. Mild hypoxia causes impaired memory and judgment, confusion, and decreased motor performance. Greater degrees of hypoxia result in obtundation, multifocal myoclonus, and sometimes focal neurological signs such as monoplegia and hemiplegia. Children with chronic cardiopulmonary disease may have an insidious alteration in behavioral state as the arterial oxygen concentration slowly declines.

Neuromuscular disorders that weaken respiratory muscles, such as muscular dystrophy, often produce nocturnal hypoventilation as a first symptom of respiratory insufficiency. This is characterized by frequent awakenings and fear of sleeping (see Chapter 7).

DIAGNOSIS. Chronic hypoxia should be considered in children with chronic cardiopulmonary disorders who become depressed or undergo personality change. Arterial oxygen pressure (Pao_2) values below 40 mm Hg are regularly associated with obvious neurological disturbances, but minor mental disturbances may occur at Pao_2 concentrations of 60 mm Hg, especially when hypoxia is chronic.

MANAGEMENT. Encephalopathy usually reverses when Pao_2 is increased, but persistent cerebral dysfunction may occur in mountain climbers after returning to sea level, and permanent cerebral dysfunction may develop in children with chronic hypoxia. As a group, children with chronic hypoxia from congenital heart disease have a lower IQ than nonhypoxic children. The severity of mental decline is related to the duration of hypoxia. Children with neuromuscular disorders who have symptoms during sleep can be treated overnight with intermittent positive-pressure ventilation (see Chapter 7).

Acute Anoxia and Ischemia

The usual circumstance in which acute anoxia and ischemia occur is cardiac arrest or sudden hypotension. Anoxia without ischemia occurs with suffocation (near-drowning, choking). Prolonged anoxia leads to bradycardia and cardiac arrest. In adults, hippocampal and Purkinje cells begin to die after 4 minutes of total anoxia and ischemia, and the outside limit of brain viability is believed to be 10 minutes. Exact timing may be difficult in clinical situations when ill-defined intervals of anoxia and hypoxia occur. Remarkable survivals are sometimes associated with near-drowning in water cold enough to lower cerebral temperature and metabolism. The pattern of hypoxic-ischemic brain injury in newborns is different and depends largely on brain maturity (see Chapter 1).

CLINICAL FEATURES. Consciousness is lost within 8 seconds of cerebral circulatory failure, but the loss may take longer when anoxia occurs without ischemia. Presyncopal symptoms of lightheadedness and visual disturbances sometimes precede loss of consciousness. Seizures and extensor rigidity follow.

Considerable effort has been made to identify predictors of the outcome after hypoxic-ischemic events. Only 13% of adults who have had a cardiac arrest regain independent function in the first year after arrest. The outcome in children is somewhat better because the incidence of preexisting cardiopulmonary disease is lower. Absence of pupillary responses on initial examination is an ominous sign; such patients do not recover independent function. Twenty-four hours after arrest, patients with poor prognoses are identified by lack of motor responses in the limbs and eyes. In contrast, a favorable outcome can be predicted for patients who rapidly recover roving or conjugate eye movements and limb withdrawal from pain. Children who are unconscious for longer than 60 days will not regain language skills or the ability to walk.

Two delayed syndromes of neurological deterioration follow anoxia. The first is *delayed postanoxic encephalopathy*, the appearance of apathy or confusion 1 to 2 weeks after apparent recovery. This is followed by motor symptoms, usually rigidity or spasticity, and may progress to coma or death. Demyelination is the suggested mechanism. The other syndrome is *postanoxic action myoclonus*. This usually follows a severe episode of anoxia and ischemia caused by cardiac arrest. All voluntary activity initiates disabling myoclonus (see Chapter 14). Symptoms of cerebellar dysfunction are also present.

DIAGNOSIS. Cerebral edema is prominent during the first 72 hours after severe hypoxia. CT during that time shows decreased density with loss of the differentiation between gray and white matter. Severe, generalized loss of density on the CT correlates with a poor outcome. An EEG that shows a burst-suppression pattern or absence of activity is associated with a poor neurological outcome or death; lesser abnormalities are not useful in predicting the prognosis.

MANAGEMENT. The principles of treating patients who have sustained hypoxic-ischemic encephalopathy do not differ substantially from the principles of caring for other comatose patients. Oxygenation, circulation, and blood glucose concentration must be maintained. Intra-

cranial pressure must be lowered sufficiently to allow satisfactory cerebral perfusion (see Chapter 4). Seizures are managed with anticonvulsant drugs (see Chapter 1). Anoxia is invariably associated with lactic acidosis, and acid-base balance must be restored.

Barbiturate coma is frequently used to slow cerebral metabolism, but neither clinical nor experimental evidence indicates a beneficial effect following cardiac arrest or near-drowning. Hypothermia prevents brain damage during the time of hypoxia and ischemia but has questionable value after the event. Corticosteroids do not improve neurological recovery in patients with global ischemia following cardiac arrest. Postanoxic action myoclonus sometimes responds to valproate.

Persistent Vegetative State

The term *persistent vegetative state* (PVS) is used to describe patients who, after recovery from coma, return to a state of wakefulness without cognition. PVS is a form of eyes-open permanent unconsciousness with loss of cognitive function and awareness of the environment but preservation of sleep-wake cycles and vegetative function. Survival is indefinite with good nursing care. The usual causes, in order of frequency, are anoxia and ischemia, metabolic or encephalitic coma, and head trauma. Anoxia-ischemia has the worst prognosis. Children who remain in a PVS for 3 months do not regain functional skills.

The American Academy of Neurology has adopted the policy that all medical treatment, including the provision of nutrition and hydration, may be ethically discontinued when a patient's condition has been diagnosed as PVS, it is clear that the patient would not want to be maintained in this state, and the family agrees to discontinue therapy.

Brain Death

Various standards for the diagnosis of brain death have been proposed, but the guidelines suggested by the American Academy of Neurology (1995) are generally accepted. The important features of the report are summarized in Table 2-5. The Academy urged caution in applying the criteria to children younger than 5 years, but subsequent experience supports the validity of the standards in the newborn and through childhood. Absence of cerebral blood flow is the earliest and most definitive proof of brain death. EEG activity may still be present 24 hours after

Table 2-5
Diagnostic Criteria for the Clinical Diagnosis of Brain Death

Prerequisites
Cessation of all brain function
Proximate cause of brain death is known
Condition is irreversible

Cardinal Features
Coma
Absent brainstem reflexes
    Pupillary light reflex
    Corneal reflex
    Oculocephalic reflex
    Oculovestibular reflex
    Oropharyngeal reflex
Apnea (established by formal apnea test)

Confirmatory Tests (optional)
Cerebral angiography
Electroencephalography
Radioisotope cerebral blood flow study
Transcranial doppler ultrasonography

cessation of cerebral blood flow but subsequently becomes isoelectric.

Infectious Disorders

Bacterial Infections

Cat Scratch Disease

Cat scratch disease is caused by *Bartonella (Rochalimaea) henselae,* a gram-negative bacillus that is transmitted by a cat scratch and perhaps by cat fleas (Marra, 1995). It is the most common cause of chronic benign lymphadenopathy in children and young adults. The estimated incidence in the United States is 22,000 per year, and 80% of cases occur in children less than 12 years of age.

CLINICAL FEATURES. The major feature is lymphadenopathy proximal to the site of the scratch. Fever is present in only 60% of cases. The disease is usually benign and self-limited. Unusual systemic manifestations are oculoglandular disease, erythema nodosum, osteolytic lesions, and thrombocytopenic purpura. The most common neurological manifestation is encephalopathy. Rare cases of transverse myelitis, radiculitis, cerebellar ataxia, and neuroretinitis have been reported.

Encephalitis occurs in less than 1% of patients with cat scratch disease. The mechanism is unknown, but it may be caused by direct infection or vasculitis. The male-to-female ratio is

2:1. Only 17% of cases occur in children less than 12 years old and 15% in children 12 to 18 years old. The frequency of fever and the site of the scratch are no different in patients with cat scratch disease encephalitis compared to those who had the disease without encephalitis. The initial and most prominent feature is a decreased state of consciousness ranging from lethargy to coma. Seizures occur in 46% of cases and combative behavior in 40%. Focal findings are rare.

DIAGNOSIS. The diagnosis requires local lymphadenopathy, contact with a cat, and an identifiable site of inoculation. Enzyme-linked immunosorbent assay (ELISA) tests and polymerase chain reaction (PCR) amplification from infected tissues are available for diagnosis. The cerebrospinal fluid is normal in 70% of cases. Lymphocytosis in the cerebrospinal fluid, when present, does not exceed 30 cells/mm^3. The EEG is diffusely slow, and the cranial magnetic resonance imaging (MRI) or CT is normal.

MANAGEMENT. All affected children recover completely, 50% within 4 weeks. Intravenous gentamicin (5 to 7 mg/kg/day) or oral trimethoprim (10 mg/kg twice daily) and sulfamethoxazole (100 mg/kg twice daily) may speed recovery in children with severe encephalopathy.

Gram-Negative Sepsis

CLINICAL FEATURES. The onset of symptoms in gram-negative sepsis may be explosive and is characterized by fever or hypothermia, chills, hyperventilation, hemodynamic instability, and mental changes (irritability, delirium, or coma). Neurological features may also include asterixis, tremor, and multifocal myoclonus. Multiple organ failure follows (1) renal shutdown caused by hypotension, (2) hypoprothrombinemia caused by vitamin K deficiency, (3) thrombocytopenia caused by nonspecific binding of immunoglobulin, (4) disseminated intravascular coagulation with infarction or hemorrhage in several organs, and (5) progressive respiratory failure.

DIAGNOSIS. Sepsis should always be considered in the differential diagnosis of shock, and blood cultures must be obtained. When shock is the initial feature, gram-negative sepsis is likely. In *Staphylococcus aureus* infections, shock is more likely to occur during the course of the infection and not as an initial feature. The cerebrospinal fluid is usually normal or may have an elevated concentration of protein. MRI or CT of the brain is normal early in the course and shows edema later on.

MANAGEMENT. Septic shock is a medical emergency. Antibiotic therapy should be initiated promptly at maximal doses (see Chapter 4). Hypotension must be treated by restoration of intravascular volume, and each factor contributing to coagulopathy must be addressed. Mortality is high even with optimal treatment.

Hemorrhagic Shock Encephalopathy Syndrome

The hemorrhagic shock and encephalopathy syndrome is presumed to be caused by bacterial sepsis, but this has not been proven.

CLINICAL FEATURES. Most affected children are younger than 1 year of age, but cases in children up to 26 months of age have been described. One half of these children have mild prodromal symptoms of a viral gastroenteritis or respiratory illness. In the rest the onset is explosive; a previously well child is found unresponsive and having seizures. Fever of 38°C or higher is a constant feature. Marked hypotension with poor peripheral perfusion is followed by profuse watery or bloody diarrhea with metabolic acidosis and compensatory respiratory alkalosis. Disseminated intravascular coagulopathy develops, and bleeding occurs from every venipuncture site. The mortality rate is 50%; the survivors have mental and motor impairment.

DIAGNOSIS. The syndrome resembles toxic shock syndrome, gram-negative sepsis, heat stroke, and Reye syndrome. Abnormal renal function occurs in every case, but serum ammonia concentrations remains normal, hypoglycemia is unusual, and blood cultures yield no growth.

Cerebrospinal fluid is normal except for increased pressure. CT shows small ventricles and loss of sulcal marking caused by cerebral edema. The initial EEG background is diffusely slow or may be isoelectric. A striking pattern called *electric storm* evolves over the first hours or days. Runs of spikes, sharp waves, or rhythmic slow waves that fluctuate in frequency, amplitude, and location characterize the pattern.

MANAGEMENT. Affected children require intensive care with ventilatory support, volume replacement, correction of acid-base and coagulation disturbances, anticonvulsant therapy, and control of cerebral edema.

Toxic Shock Syndrome

Toxic shock syndrome is a potentially lethal illness caused by infection or colonization with some strains of *S. aureus*.

CLINICAL FEATURES. The onset is abrupt and is characterized by high fever, hypotension, vomiting, diarrhea, myalgia, headache, and a desquamating rash. Multiple organ failure may occur during desquamation. Serious complications include cardiac arrhythmia, pulmonary edema, and oliguric renal failure. Initial encephalopathic features are agitation and confusion. These may be followed by lethargy, obtundation, and generalized tonic-clonic seizures.

Most pediatric cases have occurred in menstruating girls who use tampons, but they may also occur in children with occlusive dressings after burns or surgery, and as a complication of influenza and influenza-like illness in children with staphylococcal colonization of the respiratory tract.

DIAGNOSIS. No diagnostic laboratory test is available. The diagnosis is based on the typical clinical and laboratory findings. Over half of the patients have sterile pyuria, immature granulocytic leukocytes, coagulation abnormalities, hypocalcemia, low serum albumin and total protein concentrations, and elevated concentrations of blood urea nitrogen, transaminase, bilirubin, and creatine kinase. Cultures of specimens from infected areas yield *S. aureus*.

MANAGEMENT. Hypotension usually responds to volume restoration with physiological saline solutions. Some patients require vasopressors or fresh-frozen plasma. Antibiotic therapy should be initiated promptly with an agent effective against *S. aureus*.

Rickettsial Infections

Lyme Disease

Lyme disease is caused by a spirochete (*Borrelia burgdorferi*) and transmitted by the hard-shelled deer ticks: *Ixodes dammini* in the eastern United States, *I. pacificus* in the western United States, and *I. ricinus* in Europe. Lyme disease is now the most common vector-borne infection in the United States. Six northeastern states account for 80% of cases.

CLINICAL FEATURES. Three stages of disease are described, but this sequence is variable. The first symptom (stage 1) in 60% to 80% of patients is a skin lesion of the thigh, groin, or axilla (erythema chronicum migrans), which may be associated with fever, regional lymphadenopathy, and arthralgia. The rash begins as a red macule at the site of the tick bite and then spreads to form a red annular lesion with partial clearing, sometimes appearing as alternating rings of rash and clearing.

Neurological involvement (neuroborreliosis) develops weeks or months later when the infection becomes disseminated (stage 2). Most children have only headache, which clears completely within 6 weeks; this may be caused by mild aseptic meningitis or encephalitis. Fever may not occur. Facial palsy, sleep disturbances, and papilledema may occur, but polyneuropathies are uncommon in children. Transitory cardiac involvement (myopericarditis and atrioventricular block) may occur in stage 2.

A year or more of continual migratory arthritis begins weeks to years after the onset of neurological features (stage 3). Only one joint, often the knee, or a few large joints are affected. During stage 3 the patient feels ill. Encephalopathy with memory or cognitive abnormalities and confusional states, with normal cerebrospinal fluid, results may occur. Other psychiatric or fatigue syndromes appear less likely to be causally related (Halperin et al, 1996).

DIAGNOSIS. The spirochete can be grown on cultures from the skin rash during stage 1 of the disease. At the time of meningitis the cerebrospinal fluid may be normal at first but then shows a lymphocytic pleocytosis (about 100 cells/mm³, an elevated protein concentration, and a normal glucose concentration. *B. burgdorferi* may be cultured from the cerebrospinal fluid during the meningitis (Halperin et al, 1996).

A two-test approach is recommended to establish the diagnosis of neuroborreliosis (Garcia-Monco and Benach, 1995). The first step is to show the production of specific IgG and IgM antibodies in cerebrospinal fluid. Antibody production begins 2 weeks after infection, and IgG is always detectable at 6 weeks. The second step, to be used when the first is inconclusive, is the PCR to detect the organism.

MANAGEMENT. Either ceftriaxone (2 g once daily intravenously) or penicillin (3–4 million units intravenously every 3–4 hours) for 2–4 weeks is used to treat encephalitis. Routine use of corticosteroids is not indicated. Cerebrospinal fluid examination should be performed toward the end of the 2- to 4-week treatment course to assess the need for continuing treatment and again 6 months after the conclusion of therapy. Intrathecal antibody production may persist for years following successful treatment, and in isolation it does not indicate active disease. Patients in whom cerebrospinal fluid pleocytosis fails to resolve within 6 months, however, should be retreated.

Peripheral or cranial nerve involvement without cerebrospinal fluid abnormalities may be treated with oral agents, either doxycycline, 100 mg twice daily for 14–21 days, or amoxicillin, 500 mg every 8 hours for 10–21 days. An effective vaccine against Lyme disease is available and may be used for children who live in endemic areas (Sigal et al, 1998; Steere et al, 1998).

Rocky Mountain Spotted Fever

Rocky Mountain spotted fever is an acute tick-borne disorder caused by *Rickettsia rickettsii*. Its geographic name is a misnomer; the disease occurs in much of the United States, with a special predilection for southwestern and southeastern states.

CLINICAL FEATURES. Fever, myalgia, and rash are constant symptoms. The rash appears within 14 days of onset (average, 4 days) and may be maculopapular, petechial, or both. Headache is present in 66% of affected individuals, meningismus in 33%, focal neurological signs in 14%, and seizures in 6%.

DIAGNOSIS. *R. rickettsii* can be demonstrated by direct immunofluorescence or immunoperoxidase staining of a skin biopsy specimen of the rash. Other laboratory tests may indicate anemia, thrombocytopenia, coagulopathy, hyponatremia, and muscle tissue breakdown. Serology retrospectively confirms the diagnosis. The cerebrospinal fluid shows a mild pleocytosis.

MANAGEMENT. Treatment should be started when the diagnosis is suspected. Mortality is 20% when treatment is delayed. Oral or intravenous tetracycline (25–50 mg/kg/day) or chloramphenicol (50–75 mg/kg/day) in four divided doses or oral doxycycline (100 mg twice a day for 7 days) is effective. Treatment is continued for 2 days once the patient has become afebrile.

Viral Infections

Because encephalitis usually affects the meninges as well as the brain, the term *meningoencephalitis* may be more accurate. However, distinguishing encephalitis from aseptic meningitis is useful for viral diagnosis because most viruses cause primarily one or the other, but not both. An annual incidence of 7.4 : 100,000 for encephalitis and 10.9 : 100,000 for aseptic meningitis remained relatively constant in one Minnesota county over a 32-year period. Both conditions are more common in the summer, in childhood, and in males.

Routine childhood immunization has reduced the number of pathogenic viruses circulating in the community. Enteroviruses and herpes simplex virus are now the most common viral causes of meningitis and encephalitis in children. However, specific viral identification is established in only 15% to 20% of cases.

The classification of viruses undergoes frequent change, but a constant first step is the separation of viruses with a DNA nucleic acid core from those with an RNA core. The only DNA viruses that cause acute postnatal encephalitis in immunocompetent hosts are herpes viruses. RNA viruses causing encephalitis are myxoviruses (influenza and measles encephalitis), arboviruses (St. Louis encephalitis, eastern equine encephalitis, western equine encephalitis, and LaCrosse-California encephalitis), retroviruses (acquired immune deficiency syndrome encephalitis), and rhabdoviruses (rabies). RNA viruses (especially enteroviruses and mumps) are responsible for aseptic meningitis.

Some viruses, such as herpes simplex virus, are highly neurotropic (almost always infect the nervous system) but rarely neurovirulent (rarely cause encephalitis), whereas others, such as measles, are rarely neurotropic but are highly neurovirulent. In addition to viruses that directly infect the brain and meninges, encephalopathies may also follow systemic viral infections. These are thought to result from demyelination caused by immune-mediated responses of the brain to infection.

Aseptic Meningitis

The term *aseptic meningitis* is used to define a syndrome of meningismus and cerebrospinal fluid leukocytosis without bacterial or fungal infection. Drugs or viral infections are the usual cause. Viral meningitis is a benign, self-limited disease from which 95% of children recover completely.

CLINICAL FEATURES. Twenty percent of children have a history of antecedent respiratory infection or gastrointestinal illness. The onset of symptoms is abrupt and characterized by fever, headache, and stiff neck, except in infants who do not have meningismus. Irritability, lethargy, and vomiting are also common. "Encephalitic" symptoms are not part of the syndrome in children, but seizures and coma may occur in infants. Systemic illness is uncommon, but its presence may suggest specific viral disorders (parotitis suggestive of mumps, myalgia of coxsackie viral infection, rash of echovirus infection

and Lyme disease, diarrhea of enterovirus infection).

The acute illness usually lasts for less than 1 week, but malaise and headache may continue for several weeks. Communicating hydrocephalus is an unusual long-term sequela.

DIAGNOSIS. In most cases of aseptic meningitis the cerebrospinal fluid contains 10 to 200 leukocytes/mm^3, but cell counts of 1,000 cells/mm^3 or greater may occur with lymphocytic choriomeningitis. The response is primarily lymphocytic, but polymorphonuclear leukocytes may predominate early in the course. The protein concentration is generally between 50 and 100 mg/dl (0.5 and 1 g/L) and the glucose concentration is normal, although it may be slightly reduced in children with mumps and lymphocytic choriomeningitis.

Aseptic meningitis usually occurs in the spring or summer, and enteroviruses are responsible for most cases in children. The mumps and poliomyelitis viruses remain important causative agents in countries where immunization is not mandatory. Nonviral causes of aseptic meningitis are rare but must be considered; these include Lyme disease, Kawasaki disease, leukemia, systemic lupus erythematosus, migraine, and irritation of the meninges from blood, drugs, and contrast materials.

Individuals with a personal or family history of migraine may have attacks of severe headache associated with stiff neck and focal neurological disturbances, such as hemiparesis and aphasia. Cerebrospinal fluid examination shows a pleocytosis of 5 to 300 cells/mm^3 that is mainly lymphocytes and a protein concentration of 50 to 100 mg/dl (0.5 to 1 g/L). Whether the attacks are migraine provoked by intercurrent aseptic meningitis or represent a "meningitic" form of migraine is not known. The recurrence of attacks in some people suggests that the mechanism is wholly migrainous.

Bacterial meningitis is the major concern when a child has meningismus. Although cerebrospinal fluid examination provides several clues that differentiate bacterial from viral meningitis, antibiotic therapy should be initiated for every child with a clinical syndrome of aseptic meningitis until cerebrospinal fluid culture is negative for bacteria (see Chapter 4). This is especially true for children who received antibiotic therapy before examination of the cerebrospinal fluid.

MANAGEMENT. Children with viral meningitis or encephalitis are now routinely treated for herpes encephalitis until that diagnosis can be excluded; treatment with acyclovir is harmless. Treatment of viral aseptic meningitis is directed at the symptoms. Bed rest in a quiet environment and mild analgesics provide satisfactory relief of symptoms in most children.

Arboviral (Arthropod-Borne) Encephalitis

Arboviruses are classified on the basis of ecology rather than structure. Ticks and mosquitoes are the usual vectors, and epidemics occur in the spring and summer. Each type of encephalitis has a defined geographic area. Arboviruses account for 10% of encephalitis cases reported in the United States.

California-La Crosse Encephalitis

The California serogroup viruses, principally La Crosse encephalitis, are the most common cause of arboviral encephalitis in the United States (Rust et al, 1999). The endemic areas are the Midwest and western New York state. Most cases occur between July and September. Small woodland mammals serve as a reservoir and mosquitoes as the vector.

CLINICAL FEATURES. Most cases of encephalitis occur in children, and asymptomatic infection is common in adults. The initial feature is a flu-like syndrome that lasts for 2 or 3 days. Encephalitis is heralded by headache followed by seizures and rapid progression to coma. Focal neurological disturbances are present in 20% of cases. Symptoms begin to resolve 3 to 5 days after onset, and most children recover without neurological sequelae. Death is uncommon and occurs mainly in infants.

DIAGNOSIS. Examination of cerebrospinal fluid shows a mixed pleocytosis with lymphocytes predominating. The count is usually 50 to 200 cells/mm^3, but it may range from 0 to 600 cells/mm^3. The virus is difficult to culture, and diagnosis depends on showing a fourfold or greater increase in hemagglutination inhibition and neutralizing antibody titers between acute and convalescent sera.

MANAGEMENT. Treatment is supportive. No effective antiviral agent is available.

Eastern Equine Encephalitis

Eastern equine encephalitis is the most severe type of arboviral encephalitis.

CLINICAL FEATURES. Eastern equine encephalitis is a perennial infection of horses from New York to Florida. Human cases do not exceed five each year, and they follow epidemics in horses. The mortality rate is 30%. Wild birds serve as a reservoir and mosquitoes as a vector. Consequently, almost all cases occur during the summer months.

Onset is usually abrupt and characterized by high fever, headache, and vomiting, followed by drowsiness, coma, and seizures. The longer the duration of nonneurological prodromal symptoms, the better the outcome. In infants, seizures and coma are often the first manifestations. Signs of meningismus are usually present in older children. Children usually survive the acute encephalitis, but mental impairment, seizures, and disturbed motor function can be expected in survivors.

DIAGNOSIS. The cerebrospinal fluid pressure is usually elevated, and examination reveals 200 to 2,000 leukocytes/mm^3, of which half are polymorphonuclear leukocytes. MRI shows focal lesions in the basal ganglia and thalamus (Deresiewicz et al, 1997). Diagnosis relies on showing a fourfold or greater rise in complement fixation and neutralizing antibody titers between acute and convalescent sera.

MANAGEMENT. Treatment is supportive. No effective antiviral agent is available.

Japanese B Encephalitis

Japanese B encephalitis is a major form of encephalitis in Asia and is an important health hazard to nonimmunized travelers during summer months. The virus cycle is among mosquitoes, pigs, and birds.

CLINICAL FEATURES. The initial features are malaise, fever, and headache or irritability lasting for 2 to 3 days. These are followed by meningismus, confusion, and delirium. During the second or third week, photophobia and generalized hypotonia develop. Seizures may occur at any time. Finally, rigidity, a mask-like facies, and brainstem dysfunction ensue. Mortality rates are very high among indigenous populations and lower among Western travelers, probably because of a difference in the age of the exposed populations.

DIAGNOSIS. Examination of the cerebrospinal fluid shows pleocytosis (20 to 500 cells/mm^3). The cells are initially mixed, but later lymphocytes predominate. The protein concentration is usually between 50 and 100 mg/dl (0.5 and 1 mg/L), and the glucose concentration is normal. Diagnosis depends on demonstrating a fourfold or greater elevation in the level of complement-fixing antibodies between acute and convalescent sera.

MANAGEMENT. Treatment is supportive. No effective antiviral agent is available, but immunization with an inactivated vaccine protects against encephalitis in more than 90% of individuals.

St. Louis Encephalitis

St. Louis encephalitis is endemic in the western United States and epidemic in the Mississippi valley and the Atlantic states. It is the most common cause of epidemic viral encephalitis in the United States. The vector is a mosquito, and birds are the major reservoir.

CLINICAL FEATURES. Most infections are asymptomatic. The spectrum of neurological illness varies from aseptic meningitis to severe encephalitis leading to death. The mortality rate is low. Headache, vomiting, and states of decreased consciousness are the typical features. A slow evolution of neurological symptoms, the presence of generalized weakness and tremor, and the absence of focal findings and seizures favor a diagnosis of St. Louis encephalitis over herpes simplex encephalitis. The usual duration of illness is 1 to 2 weeks. Children usually recover completely, but adults may be left with mental or motor impairment.

DIAGNOSIS. Cerebrospinal fluid examination reveals a lymphocytic pleocytosis (50 to 500 cells/mm^3) and a protein concentration between 50 and 100 mg/dl (0.5 and 1 g/L). The glucose concentration is normal.

The virus is difficult to grow on culture, and diagnosis requires a fourfold or greater increase in complement fixation and hemagglutination inhibition antibody titers between acute and convalescent sera.

MANAGEMENT. Treatment is supportive. No effective antiviral agent is available.

Western Equine Encephalitis

CLINICAL FEATURES. Western equine encephalitis is a rare disorder. Wild birds serve as the reservoir and mosquitoes as the vector. All recent cases have been reported from North Dakota, South Dakota, and Canada. Between 20% and 30% of cases occur in infants.

In infants the infection is characterized by irritability, fever, meningismus, bulging of the fontanelles, seizures, and coma. Older children may have a flu-like syndrome before symptoms of meningoencephalitis develop. The initial symptom is usually behavioral change, including delirium, which is followed by drowsiness and coma. The EEG shows focal abnormalities that lateralize to one temporal lobe and suggest herpes encephalitis.

Symptoms last for 1 to 2 weeks, and although the overall mortality rate is 10%, most fatalities are infants. Fifty percent of surviving infants have permanent mental impairment and seizures.

DIAGNOSIS. Cerebrospinal fluid pleocytosis is first a mixture of polymorphonuclear leukocytes and lymphocytes and then lymphocytes alone. The protein concentration is between 50 and 100 mg/dl (0.5 and 1 g/L). Diagnosis relies on showing a fourfold or greater rise in complement-fixing or neutralizing antibodies between acute and convalescent sera.

MANAGEMENT. Treatment is supportive. The child should be treated for herpes encephalitis until a definitive diagnosis is made. No effective antiviral agent is available for western equine encephalitis.

Herpes Simplex Encephalitis

Two similar strains of herpes simplex virus (HSV) are pathogenic to humans. HSV-1 is associated with orofacial infections and HSV-2 with genital infections. Both are worldwide in distribution. Forty percent of children have antibodies to HSV-1, but antibodies to HSV-2 are not routinely detected until puberty. HSV-1 is the important causative agent of acute herpes simplex encephalitis after the newborn period and HSV-2 of encephalitis in the newborn (see Chapter 1).

Initial orofacial infection with HSV-1 may be asymptomatic. The virus replicates in the skin, infecting nerve fiber endings and then the trigeminal ganglia. Further replication occurs within the ganglia before the virus enters a latent stage during which it cannot be recovered from the ganglia. Reactivation occurs during times of stress, especially intercurrent febrile illness. The reactivated virus ordinarily retraces its neural migration to the facial skin but occasionally spreads proximally to the brain, causing encephalitis. The host's immunocompetence maintains the virus in a latent state. An immunocompromised state results in frequent reactivation and severe, widespread infection.

HSV is the single most common cause of non-epidemic encephalitis and accounts for 10% to 20% of cases. The annual incidence is estimated at 2.3 cases per million population. Thirty-one percent of cases occur in children.

CLINICAL FEATURES. Primary infection is often the cause of encephalitis in children. Only 22% of those with encephalitis have a history of recurrent labial herpes infection. Typically the onset is acute and characterized by fever, headache, lethargy, nausea, and vomiting. Eighty percent of children show focal neurological disturbances (hemiparesis, cranial nerve deficits, visual field loss, aphasia, and focal seizures), and the remainder show behavioral changes or generalized seizures without clinical evidence of focal neurological deficits. However, both groups have focal abnormalities on neuroradiographic studies or EEG. The acute stage of encephalitis lasts for approximately a week. Recovery takes several weeks and is often incomplete.

Herpes meningitis is usually associated with genital lesions and is caused by HSV-2. The clinical features are similar to those of aseptic meningitis caused by other viruses.

DIAGNOSIS. Prompt diagnosis of herpes simplex encephalitis is important because treatment is available. Cerebrospinal fluid pleocytosis is present in 97% of cases. The median count is 130 leukocytes/mm^3 (range, 0 to 1,000). Up to 500 red blood cells/mm^3 may be present as well. The median protein concentration is 80 mg/dl (0.8 g/L), but 20% of those affected have normal protein concentrations and 40% have concentrations exceeding 100 mg/dl (1 g/L). The glucose concentration in the cerebrospinal fluid is usually normal, but in 7% of cases it is less than half of the blood glucose concentration.

In the past, the demonstration of periodic lateralizing epileptiform discharges on EEG was considered presumptive evidence of herpes encephalitis. However, MRI has proved to be a more sensitive early indicator of herpes encephalitis. T$_2$-weighted studies show increased signal intensity involving the cortex and white matter in the temporal and inferior frontal lobes (Figure 2-1). The areas of involvement then enlarge and coalesce. The identification of the organism in the cerebrospinal fluid by PCR has obviated the need for brain biopsy to establish the diagnosis (Mitchell et al, 1997).

MANAGEMENT. Most physicians begin acyclovir treatment in every child with a compatible clinical history. Treatment of HSV encephalitis with intravenous acyclovir (10 mg/kg every 8 hours for 14 days) reduces mortality from 70% in untreated patients to 25–30% (Whitley and Kimberlin, 1998). The mortality rate is highest in patients who are already in coma when treat-

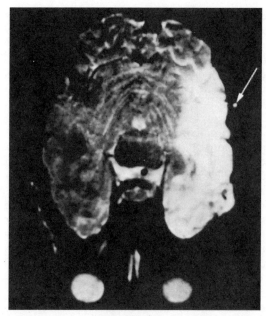

Figure 2-1. MRI image of herpes encephalitis. T$_2$-weighted image shows increased signal intensity in both temporal lobes (*arrow*).

ment is initiated. Function returns to normal in 38%.

Measles (Rubeola) Encephalitis

Compulsory immunization had almost eliminated natural measles infection in the United States, but the incidence began climbing again in 1990 because of reduced immunization rates. The risk of encephalitis from natural disease is 1:1,000. During the first 20 years of the measles vaccine program, an estimated 52 million cases of measles, 5,200 deaths, and 17,400 cases of mental retardation were prevented. The mechanism of measles encephalitis has been contested, but evidence for both direct viral infection and allergic demyelination has been presented. A chronic form of measles encephalitis (subacute sclerosing panencephalitis) is described in Chapter 5.

CLINICAL FEATURES. Measles is a neurotropic virus, and EEG abnormalities are often present even without clinical symptoms of encephalopathy. Symptoms of encephalitis usually begin 1 to 8 days after the appearance of rash but can be delayed for 3 weeks. The onset is usually abrupt and is characterized by lethargy or obtundation that may rapidly progress to coma. Generalized seizures occur in half of children. The spectrum of neurological disturbances includes hemiplegia, ataxia, and involuntary movement disorders. Acute transverse myelitis may occur as well (see Chapter 12). The incidence of neurological morbidity (mental retardation, epilepsy, and paralysis) is high but does not correlate with the severity of acute encephalitis.

Measles immunization does not cause an acute encephalopathy or any chronic brain damage syndrome. Generalized seizures may occur during the second week following immunization. These are mainly febrile seizures, and recovery is complete.

DIAGNOSIS. Examination of cerebrospinal fluid shows a lymphocytic pleocytosis. The number of lymphocytes is usually highest in the first few days but rarely exceeds 100 cells/mm³. Protein concentrations are generally between 50 and 100 mg/dl (0.5 and 1 g/L), and the glucose concentration is normal.

MANAGEMENT. Treatment is supportive. Anticonvulsant drugs usually provide satisfactory seizure control.

Postinfectious Encephalomyelitis

Demyelinating disorders that occur during or after systemic viral illnesses are called *postinfectious* and are presumed to be immune mediated. The nervous system is not thought to be infected. Either central or peripheral myelin may be affected, but whether both can be affected simultaneously has not been determined. Examples of postinfectious disorders appear in several chapters of this textbook and include the Guillain-Barré syndrome (see Chapter 7), acute cerebellar ataxia (see Chapter 10), transverse myelitis (see Chapter 12), brachial neuritis (see Chapter 13), optic neuritis (see Chapter 16), and Bell's palsy (see Chapter 17). The incidence of some postinfectious disorders is increased in immunocompromised populations, which provides further support for the immune hypothesis.

The cause-and-effect relationship between viral infection and many of these syndromes is virtually impossible to establish if 30 days is used as the latency period between viral infection and onset of neurological dysfunction. The average school-age child has four to six "viral illnesses" each year, so that 33% to 50% of children will report a viral illness 30 days before the onset of the life event. A greater than 50% incidence of viral illness 30 days before onset is not reported for any syndrome listed previously.

CLINICAL FEATURES. MRI has expanded the spectrum of clinical features associated with postinfectious encephalopathy by allowing the demonstration of small demyelinating lesions. Lethargy and weakness are at one end of the spectrum, and coma is at the other.

The encephalopathy is often preceded by lethargy, headache, and vomiting. Whether these "systemic features" are symptoms of a viral illness or of early encephalopathy is not clear. The onset of neurological symptoms is abrupt and characterized by declining consciousness and seizures. In some cases, optic neuritis, transverse myelitis, or both precedes the encephalopathy (see Chapter 12). Some children never have focal neurological signs, whereas in others the initial feature suggests a focal mass lesion.

Mortality is highest in the first week. Although recovery among survivors is variable, the degree of recovery may be astonishing.

DIAGNOSIS. Diagnosis is based on a T_2-weighted MRI scan that show a marked increase in signal intensity throughout the white matter (Figure 2-2). The lesions resolve in the weeks that follow, and no new lesions are expected. Adrenoleukodystrophy must be excluded in boys.

The cerebrospinal fluid is frequently normal. Occasional abnormalities are a mild lymphocytic pleocytosis and elevation of the protein concentration.

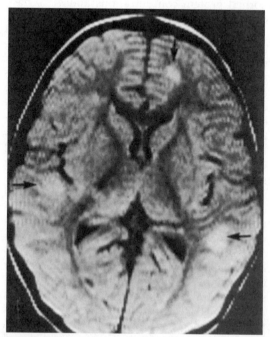

Figure 2-2. Postinfectious demyelination of the cerebral hemispheres. Areas of increased signal intensity are seen in both hemispheres (*arrows*).

MANAGEMENT. Children with severe demyelinating encephalopathies are treated with corticosteroids, despite the absence of conclusive evidence that such treatment is beneficial.

Reye Syndrome

Reye syndrome is a systemic disorder of mitochondrial function that occurs during or following viral infection. The disorder occurs more often when salicylates are administered during viral illness for relief of symptoms. Recognition of this relationship has led to decreased use of salicylates in children and a marked decline in the incidence of Reye syndrome (Belay et al, 1999).

CLINICAL FEATURES. In the United States sporadic cases are generally associated with varicella (chickenpox) or nonspecific respiratory infections; small epidemics are associated with influenza B infection. When varicella is the precipitating infection, the initial stage of Reye syndrome occurs 3 to 6 days after the appearance of rash.

The clinical course is relatively predictable and has been divided into five stages:

Stage 0: Vomiting, but no symptoms of brain dysfunction

Stage I: Vomiting, confusion, and lethargy

Stage II: Agitation, delirium, decorticate posturing, and hyperventilation

Stage III: Coma and decerebrate posturing

Stage IV: Flaccidity, apnea, and dilated, fixed pupils

The progression from stage I to stage IV may be explosive, evolving in less than 24 hours. More commonly, the period of recurrent vomiting and lethargy lasts for a day or longer. In most children with vomiting and laboratory evidence of hepatic dysfunction following varicella or respiratory infection, liver biopsy shows the features of Reye syndrome, despite normal cerebral function. This has been designated as Reye stage 0. Stages I and II represent metabolic dysfunction and cerebral edema. Stages III and IV indicate generalized increased intracranial pressure and herniation.

Focal neurological disturbances and meningismus are not part of the syndrome. Fever is not a prominent feature, and hepatomegaly occurs in one half of patients late in the course.

The outcome is variable, but as a rule, infants do worse than older children. Progression to stages III and IV at all ages is associated with a high death rate and with impaired neurological function in survivors.

DIAGNOSIS. Typical blood abnormalities are hypoglycemia, hyperammonemia, and increased concentrations of hepatic enzymes. Serum bilirubin concentrations remain normal, and jaundice does not occur. Acute pancreatitis sometimes develops and can be identified by increased concentrations of serum amylase.

The cerebrospinal fluid is normal except for increased pressure. The EEG shows abnormalities consistent with a diffuse encephalopathy.

Liver biopsy is definitive. Light microscopy shows panlobular accumulation of small intracellular lipid droplets and depletion of succinic acid dehydrogenase in the absence of other abnormalities. Electron microscopic changes include characteristic mitochondrial abnormalities, peroxisomal proliferation and swelling, proliferation of smooth endoplasmic reticulum, and glycogen depletion.

Conditions that mimic Reye syndrome are disorders of fatty acid oxidation, ornithine transcarbamylase deficiency, and valproate hepatotoxicity. Inborn errors of metabolism should be assumed and sought in any child with recurrent Reye syndrome (Table 2-4) or a family history of similar illness. Metabolic products of valproate are mitochondrial poisons that have been used to produce an experimental model of Reye syndrome.

MANAGEMENT. Children with stage I or II disease should be watched closely in a pediatric intensive care unit and treated with intravenous hypertonic (10% to 15%) glucose solution at normal maintenance volumes. Stages III and IV require treatment of increased intracranial pressure (see Chapter 4) by elevation of the head, controlled mechanical ventilation, and mannitol. Corticosteroids are of limited benefit and should not be used routinely. Some authorities continue to advocate intracranial pressure monitors and pentobarbital coma, although they have never been shown to affect the outcome. Fortunately, this once common and deadly disease has almost disappeared with discontinuation of salicylate therapy for children.

Postimmunization Encephalopathy

Three types of vaccine are in general use in the United States: live-attenuated viruses, whole or fractionated-killed organisms, and toxoids.

Live-attenuated virus vaccines (measles, mumps, rubella, varicella, and oral poliomyelitis) are intended to produce a mild and harmless infection with subsequent immunity. However, even under ideal circumstances of vaccine preparation and host resistance, symptoms of the natural disease and its known neurological complications may develop in vaccine recipients.

Whole-killed organisms (pertussis, influenza, rabies, and inactivated poliomyelitis) do not reproduce their natural disease, but are alleged to injure the nervous system by a toxic or an allergic mechanism. Whole-cell pertussis vaccine causes seizures, and while it is not established that it causes chronic brain damage, the Institute of Medicine has conceded the possibility based on the National Childhood Encephalopathy Study (Fenichel, 1999). Rabies vaccine had been an important cause of encephalomyelitis in the past, but the newer vaccine, prepared from virus grown on human diploid cells, has rarely been implicated as a cause of polyneuropathy. The older vaccine (Semple), still in use in some parts of the world, contains myelin-basic protein and is known to cause encephalomyelitis. None of the other whole-killed organism vaccines causes encephalopathy.

Toxoids are produced by the inactivation of toxins produced by bacteria. Diphtheria and tetanus toxoids are the only such vaccines now in use. Tetanus toxoid is associated with the Guillain-Barré syndrome and brachial plexitis; neither is associated with encephalopathy.

Metabolic and Systemic Disorders

Disorders of Osmolality

The number of particles in a solution determines the osmolality of a solution. Sodium salts, glucose, and urea are the primary osmoles of the extracellular space, potassium salts of the intracellular space, and plasma proteins of the intravascular space. Because cell membranes are permeable to water and osmotic equilibrium must be maintained, the volume of intracellular fluid is determined by the osmolality of the extracellular space.

Hypernatremia and hyperglycemia are the major causes of serum hyperosmolality, and hyponatremia is the main cause of serum hypoosmolality.

Diabetic Ketoacidosis

The major cause of symptomatic hyperglycemia in children is diabetic ketoacidosis. Nonketotic hyperglycemic coma, associated with mild or non–insulin-requiring diabetes, is unusual in children.

CLINICAL FEATURES. Diabetic ketoacidosis develops rapidly in children who have neglected to take prescribed doses of insulin or who have a superimposed infection. Initial features are polydipsia, polyuria, and fatigue. The child hyperventilates to compensate for metabolic acidosis. Lethargy rapidly progresses to coma. Ketoacidosis is the leading cause of death in children with diabetes, and mortality rates are still as high as 10%.

Cerebral edema is an early and almost constant feature of diabetic ketoacidosis (Hale et al, 1997). The mechanism is not established. The severity of cerebral edema correlates with changes in level of consciousness. Edema may contribute to death in some cases. Other, less common neurological complications of diabetic ketoacidosis are venous sinus thrombosis and intracerebral hemorrhage. Both are associated with focal or generalized seizures.

DIAGNOSIS. The diagnosis is based on the combination of a blood glucose level greater than 400 mg/dl (22 mmol/L), the presence of serum and urinary ketones, an arterial pH less than 7.25, and a serum bicarbonate concentration less than 15 mmol/L.

MANAGEMENT. In children with moderate to severe diabetic ketoacidosis, the rapid administration of hypotonic fluids at a time of high serum osmolality should be avoided. Fluid deficits should be replaced evenly over 48 hours. The sodium deficit should be reduced by half in the first 12 hours and the remainder eliminated over the next 36 hours. Bicarbonate ion should be given in physiological proportions.

Hypoglycemia

Symptomatic hypoglycemia after the neonatal period is usually associated with insulin use in the treatment of diabetes mellitus. Only a minority of cases are caused by sepsis and inborn errors of metabolism.

CLINICAL FEATURES. Clinical features are not precisely predictable from the blood glucose concentration. Hypoglycemia does not usually become symptomatic until blood concentrations are less than 50 mg/dl (2.8 mmol/L). The rate of fall may be important in determining the clinical features. Dizziness and tremor may occur at blood concentrations below 60 mg/dl (3.1 mmol/L) and serve as a warning of insulin overdose. Greater declines in blood glucose concentration result in confusion, delirium, and loss of consciousness. Sudden hemiplegia, usually transitory and sometimes shifting between the two sides, is a rare feature of hypoglycemia. The mechanism is unknown, and CT shows no evidence of infarction.

DIAGNOSIS. Hypoglycemia should always be suspected in diabetic children with altered mental status or decreased consciousness. The blood glucose concentration should be measured promptly.

MANAGEMENT. Diabetic children should be encouraged to carry a source of sugar for use at the first symptom of hypoglycemia. Children who are comatose from hypoglycemia should receive immediate intravenous glucose replacement. Complete recovery is the rule.

Hypernatremia

Hypernatremia is usually caused by dehydration in which water loss exceeds sodium loss and by overhydration with hypertonic saline solutions. It is a medical emergency and, if not corrected promptly, may lead to permanent brain damage and death.

CLINICAL FEATURES. Hypernatremic dehydration may be a consequence of vomiting or diarrhea, especially if water intake is restricted. Iatrogenic hypernatremia is usually caused by overzealous correction of hyponatremia. Rapid alterations in sodium concentration are much more likely to cause encephalopathy than are equivalent concentrations attained slowly. The symptoms of hypernatremia are referable to the nervous system and include irritability, lethargy progressing to coma, and seizures. The presence of focal neurological deficits suggests cerebral venous sinus thrombosis.

DIAGNOSIS. Symptomatic hypernatremia develops at sodium concentrations greater than 160 mEq/L (160 mmol/L). EEG shows the nonspecific slowing associated with metabolic encephalopathies. Focal slowing on the EEG or focal abnormalities on examination warrants CT to look for venous sinus thrombosis.

Chronic or recurrent episodes of hypernatremia may result from hypodipsia (lack of thirst), a rare condition encountered in children with congenital or acquired brain disorders. The syndrome is usually associated with a defect in secretion of antidiuretic hormone.

MANAGEMENT. Rapid water replacement can lead to cerebral edema. The recommended approach is to correct abnormalities of intravascular volume before correcting the water deficit.

Hyponatremia

Hyponatremia may result from water retention, sodium loss, or both. The syndrome of inappropriate antidiuretic hormone secretion (SIADH) is an important cause of water retention. Sodium loss results from renal disease, vomiting, and diarrhea. Permanent brain damage from hyponatremia is uncommon, but may occur in otherwise healthy children if the serum sodium concentration is allowed to remain less than 115 mEq/L for several hours.

Syndrome of Inappropriate Antidiuretic Hormone Secretion

SIADH occurs in association with several neurological disorders, including head trauma, infections, and intracranial hemorrhage.

CLINICAL FEATURES. Most patients with SIADH have a preexisting loss of consciousness from their underlying neurological disorder. In such patients hyponatremia is the only feature of SIADH. In those who are alert, lethargy develops from the hyponatremia but rarely progresses to coma or seizures.

DIAGNOSIS. Those who provide care for children with acute intracranial disorders must be vigilant for SIADH; repeated determinations of the serum sodium concentration are required. Once hyponatremia and low serum osmolality are documented, the urinary sodium concentration must be measured. The urine osmolality in SIADH is not always above the serum osmolality, but the urine is less than maximally dilute, which excludes the dilutional hyponatremia of water intoxication.

MANAGEMENT. All signs of SIADH respond to fluid restriction. An intake of 50% to 75% of daily water maintenance is generally satisfactory.

Sodium Loss

CLINICAL FEATURES. Movement of water into the brain causes *hyponatremic encephalopathy*. When the serum sodium concentration falls below 125 mEq/L (125 mmol/L), nausea, vomiting, muscular twitching, and lethargy appear. Further decline to less than 115 mEq/L (115 mmol/L) is associated with seizures and coma.

DIAGNOSIS. Hyponatremia should be recognized as a potential problem in children with vomiting or diarrhea or with renal disease. Serum and urinary sodium concentrations are both decreased.

MANAGEMENT. Hypertonic sodium chloride (514 mEq/L) is infused with the goal of increasing the serum sodium concentration to 125 to 130 mEq/L (125 to 130 mmol/L) but by no more than 25 mEq/L (25 mmol/L) in the first 48 hours. More rapid corrections are associated with seizures, hypernatremic encephalopathy, and the possibility of central pontine myelinolysis.

Endocrine Disorders

Adrenal Disorders

Adrenal hypersecretion causes agitation or depression but does not produce coma. Adrenal failure may result from sepsis, abrupt withdrawal of corticosteroid therapy, or adrenal hemorrhage. Initial symptoms are nausea, vomiting, abdominal pain, and fever. Lethargy progresses to coma and is associated with hypovolemic shock. Prompt intravenous infusion of fluids, glucose, and corticosteroids is lifesaving.

Parathyroid Disorders

The neurological features of hyperparathyroidism are all related to hypercalcemia. Weakness and myopathy are relatively common. Alterations in mental status occur in 50% of patients and include apathy, delirium, paranoia, and dementia. Apathy and delirium occur at serum calcium concentrations greater than 11 mg/dl (2.75 mmol/L), and psychosis and dementia develop at concentrations of 16 mg/dl (4.0 mmol/L) or greater.

Seizures are the main feature of hypoparathyroidism and hypocalcemia. They may be generalized or focal and are often preceded by tetany. Hypocalcemic seizures do not respond to anticonvulsant drugs and must be treated with calcium replacement.

Thyroid Disorders

Hyperthyroidism causes exhilaration bordering on mania and may be associated with seizures and chorea (see Chapter 14). Thyroid storm (crisis) is a life-threatening event characterized by restlessness, cardiac arrhythmia, vomiting, and diarrhea. Delirium is an early feature and may progress to coma.

Acquired hypothyroidism affects both the central and peripheral nervous systems. Peripheral effects include neuropathy and myopathy. Central effects are cranial nerve abnormalities, ataxia, psychoses, dementia, seizures, and coma.

Delusions and hallucinations occur in more than half of patients with long-standing disease. Myxedema coma, a rare manifestation of long-standing hypothyroidism in adults, is even less common in children. It is characterized by profound hypothermia without shivering.

Hashimoto's Encephalopathy

Hashimoto's thyroiditis is an immune-mediated disease associated with high titers of antithyroid antibodies. It is associated with myasthenia gravis and other immune-mediated disorders.

CLINICAL FEATURES. The progression of symptoms is variable but usually begins with headache and confusion that progress to stupor. Focal or generalized seizures and transitory neurological deficits (stroke-like episodes) may be an initial or a late feature. Tremulousness and myoclonus commonly occur during some stage in the illness. The encephalopathy lasts for several days and then gradually disappears. Recurrent episodes are the rule and lead to permanent neurological sequelae.

DIAGNOSIS. Hashimoto's thyroiditis should be suspected in every case of recurrent encephalopathy. The cerebrospinal fluid protein concentration is elevated, sometimes above 100 mg/dl (1 g/L), but the pressure and cell count are normal. Affected individuals are usually euthyroid. The diagnosis depends on the presence of antithyroid antibodies. Antibodies against thyroglobulin and the microsomal fraction are most common, but antibodies against other thyroid elements and other organs may be present as well.

MANAGEMENT. Corticosteroids are beneficial in ending an attack and preventing further episodes. The long-term prognosis is good (Ghika-Schmid et al, 1996).

Hepatic Encephalopathy

Children with acute hepatic failure often develop severe cerebral edema. Viral hepatitis, drugs, toxins, and Reye syndrome are the main causes of acute hepatic failure. The encephalopathy that accompanies hepatic failure is caused by hepatic cellular failure and the diversion of toxins from the hepatic portal vein into the systemic circulation. Severe viral hepatitis with marked elevation of the unconjugated bilirubin concentration may even lead to kernicterus in older children.

In children with chronic cholestatic liver disease, demyelination of the posterior columns and peripheral nerves may develop as a result of vitamin E deficiency. The major features are ataxia, areflexia, and gaze paresis, without evidence of encephalopathy (see Chapter 10).

CLINICAL FEATURES. Malaise and fatigue are early symptoms that accompany the features of hepatic failure: jaundice, dark urine, and abnormal results of liver function tests. Nausea and vomiting occur when hepatic failure is fulminant. The onset of coma may be spontaneous or induced by gastrointestinal bleeding, infection, high protein intake, and excessive use of tranquilizers or diuretics. The first features are disturbed sleep and a change in affect. These are followed by drowsiness, hyperventilation, and asterixis, a flapping tremor at the wrist when the arms are extended and the wrists flexed. Hallucinations sometimes occur during early stages, but a continuous progression to coma is more common. Seizures and decerebrate rigidity develop as the patient becomes comatose.

DIAGNOSIS. In hepatic coma, the EEG pattern is not specific but is always abnormal and suggests a metabolic encephalopathy: loss of posterior rhythm, generalized slowing of background, and frontal triphasic waves.

Biochemical markers of liver failure include a sharp rise in serum transaminase, increased prothrombin time, mixed hyperbilirubinemia, hyperammonemia, and a decline in serum albumin concentration. Abnormally high signals are seen in the pallidum using T_1-weighted MRI (Lockwood et al, 1997).

MANAGEMENT. The goal of treatment is to maintain cerebral, renal, and cardiopulmonary function until liver regeneration or transplantation can occur. Cerebral function is impaired not only by abnormal concentrations of metabolites but also by cerebral edema.

Inborn Errors of Metabolism

The inborn errors of metabolism that cause states of decreased consciousness are usually associated with hyperammonemia, hypoglycemia, or organic aciduria. Neonatal seizures are an early feature in most of these conditions (see Chapter 1), but some may not cause symptoms until infancy or childhood. Inborn errors with a delayed onset of encephalopathy include disorders of pyruvate metabolism and respiratory chain disorders (see Chapters 5, 6, 8, and 10); hemizygotes for ornithine carbamylase deficiency and heterozygotes for carbamyl phosphate synthetase deficiency (see Chapter 1); glycogen storage diseases (see Chapter 1); and primary carnitine deficiency.

Medium-Chain Acyl-CoA Dehydrogenase Deficiency

Medium-chain acyl-CoA dehydrogenase (MCAD) deficiency is a disorder of β-oxidation of fatty acids. The trait is transmitted by autosomal recessive inheritance. It is the main cause of what had been described as *primary carnitine deficiency* (Table 2-6). Carnitine has two main functions: (1) the transfer of long-chain fatty acids into the inner mitochondrial membrane to undergo β-oxidation and generate energy and (2) the modulation of the acyl-CoA/CoA ratio and the esterification of potentially toxic acyl-CoA metabolites (Pons and De Vivo, 1995). The transfer of fatty acids across the mitochondrial membrane requires the conversion of acyl-CoA to acylcarnitine and the enzyme carnitine palmitoyltransferase (CPT). If the carnitine concentration is deficient, toxic levels of acyl-CoA accumulate and impair the citric acid cycle, gluconeogenesis, the urea cycle, and fatty acid oxidation.

CLINICAL FEATURES. Affected children are normal at birth. Recurrent attacks of nonketotic hypoglycemia, vomiting, confusion, lethargy, and coma are provoked by intercurrent illness or fasting during infancy and early childhood. Cardiorespiratory arrest and sudden infant death may occur, but MCAD is not considered an important cause of the sudden infant death

---

Table 2-6
Differential Diagnosis of Carnitine Deficiency

Inborn Errors of Metabolism
Aminoacidurias
    Glutaric aciduria
    Isovaleric acidemia
    Methylmalonic acidemia
    Propionic acidemia
Disorders of pyruvate metabolism
    Multiple carboxylase deficiency
    Pyruvate carboxylase deficiency
    Pyruvate dehydrogenase deficiency
Disorders of the respiratory chain
Medium-chain acyl-CoA dehydrogenase (MCAD)
    deficiency
Phosphoglucomutase deficiency

Acquired Conditions
Hemodialysis
Malnutrition
Pregnancy
Reye syndrome
Total parenteral nutrition
Valproate hepatotoxicity

syndrome (SIDS). Between attacks the child may appear normal. In some families the deficiency causes cardiomyopathy, whereas in others it causes only mild to moderate proximal weakness (see Chapters 6 and 7). Similar clinical phenotypes are caused by deficiencies of long-chain and short-chain acyl-CoA dehydrogenase.

DIAGNOSIS. All affected children have low or absent urinary ketones during episodes of hypoglycemia and elevated serum concentrations of aspartate aminotransferase and lactate dehydrogenase. Blood carnitine concentrations are less than 20 μmol/mg noncollagen protein. The diagnosis is established by showing the enzyme deficiency or the genetic mutation.

MANAGEMENT. All affected children must avoid fasting. Dietary supplementation with L-carnitine is recommended. The initial dosage is 50 mg/kg/day, which is increased as tolerated (up to 800 mg/kg/day) until the desired blood concentration is attained. Adverse effects of carnitine include nausea, vomiting, diarrhea, and abdominal cramps. Dietary supplementation with riboflavin and glycine is also recommended, but their efficacy is less well established.

During an acute attack, a diet rich in medium-chain triglycerides and low in long-chain triglycerides should be provided in addition to carnitine. General supportive care is required for hypoglycemia and hypoprothrombinemia.

Renal Disorders

Children with chronic renal failure are at risk for acute or chronic uremic encephalopathy, dialysis encephalopathy, hypertensive encephalopathy, and neurological complications of the immunocompromised state.

Acute Uremic Encephalopathy

CLINICAL FEATURES. In children with acute renal failure, symptoms of cerebral dysfunction develop over several days. Asterixis is often the initial feature. This is followed by periods of confusion and headache, sometimes progressing to delirium and then to lethargy. Weakness, tremulousness, and muscle cramps develop. Myoclonic jerks and tetany may be present. If uremia continues, decreasing consciousness and seizures follow.

The *hemolytic-uremic syndrome* is a leading cause of acute renal failure in children younger than 5 years old. It is characterized by the combination of thrombocytopenia, uremia, and Coombs-negative hemolytic anemia. Encephalopathy is the usual initial feature, but hemiparesis and aphasia caused by thrombotic stroke can occur in the absence of seizures or altered states of consciousness. Most children recover, but may have chronic hypertension. Survivors usually have normal cognitive function, but may have hyperactivity and inattentiveness (Qamar et al, 1996).

DIAGNOSIS. The mechanism of uremic encephalopathy is multifactorial and does not correlate with concentrations of blood urea nitrogen alone. Hyperammonemia and disturbed equilibrium of ions between the intracellular and extracellular spaces are probably important factors.

Late in the course, acute uremic encephalopathy may be confused with hypertensive encephalopathy. A distinguishing feature is that increased intracranial pressure is an early feature of hypertensive encephalopathy but not of acute uremic encephalopathy. Early in the course the EEG shows slowing of the background rhythms and periodic triphasic waves.

MANAGEMENT. Hemodialysis reverses the encephalopathy and should be performed as quickly as possible after diagnosis.

Chronic Uremic Encephalopathy

CLINICAL FEATURES. Chronic uremic encephalopathy is usually caused by congenital renal hypoplasia. Renal failure begins during the first year, and encephalopathy occurs between 1 and 9 years of age. Growth failure precedes the onset of encephalopathy. Three stages are described.

Stage 1 consists of delayed motor development, dysmetria and tremor, or ataxia. Examination during this stage shows hyperreflexia, mild hypotonia, and extensor plantar responses. Within 6 to 12 months the disease progresses to stage 2.

Stage 2 is characterized by myoclonus of the face and limbs, partial motor seizures, dementia, and then generalized seizures. Facial myoclonus and lingual apraxia make speech and feeding difficult, and limb myoclonus interferes with ambulation. The duration of stage 2 is variable and may be months to years.

Stage 3 consists of progressive bulbar failure, a vegetative state, and death.

DIAGNOSIS. The diagnosis is based on clinical findings. Serial EEG shows progressive slowing and then superimposed epileptiform activity, and serial CT shows progressive cerebral atrophy. Hyperparathyroidism with hypercalcemia occurs in some children with chronic uremic encephalopathy, but parathyroidectomy does not reverse the process.

MANAGEMENT. Hemodialysis and renal transplantation have not altered the course in most patients.

Dialysis Encephalopathy

Long-term dialysis may be associated with acute, transitory neurological disturbances attributed to the rapid shift of fluids and electrolytes between intracellular and extracellular spaces. Most common are vascular headaches and seizures. Seizures usually occur toward the end of dialysis or up to 24 hours later and may be preceded by lethargy and delirium.

Progressive encephalopathies associated with dialysis are often fatal. Two important causes exist: (1) opportunistic infections in the immunodeficient host, usually caused by cytomegalovirus and mycoses in children, and (2) the dialysis dementia syndrome.

Dialysis Dementia Syndrome

CLINICAL FEATURES. The mean interval between commencement of dialysis and onset of symptoms is 4 years (range 1 to 7 years), and subsequent progression of symptoms varies from weeks to years. A characteristic speech disturbance develops either as an initial feature or later in the course. It begins as intermittent hesitancy of speech (stuttering and slurring) and may progress to aphasia. Agraphia and apraxia may be present as well. Subtle personality changes suggestive of depression occur early in the course. A phase of hallucinations and agitation may occur, and progressive dementia develops.

Myoclonic jerking of the limbs is often present before the onset of dementia. First noted during dialysis, it soon becomes continuous and interferes with normal activity. Generalized tonic-clonic seizures often develop and become more frequent and severe as the encephalopathy progresses. Complex partial seizures may be observed, but focal motor seizures are unusual.

Neurological examination reveals the triad of speech arrest, myoclonus, and dementia. In addition, symmetric proximal weakness (myopathy) or distal weakness and sensory loss (neuropathy) with loss of tendon reflexes may occur.

DIAGNOSIS. EEG changes correlate with disease progress. A characteristic early feature is the appearance of paroxysmal high-amplitude delta activity in the frontal areas, despite a normal posterior rhythm. Eventually the background becomes generally slow, and frontal triphasic waves are noted. Epileptiform activity develops in all patients with dialysis dementia and is the EEG feature that differentiates dialysis dementia from uremic encephalopathy. The activity consists of sharp, spike, or polyspike discharges that may have a periodic quality.

MANAGEMENT. Aluminum toxicity derived from the dialysate fluid is the probable cause of most cases. Removal of aluminum from dialysate prevents the appearance of new cases and progression in some established cases.

Hypertensive Encephalopathy

Hypertensive encephalopathy occurs when increases in systemic blood pressure exceed the limits of cerebral autoregulation. The result is damage to small arterioles, which leads to patchy areas of ischemia and edema. Therefore, focal neurological deficits are relatively common.

CLINICAL FEATURES. The initial features are transitory attacks of cerebral ischemia and headache. Such symptoms may be dismissed as part of uremic encephalopathy, despite the warning signs of focal neurological deficits. Headache persists and is accompanied by visual disturbances and vomiting. Seizures and diminished consciousness follow. The seizures are frequently focal at onset and then generalized. Examination reveals papilledema and retinal hemorrhages.

DIAGNOSIS. Because the syndrome occurs in children receiving long-term renal dialysis while awaiting transplantation, the differential diagnosis includes disorders of osmolality, uremic encephalopathy, and dialysis encephalopathy. A posterior cerebral edema syndrome associated with hypertensive encephalopathy is evident on MRI (Figure 2-3). Hypertensive encephalopathy can be distinguished from other encephalopathies associated with renal disease by the greater elevation of blood pressure and the presence of focal neurological disturbances.

MANAGEMENT. Hypertensive encephalopathy is a medical emergency. Treatment consists of anticonvulsant therapy and aggressive efforts to reduce hypertension. Measures to reduce cerebral edema are required in some patients.

Other Metabolic Encephalopathies

Several less common causes of metabolic encephalopathy are listed in Table 2-3. Some are

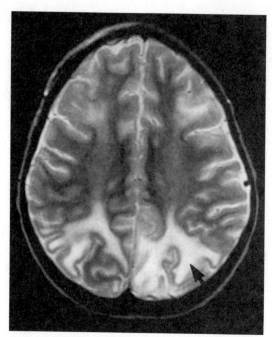

Figure 2-3. MRI in hypertensive encephalopathy. Arrow points to increased signal intensity in both occipital lobes.

attributable to derangements of a single substance, but most are multifactorial.

In 5% of children with burns covering 30% of the body surface, an encephalopathy that may be intermittent develops (burn encephalopathy). The onset may be days to weeks after the burn. Altered mental states (delirium or coma) and seizures (generalized or focal) are the major features. The encephalopathy usually cannot be attributed to a single factor.

Encephalopathies that occur during total parenteral hyperalimentation are generally due to hyperammonemia caused by excessive loads of amino acids.

Hypomagnesemia in infancy may be caused by prematurity, maternal deficiency, maternal or infant hypoparathyroidism, a high-phosphorus diet, exchange transfusion, intestinal disorders, and specific defects in magnesium absorption. These conditions are often associated with hypocalcemia. Excessive use of diuretics causes hypomagnesemia in older children. Symptoms develop when plasma magnesium concentrations are less than 1.2 mg/dl (0.5 mmol/L), and include jitteriness, hyperirritability, and seizures. Further decline in serum magnesium concentrations leads to obtundation and coma.

Deficiency of one or more B vitamins may be associated with lethargy or delirium, but only thiamine deficiency causes coma. Thiamine deficiency is relatively common in alcoholic adults and produces Wernicke encephalopathy but is uncommon in children. Subacute necrotizing encephalopathy (Leigh's disease) is a thiamine deficiency-like state in children (see Chapters 5 and 10).

Migraine

Migraine causes several neurological syndromes and is discussed in many chapters. Among its less common syndromes are a confusional state, an amnestic state, and coma.

Acute Confusional Migraine

CLINICAL FEATURES. A confused and agitated state resembling toxic-metabolic psychosis occurs as a migraine variant in children between the ages of 5 and 16 (Sheth et al, 1995). Most affected children are 10 years of age or older. The symptoms develop rapidly. The child becomes delirious and appears to be in pain but does not complain of headache. Impaired awareness of the environment, retarded responses to painful stimuli, hyperactivity, restlessness, and combative behavior are evident. The duration of an attack is usually 3 to 5 hours but may be as long as 20 hours. The child eventually falls into a deep sleep, appears normal on awakening, and has no memory of the episode. Confusional attacks tend to recur over days or months and then evolve into typical migraine episodes.

DIAGNOSIS. Migraine is always a clinical diagnosis and should be arrived at only after other possibilities are excluded. The diagnosis relies heavily on a family history of migraine, but not necessarily of confusional migraine. During or shortly after a confusional attack the EEG shows unilateral temporal or occipital slowing.

MANAGEMENT. The acute attack can be treated with intramuscular chlorpromazine, 1 mg/kg. Propranolol provides prophylaxis (see Chapter 3).

Migraine Coma

Migraine coma is a rare, extreme form of migraine.

CLINICAL FEATURES. The major features of migraine coma are (1) recurrent episodes of coma precipitated by trivial head injury and (2) apparent meningitis associated with life-threatening cerebral edema. Migraine coma occurs in kindred with familial hemiplegic migraine (see Chapter 11), but a similar syndrome may occur in sporadic cases as well. Coma develops following trivial head injury and is associated with fever. Intracranial pressure is increased because of cerebral edema. States of decreased consciousness may last for several days. Recovery is then complete.

DIAGNOSIS. Coma following even trivial head injury causes concern for intracranial hemorrhage. The initial CT scan may be normal, especially if obtained early in the course. Scans obtained between 24 and 72 hours show generalized or focal edema.

Examination of the cerebrospinal fluid reveals increased pressure and pleocytosis (up to 100 cells/mm^3). The combination of fever, coma, and cerebrospinal fluid pleocytosis suggests viral encephalitis, and herpes is a possibility if edema is localized to one temporal lobe.

MANAGEMENT. Children who have experienced migraine coma should be treated afterward with a prophylactic agent to prevent further attacks (see Chapter 3). The major treatment goal during the acute attack is to decrease intracranial pressure by reducing cerebral edema (see Chapter 4).

Transient Global Amnesia

Transient global amnesia usually occurs in adults and is characterized by sudden inability to form new memories and repetitive questioning about events, without other neurological symptoms or signs. Migraine is the probable cause when such attacks occur in children or in more than one family member (Sheth et al, 1995).

CLINICAL FEATURES. Attacks last for periods ranging from 20 minutes to several hours, and retrograde amnesia is present on recovery. Many adults with transient global amnesia have a history of migraine, and a similar syndrome may be seen in children with migraine following trivial head injury. The attacks are similar to acute confusional migraine except that the patient has less delirium and greater isolated memory deficiency.

DIAGNOSIS. A personal or family history of migraine is essential for diagnosis. The CT scan shows no abnormalities, but the EEG may show slowing of the background rhythm in one temporal lobe.

MANAGEMENT. Management is the same as for migraine with aura (see Chapter 3).

Psychological Disorders

Panic disorders and schizophrenia may have an acute onset of symptoms suggesting delirium or confusion and must be distinguished from acute organic encephalopathies.

Panic Disorder

CLINICAL FEATURES. Panic attacks were thought to be confined to adults but now are recognized to occur in adolescents and school-age children. A panic attack is an agitated state caused by anxiety. Principal features are paroxysmal dizziness, headache, and dyspnea. Hyperventilation often occurs and results in further dizziness, paresthesias, and lightheadedness. Attacks may be provoked by phobias, such as fear of going to school. They can last for minutes to hours and recur daily.

DIAGNOSIS. Panic attacks simulate cardiac or neurological disease, and many children undergo extensive and unnecessary medical evaluation before the correct diagnosis is reached. Panic disorder should be suspected in children with recurrent attacks of hyperventilation, dizziness, or dyspnea.

MANAGEMENT. Antidepressant drugs have varying degrees of efficacy. Imipramine has the best success rate. Initial dosages are less than those used for depression (0.25 mg/kg/day), but higher dosages may be needed if concurrent depression must be treated.

Schizophrenia

CLINICAL FEATURES. Schizophrenia is a disorder of adolescence or early adult life and should not be suspected in prepubertal children. Schizophrenic individuals do not have an antecedent history of an affective disorder. An initial feature is often declining work performance simulating dementia. Intermittent depersonalization (not knowing where or who one is) may occur early in the course and suggests complex partial seizures.

Thoughts move with loose association from one idea to another until they become incoherent. Delusions and hallucinations are common and usually have paranoid features. Motor activity can be either lacking, with the patient remaining stationary, or excessive and purposeless. This combination of symptoms in an adolescent may be difficult to distinguish clinically from drug encephalopathy.

DIAGNOSIS. The diagnosis is established by careful evaluation of mental status. The family may have a history of schizophrenia. Neurological and laboratory findings are normal. A normal EEG in an alert child with the clinical symptoms of an acute encephalopathy points to a psychological disturbance, including schizophrenia.

MANAGEMENT. Schizophrenia is generally considered a chemical disorder of the brain. It is incurable, but antipsychotic drugs alleviate many of the symptoms.

Toxic Encephalopathies

Accidental poisoning with drugs and chemicals left carelessly within reach is relatively common in children from ages 1 to 4. Between ages 4 and 10 there is a trough in the frequency of poisoning, which is followed by increasing frequency of intentional poisoning with substances of abuse and prescription drugs.

Immunosuppressive Drugs

Immunosuppressive drugs are used widely in children undergoing organ transplantation. The drugs themselves, secondary metabolic disturbances, and cerebral infection may cause encephalopathy at times of immunosuppression. Children being treated with amphotericin B to treat aspergillosis after bone marrow transplantation for leukemia have developed a severe encephalopathy with parkinsonian features (Mott et al, 1995).

Corticosteroid Psychosis

Daily use of corticosteroids at doses lower than 1 mg/kg may cause hyperactivity, insomnia, and anxiety. The higher dosages used for immunosuppression, generally >2 mg/kg/day, may precipitate a psychosis similar to schizophrenia or delirium. Stopping the drug reverses the symptoms.

Cyclosporine Encephalopathy

Cyclosporine, the drug most commonly used to prevent organ rejection, causes encephalopathy in 5% of recipients. The blood concentration of the drug does not correlate simply with any neurological complication. The more common syndrome consists of lethargy, confusion, cortical blindness, and visual hallucinations without any motor disturbances. A similar syndrome also occurs in children with hypertension from other causes who are not taking cyclosporine (Pavlakis et al, 1997). A second syndrome is a combination of motor symptoms (ataxia, tremor, paralysis) and altered states of consciousness and cognition.

MRI shows widespread edema and leukoencephalopathy. In children with the syndrome of visual disturbances and encephalopathy, the most intense disturbances are in the occipital lobes (see Figure 2-3). The encephalopathy clears completely when the drug is stopped. Sometimes the drug can be restarted at a lower dose without causing encephalopathy.

OKT3 Meningoencephalitis

OKT3 is an anti–T-cell monoclonal antibody used to initiate immunosuppression and to treat rejection. Up to 14% of patients develop fever and sterile meningitis 24 to 72 hours after the first injection, and up to 10% develop encephalopathy within 4 days. The encephalopathy slowly resolves over the next 2 weeks whether or not the drug is stopped.

Prescription Drugs Overdoses

Most intentional overdoses are with prescription drugs, because they are readily available. The drugs that are most likely found in homes are benzodiazepines, salicylates, acetaminophen, barbiturates, and tricyclic antidepressants. Delirium or coma may be due to toxic effects of psychoactive drugs (anticonvulsants, antidepressants, antipsychotics, and tranquilizers). The encephalopathies that occur when drugs cause disorders of osmolality or organ failure are described in the section on metabolic encephalopathies.

CLINICAL FEATURES. As a rule, toxic doses of psychoactive drugs produce lethargy, nystagmus, or ophthalmoplegia and loss of coordination. Higher concentrations cause coma and seizures. Involuntary movements may occur as an idiosyncratic or dose-related effect. Diazepam is remarkably safe, and an overdose does not cause coma or death when taken alone. Other benzodiazepines are also reasonably safe.

Tricyclic antidepressants are among the most widely prescribed drugs in the United States and account for 25% of serious overdoses. The major features of overdosage are coma, hypotension, and anticholinergic effects (flushing, dry skin, dilated pupils, tachycardia, decreased gastrointestinal motility, and urinary retention).

Seizures and myocardial depression may be present as well.

The onset of symptoms following phenothiazine or haloperidol ingestion may be delayed for 6 to 24 hours, and symptoms may be intermittent. Extrapyramidal disturbances (see Chapter 14) and symptoms of anticholinergic poisoning are prominent features. Fatalities are uncommon and probably caused by cardiac arrhythmia.

DIAGNOSIS. Most drugs can be identified in the laboratory within 2 hours. A drug screen of the urine should be performed in all cases of unidentified coma or delirium. If an unidentifiable product is found in the urine, further identification may be possible in the plasma. The blood concentration should be determined when the identity of a drug is known.

MANAGEMENT. The specificities and degree of supportive care needed depend on the drug and the severity of the poisoning. Most children need an intravenous line and careful monitoring of cardiorespiratory status. A continuous electrocardiogram (ECG) is often required because of concern for arrhythmia. Unabsorbed drug must be removed from the stomach by lavage and repeated doses of activated charcoal (30 mg every 6 hours) administered to prevent absorption and increase drug clearance. Extrapyramidal symptoms are treated with intravenous diphenhydramine, 2 mg/kg.

Poisoning

Most accidental poisonings occur in small children who ingest common household products. The ingestion is usually discovered quickly because the child becomes sick and vomits. Insecticides, herbicides, and products containing hydrocarbons or alcohol are frequently implicated. Clinical features vary depending on the agent ingested. Optimal management requires identification of constituent poisons, estimation of the amount ingested, interval since exposure, cleansing of the gastrointestinal tract, specific antidotes when available, and supportive measures.

Substance Abuse

Alcohol remains the most common substance of abuse in the United States. More than 90% of high school seniors have used alcohol one or more times, and 6% are daily drinkers. Approximately 6% of high school seniors use marijuana daily, but less than 0.1% are regular users of hallucinogens or opiates. The use of cocaine, stimulants, and sedatives has been increasing in recent years. Daily use of stimulants is reported by up to 1% of high school seniors.

CLINICAL FEATURES. The American Psychiatric Association defines the diagnostic criteria for substance abuse as (1) a pattern of pathological use with inability to stop or reduce use, (2) impairment of social or occupational functioning, which includes school performance in children, and (3) persistence of the problem for 1 month or longer.

The clinical features of acute intoxication vary with the substance used. Almost all disturb judgment, intellectual function, and coordination. Alcohol and sedatives lead to drowsiness, sleep, and obtundation. In contrast, hallucinogens cause bizarre behavior, which includes hallucinations, delusions, and muscle rigidity. Such drugs as phencyclidine (angel dust) and lysergic acid diethylamide (LSD) produce a clinical picture that simulates schizophrenia.

The usual symptoms of marijuana intoxication are euphoria and a sense of relaxation at low doses and a dream-like state with slow response time at higher doses. Very high blood concentrations produce depersonalization, disorientation, and sensory disturbances. Hallucinations and delusions are unusual with marijuana and suggest mixed-drug use.

Amphetamine abuse should be considered when an agitated state is coupled with peripheral evidence of adrenergic toxicity: mydriasis, flushing, diaphoresis, and reflex bradycardia caused by peripheral vasoconstriction.

Cocaine affects the brain and heart. Early symptoms include euphoria, mydriasis, headache, and tachycardia. Higher doses produce emotional lability, nausea and vomiting, flushing, and a syndrome that simulates paranoid schizophrenia. Life-threatening complications are hyperthermia, seizures, cardiac arrhythmia, and stroke. Associated stroke syndromes include transient ischemic attacks in the distribution of the middle cerebral artery, lateral medullary infarction, and anterior spinal artery infarction.

DIAGNOSIS. The major challenge is to differentiate acute substance intoxication from schizophrenia. Important clues are a history of substance abuse obtained from family or friends, associated autonomic and cardiac disturbances, and alterations in vital signs. Urinary and plasma screening generally detects the substance or its metabolites.

MANAGEMENT. Management of acute substance abuse depends on the substance used and the amount ingested. Physicians must be alert to the possibility of multiple drug or substance exposure. An attempt should be made to empty the gastrointestinal tract of substances taken orally. Support of cardiorespiratory function and correction of metabolic disturbances are generally required. Intravenous diazepam reduces the hallucinations and seizures produced by stimulants and hallucinogens. Standard cardiac drugs are used to combat arrhythmias.

The most vexing problem with substance abuse is generally not the acute management of intoxication, but rather breaking the habit. This requires the patient's motivation and long-term inpatient and outpatient treatment.

Trauma

Trivial head injuries, without loss of consciousness, are commonplace in children and are an almost constant occurrence in toddlers. Migraine should be suspected whenever transitory neurological disturbances (e.g., amnesia, ataxia, blindness, coma, confusion, hemiplegia) follow trivial head injuries. Important causes of significant head injuries are child abuse in infants, sports and play injuries in children, and motor vehicle accidents in adolescents.

Neonatal head injuries generally cause seizures (see Chapter 1). Loss of consciousness is the major feature of head injuries beyond the neonatal period. Mild head injuries are characterized by temporary loss of consciousness without evidence of focal neurological disturbances. Such events are usually termed *concussion*. Severe head injuries are characterized by prolonged intervals of coma associated with brain swelling and intracranial hemorrhage.

Mild and Moderate Head Injuries

CLINICAL FEATURES. A mild closed head injury is characterized by no more than brief loss of consciousness and the absence of localizing neurological signs (concussion). The child may be stunned without definite loss of consciousness. A moderate head injury is one in which the child is obtunded for several hours but is not in coma. Once consciousness is restored, the child is invariably tired and sleeps long and soundly if left undisturbed. As a rule recovery is complete, but the child may not remember the event or the period before and after it. The length of the amnestic interval correlates with the severity of injury.

Many children complain of headache and dizziness for several days or weeks following concussion (see Posttraumatic Headache in Chapter 3). They may be irritable and have memory disturbances. The severity and duration of these symptoms usually correlate with the severity of injury but sometimes seem disproportionate.

Focal or generalized seizures, and sometimes status epilepticus, may occur 1 or 2 hours following mild head injury. Seizures may even occur in children who did not lose consciousness. Such seizures rarely portend later epilepsy.

DIAGNOSIS. A cranial CT (without contrast and with windows adjusted for bone and soft tissue) should be obtained whenever loss of consciousness, no matter how brief, follows a head injury. This is probably cost-effective because it reduces the number of hospital admissions. MRI in children with moderate head injury may show foci of hypointensity in the white matter that indicate axonal injury as the mechanism of lost consciousness (Adelson and Kochanek, 1998). EEG should be performed if there is any suspicion that the head injury occurred during a seizure or if neurological disturbances are disproportionate to the severity of injury.

MANAGEMENT. Mild head injuries do not require treatment, and a child whose neurological examination and CT scan findings are normal does not require hospitalization. If the child does not need hospitalization, asking the parents to awaken the child at regular intervals and assess neurological status is unreasonable. Normal children are difficult to arouse from sleep, and a child who has had a head injury and spent several hours in an emergency department will sleep all the sounder. A child who does not need hospital observation does not need home observation.

Severe Head Injuries

The outcome following severe head injuries is usually better for children than for adults, but children less than 1 year of age have double the mortality of those between 1 and 6, and three times the mortality of those between 6 and 12. CT evidence of diffuse brain swelling on the day of injury is associated with a 53% mortality rate.

Shaking Injuries

CLINICAL FEATURES. Shaking is a common method of child abuse in infants (Duhaime et al, 1998). An unconscious infant is brought to the emergency department with bulging fontanelles. Seizures may have precipitated the hospital visit. The history is fragmentary and inconsistent among informants. Typically the child has been left in the care of a babysitter or the mother's boyfriend.

The child shows no external evidence of head injury, but ophthalmoscopic examination shows retinal and optic nerve sheath hemorrhages. Retinal hemorrhages are more common after inflicted than after accidental injuries and may be due to rotational forces. Many of the hemorrhages may be old, suggesting repeated shaking injuries. On the thorax or back the examiner may note bruises that conform to the shape of a hand where the child was held during the shaking. Healing fractures of the posterior rib cage indicate child abuse. Death may result from uncontrollable increased intracranial pressure or contusion of the cervicomedullary junction.

DIAGNOSIS. The CT shows a swollen brain but may not show subdural collections of blood if bleeding is recent. A subdural tap is both diagnostic and therapeutic.

MANAGEMENT. Bilateral subdural taps are needed to remove large collections of blood. The intention is to remove as much blood as possible. The amount available for drainage through a subdural tap is only a small percentage of the total volume in the subdural space. The goal of the subdural tap is not to remove all subdural blood, but rather to remove a sufficient quantity to relieve increased intracranial pressure and to aid reabsorptive mechanisms. Taps are repeated daily until the removable volume begins to decline; then an every-other-day schedule of subdural taps allows continued reduction of the accumulated fluid. A subdural-peritoneal shunt may be required if permanent effusion develops. Transfusion may be needed if the peripheral hematocrit value is low and falling.

Protective service must be sought to prevent further injuries. Overall, the neurological and visual outcomes among victims of shaking are poor. Most are left with a considerable handicap.

Closed Head Injuries

Supratentorial subdural hematomas are venous in origin, are frequently bilateral, and usually occur without associated skull fracture. Supratentorial epidural hematomas are usually associated with skull fracture and are described in the section on open head injuries. Epidural and subdural hematomas are almost impossible to distinguish on clinical grounds alone. Progressive loss of consciousness is a feature of both types, and both may be associated with a lucid interval between the time of injury and neurological deterioration. Posterior fossa epidural and subdural hemorrhages occur most often in newborns (see Chapter 1) and older children with posterior skull fractures.

CLINICAL FEATURES. Loss of consciousness is not always immediate; a lucid period of several minutes may intervene between injury and onset of neurological deterioration. The Glasgow Coma Scale is used widely to quantify the degree of responsiveness following head injuries (Table 2-7). Scores of 8 or less correlate well with severe injury.

The clinical features are caused by acute brain swelling and intracranial hemorrhage. Increased intracranial pressure is always present and may lead to herniation if uncontrolled. Focal neurological deficits suggest intracerebral hemorrhage.

Mortality rates in children with severe head injury are usually between 10% and 15% and have not changed substantially in the past decade. Low mortality rates are sometimes associated with higher percentages of survivors in chronic vegetative states. Duration of coma is the best guide to long-term morbidity. Perma-

---

Table 2-7
Glasgow Coma Scale*

Eye Opening (E)

Spontaneously	4
To speech	3
To pain	2
None	1

Best Motor Response (M)

Obeys	6
Localizes	5
Withdraws	4
Abnormal flexion	3
Abnormal extension	2
None	1

Verbal Response (V)

Oriented	5
Confused conversation	4
Inappropriate words	3
Incomprehensible sounds	2
None	1

* Coma score = E + M + V.

nent neurological impairment is expected when coma persists for 1 month or longer.

DIAGNOSIS. Cranial CT should be performed as rapidly as possible after closed head injuries. Typical findings are brain swelling and subarachnoid hemorrhage with blood collecting along the falx. Intracranial hemorrhage may also be detected. Immediately after injury some subdural hematomas are briefly isodense and may not be observed. Later the hematoma appears as a region of increased density, convex toward the skull and concave toward the brain. With time the density decreases.

Intracerebral hemorrhage is usually superficial but may extend deep into the brain. Frontal or temporal lobe contusion is common. Discrete deep hemorrhages without a superficial extension are not usually caused by trauma.

Children with head injuries must be kept with the neck immobilized until radiographic examination for fracture-dislocation of the cervical spine is done, because the force of a blow to the skull is frequently propagated to the neck. The child must be examined for limb and organ injury when head injury occurs in a motor vehicle accident.

MANAGEMENT. Severe head injuries should be managed in an intensive care unit. Essential support includes controlled ventilation, prevention of hypotension, and sufficient reduction in brain swelling to maintain cerebral perfusion. Methods to reduce cerebral edema are reviewed in Chapter 4. Barbiturate coma does not affect the outcome.

Acute expanding intracranial hematomas warrant immediate surgery. Small subdural collections that do not produce a mass effect can be left in place until the patient's condition is stabilized and the options are considered.

Open Head Injuries

The clinical features, diagnosis, and management of open head injuries are much the same as described for closed injuries. The major differences are the greater risk of epidural hematoma and infection and the possibility of damage to the brain surface from depression of the bone.

Supratentorial epidural hematomas are usually temporal or temporoparietal in location. The origin of the blood may be arterial (tearing of the middle meningeal artery), venous, or both. Skull fracture is present in 80% of cases. Increased intracranial pressure accounts for the clinical features of vomiting and decreased states of consciousness. Epidural hematoma has a characteristic lens-shaped appearance (Figure 2-4).

Infratentorial epidural hematoma is venous in origin and associated with occipital fracture. The clinical features are headache, vomiting, and ataxia. Skull fractures, other than linear fractures, are associated with an increased risk of infection. A fracture is referred to as depressed if the inner table fragment is displaced by at least the thickness of the skull. Depressed fractures are termed *compound* if the scalp is lacerated and *penetrating* if the dura is torn. Most skull fractures heal spontaneously. Skull fractures that do not heal are usually associated with a dural tear and feel pulsatile (Johnson and Helman, 1995). In infants, serial radiographs of the skull may suggest that the fracture is enlarging because the rapid growth of the brain causes the fracture line to spread further in order to accommodate the increasing intracranial volume. The fracture line is not being held open by a leptomeningeal cyst, and surgery is not needed.

Depressed fractures of the skull vault may injure the underlying brain and tear venous sinuses. The result is hemorrhage into the brain and subdural space. Management includes elevation of depressed fragments, debridement and closure of the scalp laceration, and systemic penicillin.

Basilar skull fractures with dural tear may result in leakage of cerebrospinal fluid from the

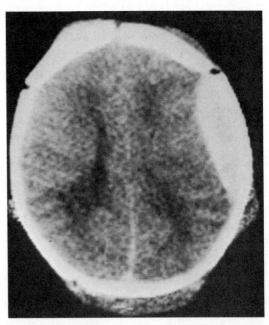

Figure 2-4. Epidural hematoma. The hematoma appears as a lens-shaped density just below the skull.

nose or ear and meningitis. Such leaks usually develop within 3 days of injury. The timing and need for dural repair are somewhat controversial, but the need for intravenous antibiotic coverage is established.

Posttraumatic Epilepsy

Posttraumatic epilepsy develops in about 50% of patients with penetrating head injuries. Half continue to have seizures as long as 15 years after injury. Two thirds have seizure onset during the first year after the injury, and 90% by 5 years, but onset is delayed by 10 to 15 years in 7%. The cause-and-effect relationship between trauma and epilepsy becomes harder to establish when the interval between the two is longer than 1 year. Patients with focal neurological deficits and large cerebral lesions immediately after injury have the greatest risk for posttraumatic epilepsy. Initial seizures are generalized in 70% to 80% of cases.

Posttraumatic epilepsy is much less common with closed head injuries. The 5-year incidence is 11.5% after severe head trauma (brain contusion, intracranial hemorrhage, or 24 hours of unconsciousness or amnesia) and 1.6% after less severe head trauma (skull fracture or 30 minutes to 24 hours of unconsciousness or amnesia). Mild head injuries (less than 30 minutes of unconsciousness or amnesia) are not associated with an increased incidence of posttraumatic epilepsy.

Vascular Disorders

Systemic Lupus Erythematosus

Although, systemic lupus erythematosus (SLE) is classified here as a vascular disorder, the pathophysiology of its neurological manifestations may be secondary to immune complex deposition in the brain rather than by vasculitis. The clinical features are consistent with a diffuse encephalopathy rather than stroke.

CLINICAL FEATURES. CNS manifestations are the initial feature of SLE in 20% of cases (Steinlin et al, 1995). Most common are neuropsychiatric disturbances (50%), seizures (20%), and headache (20%). Some degree of cognitive dysfunction can be measured in most patients, but dementia is uncommon. Depression and anxiety are relatively common. It is uncertain whether depression is caused by the disease or is a reaction to chronic illness. Corticosteroids, which

are a mainstay of treatment, may also contribute to the anxiety. Frank psychosis, as defined by impaired reality testing and hallucinations, occurs in less than 15% of patients.

DIAGNOSIS. The diagnosis of SLE is usually established by other criteria before the development of encephalopathy. Patients with encephalopathy usually have high serum titers of anti-DNA and lymphocytotoxic antibodies and high cerebrospinal fluid titers of antineural antibodies. This further supports the concept that the encephalopathy is immune mediated.

MANAGEMENT. Some features of the encephalopathy can be treated symptomatically, but immunosuppressive therapy directed at the underlying disorder is the main therapeutic modality.

References

Adelson PD, Kochanek PM. Head injury in children. *J Child Neurol* 1998;13:2–15.

American Academy of Neurology. Practice parameters for determining brain death in adults (summary statement). *Neurology* 1995;45:1012–1014.

Belay ED, Bresee JS, Holman RC, et al. Reye's syndrome in the United States from 1981 through 1987. *N Engl J Med* 1999;340:1377–1382.

Deresiewicz RL, Thaler SJ, Hsu L, et al. Clinical and neuroradiologic manifestations of eastern equine encephalitis. *N Engl J Med* 1997;336:1867–1874.

Duhaime A-C, Christian CW, Rorke LB, et al. Nonaccidental head injury in infants—the "shaken baby syndrome." *N Engl J Med* 1998;338:1822–1829.

Fenichel GM. Assessment: Neurologic risk of immunization. Report of the Therapeutics and Technology Assessment Subcommittee of the American Academy of Neurology. *Neurology* 1999;52:1546–1552.

Garcia-Monco JC, Benach JL. Lyme neuroborreliosis. *Ann Neurol* 1995;37:691–702.

Ghika-Schmid F, Ghika J, Regli F, et al. Hashimoto's myoclonic encephalopathy: An underdiagnosed treatable condition? *Mov Disord* 1996;11:555–562.

Hale PM, Rezvani I, Braunstein AW, et al. Factors predicting cerebral edema in young children with diabetic ketoacidosis. and new onset type I diabetes. *Acta Paediatr* 1997;86:626–631.

Halperin JJ, Logigian EL, Finkel MF, et al. Practice parameters for the diagnosis of patients with nervous system Lyme borreliosis (Lyme disease). *Neurology* 1996; 46:619–627.

Johnson DL, Helman T. Enlarging skull fractures in children. *Child Nerv Syst* 1995;11:265–268.

Leigh RJ, Zee DS. *The Neurology of Eye Movements,* 3rd ed. New York: Oxford University Press; 1999.

Lockwood AH, Weissenborn K, Butterworth RF. An image of the brain in patients with liver disease. *Curr Opin Neurol* 1997;10:525–533.

Marra CM. Neurological complications of *Bartonella henselae* infection. *Curr Opin Neurol* 1995;8:164–169.

Mitchell PS, Espy MJ, Smith TF, et al. Laboratory diagnosis of central nervous system infections with herpes simplex virus by PCR performed with cerebrospinal fluid specimens. *J Clin Microbiol* 1997;35:2873–2877.

Mott SH, Packer RJ, Vezina LG, et al. Encephalopathy with Parkinsonian features in children following bone marrow transplantations and high-dose amphotericin B. *Ann Neurol* 1995;37:810–814.

Pavlakis SG, Frank Y, Kalina P, et al. Occipital-parietal encephalopathy: A new name for an old syndrome. *Pediatr Neurol* 1997;16:145–148.

Pons R, De Vivo DC. Primary and secondary carnitine deficiency syndromes. *J Child Neurol* 1995;10(suppl 2): S8–S24.

Qamar IU, Ohali M, MacGregor DL, et al. Long-term neurologic sequelae of hemolytic uremic syndrome: A preliminary report. *Pediatr Nephrol* 1996;10:504–506.

Rust RS, Thompson WH, Matthews CG, et al. La Crosse and other forms of California encephalitis. *J Child Neurol* 1999;14:1–14.

Sheth RD, Riggs JE, Bodensteiner JB. Acute confusional migraine: A variant of transient global amnesia. *Pediatr Neurol* 1995;12:129–131.

Sigal LH, Zahradnik JM, Lavin P, et al. A vaccine consisting of recombinant *Borrelia burgdorferi* outer surface protein A to prevent Lyme disease. *N Engl J Med* 1998; 339:216–222.

Steere AC, Sikand VK, Meurice F, et al. Vaccination against Lyme disease with recombinant *Borrelia burgdorferi* outer-surface lipoprotein with adjuvant. *N Engl J Med* 1998;339:209–215.

Steinlin MI, Blaser SI, Gilday DL, et al. Neurological manifestations of pediatric systemic lupus erythematosus. *Pediatr Neurol* 1995;13:191–197.

Whitley R, Kimberlin DW. Herpes simplex viruses. *Clin Infect Dis* 1998;26:541–555.

Chapter 3
Headache

Approach to Headache

Ten percent of children aged 5 to 15 years old have migraine, and 1% have headaches. Children with migraine average twice as many days lost from school as those without migraine. Among American adolescents, 12% miss a day of school each month because of headache, and 13% of males and 20% of females have consulted a physician because of headache.

Parents seek medical attention for a child with headache not only hoping to relieve the pain but also seeking assurance that the child does not have a serious intracranial disease such as a brain tumor. Identifying the cause of headache may not be necessary if the family can be assured that headache is not a sign of serious illness. Not every headache can be explained, and the term *psychogenic* should not be used as a synonym for *idiopathic*. It is usually possible, often with the history and physical examination alone but sometimes with the aid of diagnostic studies, to distinguish headaches that are only painful from those that are harmful. This distinction is usually made by identifying the structure or structures that are generating pain and is almost always ensured by imaging the brain.

Sources of Pain

Pain-sensitive structures of the head and neck are summarized in Table 3-1. The major pain-sensitive structures inside the skull are blood vessels. Mechanisms that stimulate pain from blood vessels are vasodilatation, inflammation, and traction-displacement. Increased intracranial pressure causes pain mainly by the traction and displacement of intracranial arteries (see Chapter 4). The brain parenchyma, its ependy-mal lining, and the meninges are insensitive to pain.

The innervation of pain from supratentorial intracranial vessels is transmitted by the trigeminal nerve, whereas the first three cervical nerves transmit pain from infratentorial intracranial vessels. Arteries in the superficial portion of the dura are innervated by the ophthalmic division of the trigeminal nerve and refer pain to the eye and forehead. The middle meningeal artery is innervated by the second and third divisions of the trigeminal nerve and refers pain to the temple. Cerebral arteries are innervated by all three divisions of the trigeminal nerve and refer pain to the eye, forehead, and temple. In contrast, pain from all structures in the posterior fossa is referred to the occiput and neck.

Several extracranial structures are pain sensitive. Major scalp arteries are present around the eye, forehead, and temple and produce pain when dilated or stretched. Cranial bones are insensitive, but periosteum, especially in the sinuses and near the teeth, is painful when inflamed. The inflamed periosteum is usually tender to palpation or other forms of physical

Table 3-1
Sources of Headache Pain

Intracranial
Cerebral and dural arteries
Large veins and venous sinuses

Extracranial
Cervical roots
Cranial nerves
Extracranial arteries
Muscles attached to skull
Periosteum/sinuses

stimulation. Muscles attached to the skull are a possible source of pain. The largest groups of such muscles are the neck extensors, which attach to the occipital ridge, the masseter muscles, and the frontalis muscle. The mechanism of muscle pain is not fully understood but probably involves prolonged contraction. The extraocular muscles are a source of muscle contraction pain in patients with heterophoria. When an imbalance exists, especially in convergence, long periods of close work cause difficulty in maintaining conjugate gaze and pain is felt in the orbit.

Pain from the cervical roots and cranial nerves is generally due to mechanical traction from injury or malformation. Pain follows this nerve distribution: the neck and back of the head up to the vertex for the cervical roots and the face for the cranial nerves.

Taking the History

History taking is everything when attempting to diagnose the cause of headache. Most children, especially very young ones, are incapable of describing the quality of their pain, and in fact, such descriptions are rarely informative even when provided by older children. Terms such as "throbbing" and "splitting" are more often used to describe the intensity than the character of the pain. The more important questions have to do with the frequency, duration, and location of headache and its associated symptoms. Time of onset may indicate a stressful period for a child, such as attending school or visitation by a separated parent.

Asking a child younger than 10 years of age how often headaches occur or how long they last is rarely productive. Young children have no sense of time ("Are we almost there?"), but parents are usually quite helpful in this regard. The following four questions are useful in determining the headache pattern:

1. "Is the headache chronic but not disabling or does it occur occasionally and prevent normal activity?" The number of school days missed because of headache is a good indication of frequency, severity, and disability.

2. "What is the longest period of time that you have been headache free?" This identifies a common headache pattern in which the child has a flurry of headaches over a period of a week or two and then, after a prolonged headache-free interval, experiences another flurry of daily headaches.

3. "How many different kinds of headache do you have?" A common response is that the child has two kinds of headache: one headache is severe and causes the child to look sick (migraine), and the other is a mild headache that is almost constant but not disabling (analgesic rebound headache).

4. "What analgesics have you used and how often?" This helps establish what does and does not work and may also establish the diagnosis of analgesic rebound headache as a contributing factor.

Helpful responses to traditional questions concerning the history of headache can be obtained from children 10 years of age or older. Several typical headache patterns, when present, allow recognition of either the source or the mechanism of pain.

1. A continuous, low-intensity, chronic headache, in the absence of associated symptoms or signs, is not likely to indicate a serious intracranial disease.

2. Intermittent headaches, especially those that make the child look and feel sick, from which the child recovers completely and is normal between attacks, are likely to be migraine.

3. A severe headache of recent onset, unlike anything previously experienced, from which the child never returns to a normal baseline is probably due to significant intracranial disease.

4. Brief, intense pain lasting for seconds in an otherwise normal child will probably not be explained.

5. Periosteal pain, especially inflammation of the sinuses, is localized, and the area is tender to palpation. Sinusitis is overdiagnosed as a cause of headache, and computed tomographic (CT) evidence of sinusitis is common in children being evaluated for other reasons.

6. Cervical root and cranial nerve pain has a radiating or shooting quality.

Evaluation

Children referred to a pediatric neurologist for headache commonly arrive with a cranial CT or at least a report of a normal study. The only question asked by the primary physician was "Does this child have a brain tumor?" Unfortunately, the normal CT neither explained nor cured the headache. A routine brain imaging study on every child with chronic headache is not cost effective and is not a substitute for an adequate history and physical examination. As a rule, neuroimaging is not indicated in people with headache who have a normal neurological examination, especially when the headache is of the migraine type (Maytal et al, 1995).

Migraine

Migraine accounts for 75% of headaches in young children referred for neurological consultation. It is a hereditary disorder transmitted by autosomal dominant inheritance. A history of migraine in at least one parent is reported in 90% of cases if both parents are interviewed and in 80% if only one parent is interviewed. The prevalence of migraine is 2.5% under the age of 7 (both sexes equally affected), 5% from age 7 to puberty (female-to-male ratio of 3 : 2), 5% in postpubertal boys, and 10% in postpubertal girls. The higher incidence of migraine in pubertal girls than in boys is probably related to the triggering effect of the menstrual cycle on migraine attacks.

Approximately one quarter of children will be migraine free by age 25 years, boys significantly more often than girls, and more than half will still have headaches at age 50. Of those who become parents, 50% will have at least one child who suffers from migraine. (Bille, 1997).

Triggering Factors

Among persons with a predisposition to migraine, individual attacks are usually provoked by an idiosyncratic triggering factor. Common triggering factors are stress, exercise, head trauma, and the premenstrual decline in circulating estrogen. An allergic basis for migraine has been considered but never established.

Stress and Exercise

Migraine symptoms may first occur during stress or exercise or, more often, during a time of relaxation following a period of stress. When stress is the triggering factor, attacks are most likely to occur in school or just after returning home. Attacks rarely occur upon awakening. Children with migraine do not have a specific personality type. Migraine is just as likely in a "slug" as in an overachiever.

Head Trauma

The mechanism by which blows to the head and whiplash head movements provoke migraine attacks is unknown. Trivial blows to the head during competitive sports are significant triggering factors because they occur against a background of vigorous exercise and stress. A severe migraine attack—headache, vomiting, and transitory neurological deficits—following a head injury suggests the possibility of intracranial hemorrhage. The number of diagnostic tests can be reduced if the cause-and-effect relationship between head trauma and migraine is appreciated and the diagnosis of migraine established.

Transitory cerebral blindness, as well as other transitory neurological deficits, sometimes occurs after head trauma in children with migraine (see Chapter 16).

Menstrual Cycle

The higher rate of migraine among postpubertal girls compared either with prepubertal children of both sexes or with postpubertal boys supports the observation that hormonal changes in the normal female cycle trigger attacks of migraine. The widespread use of oral contraceptives has provided some insight into the relationship between the female hormonal cycle and migraine. Some oral contraceptives increase the frequency and intensity of migraine attacks in many women with a history of migraine and may precipitate the initial attack in genetically predisposed women who have previously been migraine free. Among women taking oral contraceptives, the greatest increase in frequency of migraine occurs at midcycle. The decline in the concentration of circulating estrogens is probably the critical factor in precipitating an attack.

Clinical Syndromes

Migraine in children can be divided into three groups: migraine with aura (classic migraine), migraine without aura (common migraine), and migraine equivalent syndromes. Migraine without aura is more than twice as common as migraine with aura in school-age children. Migraine with and without aura are variable expressions of the same genetic defect; and both kinds of attacks may occur in the same individual at different times. The main feature of migraine equivalent syndromes is a transitory disturbance in neurological function. Headache is a minor feature or is not present. These syndromes are discussed in several other chapters (Table 3-2).

A peculiar migraine equivalent that occurs mainly during adolescence or later is *ice-pick*

Table 3-2
Migraine Equivalents

Acute confusional migraine (see Chapter 2)
Basilar migraine (see Chapter 10)
Benign paroxysmal vertigo (see Chapter 10)
Cyclic vomiting
Hemiplegic migraine (see Chapter 11)
Ophthalmoplegic migraine (see Chapter 15)
Paroxysmal torticollis (see Chapter 14)
Transient global amnesia (see Chapter 2)

---

headache. A severe pain on top of the head is experienced that drives the patient to the floor. It ends as quickly as it comes. Bouts may be repeated over days or months and then remit spontaneously. Ice-pick headache ends so quickly that treatment is not required, only reassurance.

Migraine with Aura

Migraine with aura is a biphasic event. In the initial phase, a wave of excitation followed by depression of cortical function spreads over both hemispheres from back to front. This is associated with decreased regional cerebral blood flow and transitory neurological disturbances. These disturbances are caused primarily by neuronal depression rather than ischemia. The second phase is usually, but not necessarily, associated with increased blood flow in both the internal and external carotid circulations. Headache, nausea, and sometimes vomiting occur in the second phase. The mechanism of headache and nausea remains uncertain but is not explained by increased cerebral blood flow.

During an attack the main clinical features may be related only to the first phase (aura), only to the second phase, or to both. The usual features of the aura are visual aberrations: the perception of sparkling lights or colored lines, blind spots, blurred vision, hemianopia, transitory blindness, micropsia, and visual hallucinations. Visual symptoms are identified in about a third of children when specific questions are asked. They tend to be stereotyped for each child and may be perceived in one eye, in one field, or without localization.

Visual hallucinations and other visual distortions may be associated with impairment of time sense and body image. This symptom complex in migraine is called the *Alice-in-Wonderland syndrome.* More extreme disturbances in mental state—amnesia, confusion, and psychosis—are discussed in the sections on confusional migraine and transient global amnesia (see Chapter 2).

Dysesthesias of the limbs and perioral region are the next most common sensory features. Other possible features of the aura are focal motor deficits, usually hemiplegia or ophthalmoplegia, and aphasia. Such deficits, although alarming, are transitory; normal function usually returns within 24 hours and always within 72 hours.

A migraine attack may terminate at the end of the initial phase without headache. Alternatively, the initial phase may be brief or asymptomatic and headache the major symptom. The pain is usually dull at first and then becomes throbbing, pulsating, or pounding. *Severe headache that is maximal at onset is not migraine.* Pain is unilateral in approximately two thirds of patients and bilateral in the rest. It is most intense in the region of the eye, forehead, and temple. Eventually the pain becomes constant and diffuse. Most headaches last for 2 to 6 hours, and are associated with nausea and sometimes vomiting. Anorexia and photophobia are concomitant symptoms. The child looks sick and wants to lie down; I always ask the parent, "Does the child look sick?" With migraine, the answer is always "yes." Vomiting frequently heralds the end of the attack, and the fatigued child falls into a deep sleep. Normal function resumes when the child awakens.

Most children average one attack per month but may have long intervals without attacks and other intervals when attacks occur weekly. The intervals with frequent headaches are probably times of stress.

Migraine without Aura

The attacks of migraine without aura are monophasic. Headache and vomiting are the only features, and attacks are less readily identified as migrainous. The typical initial symptoms are personality change, malaise, and nausea. Recurrent vomiting may be the only feature of the attack in preschool children.

The headache may be unilateral and pounding, but more often the child has difficulty localizing the pain and describing its quality. When the headache is prolonged, the pain is not of uniform intensity; instead, intermittent severe headaches are superimposed on a background of chronic discomfort in the neck and other pericranial muscles. The pain is aggravated by physical activity. Migraine without aura may be difficult to separate from other headache syndromes or from intercurrent illness. The important clue is that the child appears sick, wants to lie down, and is sensitive to light and sound. Nausea and vomiting may occur repeatedly, need not herald the termination of the attack, and can be more prominent than the headache.

Diagnosis

The diagnosis of migraine is based on the clinical features; migraine is one of the few remaining neurological disorders in which the physician cannot stumble on the diagnosis by imaging the brain. Salient features are a family history of migraine and some combination of recurrent headache, nausea, or neurological disturbances, especially if the symptoms are relieved by sleep. The physician should be reluctant to make the diagnosis if questioning of both biological parents does not elicit a family history of migraine. *When obtaining the history be certain that you are speaking with the biological parents.* A history of motion sickness is obtained in almost one half of children with migraine. The significance of this association is uncertain; the incidence of motion sickness in the general population approaches 100%, depending on the amount of motion.

Diagnostic tests are unnecessary when the diagnosis of migraine can be clearly established on the basis of the family history and clinical features. Brain imaging is indicated only when there is uncertainty. The only reason to obtain an electroencephalogram (EEG) in children with migraine-like headaches is to exclude the possibility of benign occipital epilepsy (see Chapter 1).

Management

The essential caveat for the treatment of migraine is that irrespective of treatment, about half of affected children have more than a 50% reduction in headache frequency in the 6 months following the initial visit to a neurologist. This is consistent with the experience of most blinded, controlled trials of drug therapy, in which the placebo success rate is usually 50%. Once the child's parents are convinced that the headache is due to migraine and not brain tumor, they are less anxious, the child is more relaxed, and headaches either decrease in frequency or are discussed less often. The therapeutic efficacy of neurological consultation has the dual effect of making drug evaluation difficult and reinforcing the neurologist's belief that the drug regimen selected is useful.

The two approaches to migraine therapy are treatment of the acute attack and prophylaxis. Whichever approach is selected, the patient and family must be told that the migraine will not go away and that they will need to learn how to live with it. After all, migraine is not a temporary condition; it is often lifelong.

1. Instruct the patient and the parents to avoid, when possible, activities that are known to trigger attacks.

2. When an attack occurs, give in to it. Take medication and go to bed; do not try to maintain activity.

3. Do not use narcotics or other addictive drugs to treat severe attacks.

4. Sleep ends the attack. Any medication that puts the child to sleep will end the attack.

Treating the Acute Attack

The two main symptoms of a migraine attack are headache and nausea. Nonprescription analgesics and nonsteroidal anti-inflammatory drugs, especially ibuprofen, are more effective than placebo in controlling pain (Hämäläinen et al, 1997) but do not prevent vomiting. The ideal treatment for migraine is sleep. I usually prescribe oral promethazine, generally 25 mg in school-age children. It relieves nausea and causes drowsiness. When the child awakens, the attack is usually over.

The *triptans,* 3,5 substituted indoles, selective serotonin agonists, were developed during the 1990s to abort the acute migraine attack. They are considerably more expensive than promethazine but do not cause sedation when performance must be maintained. The first member of this group was sumatriptan. It was initially administered by subcutaneous injection. At a dose of 0.06 mg/kg, the severity of an attack decreased within 60 minutes in 78% of children aged 6 to 18 years (Linder, 1996). Boys respond more frequently than girls. Adverse effects include fatigue, tingling of the head and arms, and a sensation of pressure or stiffness in the neck, throat, and chest. The oral compound (sumatriptan succinate) was introduced later, and while a dosing schedule for children is not established, 25 mg of the oral preparation is safe and effective in most school-age children. Other oral triptans include naratriptan and zolmitriptan. Their increased efficacy compared to sumatriptan has not been established (Goadsby, 1998).

A sumatriptan nasal spray is now available; it may be the most effective mode of administration (Ryan et al, 1997). It takes effect 15 minutes after administration at a dose of 10–20 mg in adults. A dosing schedule for children has not been established.

Dihydroergotamine (DHE) is available as an intranasal preparation and is useful when nausea and vomiting limit the use of oral medications or when other medications are ineffective.

Migraine Prophylaxis

An extraordinarily large number of agents with diverse pharmacological properties have been administered daily to prevent migraine attacks. I suggest prophylactic agents only for children who miss school more than once each month. The most commonly used drugs are propranolol, valproate, calcium channel blocking agents, cyproheptadine, and amitriptyline. Cyproheptadine is commonly used by pediatricians but is no better than placebo in controlled clinical trials. Valproate is effective in adults but not in children. In contrast, propranolol is consistently better than placebo and should be considered the preferred drug for migraine prophylaxis (Silberstein, 1996). Calcium channel blocking agents are widely used but have not been studied rigorously in large, controlled trials.

Propranolol

Propranolol is a β-adrenergic blocking agent that was serendipitously found useful in preventing migraine attacks in patients being treated for cardiovascular disease. It decreases headache frequency by at least half in 80% of patients. The mechanism of action is probably central and not β-adrenergic blockade. Propranolol must have central action because it causes depression. Other β-adrenergic blocking agents have not been studied in migraine and should not be used.

The dosage in children is 2 mg/kg in three divided doses. Because depression is a dose-related adverse reaction and because lower doses may be effective, treatment should be started at 1 mg/kg/day. Depression is the most common reason to discontinue therapy, and parents should be warned of this reaction when the drug is started. The drug should not be used in children with asthma because it may provoke an attack. Hypotension and pulse rate reduction do not occur in children with normal cardiovascular systems. The maintenance dose of the sustained-release tablet is one third greater than that of the short-acting preparation. Plasma levels of propranolol are not useful in determining the effective dose for migraine.

People who respond to propranolol do not develop tolerance. However, if the drug is abruptly stopped after 6 to 12 months of therapy, some individuals will have rebound headaches of increased frequency. Others will continue to show the benefits achieved during therapy.

Calcium Channel Blocking Agents

Calcium channel blocking agents are vasodilators that prevent the influx of calcium into vascular smooth muscle. They have been used extensively for coronary artery disease and are effective dilators of the cerebral vasculature.

In general, the efficacy of this class of drugs remains uncertain. Clinical trials have involved small numbers of patients, and the results have not always been consistent. Flunarizine is considered the most promising agent for migraine prophylaxis, but an oral form is not available in the United States. Nifedipine is of questionable value and may cause headache. Verapamil in doses of 80–120 mg three times a day reduces the frequency of migraine with aura, but it is not as useful in common migraine. Calcium channel blocking agents as a group have little or no toxicity in children with normal cardiovascular systems.

Cluster Headache

Cluster headache is uncommon in children. It occurs mainly in boys and rarely affects other family members (Russell et al, 1995). Cluster headache must be distinguished from chronic paroxysmal hemicrania and hemicrania continua (see following section on Indomethacin Responsive Headache).

CLINICAL FEATURES. The onset is almost exclusively after age 10. Clusters of headaches recur over periods of weeks or months separated by intervals of 1 to 2 years. A cluster of daily attacks lasting for 4 to 8 weeks may occur once or twice a year, often in the autumn or spring. Headaches do not occur in the interim.

Headache is the initial feature, often beginning during sleep. The pain occurs in bursts lasting for 30 to 90 minutes and is repeated two to six times each day. It is always unilateral and affects the same side of the head in each attack.

It begins behind and around one eye and then spreads to the entire hemicranium. During an attack the affected individual cannot lie still but typically walks the floor in anguish; this feature is important in distinguishing cluster headache from migraine, in which the child wants to go to bed. Pain is intense and may be described as throbbing or constant. The scalp may seem edematous and tender. One third of individuals with cluster headache experience sudden intense jabs of pain suggesting tic douloureux. Nausea and vomiting do not occur, but symptoms of hemicranial autonomic dysfunction—injection of the conjunctiva, tearing of the eye, Horner's syndrome, sweating, flushing of the face, and stuffiness of the nose—develop ipsilateral to the headache.

DIAGNOSIS. The diagnosis of cluster headache is established on the basis of the clinical features alone and is not aided by laboratory studies.

MANAGEMENT. The management of cluster headache consists of suppressing recurrences of a bout in progress and relieving acute pain. Prednisone suppresses bouts of cluster headache. An initial dose of 1 mg/kg is administered for the first 5 days and then tapered over the following 2 weeks. If headaches reappear during the tapering process, the dose is increased and maintained at a level sufficient to keep the patient headache free. If the bout of cluster headache is prolonged, the prednisone dosage should be tapered before the appearance of adverse side effects.

The acute attacks can be treated with sumatriptan, by oxygen inhalation, or by a combination of the two. Sumatriptan is given as a 6 mg injection in adults; the dosage in children is not established. Inhalation of 100% oxygen at a rate of 8 to 10 L/min relieves an acute attack in most patients. Lithium is useful for patients with a chronic form of cluster headache in which the headache never ceases. Increasing doses are used to achieve a blood concentration of 1.2 mEq/L (1.2 mmol/L). Most patients have at least a partial response to lithium, but only 50% are relieved completely. The beneficial effect of lithium is enhanced by the addition of daily oral ergotamine.

Indomethacin Responsive Headache

Indomethacin-responsive headache syndromes are a group of seemingly unrelated headache disorders that respond to indomethacin and to nothing else. The syndromes include chronic paroxysmal hemicrania, hemicrania continua, and benign exertional headache.

Chronic Paroxysmal Hemicrania

CLINICAL FEATURES. As with cluster headache, the main features of chronic paroxysmal hemicrania are unilateral throbbing pain associated with ipsilateral autonomic features. However, the painful attack is briefer in duration but more frequent than in cluster headache (Goadsby and Lipton, 1997). Attacks last for weeks to months and are separated by remissions that last for months to years. The pain is located in the frontal and retro-orbital regions and is accompanied by conjunctival injection and tearing.

DIAGNOSIS. The diagnosis is based on the clinical features and is not aided by laboratory studies.

MANAGEMENT. Chronic paroxysmal hemicrania responds to indomethacin. The typical adult dosage is 75 mg/day. Larger dosages may be needed in successive attacks. Acetazolamide may prove successful when indomethacin fails.

Hemicrania Continua

CLINICAL FEATURES. Hemicrania continua is a continuous unilateral headache of moderate severity. Autonomic symptoms may be associated but are not prominent. Some patients have continuous headaches lasting for weeks to months separated by pain-free intervals; others never experience remissions. The episodic form may later become continuous.

DIAGNOSIS. The diagnosis is established by the clinical features. Other causes of chronic headache, such as increased intracranial pressure and chronic use of analgesics, must be excluded.

MANAGEMENT. The headaches usually respond to indomethacin at dosages of 25 to 250 mg/day.

Benign Exertional Headache

Exertion, especially during competitive sports, is a known trigger for migraine in predisposed individuals (see Migraine earlier in this chapter). Persons who do not have migraine may also experience headaches during exercise. Headache during sexual intercourse may be a form of exertional headache, and such individuals often experience the same headache during exercise.

CLINICAL FEATURES. Effort headaches tend to be acute and severe, starting early in the course of exercise, while exertion headaches tend to start later and last longer. Both may be throbbing and bitemporal. Headache may occur during prolonged sexual arousal, as well as during sexual intercourse.

More than one kind of headache is associated with sexual intercourse. A dull headache, primarily occipital but also in a band distribution, may be experienced as sexual excitement increases. This is probably caused by excessive contraction of head and neck muscles. It is not incapacitating and does not disrupt sexual activity. A more severe and dangerous headache is one that occurs just before and at the moment of orgasm. This headache, caused by sudden increase in blood pressure, is similar to the headache associated with pheochromocytoma. Blood pressure elevation during orgasm is considerable and can be associated with subarachnoid hemorrhage in adolescents with arteriovenous malformations.

DIAGNOSIS. The association between exertion and headache is easily recognized. Medical consultation is seldom requested unless the patient is a competitive athlete whose performance is impaired.

MANAGEMENT. Exertional headache can sometimes be prevented by taking indomethacin before activities known to induce benign exertional headache. The prophylactic use of indomethacin, 25 mg three times a day, or propranolol, 1 to 2 mg/kg/day, also reduces the incidence of attacks.

Chronic Low-Grade Headaches

These are constant or intermittent daily headaches. The child is not sick and usually continues normal activity but is constantly complaining of headache. The two most common causes of chronic low-grade headache are excessive use of analgesics and caffeine (Warner et al, 1998).

Analgesic Rebound Headache

CLINICAL FEATURES. Analgesic rebound is one of the more common causes of chronic headache in people of all ages. Individuals with migraine are especially predisposed to analgesic rebound headaches (*extended migraine*). The term refers to a vicious cycle of headache–analgesic use–headache when the analgesic effect wears off–more analgesic use. The pain is generalized, of low intensity, and dull. It interferes with but

does not prevent routine activities and is not aggravated by activity (Symon, 1998).

DIAGNOSIS. Any child who is taking nonprescription analgesics every day, or even most days, should be assumed to have analgesic rebound headache.

MANAGEMENT. All analgesic use must be stopped; caffeine should be avoided as well. Bedtime amitriptyline (10 mg) often helps the transition to the analgesic-free state. The first few days may be difficult, but a positive effect is noted within weeks and reinforces the recommended management. During the first months, a headache calendar should be kept so that the decline in headache frequency is documented.

Caffeine Headache

CLINICAL FEATURES. Many children, especially adolescents, drink large volumes of carbonated beverages containing caffeine each day. The amount of caffeine in many popular beverages is equivalent to that in a cup of brewed coffee. The exact mechanism of the caffeine headache is not established; it could be a withdrawal effect or a direct effect of caffeine. Individuals who regularly drink large amounts of caffeine-containing beverages often notice a dull frontotemporal headache an hour or more after the last use. More caffeine is taken to relieve the headache, and caffeine addiction is initiated. Withdrawal symptoms may become severe and include throbbing headache, anxiety, and malaise.

DIAGNOSIS. Most people associate caffeine with coffee and are unaware of the caffeine content of soft drinks. In addition to coffee, tea, and colas, other popular drinks with a high caffeine content are deceptive because they do not have a cola color. Adolescent girls frequently use diet colas as a substitute for food and become caffeine dependent.

MANAGEMENT. Caffeine addiction, like other addictions, is often hard to break. Most patients require abrupt cessation. As in analgesic rebound headache, 10 mg of amitriptyline at bedtime for the first month may be useful in breaking the cycle.

Posttraumatic Headache

Several different kinds of headache are associated with head trauma. Forty percent of people experience a vascular headache the first day or two after head injury. It is a diffuse, pounding headache made worse by movement of the head or by coughing and straining. Dizziness may be associated. Posttraumatic vascular headaches subside spontaneously. Prolonged posttraumatic headaches are analgesic rebound headaches.

CLINICAL FEATURES. The individual sustains a head injury, with or without loss of consciousness, or a whiplash injury. CT scans of the head or neck do not reveal intracranial or vertebral injury. Head and/or neck pains are experienced immediately, for which analgesics are prescribed—first a narcotic and then a nonprescription analgesic. A dull daily headache develops, for which a variety of analgesic medications are used without relief.

DIAGNOSIS. In the absence of imaging evidence of intracranial or vertebral injury, chronic low-grade head or neck pain without evidence of neurological abnormality on examination should be considered to be an analgesic rebound headache.

MANAGEMENT. See previous discussion of Analgesic Rebound Headache.

Chronic Tension Headache

The term *tension headache* is time honored and suggests that the headache is caused by stress. This is usually true with regard to episodic tension headaches (see section on Pain from Other Cranial Structures that follows), but the mechanism of chronic tension headache is less well established and is probably multifactorial. A family history of chronic tension headache is often obtained, and about half of adults with chronic tension headache date the onset to childhood.

CLINICAL FEATURES. Individuals with chronic headache of any cause may be depressed and anxious. Pain is almost always bilateral and diffuse, and the site of most intense pain may shift during the course of the day. Much of the time, the headache is dull and aching; sometimes it is more intense. Headache is generally present upon awakening and may continue all day but is not aggravated by routine physical activity. Most children describe an undulating course characterized by long periods in which headache occurs almost every day and shorter intervals when they are headache free.

Nausea, vomiting, photophobia, phonophobia, and transitory neurological disturbances are not associated with chronic tension headache. When these features are present, they usually occur only a few times a month and suggest intermittent migraine against a background of chronic tension headache. The neurological examination is normal.

DIAGNOSIS. The diagnosis of chronic tension headache is to some extent a diagnosis of exclusion. Common causes of chronic headache in children that must be distinguished are migraine and analgesic withdrawal headache. Both may coexist with chronic tension headache. Increased intracranial pressure must also be considered and excluded by brain imaging in appropriate cases. The management of chronic tension headache is often easier when the specter of brain tumor has been laid to rest.

MANAGEMENT. Chronic tension headache is by definition difficult to treat or it would not be a chronic headache. Most children have tried and received no benefit from several nonprescription analgesics before coming to a physician, and analgesic rebound headache often complicates management. The use of more powerful analgesics or analgesic-muscle relaxant combinations has limited value and generally adds upset stomach to the child's distress.

It is not always clear that a child with chronic tension headache is experiencing stress. When a stressful situation is identified (e.g., divorce of the parents, custody battle, unsuitable school placement, physical or sexual abuse), the headache cannot be managed without resolution of the stress.

Headaches Associated with Drugs and Foods

Many psychotropic drugs, analgesics, and cardiovascular agents cause headache. Cocaine use produces a migraine-like headache in individuals who do not have migraine at other times. Drug-induced headache should be suspected in a child who has headache following the administration of any drug. These headaches tend to be intermittent rather than daily.

Food Additives

CLINICAL FEATURES. Chemicals are added to foods as preservatives and to enhance their appearance. Ordinarily their concentration is low, and adverse effects occur only in individuals who are genetically sensitive. Nitrites are powerful vasodilators used to enhance the appearance of cured meats such as hot dogs, salami, bacon, and ham. Diffuse, throbbing headaches may occur just after ingestion.

Monosodium glutamate (MSG) is used primarily in Chinese cooking and may cause generalized vasodilatation. Sensitive individuals develop a throbbing bitemporal headache and a band headache, sometimes associated with pressure and tightness of the face and a burning sensation over the body. Symptoms occur 20 minutes after MSG ingestion.

DIAGNOSIS. The association between ingestion of a specific food and headache is quickly evident to the patient.

MANAGEMENT. Headache can be prevented only by avoiding the offending chemical. This is not easy; prepared foods often do not contain a list of all additives.

Marijuana

Marijuana is a peripheral vasodilator and causes a sensation of warmth, injection of the conjunctivae, and sometimes frontal headache. The headache is mild and ordinarily is experienced only during marijuana use. However, marijuana metabolites remain in the blood for several days, and chronic headaches occur in children who are regular users.

Vasculitis

Headaches caused by vasculitis, especially temporal arteritis, are important in the differential diagnosis of vascular headaches in adults. Cerebral vasculitis is uncommon in children and usually occurs as part of a collagen vascular disease, as a result of hypersensitivity, or as part of an infection of the nervous system.

Connective Tissue Disorders

Headache is a feature of systemic lupus erythematosus (SLE) and mixed connective tissue disease. In patients with connective tissue disease, it is not clear that neurological symptoms, including headache, are caused by vasculitis of the cerebral arteries.

CLINICAL FEATURES. Severe headache occurs in up to 10% of children with SLE. It may occur in the absence of other neurological manifestation and can be the initial feature of SLE.

Mixed connective tissue disease is a syndrome with features of lupus erythematosus, scleroderma, and polymyositis. Its course is usually less severe than that of lupus. Thirty-five percent of people with mixed connective tissue disease

report vascular headaches. The headaches are moderate and generally do not interfere with activities of daily living. They may be unilateral or bilateral but are generally throbbing. More than half of patients report a visual aura, and some have nausea and vomiting. Some of these children may be experiencing migraine aggravated by the underlying vasculitis; in others, the headache may be caused by the vasculitis itself.

DIAGNOSIS. The diagnosis of connective tissue disease depends on the combination of a compatible clinical syndrome and the demonstration of antinuclear antibodies in the blood. The presence of antinuclear antibodies in a child with headache who has no systemic symptoms of connective tissue disease should suggest the possibility of a hypersensitivity reaction.

MANAGEMENT. Children with connective tissue disease are ordinarily treated with corticosteroids. In many cases, headaches develop while the child is already taking corticosteroids; this is not an indication to increase the dose. Headache is not a disabling symptom, it does not indicate a generalized encephalopathy, and it should be treated with analgesics.

Hypersensitivity Vasculitis

The important causes of hypersensitivity vasculitis in children are serum sickness, Henoch-Schonlein purpura (see Chapter 11), amphetamine abuse, and cocaine abuse. Children with serum sickness or Henoch-Schonlein purpura have systemic symptoms that precede the headache. Persistent headache and behavioral changes are often the only neurological consequences of Henoch-Schonlein purpura. In contrast, substance abuse can cause a cerebral vasculitis in the absence of systemic symptoms. The features are headache, encephalopathy, focal neurological deficits, and subarachnoid hemorrhage.

Hypertension

A sudden rise in systemic blood pressure causes the explosive, throbbing headache associated with orgasm and pheochromocytoma. Children with chronic hypertension may have low-grade occipital headache on awakening that diminishes as they get up and begin activity or frontal throbbing headache during the day. However, most children with chronic hypertension are asymptomatic. The development of chronic headache in children with renal disease should not be ascribed to hypertension (see Chapter 2). Instead, alternative causes must be pursued. Headaches are common in patients undergoing dialysis and may be due to psychological tension, the precipitation of migraine attacks, and dialysis itself. *Dialysis headache* begins a few hours after the procedure is terminated and is characterized by mild bifrontal throbbing headache, which may be associated with nausea and vomiting.

Pain from Other Cranial Structures

Eyestrain

CLINICAL FEATURES. Prolonged ocular near-fixation in a child with a latent disturbance in convergence may cause dull, aching pain behind the eyes that is quickly relieved when the eyes are closed. The pain is of muscular origin and is caused by the continuous effort to maintain conjugate gaze. If work is continued despite ocular pain, episodic tension headache may develop.

DIAGNOSIS. Children who complain of eyestrain are often thought to have refractive errors, and eyeglasses are fitted. However, refractive errors do not cause eyestrain in children, as presbyopia does in adults.

MANAGEMENT. Resting the eyes relieves eyestrain.

Episodic Tension Headache

CLINICAL FEATURES. Episodic tension headache is common in people of all ages and both sexes. It is generally brought on by fatigue, exertion, and temporary life stress. The mechanism is probably prolonged contraction of muscles attached to the skull. The pain is described as constant, aching, and tight. It is localized mainly to the back of the head and neck, sometimes becomes diffuse, and may be described as a constricting band around the head. Nausea, vomiting, photophobia, and phonophobia are not present.

Headaches usually last for periods ranging from 30 minutes to all day. One episode may last for several days, with some waxing and waning, but not for a week.

DIAGNOSIS. Episodic tension headache should be differentiated from chronic tension, which has similar clinical features but persists for weeks, months, or years. Most episodic tension

headaches are self-diagnosed, and the individual rarely seeks medical attention.

MANAGEMENT. Rest, relaxation, warm compresses to the neck, and nonprescription analgesics relieve pain.

Sinusitis

When questioned about migraine symptoms, most parents identify their own episodic headache, preceded by scintillating scotoma and followed by nausea and vomiting, as sinusitis. This diagnosis is favored by physicians and patients to describe chronic or episodic headaches and is usually wrong.

CLINICAL FEATURES. Children with sinusitis are usually sick. They are febrile, feel stuffy, and have difficulty maintaining a clear airway. Localized tenderness is present over the infected frontal or maxillary sinuses, and inflammation of the ethmoidal or sphenoidal sinuses causes deep midline pain behind the nose. Pain is exaggerated by blowing the nose or by quick movements of the head, especially bending forward. Concurrent vascular headache caused by fever is common.

DIAGNOSIS. Radiographs reveal clouding of the sinuses and sometimes a fluid level. CT of the skull is exceptionally accurate in identifying sinusitis but is usually an unnecessary expense. It is impressive how often CT of the head, performed for reasons other than headache, shows radiographic evidence of asymptomatic sinusitis. Clearly, radiographic evidence of sinusitis does not necessarily explain a patient's headache.

MANAGEMENT. The primary objective of treatment is to allow the sinus to drain. This is usually accomplished with decongestants, but sometimes surgery is required. Antibiotics have limited usefulness if drainage is not established.

Temporomandibular Joint Syndrome

The temporomandibular joint (TMJ) syndrome does not cause chronic generalized daily headache. The pain is unilateral and centered over and below the TMJ (Rothner, 1995).

CLINICAL FEATURES. TMJ syndrome is not generally recognized as a disease of childhood but occurs in children as young as 8 years old. The duration of symptoms before diagnosis may be as long as 5 years and averages 2 years. The primary disturbance is an arthritis of the TMJ that causes localized pain in the lower face and crepitus in the joint. Because of pain on one side, chewing is performed on the opposite side. Unfortunately, this has the unwanted effect of overuse of the affected side. The overused masseter muscle becomes tender; a muscle contraction headache ensues and is felt on the side of the face and at the vertex. The cause of arthritis is generally attributed to bruxism or dental malocclusion, but a prior injury of the jaw accounts for one third of TMJ syndromes in children.

DIAGNOSIS. Radiographs of the TMJ usually show some internal derangement of the joint and may show degenerative arthritis. Magnetic resonance imaging (MRI) using surface coils is considered the most effective technique to show the disturbed joint architecture.

MANAGEMENT. Treatment for TMJ syndrome based on controlled experiments has not been established. Placebos provide considerable benefit, and extensive oral surgery is not indicated. Nonsteroidal anti-inflammatory agents, application of heat to the tense muscles, and dental splints may prove useful.

Whiplash and Other Neck Injuries

Whiplash and other neck injuries cause pain by rupturing cervical disks, damaging soft tissue, injuring occipital nerves, and causing excessive muscle contraction. The muscles contract in an effort to splint the area of injury and thereby reduce further tissue damage.

CLINICAL FEATURES. Constant contraction of the neck extensors causes a dull, aching pain not only in the neck but also in the shoulders and upper arms. This may persist for up to 3 months after the injury. The head is generally kept in a fixed position. Nausea and vomiting are not associated symptoms.

DIAGNOSIS. Following any neck or head injury, radiographs of the cervical spine are needed to determine the presence of fracture or dislocation. Shooting pains that radiate either to the occiput or down the arm and into the fingers suggest the possibility of disk herniation and require further study with MRI or CT.

MANAGEMENT. Warn the patient and family at the onset that prolonged head and neck pain is expected after injury and does not indicate a serious condition. The pain is relieved in part by lying or sitting with the head supported, by superficial application of heat to the painful muscles, by muscle relaxants, and by the use of nonnarcotic analgesics. *Pain that persists after 3 months and also affects the head is caused by analgesic rebound headache.*

Seizure Headache

Diffuse headache caused by vasodilatation of cerebral arteries is a frequent occurrence following a generalized tonic-clonic convulsion. In patients who have both epilepsy and migraine, one can trigger the other; frequently, headache and seizure occur concurrently. Approximately 1% of epileptic patients report headache as a seizure manifestation (*seizure headache*). Most patients with seizure headaches are known epileptics, but in some children, headache is the only feature of their seizure disorder. This is very uncommon.

CLINICAL FEATURES. Headache is part of several epilepsy syndromes, the most common one in children being benign occipital epilepsy (see Chapter 1). The sequence of events suggests migraine.

I have seen one eloquent adolescent who complained of paroxysmal "head pain that is not like other headaches" that was associated with EEG evidence of generalized epileptiform activity. The head pain was relieved by anticonvulsants.

Headache may also occur as a seizure manifestation in patients known to have a seizure disorder. Such individuals usually have a long history of partial or generalized seizures before headache becomes part of the syndrome. Associated ictal events depend on the site of the cortical focus and may include auditory hallucinations, visual disturbances, vertigo, déjà vu, and focal motor seizures. Headache may be the initial feature of the seizure or can follow other partial seizure manifestations, such as déjà vu and vertigo. The headache may be described as throbbing, sharp, or without an identified quality. Complex partial seizures, simple partial seizures, or generalized tonic-clonic seizures follow the headache phase. Spike foci in patients with seizure headaches are usually temporal in location.

Two children with seizure headaches were studied with depth electrodes before surgery. Both had seizure activity confined to the right hippocampus and amygdala during seizure headaches. In one, pain was localized to the vertex and was associated with shortness of breath and lightheadedness. At times the seizure progressed to aphasia, but consciousness was preserved. The other child had frequent attacks of dizziness and tinnitus associated with the sudden onset of pain in the temporal region. The pain lasted for 30 to 60 seconds. Temporal lobe surgery provided complete relief of seizure activity in both patients.

DIAGNOSIS. EEG is not indicated for children with chronic headaches. Interictal discharges, especially rolandic spikes, do not indicate that the headaches are a seizure manifestation, only that the child has a genetic marker for epilepsy. EEG may be warranted in children with paroxysmal headaches that are clearly not migraine. If interictal spike discharges are seen, an effort should be made to record a seizure headache with an ambulatory EEG monitor. The observation of continuous epileptiform activity during a headache provides reassurance that the headache is a seizure manifestation and that anticonvulsant drugs are indicated.

MANAGEMENT. The response to anticonvulsant therapy is usually considered diagnostic as well as therapeutic. Because the seizure focus is usually cortical and most often in the temporal lobe, carbamazepine or phenytoin is recommended.

References

Billie B. A 40-year follow-up of school children with migraine. *Cephalgia* 1997;17:488–491.

Goadsby PJ. A triptan too far? *J Neurol Neurosurg Psychiatry* 1998;64:143–147.

Goadsby PJ, Lipton RB. A review of paroxysmal hemicranias, SUNCT syndrome and other short lasting headaches with autonomic features, including new cases. *Brain* 1997;120:193–209.

Hämäläinen ML, Hoppu K, Valkeila E, et al. Ibuprofen or acetaminophen for the acute treatment of migraine in children: A double-blind, randomized, placebo-controlled, crossover study. *Neurology* 1997;48:103–107.

Linder SL. Subcutaneous sumatriptan in the clinical setting: The first 50 consecutive patients with acute migraine in a pediatric neurology office practice. *Headache* 1996; 36:419–422.

Maytal J, Bienkowski RS, Patel M, et al. The value of imaging in children with headaches. *Pediatrics* 1995; 96:413–416.

Rothner AD. Miscellaneous headache syndromes in children and adolescents. *Semin Pediatr Neurol* 1995;21:59–164.

Russell MB, Andersson PG, Thomsen LL. Familial occurrence of cluster headache. *J Neurol Neurosurg Psychiatry* 1995;58:341–343.

Ryan R, Elkind A, Baker CC, et al. Sumatriptan nasal spray for the acute treatment of migraine: Result of two clinical studies. *Neurology* 1997;49:1225–1230.

Silberstein SD. Divalproex sodium in headache: Literature review and guidelines. *Headache* 1996;36:547–555.

Symon DNK. Twelve cases of analgesic headache. *Arch Dis Child* 1998;78:555–556.

Warner JS, Vasconcellos E, Pina-Garza JE, et al. Daily headaches in adolescents and children. *J Child Neurol* 1998;38:636 (abstract).

Chapter 4
Increased Intracranial Pressure

PATIENTS DO NOT come to a physician complaining of increased intracranial pressure (Table 4-1). Most often it is brought to attention because of headache, vomiting, personality change, and alterations in states of consciousness. Less frequently, the initial complaint is diplopia or the observation that one or both eyes are turning in. Some children are referred for neurological consultation because a primary physician believes the child has papilledema. Conditions causing increased intracranial pressure are described elsewhere in the book, especially in chapters on altered states of consciousness, headache, ataxia, and disorders of ocular motility. This chapter is restricted to conditions in which symptoms of increased intracranial pressure are initial and prominent features.

Table 4-1
Features of Increased Intracranial Pressure

In Infants
Bulging fontanelle
Failure to thrive
Impaired Upward Gaze (setting-sun sign)
Large head (see Chapter 18)
Shrill cry

In Children
Diplopia (see Chapter 15)
Headache (see Chapter 3)
Mental changes
Nausea and vomiting
Papilledema

Pathophysiology

Normal intracranial pressure in the resting state is approximately 10 mm Hg (136 mm H_2O). Pressures greater than 20 mm Hg are considered abnormal. Once the cranial bones fuse during childhood, a rigid box envelopes the contents of the skull. Intracranial pressure is then the sum of the individual pressures exerted by the brain, blood, and cerebrospinal fluid. An increase in the volume of any one of these components must be accommodated by an equivalent decrease in the size of one or both of the other compartments if intracranial pressure is to remain constant. Because cerebral blood flow must be kept relatively constant to provide oxygen and nutrients, the major adaptive mechanisms available to relieve pressure are the compressibility of the brain and the rapid reabsorption of cerebrospinal fluid by arachnoid villi. Infants and young children, in whom the cranial bones are still unfused, have the additional adaptive mechanism of spreading the cranial bones apart to increase cranial volume.

Cerebrospinal Fluid

The choroid plexus accounts for at least 70% of cerebrospinal fluid production, and the transependymal movement of fluid from the brain to the ventricular system accounts for the remainder. The average volumes of cerebrospinal fluid are 90 ml in children from 4 to 13 years of age and 150 ml in adults. The rate of formation is approximately 0.35 ml/min or 500 ml/day. Therefore approximately 14% of total volume turns over every hour. The rate at which cerebrospinal fluid is formed remains relatively constant and declines only slightly as cerebrospinal fluid pressure increases. In contrast, the rate of absorption increases linearly as cerebrospinal fluid pressure exceeds 7 mm Hg. At a pressure of 20 mm Hg, the rate of absorption is three times the rate of formation.

Therefore impaired absorption, not increased formation, is the usual mechanism of progressive hydrocephalus. Choroid plexus papilloma is the only pathological process in which formation can sometimes overwhelm absorption. When absorption is impaired, efforts to decrease the formation of cerebrospinal fluid are not likely to have a significant effect on volume.

Cerebral Blood Flow

Systemic arterial pressure is the primary determinant of cerebral blood flow. Normal cerebral blood flow remains remarkably constant from birth to adult life and is generally 50 to 60 ml/min/100 g brain weight. Blood vessels on the surface and at the base of the brain are more richly innervated by autonomic nerve fibers than are vessels of any other organ. These nerve fibers allow the autoregulation of cerebral blood flow. *Autoregulation* refers to a buffering effect by which cerebral blood flow remains constant despite changes in systemic arterial perfusion pressure. Alterations in the arterial blood concentration of carbon dioxide have an important effect on total cerebral blood flow. Hypercarbia dilates cerebral blood vessels and increases blood flow, whereas hypocarbia constricts cerebral blood vessels and decreases flow. Alterations in blood oxygen content have the reverse effect, but are less potent stimuli for vasoconstriction or vasodilatation than are alterations in the blood carbon dioxide concentration.

Cerebral perfusion pressure is the difference between mean systemic arterial pressure and intracranial pressure. It can be reduced to dangerous levels either by reducing systemic arterial pressure or by increasing intracranial pressure. The autoregulation of the cerebral vessels is lost when cerebral perfusion pressure falls below 50 cm H_2O or severe acidosis is present. Increased intracranial blood volume can be caused by arterial vasodilatation or by obstruction of cerebral veins and venous sinuses. Increased intracranial blood volume, like increased cerebrospinal fluid volume, results in increased intracranial pressure.

Cerebral Edema

Cerebral edema is an increase in the brain's volume caused by an increase in its water and sodium content. Edema may be localized or generalized; when generalized, it increases intracranial pressure. Cerebral edema is generally categorized as *vasogenic, cytotoxic,* or *interstitial.*

Vasogenic edema is caused by increased capillary permeability and is encountered with brain tumor, abscess, trauma, and hemorrhage. The fluid is located primarily in the white matter and responds to treatment with corticosteroids. Osmotic agents have no effect on vasogenic edema, but they can decrease the volume of normal brain tissue and in that way reduce total intracranial pressure.

Cytotoxic edema, caused by swelling of neurons, glia, and endothelial cells, constricts the extracellular space. It is usually caused by hypoxia, ischemia, or infection of the nervous system. Corticosteroids do not decrease edema, but osmotic agents may relieve intracranial pressure by reducing brain volume.

Transependymal movement of fluid causes interstitial edema from the ventricular system to the brain. This occurs when cerebrospinal fluid absorption is blocked and the ventricles are enlarged. The fluid collects chiefly in the periventricular white matter. Agents intended to reduce cerebrospinal fluid production, such as acetazolamide and furosemide, may be useful. Corticosteroids and osmotic agents are not effective.

Mass Lesions

Mass lesions (e.g., tumor, abscess, hematoma, arteriovenous malformation) increase intracranial pressure by occupying space at the expense of other intracranial compartments, provoking cerebral edema, blocking the circulation and absorption of cerebrospinal fluid, increasing blood flow, and obstructing venous return.

Symptoms and Signs

The clinical features of increased intracranial pressure depend on the child's age and the rate at which pressure increases. Newborns and infants present a special case because increased pressure can be partially vented by expanding the volume of the skull. The rate of intracranial pressure increase is important at all ages. Intracranial structures accommodate slowly increasing pressure remarkably well, but sudden changes are intolerable and result in some combination of headache, personality change, and states of decreasing consciousness.

Increased Intracranial Pressure in Infancy

Measurement of head circumference and palpation of the anterior fontanelle are readily available methods of assessing intracranial volume and pressure rapidly. Head circumference is measured by determining its greatest anteroposterior circumference. Normal standards are different for premature and full-term newborns. Normal head growth in the term newborn is 2 cm/month for the first 3 months, 1 cm/month for the second 3 months, and 0.5 cm/month for the next 6 months. Excessive head growth is a major feature of increased intracranial pressure throughout the first year and even up to 3 years of age. However, normal head growth does not preclude the presence of increased intracranial pressure. In posthemorrhagic hydrocephalus, considerable ventricular dilatation precedes any measurable change in head circumference by compressing the brain parenchyma.

The palpable tension of the anterior fontanelle is an excellent measure of intracranial pressure. In a quiet child, a fontanelle that bulges above the level of the bone edges and is sufficiently tense to cause difficulty in determining where bone ends and fontanelle begins is abnormal and indicates increased intracranial pressure. A full fontanelle, which is clearly distinguishable from the surrounding bone edges, may indicate increased intracranial pressure but can also be caused by crying, edema of the scalp, subgaleal hemorrhage, and extravasation of intravenous fluids. The normal fontanelle is clearly demarcated from bone edges, falls below the surface, and pulsates under the examining finger.

Although the size of the anterior fontanelle and its rate of closure are variable, increased intracranial pressure should be suspected when the metopic and coronal sutures are sufficiently separated to admit a fingertip.

When the separation of cranial sutures is no longer sufficient to decompress increased intracranial pressure, the infant experiences lethargy and vomiting and fails to thrive. Palsies of the sixth cranial nerve, impaired upward gaze (setting sun sign), and disturbances of blood pressure and pulse may ensue. Papilledema is uncommon.

Increased Intracranial Pressure in Children

Headache

Headache is one of the more common symptoms of increased intracranial pressure at all ages. Traction and displacement of intracranial arteries are the major causes of headache from increased intracranial pressure (see Chapter 3). As a rule, pain fibers from supratentorial intracranial vessels are innervated by the trigeminal nerve and pain is referred to the eye, forehead, and temple. In contrast, cervical nerves innervate infratentorial intracranial vessels, and pain is referred to the occiput and neck.

When increased intracranial pressure is generalized, as may occur from cerebral edema or obstruction of the ventricular system, headache is generalized and more often prominent in the morning on awakening and rising to a standing position. Pain is constant but may vary in intensity. Coughing, sneezing, straining, and other maneuvers that transiently increase intracranial pressure exaggerate the headache. The quality of the pain is often difficult to describe. Vomiting in the absence of nausea, especially on arising in the morning, is often a concurrent feature.

In the absence of generalized increased intracranial pressure, localized, or at least unilateral, headache can occur if a mass causes traction on contiguous vessels.

In children younger than 10 years old, symptoms of increased intracranial pressure can be temporarily relieved by the separation of sutures. Such children may have a symptom-free interval of several weeks following weeks or months of chronic headache and vomiting. The relief of pressure is temporary, and symptoms return with their prior intensity. An intermittent course of symptoms should not direct attention away from the possibility of increased intracranial pressure.

Any individual who was previously well and then experiences an acute, intense headache described as "the worst headache I ever had in my life" has probably suffered a subarachnoid hemorrhage. A small hemorrhage may not cause loss of consciousness but still produces sufficient meningeal irritation to cause intense headache and some stiffness of the neck. Fever may be present.

Diplopia and Strabismus

Paralysis of one or both abducens nerves is a relatively common feature of generalized increased intracranial pressure and may be a more prominent feature than headache in children with idiopathic intracranial hypertension (pseudotumor cerebri).

Papilledema

Papilledema is passive swelling of the optic disk caused by increased intracranial pressure (Table

4-2). *Extension of the arachnoid sheath of the optic nerve to the retina is essential for the production of papilledema. This does not occur in a small percentage of people, and they can have severe increased intracranial pressure without papilledema.* The edema is usually bilateral and, when unilateral, suggests a mass lesion behind the affected eye. Early papilledema is asymptomatic, and only when it is advanced does the patient experience transitory obscuration of vision. Preservation of visual acuity differentiates papilledema from primary optic nerve disturbances such as optic neuritis, in which visual acuity is always profoundly impaired early in the course (see Chapter 16).

The observation of papilledema in a child with headache or diplopia confirms the diagnosis of increased intracranial pressure. However, the diagnosis of papilledema is not always easy, and congenital variations of disk appearance may confuse the issue. The earliest sign of papilledema is loss of spontaneous venous pulsations in the vessels around the disk margin. Spontaneous venous pulsations are said to occur in approximately 80% of normal adults, but this rate is closer to 100% in children. Spontaneous venous pulsations cease when intracranial pressure exceeds 200 mm H$_2$O. Therefore, papilledema is not present if spontaneous venous pulsations are present, no matter how obscure the disk margin may appear to be. Conversely, when spontaneous venous pulsations are lacking in children, papilledema should be suspected even though the disk margin is flat and well visualized.

As edema progresses, the disk swells and is raised above the plane of the retina, causing obscuration of the disk margin and tortuosity of the veins (Figure 4-1). Associated features include small flame-shaped hemorrhages and nerve fiber infarcts known as *cotton wool* (Figure 4-2). If the process continues, the retina sur-

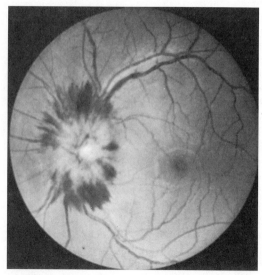

Figure 4-1. Acute papilledema. The optic disk is swollen, and peripapillary nerve fiber layer hemorrhages are evident.

rounding the disk becomes edematous so that the disk appears greatly enlarged and retinal exudates radiate from the fovea. Eventually, the hemorrhages and exudates clear, but optic atrophy ensues and blindness may be permanent. Even if increased intracranial pressure is relieved during the early stages of disk edema, 4 to 6 weeks is required before the retina appears normal again.

Congenitally elevated disks, usually caused by hyaline bodies (drusen) within the nerve

---

Table 4-2
Differential Diagnosis of a Swollen Disk

Congenital disk elevation
Increased intracranial pressure
Ischemic neuropathy
Juvenile diabetes
Optic glioma
Papillitis
Retinitis
Retrobulbar mass
Uveitis

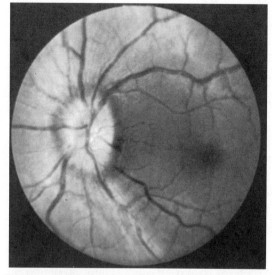

Figure 4-2. Established papilledema. The optic disk is elevated, and opacification of the nerve fiber layer can be seen around the disk margin and retinal folds (Paton lines) temporally.

head, give the false impression of papilledema. The actual drusen are not observable during the first decade, and therefore only the elevated nerve head is apparent. Drusen continue to grow and can be seen in older children and in their parents (Figure 4-3). Drusen are inherited as an autosomal dominant trait and occur more often in Europeans than other ethnic groups. Anomalous nerve head elevations can be easily distinguished from papilledema because spontaneous venous pulsations are present.

Herniation Syndromes

Increased intracranial pressure may cause portions of the brain to shift from their normal location into other compartments, compressing structures already occupying that space. Such shifts may occur under the falx cerebri, through the tentorial notch, and through the foramen magnum (Table 4-3).

Lumbar puncture is generally contraindicated in patients with increased intracranial pressure because of the fear that a change in fluid dynamics will cause herniation. It is especially hazardous when pressure between cranial compartments is unequal. This prohibition is relative, and early lumbar puncture is the rule in infants and children with suspected infections of the nervous system despite the presence of increased intracranial pressure. In other situations, lumbar puncture is rarely essential for diagnosis, but it is usually accomplished safely in

Table 4-3
Herniation Syndromes

Unilateral (Uncal) Transtentorial Herniation
Decerebrate rigidity
Declining consciousness
Dilated and fixed pupil
Homonymous hemianopia
Increased blood pressure, slow pulse
Respiratory irregularity

Bilateral (Central) Transtentorial Herniation
Decerebrate or decorticate rigidity
Declining consciousness
Impaired upward gaze
Irregular respiration
Pupillary constriction or dilatation

Cerebellar (Downward) Herniation
Declining consciousness
Impaired upward gaze
Irregular respirations
Lower cranial nerve palsies
Neck stiffness or head tilt

the absence of papilledema. People at increased risk of herniation following lumbar puncture can be defined by the following computed tomography (CT) criteria: lateral shift of midline structures, loss of the suprachiasmatic and basilar cisterns, obliteration of the fourth ventricle, and obliteration of the superior cerebellar and quadrigeminal plate cisterns.

Falx Herniation

Herniation of one cingulate gyrus under the falx cerebri is common when one hemisphere is enlarged. The major feature is compression of the internal cerebral vein and the anterior cerebral artery, resulting in still greater increased intracranial pressure because of reduced venous outflow and arterial infarction.

Unilateral (Uncal) Transtentorial Herniation

The tentorial notch allows structures to pass from the posterior to the middle fossa. Normally it is filled with the brainstem, the posterior cerebral artery, and the third nerve. Unilateral transtentorial herniation characteristically occurs when enlargement of one temporal lobe causes the uncus or hippocampus to bulge into the tentorial notch. Falx herniation is usually an associated feature. Because intracranial pressure must be considerable to cause such a shift, consciousness is decreased even before the actual hernia-

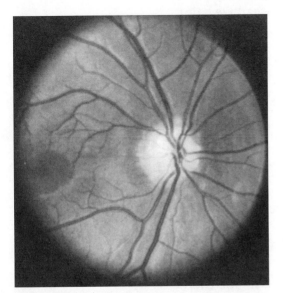

Figure 4-3. Drusen. The disk margin is indistinct, the physiological cup is absent, and yellowish globular bodies are present on the surface.

tion and continues to decline as the brainstem is compressed. Direct pressure on the oculomotor nerve causes ipsilateral dilatation of the pupil; sometimes the contralateral pupil is dilated because the displaced brainstem compresses the opposite oculomotor nerve against the incisura of the tentorium. Contralateral homonymous hemianopia occurs (but is impossible to test in an unconscious patient) because of compression of the ipsilateral posterior cerebral artery. With further pressure on the midbrain, both pupils become dilated and fixed, respirations become irregular, decerebrate posturing is noted, and death results from cardiorespiratory collapse.

Bilateral (Central) Transtentorial Herniation

Central herniation is usually associated with generalized cerebral edema. Both hemispheres are displaced downward, and the diencephalon and midbrain are pushed caudad through the tentorial notch. The diencephalon becomes edematous, and the pituitary stalk may be avulsed. The clinical features are states of decreasing consciousness, pupillary constriction and then dilatation, impaired upward gaze, irregular respiration, disturbed control of body temperature, decerebrate or decorticate posturing, and death.

Cerebellar Herniation

Increased pressure in the posterior fossa may cause upward herniation of the cerebellum through the tentorial notch or downward displacement of one or both cerebellar tonsils through the foramen magnum. Upward displacement causes compression of the midbrain, resulting in impairment of upward gaze, dilated or fixed pupils, and respiratory irregularity. Downward cerebellar herniation causes compression of the medulla, resulting in states of decreasing consciousness, impaired upward gaze, and lower cranial nerve palsies. One of the earliest features of cerebellar herniation into the foramen magnum is neck stiffness or head tilt as an effort is made to relieve the pressure by enlarging the surface area of the foramen magnum.

Medical Treatment

Several measures to lower increased intracranial pressure are available, even in circumstances

Table 4-4
Medical Measures to Decrease Intracranial Pressure

Corticosteroids
Elevation of head
Glycerol
Hyperventilation
Hypothermia
Mannitol
Osmotic diuretics
Pentobarbital coma

where surgical intervention is required (Table 4-4).

Monitoring Intracranial Pressure

The enthusiasm for continuous monitoring of intracranial pressure in children is declining. Despite advances in technology, the effect of pressure monitoring on the outcome is questionable. It has no value in children with hypoxic-ischemic encephalopathies and has marginal value in children with other kinds of encephalopathies. Head injury is the most common indication for monitoring. As a general rule, patients who are able to follow simple commands do not need to be monitored. The symptoms and prognosis of increased intracranial pressure depend more on its cause than on the level of pressure attained.

Head Elevation

Elevating the head of the bed 30 to 45 degrees above horizontal decreases intracranial pressure by improving jugular venous drainage. Systemic blood pressure is not affected, so the overall result is increased cerebral perfusion.

Hyperventilation

Intracranial pressure is reduced within seconds of the initiation of hyperventilation. The mechanism is vasoconstriction resulting from hypercarbia. The goal is to lower the arterial pressure of carbon dioxide to 25–30 mm Hg. Further reduction may cause ischemia and is contraindicated. Hyperventilation should be avoided in patients with head trauma.

Osmotic Diuretics

Mannitol is the osmotic diuretic most widely used in the United States. Mannitol, 0.25 g/kg, is given intravenously as a 20% solution. Mannitol exerts its beneficial effects as a plasma expander and as an osmotic diuretic. It is entirely excreted by the kidneys, and large doses may cause renal failure, especially when nephrotoxic drugs are used concurrently. Serum osmolarity is generally kept below 320 mOsm, and adequate intravascular volume is maintained.

Corticosteroids

Corticosteroids such as dexamethasone are effective in the treatment of vasogenic edema. The intravenous dosage is 0.1 to 0.2 mg/kg every 6 hours. Onset of action is 12 to 24 hours, and peak action may be delayed even longer. The mechanism is uncertain. Cerebral blood flow is not affected. Corticosteroids are most useful for reducing edema surrounding mass lesions and are not useful in the treatment of severe head injury.

Hypothermia

Hypothermia decreases cerebral blood flow and is frequently used concurrently with pentobarbital coma. Body temperature is generally kept between 27° and 31° C. It is not clear how much is gained by hypothermia in addition to other measures that decrease cerebral blood flow, such as head elevation, hyperventilation, and pentobarbital coma.

Pentobarbital Coma

Barbiturates reduce cerebral blood flow, decrease edema formation, and lower the brain's metabolic rate. These effects do not occur at anticonvulsant plasma concentrations but require brain concentrations sufficient to produce a burst-suppression pattern on the electroencephalogram (EEG). Barbiturate coma is particularly useful in patients with increased intracranial pressure resulting from disorders of mitochondrial function such as Reye syndrome. Pentobarbital is preferred to phenobarbital (see Chapter 1).

Hydrocephalus

Hydrocephalus is a condition marked by an excessive volume of intracranial cerebrospinal fluid. It is termed *communicating* or *noncommunicating*, depending on whether or not the cerebrospinal fluid communicates between the ventricular system and the subarachnoid space. Congenital hydrocephalus occurs in approximately one birth per thousand. It is generally associated with other congenital malformations and may be caused by genetic disturbances or intrauterine disorders such as infection and hemorrhage. Often, no cause can be determined. Congenital hydrocephalus is discussed in Chapter 18 because its initial feature is almost always macrocephaly.

Acquired hydrocephalus may be caused by brain tumor, intracranial hemorrhage, or infection. Solid brain tumors generally produce hydrocephalus by obstructing the ventricular system, whereas nonsolid tumors such as leukemia impair the reabsorptive mechanism in the subarachnoid space.

Intracranial hemorrhage and infection may produce communicating and noncommunicating hydrocephalus and also may increase intracranial pressure through the mechanisms of cerebral edema and impaired venous return. Because several factors contribute to increased intracranial pressure, the discussion of acquired hydrocephalus is categorized by cause in the sections that follow.

Brain Tumors

Primary tumors of the posterior fossa and middle fossa are discussed in Chapters 10, 15, and 16 (Table 4-5). This section deals with tumors of the cerebral hemispheres. Supratentorial tumors comprise approximately half of brain tumors in children. They occur more commonly in children less than 2 years of age and again in adolescents.

Choroid Plexus Papilloma

Choroid plexus papilloma is an unusual tumor, representing less than 2% of childhood brain tumors (Costa et al, 1997). It generally occurs during infancy and may be present at birth.

CLINICAL FEATURES. Choroid plexus tumors are usually located in one lateral ventricle but may also arise in the third ventricle. The main features are those of increased intracranial pressure from hydrocephalus. Communicating hydrocephalus is sometimes caused by excessive production of cerebrospinal fluid by the tumor, but noncommunicating hydrocephalus caused by obstruction of the ventricular foramen is the rule. If the tumor is pedunculated, its movement may cause intermittent ventricular obstruction

Table 4-5
Brain Tumors in Children

Hemispheric Tumors
Choroid plexus papilloma
Glial tumors
    Astrocytoma
    Ependymoma
    Oligodendroglioma
    Primitive neuroectodermal tumors
Pineal region tumors
    Pineal-parenchymal tumors
        Pineoblastoma
        Pineocytoma
    Germ cell tumors
        Embryonal cell carcinoma
        Germinoma
        Teratoma
    Glial tumors
        Astrocytoma
        Ganglioglioma
Other tumors
    Angiomas
    Dysplasia
    Meningioma
    Metastatic tumors

Middle Fossa Tumors
Optic glioma (see Chapter 16)
Sellar and parasellar tumors (see Chapter 16)

Posterior Fossa Tumors
Astrocytoma (see Chapter 10)
Brainstem glioma (see Chapter 15)
Ependymoma (see Chapter 10)
Hemangioblastoma (see Chapter 10)
Medulloblastoma (see Chapter 10)

by a ball-valve mechanism. The usual course is one of rapid progression, with only a few weeks from first symptoms to diagnosis.

Infants with choroid plexus tumors usually have macrocephaly and are thought to have congenital hydrocephalus. Older children have nausea, vomiting, diplopia, headaches, and weakness. Papilledema is the rule.

DIAGNOSIS. Because affected children show clear evidence of increased intracranial pressure, CT is usually the first test performed. The tumor is visualized within one ventricle as a mass of increased density with marked contrast enhancement. Hydrocephalus of one or both lateral ventricles is visualized as well. Because choroid plexus papillomas are highly vascular, angiography should be considered before surgery. Many tumors bleed spontaneously, and the spinal fluid may be xanthochromic or grossly bloody. The concentration of protein in the cerebrospinal fluid is usually elevated.

MANAGEMENT. Complete surgical extirpation is the treatment of choice. The 5-year survival rate is 50%, with most deaths occurring within 7 months of surgery. Operative mortality may be high because the tumor has a tendency to hemorrhage. If the tumor is removed completely, hydrocephalus is relieved without the need of a shunt and recurrences are unusual.

Glial Tumors

Tumors of glial origin comprise approximately 40% of supratentorial tumors in infants and children. The common glial tumors of childhood in order of frequency are astrocytoma, ependymoma, and oligodendroglioma. A mixture of two or more cell types is the rule. Oligodendroglioma occurs exclusively in the cerebral hemispheres, whereas astrocytoma and ependymoma may be found in either a supratentorial or an infratentorial location.

Oligodendroglioma is generally not encountered until adolescence. These tumors grow slowly and tend to calcify. The initial symptom is usually a seizure rather than increased intracranial pressure.

Astrocytoma

Hemispheric astrocytomas are graded by histological appearance into three classes: low-grade, anaplastic, and glioblastoma multiforme. Anaplastic tumors and glioblastoma multiforme are referred to as *high-grade tumors*. Glioblastoma multiforme accounts for fewer than 10% of childhood supratentorial astrocytomas and is more likely to occur in adolescence than in infancy. High-grade tumors may evolve from low-grade tumors.

CLINICAL FEATURES. The initial features of glial tumors in children depend on location and may include seizures, hemiparesis, and movement disorders affecting one side of the body. Seizures are the most common initial feature of low-grade gliomas. Tumors infiltrating the basal ganglia and internal capsule are less likely to cause seizures than those closer to cortical structures. A mass effect may not be present early in the course because slow-growing, infiltrating tumors can be accommodated by surrounding neural structures. Such tumors may cause only seizures for several years before causing weakness of the contralateral limbs.

Headache is a relatively common complaint and may be focal if the tumor is producing localized displacement of vessels without increasing intracranial pressure. A persistent focal headache usually correlates well with tumor location.

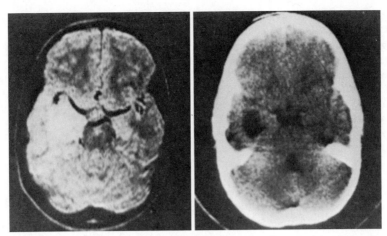

Figure 4-4. Low-grade glioma. MRI (*left*) reveals an area of increased signal intensity in the right temporal lobe, which appears as a cystic lesion on CT (*right*).

Symptoms of increased intracranial pressure, generalized headache, nausea, and vomiting are initial features of hemispheric astrocytoma in only a third of children but are common at the time of diagnosis. Intracranial pressure is likely to increase when rapidly growing tumors provoke edema of the hemisphere. A mass effect is produced that causes collapse of one ventricle, shift of midline structures, and pressure on the aqueduct. When herniation occurs, or when the lateral ventricles are dilated because of pressure on the aqueduct, the early features of headache, nausea, vomiting, and diplopia are followed by generalized weakness or fatigability, lethargy, and declining consciousness.

Papilledema occurs in children with generalized increased intracranial pressure; however, in those under 2 years of age, macrocephaly may develop instead. When papilledema is present, abducens palsy is usually an associated symptom. Other neurological findings depend on the site of the tumor and may include hemiparesis, hemisensory loss, or homonymous hemianopia.

DIAGNOSIS. Magnetic resonance imaging (MRI) is always preferable to CT when tumor is suspected. Low-grade gliomas appear as low-density or cystic areas that are enhanced when contrast material is injected (Figure 4-4). Cerebral edema is identified as a low-density area surrounding the tumor that does not show contrast enhancement.

High-grade gliomas have patchy areas of low and high density, sometimes evidence of hemorrhage, and cystic degeneration. Marked contrast enhancement is noted, often in a ring pattern. When a mass effect is present, MRI shows a shift of midline structures, deformity of the ipsilateral

ventricle, and swelling of the affected hemisphere with obliteration of sulcal markings (Figure 4-5). A mass effect is identified in half of low-grade astrocytomas and in almost all high-grade tumors.

MANAGEMENT. All children with increased intracranial pressure caused by hemispheric astrocytoma should be treated with dexamethasone to reduce vasogenic cerebral edema. Headache and nausea are frequently relieved within 24 hours, and neurological deficits are often improved as well. Surgical resection of the tumor is the next step in treatment. Complete removal

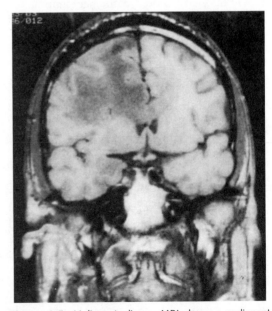

Figure 4-5. Malignant glioma. MRI shows a malignant astrocytoma invading the corpus callosum.

is rarely possible, except with cystic cerebral astrocytoma, which resembles cerebellar astrocytomas in having a mural nodule within the cyst. In these tumors, the 5-year survival rate following surgery alone is 90%.

Children with low-grade astrocytomas of the cerebral hemisphere have a 20-year survival rate of 85% after surgical resection alone (Pollack et al, 1995). Postoperative radiotherapy impairs cognition without increasing survival. Postoperative radiation is recommended for anaplastic astrocytomas. Children with anaplastic astrocytomas have less than a 30% 5-year survival rate even with radiotherapy, and those with glioblastoma multiforme have less than a 3% 5-year survival.

Because the 5-year survival rate of children with high-grade astrocytomas is poor, several chemotherapy protocols are being tried (Packer, 1999).

Ependymoma

Ependymomas are tumors derived from cells that line the ventricular system, and they may be found in either a supratentorial or an infratentorial location. Infratentorial ependymoma is discussed in Chapter 10 because the initial symptom is often ataxia. However, symptoms of increased intracranial pressure are the first feature in 90% of children with posterior fossa ependymoma, and papilledema is present in 75% at the time of initial examination. Approximately 60% of children with ependymoma are younger than 5 years old at the time of diagnosis, and only 4% are older than 15 years. As a rule, children with infratentorial ependymoma are younger than children with supratentorial ependymoma.

The expected location of supratentorial ependymoma is in relation to the third and lateral ventricles. However, ependymal tumors may arise within the hemispheres at a site distant from the ventricular system. Such tumors are thought to be derived from ependymal cell rests.

CLINICAL FEATURES. Symptoms of increased intracranial pressure are less prominent with supratentorial tumors than with infratentorial tumors. Common manifestations are focal weakness, seizures, and visual disturbances. Papilledema is a common physical finding in all patients with ependymoma. Hemiparesis, hyperreflexia, and hemianopia are typical features, but some children show only ataxia. The duration of symptoms before diagnosis averages only 7 months but can be as little as 1 month for

malignant tumors and as long as several years for low-grade tumors.

DIAGNOSIS. Tumor density on CT is usually greater than brain density, and contrast enhancement is present. Small cysts within the tumor are relatively common. Approximately one third of supratentorial ependymomas contain calcium.

Tumors within the third ventricle cause marked dilatation of the lateral ventricles, with edema of the hemispheres and obliteration of sulcal markings. High-grade tumors are likely to seed the subarachnoid space, producing metastases in the spinal cord and throughout the ventricular system. In such cases, tumor cells may line the lateral ventricles and produce a "cast" of contrast enhancement around the ventricles.

MANAGEMENT. Complete surgical resection is possible in only 30% of cases. Even after complete resection, the 5-year rate of progression-free survival is between 60% and 80%. Survival relates directly to the effectiveness of surgical removal followed by either radiation therapy or chemotherapy (Pollack et al, 1995). Neuraxis radiation therapy is not recommended unless leptomeningeal disease is already present at the time of diagnosis. No chemotherapy protocol has proven useful.

Primitive Neuroectodermal Tumors

Primitive neuroectodermal tumors (PNET) are tumors of childhood consisting of small, undifferentiated, darkly staining cells that have neuronal, glial, and mesenchymal elements. Medulloblastoma is now classified as an infratentorial PNET. This section deals with supratentorial PNET tumors. Medulloblastoma is dealt with in Chapter 10.

CLINICAL FEATURES. Age at onset may be anytime during childhood but is usually the first decade. Males and females are affected equally. Because these tumors are highly malignant, the progression of symptoms is rapid and the time to diagnosis is usually less than 3 months. Approximately half of children show features of increased intracranial pressure. Other manifestations are determined by the tumor site. Two thirds of tumors are located in the frontal or parietal lobe. Seizures, monoparesis, hemiplegia, and ophthalmoplegia are initial features in approximately 10% of patients. Hydrocephalus or head enlargement is unusual early in the course.

DIAGNOSIS. On CT, PNET are high-density lesions that enhance and produce hydrocephalus. The tumor mass is surrounded by cerebral edema, and midline structures are frequently shifted under the falx. MRI shows homogeneous to mixed signal intensity in the tumor. On T_2-weighted images, the lesions are nearly isointense to brain parenchyma, but they enhance intensely after contrast administration.

MANAGEMENT. Cerebral edema may be relieved by the use of dexamethasone. Complete tumor resection is attempted but rarely accomplished. PNETs are radiosensitive and may respond transiently to chemotherapy. Radiation of the entire craniospinal axis is required. Survival is usually less than 1 year. Several chemotherapeutic trials are ongoing.

Pineal Region Tumors

Tumors in the pineal region may be derived from several histological types. Germ cell tumors are the most common, followed by tumors of the pineal parenchyma. The incidence of pineal region tumors is 10 times higher in Japan than in the United States or Western Europe. Pineal region tumors are more common in boys than in girls and generally become symptomatic during the second decade.

CLINICAL FEATURES. Because pineal region tumors are in a midline location, where they can invade or compress the third ventricle or aqueduct, symptoms of increased intracranial pressure are common. The first symptoms may be acute and accompanied by midbrain dysfunction. Midbrain dysfunction resulting from pressure by pineal region tumors on the periaqueductal gray is usually referred to as *Parinaud syndrome*: loss of pupillary light reflex, supranuclear palsy of upward gaze with preservation of downward gaze, and retraction-convergence nystagmus when upward gaze is attempted. Eventually, paralysis of both upward and downward gaze and loss of accommodation may occur.

Tumors growing into or compressing the anterior hypothalamus produce loss of vision, diabetes insipidus, precocious puberty, and emaciation. Precocious puberty occurs almost exclusively in males. Extension of tumor into the posterior fossa produces multiple cranial neuropathies and ataxia, and lateral extension causes hemiparesis.

DIAGNOSIS. Pineal germinomas are well circumscribed and relatively homogeneous. On MRI, they are of low signal intensity on T_2-weighted images, and they enhance markedly with intravenous contrast. Teratomas appear lobulated and have both hyperdense and multicystic areas. Calcification may be present, and contrast enhancement is not uniform. Tumors that spread into the ventricular system and have intense contrast enhancement are likely to be malignant. Tumors that contain abundant amounts of calcium are likely to be benign.

Asymptomatic nonneoplastic pineal cysts are sometimes identified by CT or MRI in children who are being imaged for other reasons. These are developmental variants of the pineal gland that may contain calcium. Only rarely do they grow to sufficient size to obstruct the aqueduct or cause a Parinaud syndrome.

MANAGEMENT. Stereotactic biopsy is essential to establish the histological type and plan therapy. Ventricular drainage may be needed to relieve hydrocephalus. Germinomas are highly radiosensitive, and 5-year survival rates of 50% to 80% are reported. Other tumors of the pineal region are less radiosensitive. Complete surgical removal of pineal region tumors was discouraged in the past because mortality and morbidity rates were prohibitively high. Improved surgical techniques now allow successful removal in many cases.

Other Tumors

Cerebral metastatic disease is unusual in childhood. Tumors that produce cerebral metastases most frequently are osteogenic sarcoma and rhabdomyosarcoma in patients younger than 15 years old and testicular germ cell tumors after age 15. The cerebral hemispheres are affected more often than posterior fossa structures. Pulmonary involvement always precedes cerebral metastasis. Brain metastasis is rarely present at the time of initial cancer diagnosis.

Meningioma is uncommon in children. The initial features may be focal neurological signs, seizures, or increased intracranial pressure (Mallucci et al, 1996).

Intracranial Arachnoid Cysts

Primary arachnoid cysts are cavities that are within the arachnoid and are filled with cerebrospinal fluid. The cause of cyst formation is uncertain, but cysts are generally considered a minor disturbance in arachnoid formation and not a pathological process. Arachnoid cysts are identified in 0.5% of postmortem examinations:

two thirds are supratentorial and one third are infratentorial.

CLINICAL FEATURES. Most cysts are asymptomatic structures identified by CT or MRI. Deciding whether the cyst is the cause of the symptom for which the imaging study was ordered is sometimes a problem. Subarachnoid cysts are usually present from infancy, but may develop, or at least enlarge enough to be detected, during adolescence.

Large cysts can produce symptoms by compressing adjacent structures or by increasing intracranial pressure. Focal neurological disturbances vary with the location but are most often hemiparesis or seizures when the cyst is supratentorial and ataxia when infratentorial. Compression of the parietal lobe from early infancy may result in undergrowth of contralateral limbs.

Increased intracranial pressure can be caused by mass effect or hydrocephalus and is associated with cysts in all locations. Manifestations include macrocephaly, headache, and behavioral change.

DIAGNOSIS. It has become common for children with headache, learning or behavioral disorders, and suspected seizures to undergo imaging studies of the brain. Many have incidental arachnoid cysts. A cause-and-effect relationship should be considered only if the cyst is large and if it clearly explains the symptoms. Positron emission tomography (PET) may be useful in deciding whether an arachnoid cyst is having a pressure effect on the brain. Brain compression sufficient to disturb function is characterized by hypometabolism in the surrounding brain.

MANAGEMENT. Simple drainage of the cyst often results in reaccumulation of fluid and recurrence of symptoms. Superficial cysts can be excised and deeply located cysts shunted into the peritoneal space.

Intracranial Hemorrhage

Head Trauma

Head trauma is a major cause of intracranial hemorrhage from the newborn period through childhood and adolescence. It is associated with intracerebral hemorrhage, subarachnoid hemorrhage, subdural hematoma, and epidural hematoma. Increased intracranial pressure is a constant feature of intracranial hemorrhage and also occurs from cerebral edema following concussion without hemorrhage. Intracranial hem-

orrhage from head trauma is discussed in Chapter 2.

Intraventricular Hemorrhage in the Newborn

Intraventricular hemorrhage is primarily a disorder of live-born premature newborns with respiratory distress syndrome. The autoregulation of cerebral blood flow, which meets local tissue needs by altering cerebrovascular resistance, is impaired in premature newborns with respiratory distress syndrome. During episodes of systemic hypotension, cerebral blood flow is decreased and the potential for cerebral infarction exists. Such infarctions usually occur symmetrically in the white matter adjacent to the lateral ventricles and are termed *periventricular leukomalacia* (Volpe, 1998).

During episodes of systemic hypertension, cerebral blood flow increases. Hemorrhage occurs first in the subependymal germinal matrix and then bursts through the ependymal lining into the lateral ventricle. Such hemorrhages are called *periventricular-intraventricular hemorrhages*. The predilection of the germinal matrix for hemorrhage during episodes of increased cerebral blood flow has not been fully explained. The likely explanation is prior ischemic injury that weakens the capillary walls and their supporting structures, making them vulnerable to rupture during episodes of increased cerebral blood flow.

Intraventricular hemorrhage also occurs in full-term newborns, but the mechanism of hemorrhage at term is different from that before term.

Periventricular-Intraventricular Hemorrhage in Premature Newborns

The incidence of periventricular-intraventricular hemorrhage (PIVH) in premature newborns whose birth weight is less than 2,000 g has been declining. The reason for the decline is not fully explained but is probably attributable to advances in ventilatory care. PIVH is still identified in approximately 20% of premature newborns with a birth weight of less than 1,500 g (Roland and Hill, 1997) and in more than half of premature newborns with birth weights between 500 and 700 g.

I. Isolated subependymal hemorrhage

II. Intraventricular hemorrhage without ventricular dilatation

III. Intraventricular hemorrhage with ventricular dilatation

IV. Intraventricular hemorrhage with ventricular dilatation and hemorrhage into the parenchyma of the brain

Hemorrhage into the parenchyma of the brain (grade IV) is a coexistent process caused by hemorrhagic infarction (*periventricular hemorrhagic infarction*) and is not an extension of the first three grades of intraventricular hemorrhage.

CLINICAL FEATURES. Routine ultrasound examinations are now the standard of care for all newborns whose birth weight is 1,800 g or less. Ultrasound often shows PIVH in newborns in whom there was no clinical suspicion of hemorrhage. Among this group, some have blood in the cerebrospinal fluid and others have clear cerebrospinal fluid. Only newborns with grade III or IV hemorrhage have predictable clinical features.

In some premature newborns, PIVH produces rapid neurological deterioration characterized by decreasing states of consciousness, severe hypotonia, and respiratory insufficiency. Within minutes to hours the infant shows obvious evidence of increased intracranial pressure: bulging fontanelle, decerebrate posturing, loss of pupillary reflexes, and respiratory arrest. Hypothermia, bradycardia, hypotension, and a 10% fall in the hematocrit may be associated features.

More commonly the hemorrhage is manifested by stepwise progression of symptoms over a period of hours or even days. The initial symptoms are subtle and include a change in behavior, diminished spontaneous movement, and either an increase or a decrease in appendicular tone. The fontanelles remain soft, and vital signs are stable. These first symptoms may correspond to grade I hemorrhage. Some newborns then become stable and have no further difficulty. Others undergo clinical deterioration characterized by hypotonia and declining consciousness. This deterioration probably corresponds to the presence of blood in the ventricles. The child becomes lethargic or obtunded and then may stabilize. If continued bleeding causes acute ventricular dilatation, apnea and coma follow. Seizures occur when blood dissects into the cerebral parenchyma.

Newborns with PIVH are at risk for progressive hydrocephalus. The likelihood is much greater among children with grade III or IV hemorrhage. Initial ventricular dilatation is probably due to plugging of the arachnoid villi and impaired reabsorption of cerebrospinal fluid. The ventricles can enlarge by compressing the brain without causing a measurable change in head circumference. Therefore weekly ultrasound studies are imperative to follow the progression of hydrocephalus.

DIAGNOSIS. Ultrasound is the standard for the diagnosis of intraventricular hemorrhage in the newborn. Ultrasound is preferred over other brain imaging techniques because it can be performed in the intensive care nursery, study time is briefer, and no radiation is involved. MRI during infancy or childhood is useful to show the extent of brain damage from the combination of periventricular leukomalacia and PIVH.

PREVENTION. Prevention is the best treatment for PIVH. This can be accomplished, to a great extent, by preventing prematurity and by delivering premature newborns at specialized perinatal centers (Table 4-6). A premature newborn transported to an intensive care nursery has a far greater chance of hemorrhage than a fetus transported to the delivery room in utero. Normal tension of carbon dioxide and oxygen, normal osmolality and viscosity, normal perfusion pressure without episodic hypertension from undue stimulation, and good ventilatory control in the early hours postpartum can best be maintained in a specialized neonatal unit.

Muscle paralysis with pancuronium bromide in ventilated premature newborns reduces the incidence and severity of PIVH by stabilizing fluctuations of cerebral blood flow velocity. Phenobarbital may dampen fluctuations of systemic blood pressure and cerebral blood flow, and indomethacin inhibits prostaglandin synthesis,

---

Table 4-6
Prevention of Periventricular-Intraventricular Hemorrhage

Antenatal
Delivery in specialized center
Prevention of prematurity

Postnatal
Avoidance of rapid volume expansion
Correction of coagulation abnormalities
Maintenance of stable systemic blood pressure
Muscle paralysis of ventilated premature newborns
Potential pharmacological agents
   Indomethacin
   Phenobarbital

thereby regulating cerebral blood flow. The efficacy of both agents is inconclusive.

Extension of hemorrhage occurs in 20% to 40% of cases. Serial ultrasounds are needed for early diagnosis of posthemorrhagic hydrocephalus that develops in 10% to 15% of premature newborns with PIVH. Factors that influence the management of posthemorrhagic hydrocephalus are the rate of progression, ventricular size, and intracranial pressure. The hydrocephalus ultimately arrests or regresses in 50% of children and progresses to severe hydrocephalus in the remainder. Rapid ventricular enlargement requires intervention in less than 4 weeks.

MANAGEMENT. Once intraventricular hemorrhage has occurred, treatment is directed at preventing or stabilizing progressive posthemorrhagic hydrocephalus. The efficacy of treatment for posthemorrhagic hydrocephalus is difficult to assess because the role of ventricular dilatation in causing chronic neurological impairment is not established. Newborns with progressive posthemorrhagic hydrocephalus have also experienced asphyxial encephalopathy, germinal matrix hemorrhage, and periventricular leukomalacia. Neurological morbidity correlates better with the degree of parenchymal damage than with ventricular size.

The definitive treatment is placement of a ventriculoperitoneal shunt. However, early shunt placement, while the ventricles still contain blood, has a high incidence of shunt failure and infection. Therefore, temporizing measures are often needed. These measures include cerebrospinal fluid drainage by serial lumbar punctures, external ventriculostomy, and drugs that reduce cerebrospinal fluid production (carbonic anhydrase inhibitors and diuretics [acetazolamide and furosemide]).

Intraventricular Hemorrhage at Term

Unlike intraventricular hemorrhage in the premature newborn, which originates almost exclusively from the germinal matrix, intraventricular hemorrhage at term may originate from the veins of the choroid plexus, from the germinal matrix, or both.

CLINICAL FEATURES. Full-term newborns with intraventricular hemorrhage may be divided into two groups. More than half are delivered with difficulty, frequently in the breech position, and have suffered some degree of intrauterine asphyxia. These newborns are usually bruised and require resuscitation. At first they appear to be improving, and then multifocal seizures occur on the second day postpartum. The fontanelle is tense, and the cerebrospinal fluid is bloody.

The other half has experienced neither trauma nor asphyxia and appears normal at birth. During the first hours postpartum, however, apnea, cyanosis, and a tense fontanelle develop. The mechanism of hemorrhage is not understood. Posthemorrhagic hydrocephalus is common in both groups, and 35% require shunt placement.

DIAGNOSIS. Ultrasound is as useful for diagnosis of intraventricular hemorrhage in full-term newborns as in premature newborns.

MANAGEMENT. Full-term newborns with intraventricular hemorrhage are treated in the same manner as premature newborns with intraventricular hemorrhage.

Arterial Aneurysms

Arterial aneurysms are vestiges of the embryonic circulation and are present in a rudimentary form before birth. Only rarely do they rupture during childhood. Symptomatic arterial aneurysms in childhood may be associated with coarctation of the aorta or polycystic kidney disease. Aneurysms tend to be located at the bifurcation of major arteries at the base of the brain.

CLINICAL FEATURES. Subarachnoid hemorrhage is usually the first feature of a ruptured aneurysm. The initial symptoms may be catastrophic: sudden loss of consciousness, tachycardia, hypotension, and evidence of increased intracranial pressure, but in most patients the first bleeding is a "warning leak" that may go unrecognized. The warning leak is characterized by severe headache, stiff neck, and low-grade fever. Occasionally aneurysms produce neurological signs by exerting pressure on adjacent cranial nerves. The oculomotor nerve is most frequently affected, resulting in disturbances of gaze and pupillary function.

Physical activity is not related to the time of rupture. Aneurysmal size is the main predictor of rupture; those smaller than 1 cm in diameter have a low probability of rupture.

The patient's state of consciousness is the most important predictor of survival. Approximately 50% of patients die during the first hospitalization, some from the initial hemorrhage during the first 14 days. Untreated, another 30% die from recurrent hemorrhage in the next 10 years.

Unruptured aneurysms may cause acute severe headache without nuchal rigidity. The mechanism of headache may be aneurysmal thrombosis or localized meningeal inflammation.

DIAGNOSIS. On the day of aneurysmal rupture, CT shows intracranial hemorrhage in all patients, but the blood is rapidly reabsorbed and can be demonstrated in only two thirds on the fifth day. Most aneurysms can be visualized by standard MRI or by MRI angiography (MRA).

Lumbar puncture is often performed because the stiff neck, headache, and fever suggest bacterial meningitis. The fluid is usually grossly bloody and therefore indicative of subarachnoid hemorrhage. Unfortunately, blood in the cerebrospinal fluid is often attributed to a traumatic tap when time is not taken to centrifuge the fluid and examine it for xanthochromia. Once a diagnosis of subarachnoid hemorrhage is established, all vessels must be visualized in order to determine the aneurysmal site and the presence of multiple aneurysms. Four-vessel cerebral arteriography had been the standard imaging study, but improved MRA technology may replace angiography.

MANAGEMENT. The definitive treatment is surgical clipping and excision of the aneurysm. Early surgery is recommended in conscious patients to prevent rebleeding (Olafsson et al, 1997). Cerebral vasospasm and ischemia are the leading causes of death and disability among survivors of an initial aneurysm rupture. Pharmacological means to prevent rebleeding are becoming less important as early operative intervention is practiced. Medical therapy for the prevention and treatment of vasospasm includes a regimen of volume expansion and induced systemic hypertension. Nimodipine is effective for the prevention of delayed ischemia.

The 6-month survival rate in patients who are conscious at the time of admission is approximately 86%. In contrast, only 20% of patients who are comatose on admission are alive 6 months later.

Arteriovenous Malformations

Approximately 0.1% of children have an arteriovenous malformation, of which 12% to 18% become symptomatic in childhood (Menovsky and van Overbeeke, 1997). No familial occurrence has been documented. Two types of malformations are described. One type arises early in gestation from an abnormal communication between primitive choroidal arteries and veins.

Such malformations are in the midline and give rise to the vein of Galen malformation, malformations involving the choroid plexus, and shunts between cerebellar arteries and the straight sinus. The other type arises later in gestation or even after birth between superficial arteries and veins and results in an arteriovenous malformation within the parenchyma of the cerebral hemisphere. The vessels of the scalp, skull, and dura are interconnected, causing anastomotic channels between the extracranial and intracranial circulations to remain patent. Approximately 90% of arteriovenous malformations are supratentorial and 10% are infratentorial.

Deep Midline Malformations

Large deep midline malformations, especially those involving the great vein of Galen, produce hydrocephalus and cardiac failure during infancy. They rarely bleed (Meyers et al, 2000). These malformations are discussed in Chapter 18.

CLINICAL FEATURES. Small, deep midline malformations are rarely symptomatic in childhood. The initial feature is often caused by bleeding into the parenchyma of the brain or into the subarachnoid space. Bleeding occurs when secondary venous changes reroute the drainage to the pial veins. Because the bleeding is from the venous rather than the arterial side of the malformation, the initial symptoms are not as catastrophic as with arterial aneurysms. Symptoms may evolve over several hours, and no characteristic clinical syndrome has been established. Most patients describe sudden severe headache, neck stiffness, and vomiting. Fever is frequently an associated symptom. The presence of focal neurological deficits depends on the location of the malformation and may include hemiparesis, sensory disturbances, and oculomotor palsies. Many patients recover completely from the first hemorrhage; the risk of recurrent hemorrhage is small.

DIAGNOSIS. Most arteriovenous malformations are easily visualized on MRI or CT with contrast enhancement. The degree of ventricular enlargement is shown by either study. Four-vessel arteriography is required to define all arterial and venous channels, but may be replaced by MRA as the technology improves.

MANAGEMENT. Microsurgical excision should be performed whenever feasible. Deep midline malformations are usually managed by venous embolization. The results vary with the size and location of the malformation.

Supratentorial Malformations

CLINICAL FEATURES. Among children with arteriovenous malformations in and around the cerebral hemispheres, the initial feature is intracranial hemorrhage in half and seizures in the other half. Recurrent vascular headache may precede the onset of hemorrhage and seizures or may develop concurrently. Headaches are usually unilateral but may not occur consistently on the same side. In some patients the headaches have a migraine quality: scintillating scotoma and unilateral throbbing pain. The incidence of such migraine-like headaches in patients with arteriovenous malformations does not appear to be greater than in the population at large. The malformation probably provokes a migraine attack in people who are genetically predisposed.

Most patients who have seizures have at least one focal seizure, but among the seizures associated with arteriovenous malformations, half are focal and half are generalized. No specific location of the malformation is associated with a higher incidence of seizures. However, small superficial malformations, especially in the centroparietal region, are associated with the highest incidence of hemorrhage. Hemorrhage may be only subarachnoid or may dissect into the brain parenchyma.

DIAGNOSIS. MRI and contrast-enhanced CT provide excellent visualization of the malformation in most children. Four-vessel arteriography is required to define all arterial and venous channels, but it may be replaced by MRA as the technology improves.

MANAGEMENT. The photon knife is becoming the standard of treatment for small malformations. Other options for management include microsurgical excision and embolization. Superficial malformations are more accessible for direct surgical excision than those deep in the midline. In considering treatment modes, the physician must balance the decision to do something against the decision to do nothing based on the likelihood of further bleeding and the morbidity due to intervention.

Cocaine Abuse

Intracranial hemorrhage is associated with cocaine abuse, especially crack, in young adults. The hemorrhages may be subarachnoid or intracerebral in location and are thought to be caused by sudden transitory increases in systemic blood pressure.

Infectious Disorders

Infections of the brain and meninges produce increased intracranial pressure by causing cerebral edema, by obstructing the flow and reabsorption of cerebrospinal fluid, and by impairing venous outflow. Symptoms of increased intracranial pressure are frequently the initial features of bacterial and fungal infections and may also be the initial feature of viral encephalitis. However, viral infections are more likely to cause seizures, personality change, or decreased consciousness and therefore are discussed in Chapter 2.

Bacterial Meningitis

The offending organism and the clinical features of bacterial meningitis vary with age (Table 4-7). Therefore it is useful to discuss the syndromes of bacterial meningitis by age group: newborn, infants and young children (28 days to 5 years), and school-age children.

Meningitis in the Newborn

Meningitis occurs in approximately 1 per 2,000 term newborns and 3 per 1,000 premature newborns and accounts for up to 4% of all neonatal deaths. It is a consequence of septicemia, and organs other than the brain are infected. Maternal infection is the main risk factor for sepsis and meningitis.

An early-onset (first 5 days) and a late-onset (after 5 days) pattern of meningitis have been identified in newborns. In early-onset meningitis

Table 4-7
Most Common Organisms Responsible for Bacterial Meningitis

Newborn
Escherichia coli
Group B *Streptococcus*
Listeria monocytogenes
Other enterobacteriaceae

Infancy and Preschool
Haemophilus influenzae
Mycobacterium tuberculosis
Neisseria meningitidis
Streptococcus pneumoniae

School Age
Mycobacterium tuberculosis
Neisseria meningitides
Streptococcus pneumoniae

the infection is acquired at the time of delivery, and the responsible organisms are almost always *Escherichia coli* or group B *Streptococcus*. The child becomes symptomatic during the first week, and the mortality rate is 20% to 50%. In late-onset meningitis the infection is acquired postnatally, and symptoms may begin as early as the fourth day postpartum but usually begin after the first week. Newborns requiring intensive care are specifically at risk for late-onset meningitis because infection is introduced by instrumentation. The responsible organisms are not only *E. coli* and group B *Streptococcus*, but also enterococci, gram-negative enteric bacilli (*Pseudomonas* and *Klebsiella*), and *Listeria monocytogenes*. The mortality rate is 10% to 20%.

CLINICAL FEATURES. Newborns infected in utero or during delivery may experience respiratory distress and shock within 24 hours of birth. Other features that may be associated with septicemia include hyperthermia, hypothermia, jaundice, hepatomegaly, lethargy, anorexia, and vomiting.

In meningitis of late onset the clinical manifestations are variable. Initial symptoms are usually nonspecific and include lethargy, disturbed feeding, and irritability. As the meningitis worsens, hyperthermia, respiratory distress or apnea, and seizures are present in about half of newborns, but bulging of the fontanelle occurs in only a quarter, and nuchal rigidity is unusual. Shock is the usual cause of death.

DIAGNOSIS. The diagnosis of septicemia and meningitis in the newborn is often difficult to establish on the basis of symptoms. Lumbar puncture must be prompted by the first suspicion of septicemia. Even in the absence of infection the cerebrospinal fluid of febrile newborns contains an average of 11 leukocytes/mm³, with a range of 0 to 20. Less than 6% are polymorphonuclear leukocytes. The protein concentration has a mean value of 84 mg/dl (0.84 g/L),

with a range from 40 to 130 mg/dl (0.4 to 1.3 g/L), and the glucose concentration has a mean value of 46 mg/dl (0.46 g/L), with a range from 36 to 56 mg/dl (0.36 to 0.56 g/L).

In newborns with meningitis the leukocyte count is usually in the thousands, and the protein concentration may vary from less than 30 mg/dl (0.3 g/L) to more than l,000 mg/dl (10 g/L). A Gram-stained smear of cerebrospinal fluid permits identification of an organism in less than half of cases. Even when the smear is positive, identification may be inaccurate.

Rapid detection of bacterial antigens by immunoelectrophoresis, latex agglutination, and radioimmunoassays also may be useful (Trujillo and McCracken, 1997).

MANAGEMENT. Treatment is initiated with the first suspicion of sepsis. Laboratory confirmation is not required. The choice of initial antibiotic coverage varies but usually includes ampicillin and either gentamicin or cefotaxime. All antibiotics are administered intravenously in divided doses (Table 4-8). If an organism is grown on culture, specific therapy is initiated.

E. coli is best treated with ampicillin and cefotaxime, group B *Streptococcus* with penicillin or ampicillin, and *Klebsiella pneumoniae* with cefotaxime and an aminoglycoside. *Pseudomonas* is difficult to eradicate, and combined intravenous and intrathecal therapy may be required. Carbenicillin and gentamicin are preferred for intravenous use.

Neonatal meningitis is treated for at least 2 weeks beyond the time the cerebrospinal fluid becomes sterile. Two days after antibiotic therapy is discontinued, the cerebrospinal fluid should be cultured again. If the culture is positive for bacteria, a second course of therapy is indicated.

Citrobacter diversus infections often cause a hemorrhagic necrosis of the brain, with liquefaction of the cerebral white matter and abscess

Table 4-8
Intravenous Antibiotic Dosages for Newborns

Drug	0–7 Days	8–28 Days
Ampicillin	100–150 mg/kg/day (q12h)	150–200 mg/kg/day (q8h)
Cefotaxime	100 mg/kg/day (q8h)	150–200 mg/kg/day (q8h)
Ceftaxidime	60 mg/kg/day (q12h)	90 mg/kg/day (q8h)
Gentamicin	5 mg/kg/day (q12h)	7.5 mg/kg/day (q8h)
Methacillin	100–150 mg/kg/day (q8h)	15–200 mg/kg/day (q6h)
Penicillin G	100,000–150,000 U/kg (q12h)	150,000–400,000 U/kg/day (q8h)
Vancomycin	20 mg/kg/day (q12h)	40–60 mg/kg/day (q6h)

formation. These abscesses are readily identified on CT. Surgical drainage is seldom indicated and could cause further damage to the overlying preserved cortex.

Mortality is between 20% and 30% and is highest for gram-negative infections. The type of infecting organism and the gestational age of the infant are the main variables that determine mortality. Permanent neurological sequelae occur in 30% to 50% of survivors and include hydrocephalus, cerebral palsy, epilepsy, mental retardation, and deafness. Even when the head circumference is normal, follow-up CT is often needed to exclude underlying hydrocephalus.

Meningitis in Infants and Young Children

For children 6 weeks to 3 months of age, group B *Streptococcus* remains a leading cause of meningitis and *E. coli* becomes less common. The other important organism is *Neisseria meningitidis* (Riordan et al, 1995). *H. influenzae*, which had been an important pathogen after 3 months of age, has almost disappeared because of routine immunization. *Streptococcus pneumoniae* and *Neisseria meningitides* are now the principal causes of meningitis in children older than 1 month (Quagliarello and Scheld, 1997).

CLINICAL FEATURES. The onset of meningitis may be insidious or fulminating. The typical clinical findings include fever, irritability, and neck stiffness. A bulging fontanelle is noted in young infants. Headache, vomiting, and lethargy are the initial features after the fontanelle has closed. Seizures occur in about a third of children with meningitis. They usually occur during the first 24 hours of illness and may be the initial feature that brings the child to medical attention. Once seizures have occurred, the state of consciousness declines. Seizures can be focal or generalized and may be difficult to control.

Examination reveals a sick and irritable child who resists being touched or moved. Ophthalmoscopic findings are usually normal or show only minimal papilledema. Focal neurological signs are unusual except in tuberculous meningitis or in cases when abscess formation has occurred.

The rapidity with which neurological function declines depends on the severity of cerebral edema and cerebral vasculitis. Death may ensue from brainstem compression caused by transtentorial herniation. Peripheral vascular collapse can result from brainstem herniation, endotoxic shock, or adrenal failure. Sixty percent of children with meningococcemia have a characteristic petechial or hemorrhagic rash. The rash, although generalized, is most prominent below the waist.

Neck stiffness, characterized by limited mobility and pain on attempted flexion of the head, is caused by meningeal irritation. Other signs of meningeal irritation are those of Kernig and Brudzinski. Both are tested with the patient supine. The *Kernig sign* is marked by pain and resistance to extending the knee with the leg flexed at the hip; the *Brudzinski sign* is spontaneous flexion at the hips when the neck is passively flexed. These signs of meningeal irritation can be noted in subarachnoid hemorrhage as well as in infectious meningitis.

DIAGNOSIS. Lumbar puncture and examination of the cerebrospinal fluid are essential for the diagnosis of bacterial meningitis. However, because bacterial meningitis is often associated with septicemia, cultures of the blood, urine, and nasopharynx are indicated as well. The peripheral white blood cell count, especially immature granulocytes, is usually increased. Peripheral leukocytosis is much more common in bacterial than in viral infections but does not rule out viral meningitis. The platelet count is important because some infections are associated with thrombocytopenia. The blood glucose concentration must be measured concurrently for proper evaluation of the cerebrospinal fluid concentration of glucose. Serum electrolytes, especially sodium, should be measured as well. Inappropriate antidiuretic hormone secretion is present in the majority of patients with acute bacterial meningitis. A tuberculin skin test should be administered to every child at risk for tuberculous meningitis.

Lumbar puncture must be performed as quickly as possible when bacterial meningitis is suspected. It has become routine to perform a cranial CT before doing a lumbar puncture, a routine that is of questionable value medically and adds considerably to the cost of care. When the need for CT scanning significantly delays lumbar puncture, blood cultures should be obtained and antibiotic therapy administered. Generalized increased intracranial pressure is always part of acute bacterial meningitis and is not a contraindication to lumbar puncture.

Information to be derived from the procedure includes opening and closing pressures, appearance, white blood cell count with differential count, red blood cell count, concentrations of glucose and protein, and identification of microorganisms as shown by Gram stain and culture. The characteristic findings are increased pressure, a cloudy appearance, a cellular response of several thousand polymorphonuclear leukocytes, a reduction in the concentration of glucose to less than half of that in the plasma, and an elevated protein concentration. However, the expected findings of bacterial meningitis may vary with the organism, the timing of the lumbar puncture, the prior use of antibiotics, and the immunocompetence of the host.

MANAGEMENT. Antimicrobials and dexamethasone should be administered immediately. Treatment should not be delayed until after the results of lumbar puncture are obtained. Dexamethasone is administered at the rate of 15 mg/kg every 6 hours for 2 days (McIntyre et al, 1997). Children treated with dexamethasone become afebrile more quickly and have an improved neurological outcome and a lower incidence of postmeningitic deafness.

Ampicillin and a cephalosporin (cefotaxime, ceftriaxone, and cefuroxime) are now considered the therapy of choice in the initial treatment of meningitis. Gram stain identification is useful but can be misleading, and the final choice of antibiotic therapy should await the results of culture and antibiotic sensitivity.

Several special cases exist in the choice of initial antimicrobials to treat bacterial meningitis. Meningitis in children with a ventricular shunt in place is usually caused by a staphylococcal species, and nafcillin may be added to the preceding choices or given alone if gram-positive cocci are present on smear. Anaerobic and aerobic organisms frequently cause meningitis secondary to chronic sinusitis or dental infection. Penicillin G and chloramphenicol are therefore reasonable choices for initial therapy, although cefotaxime may be needed for some gram-negative organisms not covered by chloramphenicol. Meningitis following trauma is usually caused by *S. pneumoniae*, whereas meningitis following neurosurgical procedures may be due to either streptococcal or staphylococcal organisms. Gram-negative organisms may be responsible as well, and a combination of penicillin G and cefotaxime is recommended.

Once a specific organism is identified, an appropriate antibiotic or combination of antibiotics is then chosen (Table 4-9).

The outcome for infants and children with bacterial meningitis depends on the infecting organism and the speed with which appropriate antibiotic therapy is initiated. Ten percent of children have persistent bilateral or unilateral hearing loss following bacterial meningitis, and 4% have neurological deficits. The incidence of

Table 4-9
Intravenous Antibiotic Dosages for Children

Drug	Dosage
Amikacin	20–30 mg/kg/day (q8h)
Ampicillin	200–300 mg/kg/day (q6h)
Cefotaxime	200 mg/kg/day (q6h)
Ceftriaxone	80–100 mg/kg/day (q12h)
Ceftrazidime	125–150 mg/kg/day (q8h)
Chloramphenicol	75–100 mg/kg/day (q6h)
Gentamicin	7.5 mg/kg/day (q8h)
Penicillin G	250,000 units/kg/day (q6h)
Tobramycin	6 mg/kg/day (q8h)
Vancomycin	40–60 mg/kg/day (q6h)

hearing loss is 31% following infection with *S. pneumoniae* and 6% with *H. influenzae*. Hearing loss occurs early and is probably not related to the choice of antibiotic. Children with neurological deficits are at risk for epilepsy.

Meningitis in School-Age Children

S. pneumoniae and *N. meningitidis* account for most cases of bacterial meningitis in previously healthy school-age children in the United States, whereas *Mycobacterium tuberculosis* is a leading cause of meningitis in economically deprived populations. The symptoms of bacterial meningitis in school-age children do not differ substantially from those encountered in preschool children. The reader is referred to the previous section on clinical features and treatment.

In one retrospective study of children who had been treated for bacterial meningitis in the 1980s, 8.5% had major neurological deficits (mental retardation, seizures, hydrocephalus, cerebral palsy, blindness, or hearing loss) and 18.5% had learning disabilities (Grimwood et al, 1995).

Special Circumstances

Pneumococcus

Conditions associated with pneumococcal meningitis are otitis media, skull fractures, and sickle cell disease. Pneumovax is recommended for children with asplenia and chronic illnesses. Penicillin G and ampicillin are equally effective in treating meningitis caused by penicillin-sensitive strains of *S. pneumoniae*. Organisms resistant to both penicillin and ceftriaxone are treated with ceftriaxone combined with vanco-mycin.

Meningococcus

Vaccination is recommended for children with complement deficiency or asplenia. Prophylaxis for meningococcal meningitis is recommended for all household members who may have had saliva-exchange contact. A 2-day course of oral rifampin, 10 mg/kg every 12 hours for children 1 month to 12 years old and 5 mg/kg every 12 hours for infants younger than 1 month of age.

Tuberculous Meningitis

Worldwide, tuberculosis remains a leading cause of morbidity and death in children. In the United States, it represents less than 5% of bacterial meningitis cases in children but occurs with higher frequency where sanitation is poor. Children are infected by inhalation of the organism from adults. Tuberculosis occurs first in the lungs and is then disseminated to other organs within 6 months.

CLINICAL FEATURES. The peak incidence of tuberculous meningitis is between 6 months and 2 years of age. The first symptoms tend to be more insidious than with other bacterial meningitides, but they sometimes progress in a fulminating fashion. Tuberculous meningitis, unlike fungal meningitis, is not a cause of chronic meningitis. If not treated, a child with tuberculous meningitis will die within 3 to 5 weeks.

Most often, fever develops first and the child becomes listless and irritable. Irritability may be caused in part by headache, which is a common feature. Vomiting and abdominal pain are sometimes associated symptoms. Headache and vomiting increase in frequency and severity and are accompanied by signs of meningismus during the second week after onset of fever. Cerebral infarction occurs in 30% to 40% of affected children. Seizures may occur early, but more often they occur after meningismus is established. Consciousness declines progressively, and focal neurological deficits are noted. Most common are cranial neuropathies and hemipareses. Papilledema occurs relatively early in the course.

DIAGNOSIS. Tuberculosis must be considered in any child with a household contact. General use of tuberculin skin testing in children is critical to early detection. In the early stages, children with tuberculous meningitis may have only fever. The peripheral white blood cell count is generally elevated to between 10,000 and 20,000 cells/mm^3. Hyponatremia and hypochloremia are frequently present because of inappropriate secretion of antidiuretic hormone. The cerebrospinal fluid is usually cloudy and increased in pressure. The leukocyte count in the cerebrospinal fluid may range from 10 to 250 cells/mm^3 and rarely exceeds 500. Lymphocytes predominate. The glucose concentration declines throughout the course of the illness and is generally less than 35 mg/dl (1.8 mmol/L). Conversely, the protein concentration increases steadily and is usually greater than 100 mg/dl (1 g/L).

Smears of cerebrospinal fluid stained by the acid-fast technique generally demonstrate the bacillus. Recovery of the organism from the cerebrospinal fluid is not always successful even when guinea pig inoculation is used. Newer diagnostic tests include a polymerase chain reaction (PCR) technique with reported sensitivities of 70% to 75% and enzyme-linked immunosorbent assay (ELISA) and radioimmunoassay tests for antimycobacterial antigens in the cerebrospinal fluid.

MANAGEMENT. The prognosis for survival and for neurological recovery is enhanced by early treatment. Once a child's skin test is positive for the organism, isoniazid therapy is initiated even if the child is asymptomatic. Complete neurological recovery is unlikely once the child becomes comatose. Mortality rates of 20% are recorded even when treatment is initiated early.

The recommended initial drug regimen for treatment of tuberculous meningitis in the first 2 months is isoniazid, 20 mg/kg/day orally up to 500 mg/day; streptomycin, 20 mg/kg/day intramuscularly up to 1 g/day until drug susceptibility is known; rifampin, 15 mg/kg/day orally up to 600 mg/day, and pyrazinamide, 30 mg/kg/day. Isoniazid and rifampin are continued for an additional 10 months. The use of corticosteroids to reduce inflammation is appropriate to reduce inflammation and cerebral edema.

Communicating hydrocephalus is a common complication of tuberculous meningitis because of impaired reabsorption of cerebrospinal fluid. The size of the ventricles must be assessed by CT at periodic intervals and whenever unexplained deterioration of mental function occurs. Before the infection is brought under control, communicating hydrocephalus may be treated by repeated lumbar punctures and acetazolamide. In many cases, obstructive hydrocephalus develops later; in those cases, a surgical shunt is required.

Brain Abscess

The factors commonly predisposing to pyogenic brain abscess in children are meningitis, chronic otitis media, sinusitis, and congenital heart disease. Brain abscesses in the newborn are almost always the result of meningitis caused by *C. diversus* and other species of Enterobacteriaceae. Pyogenic abscesses in children younger than 5 months old but beyond the neonatal period are uncommon, and most often occur in children with hydrocephalus and shunt infection. The organisms most often responsible are species of *Staphylococcus*.

After 5 months of age the infecting organisms are diverse, and many abscesses contain a mixed flora. Coagulase-positive *S. aureus* and anaerobic *Streptococcus* are the organisms most frequently recovered, but no organism is recovered in up to 20% of cases.

CLINICAL FEATURES. The clinical features of brain abscess, like those of any other space-occupying lesion, depend on the age of the child and the location of the mass. Encapsulation of the abscess is preceded by a period of cerebritis characterized by fever, headache, and lethargy. Seizures may also occur, but in the absence of seizures the initial symptoms may not be severe enough to arouse suspicion of cerebral infection. If the period of cerebritis is not recognized, the initial clinical manifestations are the same as those of other mass lesions. Infants have abnormal head growth, a bulging fontanelle, failure to thrive, and sometimes seizures. Older children show signs of increased intracranial pressure and focal neurological dysfunction. Fever is present in only 60% of cases, and meningeal irritation is relatively uncommon. Therefore, on the basis of clinical features alone, pyogenic brain abscess is difficult to separate from other mass lesions such as brain tumor. About 80% of abscesses are in the cerebral hemispheres. Hemiparesis, hemianopia, and seizures are the usual clinical features. Cerebellar abscess most often results from chronic otitis and is manifest as nystagmus and ataxia.

DIAGNOSIS. The combination of headache and papilledema, with or without focal neurological dysfunction, suggests the possibility of a mass lesion and calls for CT. Most abscesses appear as an area of decreased density surrounded by a rim of intense enhancement referred to as a *ring lesion*. This lesion, although characteristic, is not diagnostic. Malignant brain tumors may have a similar appearance. Ring enhancement occurs during the late stages of cerebritis, just before capsule formation. After the capsule forms, the diameter of the ring decreases and the center becomes more hypodense. Multiple abscesses may be present.

MANAGEMENT. The development of CT has altered the management of cerebral abscess. Previously, surgical drainage was initiated as soon as abscess formation was identified. Now even encapsulated abscesses are treated medically and the patient's progress is followed with serial scans.

The initial step in treatment is to reduce brain swelling by the use of corticosteroids. This is followed by an intravenous antibiotic regimen that generally includes a penicillinase-resistant penicillin such as methicillin, 300 mg/kg/day, and chloramphenicol, 100 mg/kg/day. This combination is selected for its effectiveness against *Staphylococcus* and mixed gram-negative organisms. If an organism can be identified by culture of spinal fluid or blood, more specific antibiotic therapy is selected. In general, penicillin G is preferable to ampicillin if penicillin-sensitive organisms are recovered.

If medical therapy does not resolve the abscess, surgical drainage is necessary. Even in such cases, prolonged medical therapy before surgery increases the success of total excision.

Subdural and Epidural Empyema

Meningitis in infants and sinusitis in older children are the most common factors causing infection in the subdural space. The subdural space is sterile in children with bacterial meningitis but can become contaminated by organisms if a subdural tap is performed before the subarachnoid space is sterilized with antibiotics or by secondary thrombophlebitis of perforating cerebral veins. In older children, subdural and epidural abscesses are usually caused by penetrating head injuries or chronic mastoiditis.

Infections of the subdural space are difficult to contain and may extend over an entire hemisphere.

CLINICAL FEATURES. Subdural empyema produces increased intracranial pressure because of mass effect, cerebral edema, and vasculitis. Vasculitis leads to thrombosis of cortical veins, resulting in focal neurological dysfunction as well as increased intracranial pressure. Children with subdural infections are very sick. They have headache, fever, vomiting, seizures, and states of decreasing consciousness. Unilateral and alternating hemipareses are common. Children who are comatose have papilledema.

DIAGNOSIS. Subdural empyema should be suspected in children with meningitis whose condition declines after an initial period of recovery or in children who continue to have increased intracranial pressure of uncertain cause. Examination of the cerebrospinal fluid may not be helpful; sometimes the fluid is normal. The usual abnormality is a mixed cellular response, generally less than 100 cells/mm^3, with a lymphocytic predominance. The glucose concentration is normal, and the protein concentration is only mildly elevated.

CT is particularly helpful in showing a subdural or epidural abscess. The infected collection appears as a lens-shaped mass of increased lucency just beneath the skull. A shift of midline structures is generally present.

In infants, subdural puncture can provide a specimen of the abscess for identification of the organism. Subdural puncture can also be used to drain much of the abscess.

MANAGEMENT. The child with subdural or epidural empyema must be treated with corticosteroids to decrease intracranial pressure, antibiotics to eradicate the organisms, and anticonvulsants for seizures. Surgical drainage of subdural empyema was once considered an absolute necessity; it now appears that some patients can be treated medically, using CT to monitor progress.

Fungal Infections

Fungi exist in two forms: molds and yeasts. Molds are filamentous and divided into segments by hyphae. Yeasts are unicellular organisms surrounded by a thick cell wall and sometimes a capsule. Several fungi exist as yeast in tissue but are filamentous when grown in culture. Such fungi are said to be dimorphic. The common fungal pathogens are listed in Table 4-10.

Table 4-10
Common Fungal Pathogens

Yeast Forms
Candida
Cryptococcus neoformans

Dimorphic Forms
Blastomyces dermatitidis
Coccidioides immitis
Histoplasma capsulatum

Mold Forms
Aspergillus species

Fungal infections of the central nervous system may cause an acute, subacute, or chronic meningitis; solitary or multiple abscesses; and granulomas. Fungal infections of the nervous system are most common in children who are immunosuppressed, especially those with leukemia or acidosis. Fungal infections also occur in children who are immunocompetent. *Cryptococcus neoformans* and *Coccidioides immitis* are the leading causes of fungal meningitis in immunocompetent children.

Candidal Meningoencephalitis

Candida is a common inhabitant of the mouth, vagina, and intestinal tract. Ordinarily it causes no symptoms; however, it can multiply and become an important pathogen in children who are immunosuppressed, taking multiple antibiotics, suffering from debilitating diseases, transplant recipients, and critically ill neonates being treated with long-term vascular catheters. The most common sites of infection are the mouth (thrush), skin, and vagina. Candidal meningitis is almost unheard of in normal nonhospitalized children.

CLINICAL FEATURES. *Candida* reaches the brain and other organs by vascular dissemination. The brain is less often involved than other organs, and the prominent features of candidal sepsis include fever, lethargy, and vomiting. Hepatosplenomegaly and arthritis may be present.

Cerebral involvement can be in the form of meningitis, abscess formation, or both. The clinical features of meningoencephalitis are fever, vomiting, meningismus, papilledema, and seizures leading to states of decreased consciousness. In some individuals, a single large cerebral abscess forms that causes focal neurological dysfunction and papilledema.

DIAGNOSIS. Cerebral candidiasis should be suspected when unexplained fever develops in children with risk factors for disseminated disease. The organism can be isolated from blood, joint effusion fluid, or cerebrospinal fluid. When meningitis is present, a predominantly neutrophilic response is present in the cerebrospinal fluid associated with a protein concentration that is generally 100 mg/dl (1 g/L). The glucose concentration is only slightly reduced. Children who have a candidal abscess rather than meningitis are likely to have normal or near-normal cerebrospinal fluid. A mass lesion resembling a pyogenic abscess or tumor is seen on CT.

MANAGEMENT. When candidal infections develop in children because of indwelling vascular catheters, the catheter must be removed. Amphotericin B and flucytosine are used together and thought to have a synergistic effect. Dosages are the same as for other fungal infections, and the drugs should be administered for 6 to 12 weeks, depending on the efficacy of therapy and the presence of adverse reactions.

Coccidioidomycosis

C. immitis is endemic in the San Joaquin Valley of California and all southwestern states. Infection is caused by inhalation; almost 90% of individuals become infected within 10 years of moving into an endemic area. Only 40% of patients become symptomatic; the other 60% are identified only by a positive skin test.

CLINICAL FEATURES. Malaise, fever, cough, myalgia, and chest pain follow respiratory infection. The pulmonary infection is self-limited. The fungus is disseminated from the lung to other organs in only 1 person in 400. The dissemination rate is considerably higher in infants than in older children and adults.

Coccidioidal meningitis is almost always caused by hematogenous spread from lung to meninges but sometimes occurs by direct extension following infection of the skull. Symptoms of meningitis develop 2 to 4 weeks after respiratory symptoms begin. The main features are headache, apathy, and confusion. These symptoms may persist for weeks or months without concurrent seizures, meningismus, or focal neurological disturbances. If the meningitis is allowed to become chronic, hydrocephalus eventually develops because the basilar meningitis prevents reabsorption of cerebrospinal fluid.

DIAGNOSIS. Coccidioidal meningitis should be suspected in patients living in endemic areas when headache develops following an acute respiratory infection. Skin hypersensitivity among individuals living in an endemic area is not helpful, because a large percentage of the population is exposed and has a skin test positive for the organism. The cerebrospinal fluid generally demonstrates increased pressure and a lymphocytic cellular response of 50 to 500 cells/mm³. Eosinophils are frequently present as well. The protein concentration ranges from 100 to 500 mg/dl (1 to 5 g/L), and the glucose concentration is less than 35 mg/dl (1.8 mmol/L). The diagnosis is confirmed by isolation of the fungus, but this is often difficult to accomplish.

Complement-fixing antibodies in the cerebrospinal fluid are detected in 70% of cases, and positive culture results in less than half.

Table 4-11
Dosage Schedule for Amphotericin B

Amphotericin B is first administered intravenously in a single test dose of 0.1 mg/kg (not to exceed 1 mg) over at least 20 minutes to assess the child's temperature and blood pressure responses. If the response is acceptable, the first therapeutic dose of 0.25 mg/kg is administered over 2 hours the same day as the test dose. The dose is increased in daily increments of 0.1 to 0.25 mg/kg, depending on the severity of infection, until the daily maintenance dose of 1 mg/kg is achieved. In life-threatening situations, daily dosages of 1.25 to 1.5 mg/kg may be needed.

MANAGEMENT. Amphotericin B is the drug of choice for coccidioidal meningitis. It must be administered both intravenously (Table 4-11) and intrathecally. The initial intrathecal dose is 0.1 mg for the first three injections and is then increased to 0.25 to 0.5 mg three or four times each week. Treatment must be prolonged, and some recommend that weekly intrathecal injections be continued indefinitely. Adverse reactions to intrathecal administration include aseptic meningitis and pain in the back and legs. Miconazole may be administered intravenously and intrathecally to patients unable to tolerate high doses of amphotericin B.

Cryptococcal Meningitis

C. neoformans is carried by birds, especially pigeons, and is widely disseminated in soil. Human infection is acquired by inhalation. The organism is disseminated in the blood but has a predilection for the central nervous system. It is an important cause of subacute and chronic meningoencephalitis.

CLINICAL FEATURES. Cryptococcal meningitis is uncommon before age 10, and perhaps only 10% of cases occur before age 20. Males are affected more often than females. Most children with cryptococcal meningitis are immunocompetent.

The first symptoms are usually insidious; chronic headache is the major feature. The headache waxes and wanes, but eventually becomes continuous and associated with nausea, vomiting, and lethargy. Body temperature may remain normal, especially in older children and adults, but younger children often have low-grade fever. Personality and behavioral changes are relatively common. The child becomes moody, listless, and sometimes frankly psychotic. Increased intracranial pressure is characterized by blurred vision, diplopia, and papilledema. Seizures and focal neurological dysfunction are not early features but are signs of vasculitis, hydrocephalus, and granuloma formation.

DIAGNOSIS. The diagnosis of cryptococcal meningitis is often missed even when suspected. The cerebrospinal fluid may be normal but more often shows an increased opening pressure and a lymphocytic leukocytosis that generally averages fewer than 100 cells/mm^3. The protein concentration is almost always elevated, generally greater than 100 mg/dl (1 g/L), and the glucose concentration is usually less than 40 mg/dl (2 mmol/L).

The diagnosis of cryptococcal meningitis relies on detection of cryptococcal polysaccharide antigen by latex agglutination, demonstration of the organism in India ink preparations of cerebrospinal fluid, or cerebrospinal fluid culture. Approximately 50% of India ink preparations and 75% of culture results are positive. The latex agglutination test for cryptococcal polysaccharide antigen is sensitive and specific for cryptococcal infection.

MANAGEMENT. The treatment of choice is intravenous amphotericin B (0.3–0.5 mg/kg/day) combined with oral flucytosine (150 mg/kg/day) in four divided doses (Sanchez and Noskin, 1996). Amphotericin B is given intravenously diluted with 5% dextrose and water in a drug concentration no greater than 1 mg/10 ml of fluid. Nephrotoxicity is the limiting factor in achieving desirable blood levels. The intravenous regimen is generally the same for all fungal infections of the nervous system and is summarized in Table 4-11. The total dose varies with the response and the side effects but is usually in the range of 1,500 to 2,000 mg/1.7 m^2 of body surface. Therapy must be continued for 4–6 weeks.

The toxic effects include chills, fever, nausea, and vomiting. Anemia and nephrotoxicity must be monitored with frequent blood counts and urinalyses. Renal impairment is manifested by the appearance of cells or casts in the urine, an elevated blood urea nitrogen concentration, and decreased creatinine clearance. When renal impairment occurs, the drug must be discontinued and restarted at a lower dose.

Cytopenia limits the use flucytosine. Seriously ill patients, treated late in the course of the disease, should also be given intrathecally administered amphotericin B and miconazole.

A decline of the agglutination titer in the cerebrospinal fluid is used to follow the efficacy of therapy. Periodic CT is necessary to monitor for the development of hydrocephalus.

Other Fungal Infections

Histoplasmosis is endemic in the central United States and causes pulmonary infection. Miliary spread is unusual. Neurological histoplasmosis may take the form of leptomeningitis, focal abscess, or multiple granulomas. Blastomycosis is primarily a disease of North America. It reaches the brain by hematogenous spread from the lungs and produces multiple abscesses that give the appearance of metastatic disease on CT. The cellular response in the cerebrospinal fluid is markedly increased when fungi produce meningitis and may be normal or only mildly increased when abscess formation occurs. Amphotericin B is the mainstay of therapy for fungal infections; itraconazole is used in combination with amphotericin B against *Histoplasma capsulatum*.

Idiopathic Intracranial Hypertension (Pseudotumor Cerebri)

The term *idiopathic intracranial hypertension* (IIH) is used to characterize a syndrome of increased intracranial pressure, normal cerebrospinal fluid content, and a normal brain with normal or small ventricles on brain imaging studies. The syndrome may have an identifiable underlying cause or may be idiopathic. A specific cause can usually be found in children younger than 6 years of age, while most idiopathic cases occur after age 11. Some causes of IIH are listed in Table 4-12. A cause-and-effect relationship has not been established in all of these conditions. The most frequent causes are otitis media, head trauma, the use of certain drugs and vitamins, and feeding following malnutrition.

CLINICAL FEATURES. Both sexes are affected equally and many affected children are overweight. The initial features are headache (63%), vomiting (43%), and diplopia (36%). Young children may have only irritability, somnolence, or apathy. Less common symptoms are transitory visual obscurations, neck stiffness, tinnitus, paresthesias, and ataxia. Most children are not acutely ill, and mentation is normal.

Neurological examination is unremarkable except for papilledema and abducens nerve palsy. No signs of focal neurological dysfunction are observed. The major concern is for vision. If the syndrome is left untreated, some

Table 4-12
Causes of Idiopathic Intracranial Hypertension

Drugs
Corticosteroid withdrawal
Nalidixic acid
Oral contraceptives
Tetracycline
Thyroid replacement
Vitamin A

Systemic Disorders
Guillain-Barré syndrome
Iron deficiency anemia
Leukemia
Polycythemia vera
Protein malnutrition
Systemic lupus erythematosus
Vitamin A deficiency
Vitamin D deficiency

Head Trauma

Infections
Otitis media
Sinusitis

Metabolic Disorders
Adrenal insufficiency
Diabetic ketoacidosis (treatment)
Galactosemia
Hyperadrenalism
Hyperthyroidism
Hypoparathyroidism
Pregnancy

children have progressive papilledema and optic atrophy. Loss of vision may be rapid and severe. Early diagnosis and treatment are therefore essential to preserve vision.

DIAGNOSIS. Pseudotumor cerebri is a diagnosis of exclusion. If a child has headache and papilledema, a brain imaging study is needed to exclude a mass lesion or hydrocephalus. The results of imaging studies are usually normal in children with pseudotumor cerebri. In some the ventricles are small and the normal sulcal markings are obliterated. Visual fields, with special attention to the size of the blind spot, must be assessed at baseline and the assessment repeated after treatment is initiated.

Underlying causes of pseudotumor cerebri must be excluded by careful history and physical examination. Ordinarily these causes are easily identified.

MANAGEMENT. The goals of therapy are to relieve headache and preserve vision. A single lumbar puncture, with the closing pressure reduced to half of the opening pressure, is sufficient to reverse the process in many cases. The mechanism by which this is effective is unknown, but a transitory change in cerebrospinal fluid dynamics seems sufficient to readjust the pressure.

Children with pseudotumor cerebri are commonly treated with acetazolamide, 10 mg/kg/day, following the initial lumbar puncture. Whether this is an important addition to lumbar puncture is not clear. If symptoms return, lumbar puncture should be repeated on subsequent days. Serial lumbar punctures are sometimes needed.

Occasionally children continue to have increased intracranial pressure and evidence of progressive optic neuropathy despite the use of lumbar puncture and acetazolamide. In such patients, studies should be repeated to look for a cause other than idiopathic pseudotumor cerebri. If none is found, lumboperitoneal shunt may be needed. Optic nerve fenestration relieves papilledema but does not relieve increased intracranial pressure.

References

Costa JM, Ley L, Claramunt E, et al. Choroid plexus papillomas of the III ventricle in infants. Report of three cases. *Child Nerv Syst* 1997;13:244–249.

Grimwood K, Anderson VA, Bond L, et al. Adverse outcome of bacterial meningitis in school-age survivors. *Pediatrics* 1995;95:646–656.

Mallucci CL, Parkes SE, Barber P, et al. Paediatric meningeal tumors. *Child Nerv Sys* 1996;12:582–589.

McIntyre PB, Berkey CS, King SM, et al. Dexamethasone as adjunctive therapy in bacterial meningitis: A meta-analysis of randomized clinical trials since 1988. *JAMA* 1997;278:925–931.

Menovsky T, van Overbeeke JJ. Cerebral arteriovenous malformations in childhood: State of the art with special reference to treatment. *Eur J Pediatr* 1997;56: 741–746.

Meyers PM, Halbach VV, Phatouros CP, et al. Hemorrhagic complications in vein of Galen malformations. *Ann Neurol* 2000;47:748–755.

Olafsson E, Hauser A, Gudmundsson G. A population-based study of prognosis of ruptured cerebral aneurysm: Mortality and recurrence of subarachnoid hemorrhage. *Neurology* 1997;48:1191–1195.

Packer RJ. Brain tumors in children. *Neurology* 1999; 56:421–425.

Pollack IF, Gerszten PC, Martinez AJ, et al. Intracranial ependymomas of childhood: Long-term outcome and prognostic factors. *Neurosurgery* 1995;37:655–667.

Quagliarello VJ, Scheld WM. Treatment of bacterial meningitis. *N Engl J Med* 1997;336:708–716.

Riordan FAI, Thomson APJ, Sills JA, et al. Bacterial meningitis in the first three months of life. *Postgrad Med J* 1995;71:36–38.

Roland EH, Hill A. Intraventricular hemorrhage and post-hemorrhagic hydrocephalus. *Clin Perinatol* 1997;24: 589–605.

Sanchez JL, Noskins GA. Recent advances in the management of opportunistic fungal infections. *Compr Ther* 1996;22:703–712.

Trujillo M, McCracken G. Neonatal meningitis. In K Roos, ed. *Central Nervous System Infectious Diseases and Therapy*. New York: Marcel Dekker; 1997: 25–44.

Volpe JJ. Neurological outcome of prematurity. *Arch Neurol* 1998;55:297–300.

Chapter 5
Psychomotor Retardation and Regression

THE DIFFERENTIAL DIAGNOSIS of psychomotor retardation (developmental delay) is quite different from that of psychomotor regression. Slow progress in the attainment of developmental milestones may be caused by either static (Table 5-1) or progressive (Table 5-2) encephalopathies. In contrast, the loss of developmental milestones previously attained usually indicates a progressive disease of the nervous system, but it may also be caused by a parental misperception of attained milestones or by the development of new clinical features from an established static disorder as the brain matures (Table 5-3).

Table 5-1
Diagnosis of Developmental Delay: No Regression

Predominant Speech Delay
Bilateral hippocampal sclerosis
Congenital bilateral perisylvian syndrome (see Chapter 17)
Hearing impairment (see Chapter 17)
Infantile autism

Predominant Motor Delay
Ataxia (see Chapter 10)
Hemiplegia (see Chapter 11)
Hypotonia (see Chapter 6)
Neuromuscular disorders (see Chapter 7)
Paraplegia (see Chapter 12)

Global Developmental Delay
Cerebral malformations
Chromosomal disturbances
Intrauterine infection
Perinatal disorders
Progressive encephalopathies (see Table 5-2)

Developmental Delay

Delayed achievement of developmental milestones is one of the more common problems evaluated by child neurologists. Two important questions must be asked: (1) Is delay restricted to specific areas of development or is it global? (2) Is development only delayed or is it also regressing?

The second question is often difficult to answer in regard to infants. Even in static encephalopathies, new symptoms such as involuntary movements and seizures may occur as the child gets older, and delayed acquisition of milestones without other neurological deficits is sometimes the initial feature of progressive disorders. However, once it is clear that milestones previously achieved have been lost or that focal neurological deficits are evolving, a progressive disease of the nervous system must be considered.

The Denver Developmental Screening Test (DDST) is an efficient and reliable method for assessing development in the physician's office. It rapidly assesses four different components of development: personal-social, fine motor adaptive, language, and gross motor. The results can be amplified by several psychometric tests, but the DDST in combination with neurological assessment provides sufficient information to initiate further diagnostic studies.

Language Delay

Normal infants and children have a remarkable facility for acquiring language during the first decade. Those who are exposed to two languages concurrently learn both. Vocalization of vowels occurs in the first month, and laughing

Table 5-2
Progressive Encephalopathy: Onset before Age 2

Acquired Immune Deficiency Syndrome Encephalopathy

Disorders of Amino Acid Metabolism
Homocystinuria (21q22)
Maple syrup urine disease
    Intermediate form
    Thiamine-responsive form
Phenylketonuria

Disorders of Lysosomal Enzymes
Ganglioside storage disorders
    GM$_1$ gangliosidosis
    GM$_2$ gangliosidosis (Tay-Sachs disease, Sandhoff disease)
Gaucher disease type II (glucosylceramide lipidosis)
Globoid cell leukodystrophy (Krabbe disease)
Glycoprotein degradation disorders
I-cell disease
Mucopolysaccharidoses
    Type I (Hurler Syndrome)
    Type III (Sanfilippo disease)
Niemann Pick disease type A (sphingomyelin lipidosis)
Sulfatase deficiency disorders
    Metachromatic leukodystrophy (sulfatide lipidoses)
    Multiple sulfatase deficiency

Carbohydrate-Deficient Glycoprotein Syndromes

Hypothyroidism

Mitochondrial Disorders
Alexander disease
Mitochondrial myopathy, encephalopathy, lactic acidosis, and stroke (see Chapter 11)
Progressive infantile poliodystrophy (Alpers disease)
Subacute necrotizing encephalomyelopathy (Leigh disease)
Trichopoliodystrophy (Menkes disease)

Neurocutaneous Syndromes
Chediak-Higashi syndrome
Neurofibromatosis
Tuberous sclerosis

Other Disorders of Gray Matter
Infantile ceroid lipofuscinosis (Santavuori-Haltia disease)
Infantile neuroaxonal dystrophy
Lesch-Nyhan disease
Progressive neuronal degeneration with liver disease
Rett syndrome

Other Disorders of White Matter
Aspartoacylase deficiency (Canavan disease)
Galactosemia: Transferase deficiency
Neonatal adrenoleukodystrophy (see Chapter 6)
Pelizaeus-Merzbacher disease

Progressive Hydrocephalus

Table 5-3
Causes of Apparent Regression in Static Encephalopathy

Increasing spasticity (usually during the first year)
New-onset movement disorders (usually during the second year)
New-onset seizures
Parental misperception of attained milestones
Progressive hydrocephalus

and squealing are well established by 5 months. At 6 months infants begin articulating consonants, usually M, D, and B. Parents translate these to mean "mama," "dada," and "bottle" or "baby," although this is not the infant's intention. These first attempts at vowels and consonants are automatic and sometimes occur even in deaf children. In the months that follow, the infant imitates many speech sounds, babbles and coos, and finally learns the specific use of "mama" and "dada" by 1 year of age. Receptive skills are always more highly developed than expressive skills, because it is necessary to decode language before it can be encoded. By 2 years of age children have learned to combine at least 2 words, understand more than 250 words, and follow many simple verbal directions.

Developmental disturbances in the language cortex of the left hemisphere that occur before 5 years of age may displace language to the right hemisphere. This does not occur in older children.

Bilateral Hippocampal Sclerosis

Both bilateral hippocampal sclerosis and *the congenital bilateral perisylvian syndrome* Cause a profound impairment of language development. The former also causes failure of cognitive capacity that mimics infantile autism (DeLong and Heinz, 1997), while the latter causes a pseudobulbar palsy (see Chapter 17). Infants with medial bilateral hippocampal sclerosis generally come to medical attention for refractory seizures. However, the syndrome emphasizes that the integrity of one medial hippocampal gyrus is imperative for language development.

Hearing Impairment

The major cause of isolated delay in speech development is a hearing impairment (see Chapter 17). Hearing loss may occur concomitantly with global developmental retardation, as in rubella embryopathy, cytomegalic inclusion disease, neonatal meningitis, kernicterus, and several genetic disorders. Hearing loss need not be profound; it can be insidious, yet delay speech development. The loss of high-frequency tones inherent in telephone conversation prevents the clear distinction of many consonants that we learn to fill in through experience; infants do not have experience in supplying missing sounds.

The hearing of any infant with isolated delay in speech development should be tested by audiometry. Crude testing in the office by slamming objects and ringing bells is inadequate. Hearing loss should be suspected in children with global retardation caused by disorders ordinarily associated with hearing loss or in retarded children who fail to imitate sounds. Other clues to hearing loss in children are excessive gesturing and staring at the lips of people who are talking.

Infantile Autism

Infantile autism is conceptualized as a developmental disorder of brain function with many different causes (Rapin 1997). These disorders have a wide range of behavioral consequences that are broadly referred to as *pervasive developmental disorders*.

CLINICAL FEATURES. The major diagnostic criteria are failure of language development, severe impairment of interpersonal relationships, a restricted repertoire of activities, and onset before 3 years of age. Failure of language development is the feature most likely to bring autistic infants to medical attention and correlates best with the outcome; children who fail to develop language before age 5 have the worst outcome. The IQ is less than 70 in most children with autism. Some autistic children show no affection to their parents or other care providers, while others are affectionate on their own terms. Autistic children do not show normal play activity; some have a morbid preoccupation with spinning objects, stereotyped behaviors such as rocking and spinning, and relative insensitivity to pain.

DIAGNOSIS. Infantile autism is a clinical diagnosis and cannot be confirmed by laboratory tests. Infants with profound hearing impairment may display autistic behavior, and hearing must always be tested. Electroencephalography (EEG) is indicated when seizures are suspected.

MANAGEMENT. Autism is not curable, but several drugs may be useful to control specific behavioral disturbances. Some aspects of the severely aberrant behavior can be improved by behavior modification techniques. However, despite the best program of treatment, these children function in a moderately to severely retarded range, even though some individuals have islands of normal or extraordinary ability (*idiot savant*).

Delayed Motor Development

Infants with delayed gross motor development but normal language and social skills are often hypotonic and may have a neuromuscular disease (see Chapter 6). Isolated delay in motor function is also caused by ataxia (see Chapter 10), mild hemiplegia (see Chapter 11), and mild paraplegia (see Chapter 12). Many such children have a mild form of cerebral palsy, sufficient to delay the achievement of motor milestones but not severe enough to cause a recognizable disturbance in cognitive function during infancy. Mild disturbances in cognitive function are more often detected when the child enters school.

Global Developmental Delay

Most infants with global developmental delay have a static encephalopathy caused by an antenatal or perinatal disturbance. However, a small percentage of infants with developmental delay and no evidence of regression have an underlying genetic disease. An exhaustive search for an underlying cause in every infant whose development is slow but not regressing is not cost effective. Factors that increase the likelihood of finding a progressive disease are an affected family member, parental consanguinity, organomegaly, and absent tendon reflexes. Unenhanced cranial magnetic resonance imaging (MRI) is a reasonable screening test in all infants with global developmental delay. It often detects a malformation or other evidence of prenatal disease and provides a diagnosis that ends the uncertainty.

Chromosomal Disturbances

Abnormalities in chromosome structure or number are the single most common cause of severe mental retardation, but they still comprise only one third of the total. Abnormalities of autosomal chromosomes are always associated with infantile hypotonia (see Chapter 6). In addition, multiple minor face and limb abnormalities are usually associated features. These abnormalities in themselves are not unusual, but they assume diagnostic significance in combination. Clinical features that suggest chromosomal aberrations are summarized in Table 5-4, and some of the more common chromosome syndromes are listed in Table 5-5.

Table 5-4
Clinical Indications for Chromosome Analysis

Genitourinary
Ambiguous genitalia
Polycystic kidney

Head and Neck
High nasal bridge
Hypertelorism or hypotelorism
Microphthalmia
Mongoloid slant (in non-Asians)
Occipital scalp defect
Small mandible
Small or fish mouth (hard to open)
Small or low-set ears
Upward slant of eyes
Webbed neck

Limbs
Abnormal dermatoglyphics
Low-set thumb
Overlapping fingers
Polydactyly
Radial hypoplasia
Rocker-bottom feet

Fragile X Syndrome

The fragile X syndrome is the most common chromosomal cause of mental retardation. Its prevalence in males is approximately 20:100,000. The name derives from a fragile site (constriction) detectable in folate-free culture medium at the Xq 27 location. The unstable fragment contains a trinucleotide repeat in the FMR1 gene that becomes larger in successive generations (*DNA amplification*), causing more severe phenotypic expression. A decrease in the repeat size to normal may also occur (Väisänen et al, 1996).

CLINICAL FEATURES. The phenotype of males is almost entirely dependent on the nature of the mutation. The phenotype of females depends on both the nature of the FMR1 mutation and random X-chromosome inactivation. Males who inherit a full fragile X mutation generally have the typical syndrome of moderate retardation (IQ 40 to 55), behavioral problems that may resemble those of autism or attention deficit disorder, and somatic abnormalities (long face, enlarged ears, and macro-orchidism). While autistic behavior is common in children with the fragile X syndrome, the clinical features of the syndrome do not usually meet the diagnostic criteria of infantile autism. About 50% of females who inherit a full fragile X mutation are mentally retarded; however, they are usually less severely affected than males with a full muta-

tion. Approximately 20% of males with a fragile X chromosome are normal, while 30% of carrier females are mildly affected. An asymptomatic male can pass the abnormal chromosome to his daughters, who are usually asymptomatic as well. The daughter's children, both male and female, may be symptomatic.

DIAGNOSIS. More than 99% of cases are detected by DNA-based testing to detect a trinucleotide repeat expansion in the FMR1 gene (Tarleton and Saul, 1998). The other 1% of patients has a deletion or point mutation.

MANAGEMENT. High-dose folic acid was formerly used to treat children with the fragile X syndrome but was not effective. Treatment today consists of pharmacological management of behavior problems and educational intervention.

Cerebral Malformations

Approximately 3% of all children have at least one major malformation, but the responsible etiological factors can be identified in only 20% of cases. Many intrauterine diseases cause destructive changes that cause malformation of the developing brain. The exposure of an embryo to infectious or toxic agents during the first weeks after conception can disorganize the delicate sequencing of neural development at a time when the brain is incapable of generating a cellular

Table 5-5
Selected Autosomal Syndromes*

Defect	Features
5p monosomy	Characteristic "cri du chat" cry
	Moonlike face
	Hypertelorism
	Microcephaly
10p trisomy	Dolichocephaly
	"Turtle's beak"
	Osteoarticular anomalies
Partial 12p monosomy	Microcephaly
	Narrow forehead
	Pointed nose
	Micrognathia
18 trisomy	Pointed ears
	Micrognathia
	Occipital protuberance
	Narrow pelvis
	Rocker-bottom feet
21 trisomy	Hypotonia
	Round flat (mongoloid) facies
	Brushfield spots
	Flat nape of neck

* Growth retardation and mental retardation are features of all autosomal chromosome disorders.

response. Alcohol, lead, prescription drugs, and substances of abuse have all been implicated in the production of cerebral malformations. Although a cause-and-effect relationship is difficult to establish in an individual case, maternal cocaine use is probably responsible for vascular insufficiency and infarction of many organs, including the brain.

Cerebral malformations should be suspected in any retarded child who is dysmorphic, has malformations of other organs, or has an abnormality of head size and shape (see Chapter 18). Noncontrast-enhanced computed tomography (CT) is satisfactory to show major malformations, but MRI is the better method to show migrational defects and is more cost-effective for diagnosis of malformations.

Intrauterine Infections

The most common intrauterine infections are human immunodeficiency virus (HIV) and cytomegalovirus. The acquired immune deficiency syndrome (AIDS) epidemic in adults is responsible for the reemergence of congenital syphilis, but it has not been associated with a concomitant increase in the incidence of intrauterine toxoplasmosis. HIV infection can occur in utero, but most infected infants are asymptomatic in the newborn period and later develop progressive disease of the brain. Therefore they are dealt with in the section on progressive encephalopathies. Rubella embryopathy has almost disappeared because of mass immunization but reappears when immunization rates decline.

Congenital Syphilis

Reported cases of congenital syphilis have increased since 1988, partly because of an actual increase in case number but also because the case definition has broadened. All stillborn infants and live infants born to a woman with a history of untreated or inadequately treated syphilis are considered to have congenital syphilis. However, this definition is questionable (Risser and Hwang, 1996).

CLINICAL FEATURES. Two thirds of infected newborns are asymptomatic and are identified only on screening tests. The more common features in symptomatic newborns and infants are condylomata lata, periostitis or osteochondritis, persistent rhinorrhea, and maculopapular rash. The onset of neurological disturbances is usually after age 2 and includes nerve deafness and mental retardation. The combination of nerve

deafness, interstitial keratitis, and peg-shaped upper incisors is the *Hutchinson triad.*

DIAGNOSIS. Nontreponemal antibody tests (Venereal Disease Research Laboratory [VDRL] and rapid plasma reagin card tests) are used for screening, and the fluorescent treponemal antibody test absorbed with nonpallidum treponemas (FTA-ABS) is used for confirmation. AIDS should be suspected in every child with congenital syphilis.

MANAGEMENT. Newborns and infants with confirmed or presumptive congenital infection should be treated intravenously with crystalline penicillin G, 100,000 to 150,000 units/kg/day in six divided doses every 8 to 12 hours for 10 to 14 days, or intramuscularly with procaine penicillin G, 50,000 units/kg once daily for 10 to 14 days.

Cytomegalic Inclusion Disease

Cytomegalovirus (CMV) is a member of the herpes virus group and produces a chronic infection characterized by long periods of latency punctuated by intervals of reactivation. CMV is the most common congenital viral infection and results either from primary maternal infection or from reactivation of virus in the mother. Cytomegalic inclusion disease is sexually transmitted in adults and causes an unapparent cervical infection. Pregnancy may cause reactivation of maternal infection, and CMV can be cultured from the urine in 1% to 2% of live-born infants in the United States. Fortunately, less than 0.05% of newborns with viruria have symptoms of cytomegalic inclusion disease.

CLINICAL FEATURES. Less than 10% of infected newborns are symptomatic. The typical clinical features are skin rash, hepatosplenomegaly, jaundice, chorioretinitis, and microcephaly with cerebral calcification. Migrational defects (lissencephaly, polymicrogyria, and cerebellar agenesis) are the main consequence of fetal infection during the first trimester. Some infants have microcephaly secondary to intrauterine infection without evidence of systemic infection at birth.

DIAGNOSIS. In symptomatic cases, virus can be cultured from throat swabs or urine, and CMV-specific IgM is present in serum. Urine culture results are also positive in asymptomatic cases. Isolation of CMV from the urine or cerebrospinal fluid indicates active infection in the newborn. Such newborns should be isolated from women of childbearing age. In infants with developmental delay and microcephaly, the diagnosis of cytomegalic inclusion disease is made by serological demonstration of prior infection and a consistent pattern of intracranial calcification.

MANAGEMENT. Much of the brain damage from congenital CMV occurs in utero and cannot be changed by postnatal treatment. The main antiviral agents used in adults are ganciclovir, cidofovir, and foscarnet. Only ganciclovir has been used in newborns.

Rubella Embryopathy

CLINICAL FEATURES. Rubella embryopathy is a multisystem disease characterized by intrauterine growth retardation, cataracts, chorioretinitis, congenital heart disease, sensorineural deafness, hepatosplenomegaly, jaundice, anemia, thrombocytopenia, and rash. Eighty percent of children with a congenital rubella syndrome have nervous system involvement. The neurological features are bulging fontanelle, lethargy, hypotonia, and seizures. Seizures may be delayed until 3 months of age.

DIAGNOSIS. Rubella embryopathy should not be considered a cause of psychomotor retardation unless the newborn has other symptoms of rubella infection.

MANAGEMENT. No treatment is available for active infection.

Toxoplasmosis

Toxoplasma gondii is a protozoan that is estimated to infect 1 per 1,000 live births in the United States each year. The symptoms of toxoplasmosis infection in the mother usually go unnoticed. Transplacental transmission of toxoplasmosis is possible only if primary maternal infection occurs during pregnancy. The rate of placental transmission is highest during the last trimester, but fetuses infected at that time are least likely to have symptoms later on. The transmission rate is lowest during the first trimester, but fetuses infected at that time have the most serious sequelae.

CLINICAL FEATURES. About 25% of infected newborns have multisystem involvement (fever, rash, hepatosplenomegaly, jaundice, and thrombocytopenia) at birth. Neurological dysfunction is manifested as seizures, altered states of consciousness, and increased intracranial pressure. The triad of hydrocephalus, chorioretinitis, and intracranial calcification is the hallmark of congenital toxoplasmosis in older children. About 8% of infected newborns, who are asymptomatic at birth, later show neurological sequelae, especially psychomotor retardation.

DIAGNOSIS. The Sabin-Feldman dye test had been the standard for diagnosis, but another useful serological test for the diagnosis of congenital toxoplasmosis in the newborn is an enzyme-linked immunosorbent assay (ELISA) that shows IgM-specific antibody to *Toxoplasma* in umbilical cord blood. The demonstration of IgM-specific antibody is essential to prove active infection in the newborn. IgG-specific antibody appears in the newborn's serum by passive transfer from the mother and does not indicate active infection. Persistence of IgG-specific antibody correlates with active infection.

In older children, the diagnosis requires not only serological evidence of prior infection but also compatible clinical features.

MANAGEMENT. A combined prenatal and postnatal treatment program for congenital toxoplasmosis can reduce the neurological morbidity (Roizen et al, 1995). When maternal acute infection is recognized by seroconversion, fetal blood and amniotic fluid are cultured and fetal blood is tested for *Toxoplasma*-specific IgM. The mother is then treated with spiramycin; if fetal infection is documented, pyrimethamine and either sulfadoxine or sulfadiazine are added to the regimen.

In newborns with clinical evidence of toxoplasmosis, pyrimethamine (Daraprim), 0.5 mg/kg, and sulfadiazine, 25 mg/kg, are administered orally every 12 hours for 1 year. Because pyrimethamine is a folic acid antagonist, folic acid, 0.1 mg/kg/day, is also given. The peripheral platelet count must be monitored regularly. Prednisone, 1 to 2 mg/kg/day, should be added to the therapy in newborns with a high protein concentration in the cerebrospinal fluid or chorioretinitis.

Perinatal Disorders

Perinatal infection, asphyxia, maternal drug use, and trauma are the main perinatal events that cause psychomotor retardation (see Chapter 1). The important infectious diseases are bacterial meningitis (see Chapter 4) and herpes encephalitis (see Chapter 1). Although the overall mortality rate for bacterial meningitis is now less than 50%, significant neurological disturbances are noted almost immediately in 50% of survivors. Mental and motor disabilities, hydrocephalus, epilepsy, deafness, and visual loss are the most common sequelae. Psychomotor retardation may be the only or the most prominent sequela. Progressive mental deterioration can occur if meningitis causes a secondary hydrocephalus.

Telling Parents Bad News

It is not possible to make bad news sound good or even half bad. The goal of telling parents that their child will be mentally retarded or otherwise neurologically impaired is that they hear and understand what you are saying. The mind must be prepared to hear bad news. It is a mistake to tell people more than they are ready to accept. Too often, parents bring their child for a second or third opinion because previous doctors "didn't tell us anything." In fact, they said too much too fast and were tuned out.

My goal for the first visit is to establish that the child's development is not normal (not a normal variation), that something is wrong with the brain, and that I share the parents' concern. Unfortunately, mothers often come alone for this critical visit and must later restate your comments to doubting fathers and grandparents. Most parents cannot handle more information than "the child is not normal" at the first consultation, and further discussion is saved for a later visit. However, probing questions should always be answered fully. Parents must never lose confidence in your willingness to be forthright. The timing of the next visit depends on the age of the child and the severity of the retardation. The more the child falls behind in reaching developmental milestones, the more ready parents will be to accept the diagnosis of mental retardation.

When the time comes to tell a mother that her child is retarded, she will cry. If she does not cry, she has not heard what you were saying or understood its implications and you have failed to communicate effectively. It is not helpful to describe mental retardation as mild, moderate, or severe. Parents want to know what the child will do. Will he walk? Need special schools? Live alone? The next question is "What can I do to help my child?" Parents must do something, and should be directed to programs that provide developmental specialists and other parents who can help them learn how to live with a chronic handicapping disorder and gain access to community resources.

Progressive Encephalopathies with Onset before Age 2

The differential diagnosis of progressive diseases of the nervous system that start before age 2 years is somewhat different from those that begin during childhood (see Table 5-6). Three questions must be answered in taking the history and performing the physical examination before laboratory diagnosis is initiated:

1. Are the clinical features referable only to the central nervous system or are other organs involved? Other organ involvement should suggest lysosomal, peroxisomal, and mitochondrial disorders.

2. Are the clinical features referable only to the central nervous system or is the peripheral nervous system involved? Nerve or muscle involvement suggests mainly lysosomal and mitochondrial disorders.

3. Does the disease affect primarily the gray matter or the white matter?

Early features of gray matter disease are personality change, seizures, and dementia. White matter disease is characterized by focal neurological deficits, spasticity, and blindness. Whether the process begins in the gray matter

---

Table 5-6
Progressive Encephalopathy: Onset after Age 2

Disorders of Lysosomal Enzymes
Gaucher disease type III (glucosylceramide lipidosis)
Globoid cell leukodystrophy (late-onset Krabbe disease)
Glycoprotein degradation disorders
    Aspartylglycosaminuria
    Mannosidosis type II
GM_2 gangliosidosis (juvenile Tay-Sachs disease)
Metachromatic leukodystrophy (late-onset sulfatide lipidoses)
Mucopolysaccharidoses types II and VII
Niemann-Pick type C (sphingomyelin lipidosis)

Infectious Disease
Acquired immune deficiency syndrome encephalopathy
Congenital syphilis
Subacute sclerosing panencephalitis

Other Disorders of Gray Matter
Ceroid lipofuscinosis
    Juvenile
    Late infantile (Bielschowsky-Jansky disease)
Heller syndrome
Huntington disease
Mitochondrial disorders
    Late-onset poliodystrophy
    Myoclonic epilepsy and ragged-red fibers (MERRF)
Progressive neuronal degeneration with liver disease
Xeroderma pigmentosum

Other Disorders of White Matter
Adrenoleukodystrophy
Alexander disease
Cerebrotendinous xanthomatosis

or the white matter, eventually clinical features of dysfunction develop in both. The EEG is usually abnormal early in the course of gray matter disease and late in the course of white matter disease. MRI shows cortical atrophy in gray matter disease and cerebral demyelination in white mater disease (Figure 5-1). Visual evoked responses and motor conduction velocities are useful in documenting demyelination, even subclinical, in the optic and peripheral nerves, respectively.

Acquired Immune Deficiency Syndrome Encephalopathy

Acquired immune deficiency syndrome (AIDS) is a human retroviral disease caused by the lentivirus subfamily now designated as human immunodeficiency virus (HIV). HIV is spread in adults by sexual contact, intravenous drug abuse, and blood transfusion. Pediatric AIDS cases result from transplacental or perinatal transmission of HIV from mothers who are intravenous drug users and prostitutes. Transmission may occur by breast-feeding. The mother may be asymptomatic when the infection is noted in the child.

CLINICAL FEATURES. Approximately 30% of children born to AIDS-infected mothers show

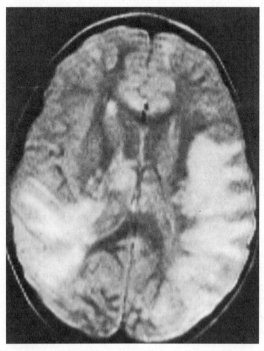

Figure 5-1. Krabbe disease. MRI shows extensive demyelination of cerebral hemispheres.

evidence of infection during the first year. As a rule, the outcome is worse when the onset of symptoms is early, and the rate of progression in the child relates directly to the severity of disease in the mother.

Children with AIDS fail to thrive and have an increased incidence of bacterial infections, but only 10% acquire opportunistic infections. The most common opportunistic infections are *Pneumocystis carinii* pneumonia, disseminated candidiasis, and disseminated *Mycobacterium avium intracellulare*. Toxoplasmosis, a common complication in adults with AIDS, is uncommon in pediatric AIDS. An immunocompromised state should be suspected in every child with an opportunistic infection.

The possible spectrum of neurological outcomes in children infected with HIV includes a static encephalopathy resulting from other prenatal and perinatal risk factors associated with drug abuse in the mother; opportunistic infection of the nervous system; HIV infection of the brain, causing a subacute encephalopathy; and HIV infection of the spinal cord, causing a transverse myelitis (see Chapter 12). AIDS experts now believe that the disease will develop in all children with HIV infection.

AIDS encephalopathy may be subacute or indolent and is not necessarily associated with failure to thrive or opportunistic infections. The onset of encephalopathy may occur from 2 months to 5 years after exposure to the virus. Ninety percent of affected infants show symptoms by 18 months of age. The encephalopathy is characterized by progressive loss of developmental milestones, microcephaly, dementia, and spasticity. Other features in less than 50% of children are ataxia, pseudobulbar palsy, involuntary movement disorders, myoclonus, and seizures. Death usually occurs a few months after the onset of AIDS encephalopathy.

DIAGNOSIS. The diagnosis of AIDS in infants born to infected mothers is complicated because all such newborns are HIV-antibody positive from passive transfer, but only 15% to 30% are HIV infected. The diagnosis of AIDS in a child less than 18 months of age who is HIV seropositive or born to an HIV-infected mother is established by a positive result on two separate determinations from one or more of the following tests: HIV culture, HIV polymerase chain reaction, or HIV antigen. Children 18 months of age or older are diagnosed as HIV infected when the HIV-antibody tests are positive by reactive enzyme immunoassay and confirmed by Western blot or immunofluorescence assay.

Treatable infections (cryptococcal meningitis, *Candida* meningitis) must be excluded before HIV encephalitis is diagnosed. The cerebrospinal fluid abnormalities are minimal and vary from patient to patient. The protein concentration is 50 to 100 mg/dl (0.5 to 1 g/L) and the glucose concentration is normal or slightly decreased, but monocytic pleocytosis is uncommon. In some children, progressive calcification of the basal ganglia is seen on CT. The mortality rate in symptomatic children is 100%.

MANAGEMENT. Combined treatment with zidovudine (azidothymidine, AZT), didanosine, and nevirapine is well tolerated and may have sustained efficacy against HIV-1 (Luzuriaga et al, 1997). Bone marrow suppression is the only important evidence of toxicity.

Disorders of Amino Acid Metabolism

Disorders of amino acid metabolism impair neuronal function by causing excessive production of toxic intermediary metabolites and reducing the production of neurotransmitters. The clinical syndromes are either an acute neonatal encephalopathy with seizures and cerebral edema (see Chapter 1) or mental retardation and dementia. Some disorders of amino acid metabolism cause cerebral malformations, such as agenesis of the corpus callosum. Although the main clinical features of aminoaciduria are referable to gray matter dysfunction (mental retardation, seizures), myelination is often profoundly delayed or defective.

Homocystinuria

The main defect responsible for mental retardation is almost complete deficiency of the enzyme cystathionine-synthase. Transmission is by autosomal recessive inheritance. Heterozygotes have partial deficiencies. Cystathionine synthase catalyzes the condensation of serine and homocysteine to form cystathionine (Figure 5-2). When the enzyme is deficient, the blood and urine concentrations of homocysteine, homocystine, and methionine are increased. It is hypermethioninemia that is detected in newborn screening programs.

CLINICAL FEATURES. Affected individuals appear normal at birth. Neurological features may be global mental retardation, cerebral thromboembolism, or both. Developmental delay occurs in half of cases, and intelligence declines progressively with age in untreated children. Most will eventually function in the mildly retarded

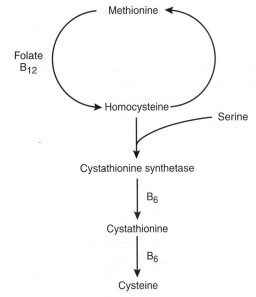

Figure 5-2. Metabolic disturbance in homocystinuria. Absence of cystathionine β-synthase (cystathionine synthetase) blocks the metabolism of homocysteine, causing the accumulation of homocystine and methionine.

range. Ataxia, dystonia, aphasia, pseudobulbar palsy, and seizures may be associated.

High plasma homocysteine concentrations adversely affect collagen metabolism and are responsible for intimal thickening of blood vessel walls, leading to arterial and venous thromboembolic disease. Cerebral thromboembolism is a life-threatening complication. Emboli may occur in infancy, may be delayed until adult life, and also occur in young adult heterozygotes (Welch and Loscalzo, 1998). Occlusion of the coronary or carotid arteries can lead to sudden death or severe neurological handicap. Thromboembolism is the first clue to the diagnosis in 15% of cases.

Dislocation of the lens, an almost constant feature of homocystinuria, typically occurs between 2 and 10 years of age but may be delayed until adult life. Almost all patients have lens dislocation by age 40. Older children have osteoporosis. The spine is affected first and most severely, resulting in scoliosis. Many children are tall and thin, with blond, sparse, brittle hair and a Marfan syndrome habitus. This habitus does not develop until middle or late childhood and serves as a clue to the diagnosis in fewer than 40% of cases.

The diagnosis should be suspected in any infant with isolated and unexplained developmental delay, since disease-specific features may not appear until later childhood. The presence of either thromboembolism or lens dislocation strongly suggests homocystinuria.

DIAGNOSIS. The concentrations of homocystine and methionine are increased in the blood and urine. Definitive diagnosis is established by showing a deficiency of cystathionine synthase either in the liver or in cultured fibroblasts.

MANAGEMENT. The administration of pyridoxine, 500 to 1,000 mg/day, reduces or eliminates the biochemical abnormalities in one third of patients. An equal number are not pyridoxine responsive, and the remainder have an intermediate response. Folate must be given concomitantly. Most patients who respond to pyridoxine probably have a low-level or mutant form of cystathionine synthase activity that is enhanced by the addition of cofactor.

The most widely used dietary treatment for homocystinuria is methionine restriction and cystine supplementation. Unfortunately, this diet is not palatable and long-term use is difficult to achieve even though it prevents mental retardation when started shortly after birth. Betaine, a methyl donor that recycles homocysteine to methionine, is recommended at a dose of 6 to 9 g/day for children who neither respond to pyridoxine nor tolerate a methionine-restricted diet.

Maple Syrup Urine Disease (Intermediate)

The three major branched-chain amino acids (BCAA) are leucine, isoleucine, and valine. In the course of their metabolism, they are first transaminated to α-ketoacids and then further catabolized by oxidative decarboxylation (see Figure 1-4). Branched-chain ketoacid (BCKA) dehydrogenase is the enzyme responsible for oxidative decarboxylation. Its deficiency is associated with at least three different phenotypes: classic, intermittent, and intermediate maple syrup urine disease. The classic and intermittent forms are characterized by acute encephalopathies with ketoacidosis (see Chapters 1 and 10). The ketoacidosis is usually milder as well. The levels of dehydrogenase enzyme activity in the intermediate and intermittent forms are approximately the same (5% to 40%), whereas activity in the classic form is zero to 2% of normal. Phenotypic differences between the intermediate and intermittent forms may be related to protein intake.

CLINICAL FEATURES. The onset of the intermediate form is late in infancy, often in association with a febrile illness or a large protein intake.

In the absence of vigorous early therapeutic intervention, moderate mental retardation results. Ataxia and failure to thrive are common. Infants with intermediate maple syrup urine disease are slow in achieving milestones and hyperactive. As children, they generally function in the moderately retarded range of intelligence. Physical development is normal except for coarse, brittle hair. The urine may have the odor of maple syrup. Acute mental changes, seizures, and focal neurological deficits do not occur.

Some infants with the intermediate form are thiamine responsive. These present primarily with moderate retardation.

DIAGNOSIS. BCAA and BCKA concentrations are elevated, though not as high as in the classic disease. A presumptive diagnosis requires the demonstration of BCAA in the urine by a ferric chloride test or the 2,4-dinitrophenylhydrazine test. Quantitative measurement of blood and urine BCAA and BCKA is diagnostic.

TREATMENT. All infants with intermediate maple syrup urine disease should be put on a protein-restricted diet. In addition, a trial of thiamine, 100 mg/day, is given to determine whether the biochemical error is thiamine responsive. If 100 mg is not effective, daily dosages up to 1 g of thiamine should be tried before the condition is designated as thiamine refractory.

Phenylketonuria

Phenylketonuria is a disorder of phenylalanine metabolism caused by partial or total deficiency of the hepatic enzyme phenylalanine hydroxylase, for which the gene is located on chromosome 12q.24.1. The deficiency is transmitted by autosomal recessive inheritance and occurs in approximately 1 per 16,000 live births. Because phenylalanine cannot be adequately hydroxylated to tyrosine, it accumulates and is transaminated to phenylpyruvic acid (Figure 5-3). Phenylpyruvic acid is oxidized to phenylacetic acid, which is excreted in the urine and causes a musty odor.

CLINICAL FEATURES. Affected children are normal at birth and would not be detected in the absence of compulsory mass screening. The screening test detects hyperphenylalaninemia, which is not synonymous with phenylketonuria (Table 5-7). Blood phenylalanine and tyrosine concentrations must be precisely determined in every newborn whose abnormality is detected by the screening test in order to differentiate classic phenylketonuria from other conditions. In newborns with classic phenylketonuria, hy-

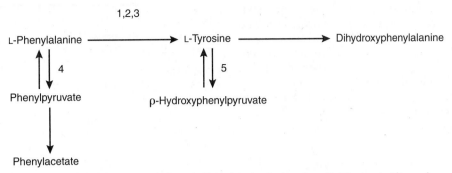

Figure 5-3. Phenylalanine metabolism. 1. Phenylalanine hydroxylase. 2. Dihydropteridine reductase. 3. Tetrahydrobiopterin. 4. Phenylalanine transaminase. 5. Tyrosine transaminase.

perphenylalaninemia develops 48 to 72 hours after initiation of milk feeding. Blood phenylalanine concentrations are 20 mg/dl or greater, and serum tyrosine levels are less than 5 mg/dl. When blood phenylalanine concentrations reach 15 mg/dl, phenylalanine spills over into the urine and the addition of ferric chloride solution (5 to 10 drops of FeCl to l ml of urine) produces a green color.

Untreated infants appear normal during the first months, but the skin may have a musty odor because of phenylacetic acid in the sweat. Developmental delay is sometimes obvious by the third month and always before the end of the first year. By the beginning of the second year, developmental regression is evident. Behavioral disturbances characterized by hyperactivity and aggressiveness are common; focal neurological deficits are unusual. Approximately 25% of affected infants have seizures. Some have infantile spasms and hypsarrhythmia; others have tonic-clonic seizures. Infants with phenylketonuria frequently have blond hair, pale skin, and blue eyes owing to diminished pigment production. Eczema is common. These skin changes are the only nonneurological features of phenylketonuria.

DIAGNOSIS. The clinical heterogeneity of classic phenylketonuria is probably due to the existence of several mutant alleles of the phenylalanine hydroxylase enzyme. Blood phenylalanine levels less than 25 mg/dl and a normal concentration of tyrosine characterize benign variants of phenylketonuria. The malignant forms of phenylketonuria are caused by disturbances in tetrahydrobiopterin. Seizures are the initial symptom and are followed by mental retardation and motor deficits. Progressive calcification of the basal ganglia occurs in untreated children.

Transitory tyrosinemia is estimated to occur in 2% of full-term newborns and in 25% of premature newborns. It is caused by a transitory deficiency of the enzyme *p*-hydroxyphenylpyruvic acid. It is a benign condition and can be distinguished from phenylketonuria because the blood concentrations of both tyrosine and phenylalanine are elevated.

MANAGEMENT. Guidelines for management were formulated by the American Academy of Pediatrics (Wappner et al, 1999). A phenylalanine-restricted diet should be started immediately in newborns with a blood phenylalanine concentration of 20 mg/dl or greater. Dietary therapy is complex, and is best undertaken and administered by physicians and nutritionists with experience in treating patients with hyperphenylalaninemia. The goal of therapy is to maintain blood phenylalanine concentrations between 4 and 6 mg/dl. Diet therapy is probably needed throughout life to prevent intellectual deterioration.

Table 5-7
Differential Diagnosis
of Hyperphenylalaninemia

Classic Phenylketonuria
Complete hydroxylase deficiency (zero to 6%)

Benign Variants
Other
Partial hydroxylase deficiency (6% to 30%)
Phenylalanine transaminase deficiency
Transitory hydroxylase deficiency

Malignant Variants
Dihydropteridine reductase deficiency
Tetrahydrobiopterin synthesis deficiency

Tyrosinemia
Transitory tyrosinemia
Tyrosinosis

Liver Disease
Galactose-l-phosphate uridylyl transferase deficiency

Tetrahydrobiopterin is a cofactor for phenylalanine hydroxylase, tyrosine hydroxylase, and tryptophan hydroxylase. Defective recycling or synthesis causes deficiency. In infants with cofactor deficiency, a phenylalanine-restricted diet reduces the blood phenylalanine concentration but does not prevent neurological deterioration. For these children, tetrahydrobiopterin administration is the therapy of choice.

Disorders of Lysosomal Enzymes

Lysosomes are cytoplasmic vesicles containing hydrolytic enzymes that degrade the products of cellular catabolism. Lysosomal enzyme disorders are caused by impaired enzyme synthesis, abnormal enzyme targeting, or a defective accessory factor needed for enzymatic processing. When lysosomal enzymes are impaired, abnormal storage of materials occurs, causing cell injury and death. One or several organs may be affected, and the clinical features depend on the organ(s) involved. Mental retardation and regression are features of many lysosomal enzyme storage diseases. In some diseases, such as acid lipase deficiency (Wolman disease) and ceramide deficiency (Farber lipogranulomatosis), mental retardation occurs, but it is neither a prominent nor an initial feature. Such disorders are omitted from this discussion.

GM$_1$ Gangliosidosis

Deficiency of the lysosomal enzyme β-galactosidase causes GM$_1$. The amount and type of residual activity determine whether the phenotype is a generalized gangliosidosis, as in GM$_1$ gangliosidosis, or visceral storage of mucopolysaccharides with little brain disease, as in Morquio B disease. The β-galactosidase gene is located on chromosome 3p, and the disease is transmitted by autosomal recessive inheritance.

Table 5-8
The Hurler Phenotype

Abdominal hernia
Coarse facial features
Corneal opacity
Deafness
Dysostosis multiplex
Mental retardation
Stiff joints
Visceromegaly

Table 5-9
Lysosomal Enzyme Disorders with a Cherry-Red Spot

Cherry-red spot myoclonus (see Chapter 1)
Farber lipogranulomatosis
GM$_1$ gangliosidosis
GM$_2$ gangliosidosis
Metachromatic leukodystrophy
Niemann-Pick disease
Sialidosis type III

CLINICAL FEATURES. The onset is between 6 and 18 months. Weakness and incoordination are noted first. Spasticity, mental retardation, and seizures follow. Psychomotor development is first slow and then regresses. Affected newborns are poorly responsive, hypotonic, and hypoactive. The Hurler phenotype is present (Table 5-8), except that the cornea is clear and a cherry-red spot of the macula is present in 50% of patients (Table 5-9). Death occurs between the ages of 3 and 7 years.

DIAGNOSIS. Infantile GM$_1$ gangliosidosis can be distinguished from Hurler syndrome by the absence of mucopolysacchariduria and the presence of a cherry-red spot. The diagnosis is established by showing enzyme deficiency in leukocytes, cultured fibroblasts, or serum.

MANAGEMENT. Treatment is not available.

GM$_2$ Gangliosidosis

These are a group of related disorders in which GM$_2$ gangliosides are stored because of deficiency of hexosaminidase A, hexosaminidase B, or the GM$_2$ activator of hexosaminidase A or B. The abnormal gene, transmitted by autosomal recessive inheritance, may be a mutation in the gene for the α-subunit on chromosome 15, the β-subunit on chromosome 5, or the glycoprotein activator for hexosaminidase (AB variant) on chromosome 5.

Tay-Sachs Disease

Tay-Sachs disease, or *infantile GM$_2$ gangliosidosis*, is caused by deficiency of hexosaminidase A due to mutation of the α locus. The gene frequency is 1:30 in Ashkenazi Jews and 1:300 in gentiles. The central nervous system is the only affected organ. The juvenile and adult forms of GM$_2$ gangliosidosis are caused by partial deficiencies of hexosaminidase A.

CLINICAL FEATURES. The typical initial symptom, between 3 and 6 months of age, is an abnormal startle reaction (Moro reflex) to noise or light. Motor regression begins between 4 and 6 months of age. The infant may be brought to medical attention because of either delayed achievement of motor milestones or loss of milestones previously attained. A cherry-red spot of the macula is present in almost every patient but is not specific for Tay-Sachs disease, because it can be seen in several storage diseases and in central retinal artery occlusion (Table 5-9). The cherry-red spot develops as retinal ganglion cells in the parafoveal region accumulate stored material, swell, and burst. The red color of the normal fundus can then be seen. Optic atrophy and blindness follow.

By 1 year of age, the infant is severely retarded, unresponsive, and spastic. During the second year, the head enlarges and seizures develop. Most children die by 5 years of age.

DIAGNOSIS. The diagnosis should be strongly suspected in any Jewish child with psychomotor retardation and a cherry-red spot of the macula. The diagnosis is established by showing deficient activity of hexosaminidase A in white blood cells or serum. Heterozygotes can be detected by the same assay. Prenatal diagnosis is possible by amniocentesis.

MANAGEMENT. Treatment is supportive.

Sandhoff Disease

In Sandhoff disease, both hexosaminidase A and B are severely deficient. The disease is transmitted by autosomal recessive inheritance and is characterized by the storage of globosides and GM_2 gangliosides in brain and viscera.

CLINICAL FEATURES. The clinical features and course of Sandhoff disease are identical to those of Tay-Sachs disease. The only difference is that organs other than the central nervous system are sometimes involved. Moderate hepatosplenomegaly may be present, and occasionally patients have bony deformities similar to those of infantile GM_1 gangliosidosis.

DIAGNOSIS. The disease should be suspected in every non-Jewish infant with a Tay-Sachs phenotype. Peripheral lymphocytes are not vacuolated, but foamy histocytes may be present in the bone marrow. The diagnosis is established in patients and carriers by showing hexosaminidase deficiency in leukocytes, cultured fibroblasts, or serum. Prenatal diagnosis can be made by the detection of N-acetylglucosaminyl oligosaccharides in amniotic fluid.

MANAGEMENT. Treatment is supportive.

Gaucher Disease Type II (Glucosylceramine Lipidosis)

Gaucher disease is transmitted by autosomal recessive inheritance. The abnormal gene is located on chromosome 1q21. Deficiency of the enzyme glucocerebrosidase (glucosylceramide β-glucosidase) causes the lysosomal storage of glucocerebrosides. Rare cases are caused by deficiency of saposin C, an enzymatic cofactor. Type I, the most common form of Gaucher disease, does not affect the nervous system. Type II is an acute and devastating infantile disorder affecting the brain and viscera. Type III, like type II, is characterized by neurovisceral storage, but the onset is in childhood and the course is slow.

CLINICAL FEATURES. Infants with Gaucher disease type II usually have symptoms of neurovisceral dysfunction before 6 months of age and frequently before 3 months of age. The initial symptoms are motor regression and cranial nerve dysfunction. Children are first hypotonic and then spastic. Head retraction is an early and characteristic sign that probably is due to meningeal irritation. Difficulties in sucking and swallowing, trismus, and oculomotor palsies are typical. Mental deterioration is rapid, but seizures are uncommon. Splenomegaly is more prominent than hepatomegaly, and jaundice is unexpected. Hypersplenism results in anemia, thrombocytopenia, and leukopenia. Death usually occurs during the first year and always by the second.

DIAGNOSIS. Diagnosis is made by enzymatic analysis of leukocytes or cultured fibroblasts. Gaucher cells can be seen on bone marrow aspirate but are not necessary for diagnosis. Carrier detection and prenatal diagnosis are available.

MANAGEMENT. Intravenous enzyme replacement therapy is effective in treating the systemic disease of types I and III. It has not been effective in stopping neurological progression (Brady, 1998).

Globoid Cell Leukodystrophy (Krabbe Disease)

Krabbe disease (galactosylceramide lipidosis) is a rapidly progressive demyelinating disorder of infants caused by deficient activity of the enzyme galactosylceramide β-galactosidase. A juvenile and an adult form of the disease also occur. It is transmitted by autosomal recessive inheritance, and the gene has been mapped to chromosome 14. Galactosylceramide is stored within multinucleated macrophages of the white matter of the central nervous system, forming globoid cells.

CLINICAL FEATURES. The median age of onset is 4 months, with a range of 1 to 7 months. Initial symptoms are irritability and hyperreactivity to stimuli. These are followed by progressive hypertonicity in the skeletal muscles. Unexplained low-grade fever is common. Psychomotor development arrests and then regresses. Within 2 to 4 months, the infant is in a permanent position of opisthotonos and has lost all previously achieved milestones. Tendon reflexes become hypoactive and disappear. Startle myoclonus and seizures develop. Blindness occurs, and before 1 year 90% of these infants are either dead or in a chronic vegetative state.

Several variant forms of globoid leukodystrophy with different clinical features are described: infantile spasm syndrome (see Chapter 1), focal neurological deficits (see Chapters 10 and 11), and polyneuropathy (see Chapter 7). The juvenile form is discussed later in this chapter.

DIAGNOSIS. MRI shows diffuse demyelination of the cerebral hemispheres (Figure 5-3). Motor nerve conduction velocity of peripheral nerves is usually prolonged, and the protein content of cerebrospinal fluid is elevated. The diagnosis is established by showing deficient activity of galactosylceramide β-galactosidase in leukocytes or cultured fibroblasts.

MANAGEMENT. Bone marrow transplantation has been shown to reverse the neurological manifestations (Krivit et al, 1998).

Glycoprotein Degradation Disorders

Glycoproteins are complex molecules composed of oligosaccharides attached to protein. Disorders of glycoprotein degradation are uncommon and resemble mild forms of mucopolysaccharidoses. All are transmitted as autosomal recessive traits. The main forms are caused by deficiency of the enzyme α-mannosidase coded on chromosome 19p and deficiency of the lysosomal enzyme α-fucosidase coded on chromosome 1p.

CLINICAL FEATURES. The clinical features are either a Hurler phenotype (Table 5.8) or a myoclonus-dementia complex. Some patients have macular degeneration (cherry-red spot). Angiokeratoma can be present. These disorders cannot be distinguished from other lysosomal storage diseases by clinical features alone.

DIAGNOSIS. The urine shows excessive excretion of oligosaccharides or glycoasparagines but not mucopolysaccharides. Biopsy of the skin and other tissues shows membrane-bound vacuoles containing amorphous material. Tissue concentrations of glycoproteins, and often glycolipids, are increased.

MANAGEMENT. Treatment is not available.

I-Cell Disease

I-cell disease (mucolipidosis II) is caused by deficiency or dysfunction of the enzyme N-acetylglucosamine phosphotransferase causing lysosomal storage of many mucolipid materials. At least three different genes are involved. The trait is transmitted by autosomal recessive inheritance. The gene maps to chromosome 4q21-q23.

CLINICAL FEATURES. I-cell disease resembles Hurler syndrome except that symptoms appear earlier, the neurological deterioration is more rapid, and mucopolysacchariduria is not present. Affected newborns are small for gestational age and may have hyperplastic gums. Coarsening of facial features and limitation of joint movements occur within the first months. The complete Hurler phenotype is present within the first year, except that corneal opacification is not seen in all cases. Gingival hypertrophy is quite striking. Death from congestive heart failure usually occurs before age 5.

DIAGNOSIS. I-cell disease should be considered in infants with the Hurler phenotype and a screening test negative for mucopolysacchariduria. The diagnosis is established by showing a specific pattern of lysosomal enzyme deficiency in fibroblasts.

MANAGEMENT. Treatment is not available.

Mucopolysaccharidoses

The mucopolysaccharidoses (MPS) are caused by a deficiency of the lysosomal enzymes responsible for catalyzing the degradation of glycosaminoglycans (mucopolysaccharides). Mucopolysaccharides are a normal component of cornea, cartilage, bone, connective tissue, and the reticuloendothelial system, and all may be affected by excessive storage. All MPS are transmitted by autosomal recessive inheritance except type-II, which is X-linked. (Wraith, 1995).

Type I MPS (Hurler Syndrome)

The Hurler syndrome is caused by absence of the lysosomal hydrolase α-L-iduronidase. It is transmitted by autosomal recessive inheritance; the gene has been mapped to chromosome 4p16.3. Dermatan sulfate and heparan sulfate cannot be fully degraded and appear in the urine. Mucopolysaccharides are stored in the cornea, collagen, and leptomeninges, and gangliosides are stored in cortical neurons.

CLINICAL FEATURES. Affected children are normal during the first year. In the second year, development is arrested and slow regression occurs. Motor dysfunction affects the corticospinal tracts and peripheral nerves. A distinctive Hurler phenotype evolves that is common to many lysosomal enzyme disorders (Table 5-8). Clouding of the cornea is present in all cases, sometimes causing complete blindness. Facial features become coarse. The child has progressive hepatosplenomegaly, umbilical hernia, and skeletal deformities that produce dwarfism, kyphoscoliosis, and limited movement of the joints. The skeletal deformities, termed *dysostosis multiplex*, produce characteristic radiographic features: hypoplasia of the lateral clavicle, rounding and sometimes hypoplasia of the thoracolumbar vertebral bodies, flaring of the pelvis with hypoplasia of the acetabula, broadening of the ribs, and widening of the diaphyses of long bones. The skull loses its convolutional markings, the sella turcica is enlarged, and the orbits are shallow. Communicating hydrocephalus may result from thickening of the leptomeninges. Death usually occurs by age 10.

DIAGNOSIS. The diagnosis is suggested by the physical and radiographic appearance, the presence of vacuolated lymphocytes, and mucopolysacchariduria. A simple screening test is the appearance of a metachromatic spot when a drop of urine is placed on paper impregnated with toluidine blue. The diagnosis is established only by showing the enzyme deficiency in leukocytes or cultured fibroblasts.

MANAGEMENT. Bone marrow transplantation is being tried with variable success in all MPS types.

Type III-MPS (Sanfilippo Disease)

Type III-MPS is distinct from other MPS because only heparan sulfate is stored in viscera and appears in the urine. Gangliosides are stored in neurons. Four different, but related, enzyme deficiencies have been implicated. All are transmitted by autosomal recessive inheritance.

CLINICAL FEATURES. The Hurler phenotype is not prominent, but hepatomegaly is present in two thirds of cases. Dwarfism does not occur. The major feature is neurological deterioration characterized by delayed motor development beginning toward the end of the second year, followed by an interval of arrested mental development and progressive dementia. Hyperactivity and sleep disorders are relatively common between the ages of 2 and 4. Most affected children are severely retarded by age 11 and dead before age 20. However, considerable variability exists, and type III-MPS should be considered even when the onset of mental regression occurs after age 5.

DIAGNOSIS. The diagnosis should be suspected in infants and children with progressive psychomotor regression and a screening test positive for mucopolysacchariduria. The presence of heparan sulfate, but not dermatan sulfate, in the urine is presumptive evidence of the disease. Definitive diagnosis requires the demonstration of enzyme deficiency in cultured fibroblasts.

MANAGEMENT. Bone marrow transplant is being tried, with variable success, in all MPS types.

Niemann-Pick Disease Type A (Sphingomyelin Lipidosis)

Niemann-Pick disease type A is caused by a deficiency of the enzyme sphingomyelinase. The trait is transmitted by autosomal recessive inheritance. Type A is the acute infantile form of Niemann-Pick disease.

CLINICAL FEATURES. The onset of the acute infantile form occurs in the first months of life. The features are feeding difficulty, failure to thrive, and hepatomegaly. Splenomegaly occurs later and is not prominent. A cherry-red spot is present in 50% of cases (Table 5-9). Psychomotor regression, characterized by postural hypotonia and loss of reactivity to the environment, occurs during the first year but may be overlooked because of the child's failure to thrive. With time, emaciation, a tendency toward opisthotonos, exaggerated tendon reflexes, and blindness develop. Seizures are uncommon.

DIAGNOSIS. The diagnosis is suggested by the clinical course. Vacuolated histiocytes are present in the bone marrow and vacuolated lymphocytes in the peripheral blood. The diagnosis is established by showing a deficiency of sphingomyelinase in leukocytes or cultured fibroblasts.

MANAGEMENT. Treatment is supportive.

Sulfatase Deficiency Disorders

Metachromatic Leukodystrophy (Sulfatide Lipidoses)

Metachromatic leukodystrophy (MLD) is a disorder of central and peripheral myelin metabolism. It is caused by deficiency of either aryl-sulfatase A (chromosome 22) or its sphingolipid activator protein B (saposin B); together they form cerebroside sulfatase. The disease is transmitted by autosomal recessive inheritance. Infantile, juvenile, and adult forms are recognized. Because peripheral neuropathy is a prominent feature of the infantile form, the condition is discussed in Chapter 7. The juvenile form affects primarily the brain and is discussed later in this chapter.

Multiple Sulfatase Deficiency

Multiple sulfatase deficiency is a rare disorder characterized by deficiency of several sulfatases (arylsulfatase A, arylsulfatase B, iduronate sulfatase, *N*-acetylgalactosamine-6-sulfate sulfatase, and heparan-*N*-sulfatase) and the accumulation of sulfatides, glycosaminoglycans, sphingolipids, and steroid sulfates in tissue and body fluids.

CLINICAL FEATURES. Development during the first year is normal, but in the second year developmental arrests and regression occurs. Ataxia and speech disturbances are also noted during the second year. Neurological deterioration is progressive. The appearance suggests an MPS: short stature, microcephaly, and facial dysmorphism. Retinal degeneration can occur as well and suggests a neuronal ceroid lipofuscinosis.

DIAGNOSIS. Sulfatase activity is deficient, but not absent, in cultured skin fibroblasts and leukocytes. If only arylsulfatase A is measured, an improper diagnosis of juvenile sulfatide lipidosis may be considered because peripheral neuropathy is not present. However, the facial dysmorphism is not consistent with either the infantile or the juvenile form of sulfatide lipidosis.

MANAGEMENT. Treatment is supportive.

Carbohydrate-Deficient Glycoprotein Syndromes

The carbohydrate-deficient glycoprotein (CDG) syndromes are a group of genetic, multisystemic diseases with major nervous system involvement (Stibler et al, 1995). They are characterized by a deficiency of the carbohydrate moiety of secretory glycoproteins, lysosomal enzymes, and probably also membrane glycoproteins. They occur mainly in northern Europeans and are transmitted by autosomal recessive inheritance. The affected organelles are not lysosomes but may be the Golgi apparatus or the endoplasmic reticulum.

CLINICAL FEATURES. Affected newborns with CDG syndrome type I seem normal except for the appearance of dysmaturity. Early infancy is characterized by failure to thrive, developmental delay, hypotonia, and multisystem failure. Neurological deterioration follows in later infancy. The main features are mental deficiency, ataxia, retinitis pigmentosa, hypotonia, and weakness. Childhood and adolescence are characterized by short stature, failure of sexual maturation, skeletal abnormalities, liver dysfunction, and polyneuropathy.

Children with CDG syndrome type II have a more profound mental retardation but no cerebellar ataxia or peripheral neuropathy, and those with CDG syndrome types III and IV have severe neurological impairment and seizures from birth.

DIAGNOSIS. Abnormal serum transferrin isoform patterns are the most constant abnormality in all CDG syndromes and are the basis for diagnosis. Each type has a distinctive pattern of abnormal serum transferrin patterns.

MANAGEMENT. Treatment is supportive.

Hypothyroidism

Congenital hypothyroidism resulting from thyroid dysgenesis occurs in 1 per 4,000 live births. It can be caused by mutations in the genes encoding thyrotropin, thyrotropin-releasing hormone, thyroid transcription factor 2, and other factors (Clifton-Bligh et al, 1998). Early diagnosis and treatment are imperative to ensure a favorable outcome. Fortunately, newborn screening is universal in the United States and detects virtually all cases.

CLINICAL FEATURES. Affected infants are usually asymptomatic at birth. Clinical features evolve insidiously during the first weeks postpartum, and their significance is not always appreciated. Frequently gestation lasts for more than 42 weeks, and birth weight is greater than 4 kg. Early clinical features include a wide-open posterior fontanelle, constipation, jaundice, poor temperature control, and umbilical hernia. The tongue is sometimes large, which makes feeding difficult. Edema of the eyes, hands, and feet may be present at birth but is often unrecognized in early infancy.

DIAGNOSIS. Radiographs of the long bones show delayed maturation, and radiographs of the skull show excessive numbers of wormian bones. The diagnosis is established by showing a low serum concentration of thyroxine (T_4) and a high serum concentration of thyroid-stimulating hormone (TSH).

MANAGEMENT. Once the diagnosis of congenital hypothyroidism is confirmed, treatment is initiated with sodium-1-thyroxine, 24 to 50 g/day. Most, if not all, of the sequelae of congenital hypothyroidism can be prevented by early treatment. Each month of delay reduces the ultimate intelligence of the infant.

Mitochondrial Disorders

Mitochondrial disorders involve pyruvate metabolism, the Krebs cycle, and respiratory complexes. Figure 8-2 depicts the five respiratory complexes, and Table 8-6 lists the disorders assigned to abnormalities in each of these complexes.

Alexander Disease

Alexander disease is a rare disorder caused by a mutation in the gene encoding NADH-ubiquinone oxidoreductase flavoprotein-1 (Schuelke et al, 1999). The gene maps to chromosome 11q13. Rosenthal fibers, the pathologic hallmark of disease, are rod-shaped or round bodies that stain red with hematoxylin and eosin and black with myelin stains. They appear as small granules within the cytoplasm of astrocytes. Rosenthal fibers are scattered diffusely in the cerebral cortex and the white matter but have a predilection for the subpial, subependymal, and perivascular regions.

CLINICAL FEATURES. The onset may be anytime from birth to early childhood. These infants show arrest and regression of psychomotor development, enlargement of the head owing to megalencephaly, spasticity, and seizures. Megalencephaly may be the initial feature. Optic atrophy does not occur. Death by the second or third year is the rule.

DIAGNOSIS. The cerebrospinal fluid is normal. The disease should be suspected in infants with macrocephaly and MRI evidence of progressive leukodystrophy affecting the deep white matter and sparing the periventricular region. Definitive diagnosis relies entirely on the postmortem demonstration of Rosenthal fibers.

MANAGEMENT. Treatment is supportive.

Subacute Necrotizing Encephalomyelopathy (Leigh Disease)

Leigh disease is a syndrome of progressive poliodystrophy primarily affecting neurons of the brainstem, thalamus, basal ganglia, and cerebellum. These pathological features can be caused by cytochrome c oxidase (COX) deficiency, as well as defects in other enzymes involved in energy metabolism (DiMauro and De Vivo, 1996). Usually the disease is transmitted by autosomal recessive inheritance, but X-linked inheritance occurs as well.

CLINICAL FEATURES. Onset occurs during the first year in 60%, during the second year in 20%, and after infancy in 20%. Children who have symptoms in early infancy have a steadily progressive course with severe disability and death. The initial symptoms are some combination of developmental delay, failure to thrive because of poor feeding or vomiting, hypotonia, and seizures. Symptoms are made worse by intercurrent infection or ingestion of a high-carbohydrate meal. Three typical, but not constant, features during infancy are respiratory disturbances, abnormal ocular motility, and hypotonia. Respiratory disturbances are at first episodic and can be characterized by Cheyne-Stokes breathing, ataxic breathing, or central hyperventilation. Respiratory distress is the usual cause of death. Ocular motility dysfunction varies from nystagmus to ophthalmoplegia. Hypotonia results from a combination of peripheral neuropathy and disturbed cerebellar function.

Children with Leigh disease caused by cytochrome c oxidase deficiency are normal during the first 8 to 12 months and then develop diarrhea, vomiting, and failure to thrive. Symptoms of neurological deterioration, similar to those described above, occur in late infancy or early childhood. The course is less rapidly progressive and symptoms are more intermittent, with exacerbations at the time of infection.

DIAGNOSIS. Blood concentrations of lactate and pyruvate are usually elevated and rise even higher at the time of clinical exacerbation. An oral glucose load causes blood lactate concentrations to double after 60 minutes.

Lesions in the brainstem and around the third ventricle may be visualized on CT and MRI. Motor nerve conduction velocities are usually slowed. When peripheral neuropathy is present, the protein content of the cerebrospinal fluid is elevated. Studies should search for COX deficiency and for disturbances in pyruvate utilization caused by deficiencies in pyruvate decarboxylase, multiple carboxylases, or pyruvate dehydrogenase. Muscle biopsy specimens have been useful for enzyme analysis in several patients.

MANAGEMENT. Children with disorders of pyruvate utilization are less likely to have acute exacerbations of illness on a carbohydrate-restricted diet. Calories should be provided primarily as lipids. Large doses of thiamine are helpful in some patients. Oral acetazolamide is useful in the treatment of cases transmitted by X-linked recessive inheritance. The mechanism of action is unknown.

Progressive Infantile Poliodystrophy (Alpers Disease)

Alpers disease was described originally as a progressive degeneration of cerebral gray matter and probably encompassed several disease processes. Deficiencies in pyruvate carboxylase activity and respiratory chain complexes I and IV have been identified in familial cases associated with mitochondrial myopathy.

CLINICAL FEATURES. The onset of symptoms is either during infancy or childhood. The disorder with infantile onset tends to be sporadic and is characterized first by delay in the achievement of developmental milestones and then by either myoclonic or tonic-clonic seizures. The first seizure can be status epilepticus. Prolonged seizures are sometimes followed by transitory hemiplegia. Psychomotor regression becomes evident, and blindness may occur.

DIAGNOSIS. Definitive diagnosis can be established only by postmortem examination. However, an elevated blood lactate concentration should suggest disturbed pyruvate utilization and prompt investigation of mitochondrial enzymes in liver and skeletal muscle. A carbohydrate load in the form of an oral glucose tolerance test may raise the blood lactate concentration to two or three times normal and worsen symptoms.

MANAGEMENT. Treatment is supportive.

Trichopoliodystrophy (Menkes Syndrome)

Menkes syndrome is a primary defect in the intestinal transport of copper (Tumer and Horn, 1997). The gene defect maps to chromosome Xq13. The symptoms are attributed to a secondary deficiency of copper-dependent enzymes, especially COX. Some patients show enzyme deficiency in muscle, brain, and liver mitochondria, others show a decreased copper concentration only in the brain.

CLINICAL FEATURES. The initial symptoms usually develop in the first 3 months. Development is first arrested and then regresses. The infant becomes lethargic and less reactive. Myoclonic seizures, provoked by stimulation, are an early and almost constant feature. By the end of the first year the infant is in a chronic vegetative state, and most die before 18 months.

The appearance of the scalp hair and eyebrows is almost pathognomonic. The hair is sparse, poorly pigmented, and wiry. The shafts break easily, forming short stubble (kinky hair). Radiographs of the long bones suggest osteogenesis imperfecta. Other facial abnormalities include abnormal fullness of the cheeks, a high-arched palate, and micrognathia.

DIAGNOSIS. Low plasma concentrations of ceruloplasmin and copper suggest the diagnosis. Gene detection confirms the diagnosis. Prenatal diagnosis is possible.

MANAGEMENT. Copper supplementation with copper histinate may prolong survival.

Neurocutaneous Syndromes

Chediak-Higashi Syndrome

CLINICAL FEATURES. Affected children are born with deficient pigment of the skin and hair. Areas of skin depigmentation form bizarre patterns that resemble giant fingerprints. Recurrent infections are prominent during infancy because of neutrophil dysfunction, with decreased bactericidal killing. Other systemic features include anemia, abnormal platelet function, bleeding, and the eventual development of lymphoreticular malignancy.

Developmental retardation, seizures, and severe peripheral neuropathy develop during the first 2 years. Symptoms of autonomic dysfunction, increased perspiration, and failure to produce overflow tears are common and may suggest dysautonomia. Death usually occurs before age 10 years.

DIAGNOSIS. The diagnosis is primarily based on the typical neurological features and pigmentary changes. Examination of the peripheral blood smear is confirmatory. The nuclei of polymorphonuclear leukocytes are pyknotic, and their cytoplasm contains large oval and fusiform granules that stain for myeloperoxidase.

MANAGEMENT. Treatment is supportive.

Neurofibromatosis Type 1

The neurofibromatoses (NF) are divided into a peripheral type (type 1) and a central type (type 2). Both are transmitted by autosomal dominant inheritance and show considerable variation in expression. The abnormal gene for neurofibromatosis type 1 (NF1) is located on chromosome 17, and its abnormal protein product is *neurofibomin*. NF1 is the most common of the neurocutaneous syndromes, occurring in approximately 1 in 3,000 individuals. Almost 50% of patients with NF1 are new mutations. New mutations are associated with increased paternal age.

Neurofibromatosis type 2 (NF2) is characterized by bilateral acoustic neuromas as well as other intracranial and intraspinal tumors (see Chapter 17).

CLINICAL FEATURES. The clinical manifestations are highly variable (Friedman and Birch, 1997). In mild cases, café au lait spots and subcutaneous neurofibromas are the only features. Axillary freckles are common.

Severely affected individuals have developmental and neoplastic disorders of the nervous system. The main central nervous system abnormalities are optic pathway glioma, intraspinal neurofibroma, dural ectasia, and aqueductal stenosis. Acoustic neuromas are not part of NF1. The usual cognitive defect is a learning disability, not mental retardation (North et al, 1997).

DIAGNOSIS. Two or more of the following features are considered diagnostic: (1) six café au lait spots more than 5 mm in diameter in prepubertal individuals or more than 15 mm in postpubertal individuals, (2) two or more neurofibromas or one plexiform neurofibroma, (3) freckling in the axillary or inguinal region, (4) optic glioma, (5) two or more iris hamartomas (Lisch nodules), (6) a distinctive osseous lesion such as sphenoid dysplasia or thinning of long bones, and (7) a first-degree relative with NF1.

MRI may provide additional diagnostic information. Areas of increased T_2 signal intensity are often present in the basal ganglia, cerebellum, brainstem, and subcortical white matter. The histology of these areas is not established, and they tend to disappear with age. It is not clear if the total burden of such areas correlates with intellectual impairment. DNA-based testing is available but unreliable.

MANAGEMENT. Management is primarily supportive: anticonvulsant drugs for seizures, surgery for accessible tumors, and orthopedic procedures for bony deformities. Routine MRI studies to screen for optic gliomas in nonsymptomatic children are not recommended.

Tuberous Sclerosis

The tuberous sclerosis complex (TSC) is transmitted by autosomal dominant inheritance and has variable phenotypic expression (Weiner et al, 1998). Two genes are responsible for TSC.

One gene (TSC1) is located at chromosome 9q34, and the other (TSC2) is near the gene for adult polycystic kidney disease at chromosome 16p13.3. No obvious phenotypic differences exist between TSC1 and TSC2.

CLINICAL FEATURES. The most common initial symptom of neurological dysfunction during infancy is seizures, especially infantile spasms (see Chapter 1). Some infants have evidence of developmental delay before the onset of seizures. The delay is often insufficient to prompt medical consultation. Most children with tuberous sclerosis who are mentally retarded eventually have seizures, and all children who have intractable seizures during the first year will be mentally retarded. Seizures and mental retardation are due to disturbed histogenesis of the brain. Neurons are decreased in number, and astrocytes are large and bizarrely shaped. Glial tumors are common in the subependymal region and may cause obstructive hydrocephalus.

In late infancy and early childhood, café au lait spots develop and an isolated raised plaque in the skin over the lower back or buttocks (Shagreen patch) is present by 15 years in 50% of affected children. During childhood, adenomata sebaceum (actually angiokeratomas) appear on the face, usually in a butterfly distribution. Other organ involvement includes retinal tumors, rhabdomyoma of the heart, renal tumors, and cysts of the kidney, bone, and lung.

The disease shortens the life expectancy. The causes of death during childhood are renal disease, cardiovascular disorders, brain tumors, and status epilepticus.

DIAGNOSIS. The diagnostic criteria for TSC (Table 5-10) were recently revised (Roach et al, 1998). Molecular testing for both genes is available on a research basis only.

MANAGEMENT. The following evaluations are recommended in children with TSC: renal ultrasonography every 1 to 3 years followed by renal CT/MRI if large or numerous renal tumors are detected; cranial CT/MRI every 1 to 3 years; echocardiography if cardiac symptoms indicate the need; and chest CT if pulmonary symptoms indicate the need.

Anticonvulsants are helpful in reducing seizure frequency but rarely provide complete control. Mental retardation is not reversible. Genetic counseling is an important aspect of patient management. Although the disease is transmitted by autosomal dominant inheritance, gene expression is so variable that neither parent may appear affected. Sporadic cases were thought to be common. However, 25% of parents without a personal or family history of tu-

Table 5-10
Diagnostic Criteria for the Tuberous Sclerosis Complex

Definite TSC: two major features or one major feature plus two minor features
Probable TSC: one major feature plus one minor feature
Possible TSC: one major feature or two or more minor features

Major Features
Cardiac rhabdomyoma, single or multiple
Cortical tuber*
Facial angiofibromas or forehead plaque
Hypomelanotic macules (three or more)
Lymphangiomyomatosis†
Multiple retinal nodular hamartomas
Nontraumatic ungual or periungual fibromas
Renal angiomyolipoma†
Shagreen patch (connective tissue nevus)
Subependymal giant cell astrocytoma
Subependymal nodule

Minor Features
Bone cysts
Cerebral white matter radial migration lines*
"Confetti" skin lesions
Gingival fibromas
Hamartomatous rectal polyps
Multiple randomly distributed pits in dental enamel
Multiple renal cysts
Nonrenal hamartoma
Retinal achromic patch

* When cerebral cortical dysplasia and cerebral white matter migration tracts occur together, they are counted as one rather than two features of TSC.
† When both lymphangiomyomatosis and renal angiomyolipomas are present, other features of tuberous sclerosis must be present before TSC is diagnosed.

berous sclerosis are shown to be affected by a careful history and physical examination, including fundoscopic examination, renal ultrasound, and cranial MRI.

Other Disorders of Gray Matter

Early-Infantile Neuronal Ceroid Lipofuscinosis (Santavuori-Haltia Disease)

The neuronal ceroid lipofuscinoses (NCLs) are a group of genetic disorders transmitted as autosomal recessive traits in which *lipofuscin* is stored in neurons and some visceral tissues. These disorders had been classified by age at onset and rapidity of progression but are now diagnosed by mutation analysis. The early infantile form (Santavuori disease) occurs primarily in Finnish people. The responsible mutation occurs in the palmitoyl protein thioesterase (PPT)

gene on chromosome 1 (Syvänen et al, 1997). This site has been designated NCL1.

The more common NCL types occur after age 2 (see section on Progressive Encephalopathies with Onset After Age 2 later in this chapter) and are caused by mutations at other sites.

CLINICAL FEATURES. Onset is usually in the second year but may be in the first. Visual impairment and myoclonus are initial features. Rapid deterioration follows and is characterized by psychomotor regression, hypotonia, ataxia, and hyperkinesia. Seizures are not prominent.

Total blindness develops between the ages of 2 and 3 years. The macula degenerats and has a brownish color, the optic disk is atrophic, and the peripheral retina is hypopigmented.

DIAGNOSIS. PPT activity is found to be deficient in fibroblasts, leukocytes, lymphoblasts, amniotic fluid cells, and chorionic villi using a new fluorimetric assay (Voznyi et al, 1999).

MANAGEMENT. Seizures and myoclonus should be treated with a combination of valproate, clonazepam, and phenobarbital (see Chapter 1). No treatment for the underlying metabolic error is available.

Infantile Neuroaxonal Dystrophy

Infantile neuroaxonal dystrophy (*Seitelberger disease*) is a disorder of axon terminals transmitted by autosomal recessive inheritance. It shares many pathological features with Hallervorden-Spatz disease (see Chapter 14) and may be an infantile form.

CLINICAL FEATURES. Affected children usually develop normally during the first year, but most do not walk independently. Motor regression is evidenced at the end of the first year as clumsiness and frequent falling. The infant is first hypotonic and hyporeflexic. Muscle atrophy may be present as well. At this stage a peripheral neuropathy is suspected, but motor nerve conduction velocity and the protein content of the cerebrospinal fluid are normal.

After the initial phase of hypotonia, symptoms of cerebral degeneration become prominent. Increasing spastic quadriparesis, optic atrophy, involuntary movements, and mental regression are evident. By 2 years of age, most children are severely handicapped. Deterioration to a vegetative state follows, and death usually occurs by age 10 years.

DIAGNOSIS. The cerebrospinal fluid is usually normal. Electromyography shows a denervation pattern consistent with anterior horn cell disease. Motor nerve conduction velocities are normal. T2-weighted MRI shows marked cerebellar atrophy with diffuse hyperintensity of the cerebellar cortex. The hyperintensity is probably due to extensive gliosis.

A definitive diagnosis requires evidence of neuroaxonal spheroids in peripheral nerve endings, conjunctiva, or brain. Neuroaxonal spheroids are large eosinophilic spheroids, caused by axonal swelling, throughout the gray matter. They are not unique to neuroaxonal dystrophy and are also seen in Hallervorden-Spatz disease, infantile GM$_2$ gangliosidosis, Niemann-Pick disease type C, and several other neurodegenerative conditions.

MANAGEMENT. Treatment is supportive.

Lesch-Nyhan Disease

Lesch-Nyhan disease is caused by a deficiency of the enzyme hypoxanthine guanine phosphoribosyltransferase. The gene map locus is chromosome Xq26-q27.2.

CLINICAL FEATURES. Affected newborns appear normal at birth, except for mild hypotonia. Delayed motor development and poor head control are present during the first 3 months. These are followed by progressive limb rigidity and torticollis or retrocollis. The progression of neurological disturbance is insidious, and many affected patients are thought to have cerebral palsy. During the second year, facial grimacing, corticospinal tract dysfunction, and involuntary movements (usually chorea but sometimes athetosis) develop.

It is not until after age 2, and sometimes considerably later, that affected children begin biting their fingers, lips, and cheeks. Compulsive self-mutilation is characteristic, but not invariable, and causes severe disfigurement. Often wrapping the hands or removing teeth is necessary to prevent further harm. In addition to self-directed aggressive behavior, aggressive behavior toward caretakers may be present. Mental retardation is constant but of variable severity. Intelligence is difficult to evaluate because of behavioral and motor disturbances.

DIAGNOSIS. Uric acid concentrations are increased in the blood and urine. Indeed, some parents note a reddish discoloration of diapers caused by uric acid. The diagnosis is established by showing that hypoxanthine guanine phosphoribosyltransferase activity is absent in erythrocytes or cultured fibroblasts.

MANAGEMENT. Allopurinol decreases the urinary concentration of uric acid and prevents the development of nephropathy. Self-mutilatory behavior may be abated by the use of levodopa or tetrabenazine. However, no treatment is available to prevent progressive degeneration of the nervous system.

Progressive Neuronal Degeneration with Liver Disease

This syndrome probably encompasses several different conditions and is sometimes referred to as *Alpers diffuse degeneration of cerebral gray matter with hepatic cirrhosis* (Harding et al, 1995). It is not the same disorder as progressive infantile poliodystrophy (Alpers), listed in this chapter as a mitochondrial disorder.

CLINICAL FEATURES. Hypotonia, failure to thrive, and developmental delay during infancy are followed by intractable seizures and liver failure. Status epilepticus is common. Death from liver failure usually occurs by age 3.

In addition to the infantile form, a similar syndrome has been described in children and adolescents. Among older children, visual hallucinations may be an initial feature. Status epilepticus and liver failure are common. Death is invariable.

DIAGNOSIS. MRI shows abnormalities in the deep gray matter as well as in the cortex. The occipital lobes are selectively involved. The diagnosis is suspected by the combination of encephalopathy and liver failure. The encephalopathy is not caused by the liver failure. The definitive diagnosis requires postmortem examination to show a patchy destruction of the cerebral cortex with predominant involvement of the occipital lobes.

MANAGEMENT. Anticonvulsant drugs are used to treat seizures, but no treatment is available for the underlying disease.

Rett Syndrome

Rett syndrome occurs only in girls, and the prevalence is estimated to be $1:10,000-1:20,000$. The syndrome can be caused by mutation in the gene encoding methyl-CpG-binding protein-2. The gene maps to chromosome Xq28. The precise mechanism of inheritance by which an X-linked disorder occurs only in females is not established (Online Mendelian Inheritance in Man, 1999).

CLINICAL FEATURES. Affected girls are normal during the first year. Developmental arrest usually begins at 12 months, but may appear as early as 5 months or as late as 18 months. The initial features are deceleration of head growth leading to microcephaly, lack of interest in the environment, and hypotonia. Within a few months, rapid developmental regression occurs and is characterized by loss of language skills, decreased use of the hands, gait ataxia, seizures, and autistic behavior. Dementia is usually severe. Although affected girls are unable to sustain interest in the environment, stimulation produces an exaggerated, stereotyped reaction consisting of jerking movements of the trunk and limbs with episodes of disorganized breathing and apnea, followed by hyperpnea. During these episodes, circumoral cyanosis and diffuse perspiration may occur. Similar episodes may also occur without stimulation but not during sleep. Such episodes are frequently interpreted as seizures, although it is not clear that they are epileptic in nature. Typical tonic-clonic seizures, partial complex seizures, or myoclonic seizures occur in most children between the ages of 1 and 3 years.

A characteristic feature of the syndrome is loss of purposeful hand movements before the age of 3. They are replaced by stereotyped activity that looks like hand wringing or washing. Repetitive blows to the face are another form of stereotyped hand movement.

The initial rapid progression is followed by a continued slower progression of neurological deterioration. Spastic paraparesis and quadriparesis are frequent endpoints.

DIAGNOSIS. Diagnosis is based entirely on the clinical features. Laboratory tests are not helpful.

MANAGEMENT. Seizures often respond to standard anticonvulsant drugs. Attempts to treat the respiratory irregularities with naloxone and magnesium sulfate have proven ineffective.

Other Disorders of White Matter

Aspartoacylase Deficiency (Canavan Disease)

Canavan disease (also called *spongy degeneration of infancy*) is transmitted by autosomal recessive inheritance. It is caused by deficiency of aspartoacylase. Different mutations account for Jewish and non-Jewish cases, but the variability of the clinical course cannot be explained by genetic heterogeneity alone (Traeger and Rapin, 1998).

CLINICAL FEATURES. Psychomotor arrest and regression occur during the first 6 months postpartum. Clinical features include decreased awareness of the environment, difficulty in feeding, irritability, and hypotonia. The initial flac-

cidity is eventually replaced by spasticity. A characteristic posture, with leg extension, arm flexion, and head retraction, is assumed, especially when the child is stimulated. Macrocephaly is noted by 6 months of age. The head continues to enlarge throughout infancy, and this growth reaches a plateau by the third year. Optic atrophy leading to blindness is noted between 6 and 10 months.

DIAGNOSIS. Abnormal excretion of N-acetylaspartic acid can be detected in the urine, and aspartoacylase activity in cultured fibroblasts is less than 40% of normal. MRI shows diffuse symmetric leukoencephalopathy even before neurological symptoms are evident. Demyelination of peripheral nerves does not occur, and the cerebrospinal fluid is normal.

MANAGEMENT. Treatment is supportive.

Galactosemia: Transferase Deficiency

Three separate inborn errors of galactose metabolism are known to produce galactosemia in the newborn, but only galactose-1-phosphate uridyltransferase deficiency produces mental retardation. The defect is transmitted by autosomal recessive inheritance, and the gene map locus is 9p13.

CLINICAL FEATURES. Affected newborns appear normal, but cataracts are already developing. The initial symptoms are provoked by the first milk feeding and include failure to thrive, vomiting, diarrhea, jaundice, and hepatomegaly. During this time some newborns have clinical features of increased intracranial pressure, probably resulting from cerebral edema. The combination of a tense fontanelle and vomiting suggests a primary intracranial disturbance and can delay the diagnosis and treatment of the metabolic error.

DIAGNOSIS. Galactosemia should be considered in any newborn with vomiting and hepatomegaly, especially when cataracts are present. The best time to test the urine for reducing substances (by the use of Clinitest tablets) is after feeding. Specific tests for glucose (Testape, Clinistix) show no abnormality. Most cases of galactosemia in newborns are now detected by routine screening tests.

MANAGEMENT. Long-term results of treatment have been disappointing; IQ is low in many cases despite early and seemingly adequate therapy consisting of a galactose-free diet. The achievement of developmental milestones is delayed during the first year, and intellectual function is moderately retarded by age 5. After age 5, truncal ataxia develops and progresses in severity. Associated with ataxia is a coarse resting tremor of the limbs. Because of the restricted diet, cataracts and hepatomegaly are not present.

Pelizaeus-Merzbacher Disease

Pelizaeus-Merzbacher disease is a rare demyelinating disorder transmitted by X-linked recessive inheritance. The gene maps to chromosome Xq22. The disease is caused by defective biosynthesis of a proteolipid protein that comprises half of the myelin sheath protein (Garbern et al, 1999). An infantile, a neonatal, and a transitional phenotype are differentiated.

CLINICAL FEATURES. The first symptoms of the neonatal form suggest spasmus nutans (see Chapter 15). The neonate has an intermittent nodding movement of the head and pendular nystagmus. Chorea or athetosis develops, psychomotor development is arrested by the third month, and regression follows. Limb movements become ataxic and tone becomes spastic, first in the legs and then in the arms. Optic atrophy and seizures are late occurrences. Death occurs by 5 to 7 years of age.

When the onset of disease is at the end of the first month or later, the symptoms are the same as in the neonatal form but the course is more prolonged and survival to adult life is relatively common.

DIAGNOSIS. MRI shows diffuse demyelination of the hemispheres with sparing of scattered small areas. The diagnosis is established by showing a deletion of the exon coding the proteolipid protein on the X chromosome. Postmortem examination shows diffuse demyelination of the cerebral and cerebellar hemispheres, with patches of normal myelin remaining. Nerve cells and axons appear normal. When survival is prolonged, myelin is completely absent in the cerebral hemispheres.

MANAGEMENT. Treatment is supportive.

Progressive Hydrocephalus

CLINICAL FEATURES. Progressive dilatation of the ventricular system may be a consequence of congenital malformations, infectious diseases, intracranial hemorrhage, or connatal tumors. Whatever the cause, the clinical features of increasing intracranial pressure are much the same. Head circumference enlarges, the anterior fontanelle feels full, and the child becomes lethargic, has difficulty feeding, and vomits. Ataxia and a spastic gait are common.

DIAGNOSIS. Progressive hydrocephalus is often insidious in premature newborns with intraventricular hemorrhage, especially when delayed progression follows initial arrest. Hydrocephalus should always be suspected in newborns and infants with excessive head growth. Head CT confirms the diagnosis.

MANAGEMENT. Ventriculoperitoneal shunt is the usual procedure to relieve hydrocephalus in newborns and small infants with primary dilatation of the lateral ventricles (see Chapter 18).

Progressive Encephalopathies with Onset after Age 2

Disorders of Lysosomal Enzymes

GM$_2$ Gangliosidosis (Juvenile Tay-Sachs Disease)

The juvenile form of Tay-Sachs disease, like the infantile form, is caused by deficiency of N-acetyl-β-hexosaminidase. The enzymatic basis of the phenotypic variability is incompletely understood.

CLINICAL FEATURES. There is no ethnic predilection. Affected children appear normal until age 3 years, but then dysarthria, language retardation, and gait disturbances develop. The gait is first ataxic and then spastic. Progressive dementia follows, and death usually occurs within the first decade. Seizures and involuntary movements may occur in some patients.

DIAGNOSIS. Enzyme deficiency is demonstrated in leukocytes and fibroblasts.

MANAGEMENT. Treatment is supportive.

Gaucher Disease Type III (Glucosylceramide Lipidosis)

The late-onset type of Gaucher disease, like other types, is caused by deficiency of the enzyme glucocerebrosidase and transmitted by autosomal recessive inheritance.

CLINICAL FEATURES. Age at onset ranges from early childhood to adult life. Hepatosplenomegaly usually precedes neurological deterioration. The most common neurological manifestations are seizures and mental regression. Mental regression varies from mild memory loss to severe dementia. Myoclonus and myoclonic seizures develop in many patients. Some combination of spasticity, ataxia, and cranial nerve dysfunction may be present as well. Vertical oculomotor apraxia, as described in Niemann-Pick disease, may occur in late-onset Gaucher disease as well.

DIAGNOSIS. Gaucher cells are present in the bone marrow and are virtually diagnostic. Confirmation requires the demonstration of deficient glucocerebrosidase activity in hepatocytes or leukocytes.

MANAGEMENT. The clinical features are modified by repeated infusions of modified acid β-glucosidase (NIH Technology Assessment Panel on Gaucher Disease, 1996).

Globoid Cell Leukodystrophy (Late-Onset Krabbe Disease)

Globoid cell leukodystrophy is caused by deficiency of the enzyme galactosylceramide β-galactosidase. The defect is transmitted by autosomal recessive inheritance. The onset of symptoms in late infancy and in adolescence can occur in the same family. The severity of the enzyme deficiency is similar in all phenotypes from early infancy to adolescence.

CLINICAL FEATURES. Neurological deterioration usually begins between the ages of 2 and 6, but may start as early as the second year or as late as adolescence. The major features are mental regression, cortical blindness, and generalized or unilateral spasticity. The initial feature may be progressive spasticity rather than dementia. Unlike the infantile form, peripheral neuropathy is not a feature of the juvenile form, and the protein content of the cerebrospinal fluid is normal. Progressive neurological deterioration results in a vegetative state.

DIAGNOSIS. MRI shows diffuse demyelination of the cerebral hemispheres. The diagnosis is established by showing the enzyme deficiency in leukocytes or cultured fibroblasts.

MANAGEMENT. Treatment is supportive.

Glycoprotein Degradation Disorders

Aspartylglycosaminuria

Aspartylglycosaminuria is a very rare condition that occurs primarily in Finnish individuals. The defect, a deficiency of the enzyme N-aspartyl-β-glucosaminidase, is transmitted by autosomal recessive inheritance. The gene maps to chromosome 4q32-q33.

CLINICAL FEATURES. Affected individuals are healthy in early infancy but later have recurrent infection, diarrhea, and inguinal hernia. During early childhood, the facial features become coarse and hepatomegaly occasionally develops. Lens opacities occur after age 10. Speech may be delayed, but mental development is otherwise

normal until age 5. Afterward, a slowly progressive regression of mental and motor skills results in severe retardation and generalized weakness.

DIAGNOSIS. Vacuolated lymphocytes are present in the peripheral blood of most patients, and a mild form of dysostosis multiplex is demonstrated radiographically. The urine does not contain mucopolysaccharides but does contain oligosaccharides. The diagnosis is established by showing enzyme deficiency in leukocytes or cultured fibroblasts.

MANAGEMENT. Treatment is supportive.

Mannosidosis Type II

CLINICAL FEATURES. The late-onset, juvenile and adult form of mannosidosis is characterized by normal early development followed by mental regression during childhood or adolescence. Dysostosis multiplex is not a prominent feature, but deafness occurs in all cases.

DIAGNOSIS. Vacuolated lymphocytes are present in peripheral blood. The urine contains oligosaccharides but not mucopolysaccharides. The diagnosis is established by showing deficient activity of β-mannosidase in cultured fibroblasts.

MANAGEMENT. Treatment is supportive.

Metachromatic Leukodystrophy (Late-Onset Lipidosis)

The juvenile form of sulfatide lipidosis, like the infantile form, is caused by a deficiency of the enzyme arylsulfatase A and is transmitted by autosomal recessive inheritance. Two groups of mutations in the gene encoding arylsulfatase A are identified as I and A. The I group generates no active enzyme, and the A group generates small amounts. Late-onset disease is associated with an I-A genotype, and the adult form with an A-A genotype correlates with the clinical phenotype.

CLINICAL FEATURES. The onset of symptoms is generally between 5 and 10 years but may be delayed until adolescence or occur as early as late infancy. The early-onset juvenile form is clinically different from the infantile form despite the age overlap. No clinical symptoms of peripheral neuropathy occur, progression is slow, and the protein content of the cerebrospinal fluid is normal.

Mental regression, speech disturbances, and clumsiness of gait are the prominent initial features. The dementia usually progresses slowly over a period 3 to 5 years but sometimes progresses rapidly to a vegetative state. A delay of several years may separate the onset of dementia from the appearance of other neurological disturbances. Ataxia may be an early and prominent manifestation. A spastic quadriplegia eventually develops in all affected children, and most have seizures. Death usually occurs during the second decade.

DIAGNOSIS. The juvenile form can overlap in age with a late-onset form that usually is manifest as psychosis or dementia. MRI demonstrates demyelination in the cerebral hemispheres. Motor nerve conduction velocities may be normal early in the course. The diagnosis is established by showing arylsulfatase A deficiency in leukocytes or cultured fibroblasts.

MANAGEMENT. Treatment is supportive.

Mucopolysaccharidoses

The mucopolysaccharidoses (MPS) result from deficiencies of enzymes involved in the catabolism of dermatan sulfate, heparan sulfate, or keratin sulfate. At least seven major types of MPS are recognized. Four of these, types I, II, III, and VII, affect the nervous system and cause mental retardation. Types I and III have their onset in infancy and are discussed in the prior section. Types II and VII ordinarily have their onset in childhood following 2 or more years of normal development.

Type II MPS (Hunter Syndrome)

This is the only MPS transmitted by X-linked inheritance. The gene maps to chromosome Xq28.

CLINICAL FEATURES. Patients with the Hunter syndrome have a Hurler phenotype (Table 5-8) but lack corneal clouding. Iduronate sulfatase is the deficient enzyme; dermatan sulfate and heparan sulfate are stored in the viscera and appear in the urine.

The Hurler phenotype may develop rapidly or evolve slowly during childhood and may not be recognized until the second decade or later. A prominent feature is the appearance of a nodular, ivory-colored lesion on the back, usually around the shoulders and upper arms. Mental regression caused by neuronal storage of gangliosides is slowly progressive, but many patients come to medical attention because of chronic hydrocephalus. Affected children survive into adult life. The accumulation of storage materials in collagen causes the entrapment of peripheral nerves, especially the median and ulnar nerves.

DIAGNOSIS. The diagnosis is suggested by the presence of mucopolysacchariduria with equal excretion of dermatan sulfate and heparan sulfate. The diagnosis is established by showing enzyme deficiency in cultured fibroblasts or serum. Prenatal diagnosis is accomplished by detecting iduronate sulfatase activity in amniotic fluid.

MANAGEMENT. Nerve entrapment and hydrocephalus can be relieved by appropriate surgical procedures. Treatment is not available for the underlying storage disease.

Type VII MPS (Sly Disease)

Sly disease is a rare disorder caused by deficiency of the enzyme β-glucuronidase. It is transmitted by autosomal recessive inheritance.

CLINICAL FEATURES. The patient has an incomplete Hurler phenotype, with hepatosplenomegaly, inguinal hernias, and dysostosis multiplex as the major features. Corneal clouding does not occur, and the face, although unusual, is not typical of the Hurler phenotype. Psychomotor retardation develops after age 2 but not in all cases.

DIAGNOSIS. Both dermatan sulfate and heparan sulfate are present in the urine, causing a screening test to be positive for mucopolysacchariduria. Specific diagnosis requires the demonstration of β-glucuronidase deficiency in leukocytes or cultured fibroblasts.

MANAGEMENT. Treatment is supportive.

Niemann-Pick Disease Type C (Sphingomyelin Lipidosis)

The chronic neuronopathic form of Niemann-Pick disease is similar to the acute infantile form except that onset is usually after age 2, progression is slower, and there is no specific racial predilection. The biochemical defect is deficient esterification of cholesterol. The defect is transmitted by autosomal recessive inheritance, and the gene maps to chromosome 18q11-12 (Patterson, 2000).

CLINICAL FEATURES. Three phenotypes are distinguished by age of onset and predominant symptoms. The early-onset form is characterized by organomegaly and rapidly progressive hepatic dysfunction during the first year, often in the first 6 months. Developmental delay is noted during the first year, and neurological deterioration (ataxia, vertical gaze apraxia, dementia) occurs between 1 and 3 years of age.

The delayed-onset form is more common than the other two and has the most stereotyped clinical features. Early development is normal. Cerebellar ataxia or dystonia is the initial feature (mean age, 3 years), and apraxia of vertical gaze and cognitive difficulties follow (mean age, 6 years). Oculomotor apraxia, in which the eyes move reflexively but not voluntarily, is unusual in children (see Chapter 15). Vertical gaze apraxia is particularly uncommon and always suggests Niemann-Pick disease type C. Progressive neurological degeneration is relentless. Dementia, seizures, and spasticity cause severe disability during the second decade. Organomegaly is seldom prominent early in the course.

The late-onset form begins in adolescence or adult life and is similar to the delayed-onset form except that the progression is considerably slower.

DIAGNOSIS. Biochemical testing shows impaired cholesterol esterification and positive filipin staining in cultured fibroblasts. Biochemical testing for carrier status is not reliable. Almost all affected children have a gene mutation, but molecular testing is not yet commercially available.

MANAGEMENT. Treatment is supportive. Bone marrow transplantation, combined bone marrow and liver transplantation, and cholesterol-lowering therapy are not effective.

Infectious Diseases

Infectious diseases are an uncommon cause of progressive dementia in childhood. Several fungal species may cause chronic meningitis characterized by personality change and some decline in higher intellectual function. *Cryptococcus* infection is especially notorious for its indolent course. However, the major features of these infections are fever and headache. Chronic meningitis is not a serious consideration in the differential diagnosis of isolated psychomotor regression.

In contrast, chronic viral infections, especially HIV (see the previous discussion of AIDS encephalopathy), may produce a clinical picture similar to that of many genetic disorders in which dementia is a prominent feature.

Subacute Sclerosing Panencephalitis

Subacute sclerosing panencephalitis (SSPE) is a form of chronic measles encephalitis that was once endemic in several parts of the world but has almost disappeared in countries that require routine measles immunization. In a nonimmunized population the average age at onset is 8 years. As a rule, children with SSPE have experienced natural infection with the rubeola virus at an early age, half before age 2 years. A concomitant infection with a second virus at the time of initial exposure to measles and immunosuppression are additional risk factors for SSPE. In the United States, incidence rates were highest in rural areas, especially in the southeastern states and the Ohio River Valley.

CLINICAL FEATURES. The first symptoms of disease are personality change and declining school performance. Personality change may consist of aggressive behavior or withdrawal, and psychological rather than medical services may be sought. However, retinal examination during this early stage shows pigmentary changes in the macula. Generalized seizures, usually myoclonic, develop next. An EEG at this time shows the characteristic pattern of periodic bursts of spike-wave complexes (approximately every 5 to 7 seconds) occurring synchronously with the myoclonic jerk. After the onset of seizures, the child shows rapid neurological deterioration characterized by spasticity, dementia, and involuntary movements. Within 1 to 6 years from the onset of symptoms, the child is in a chronic vegetative state.

DIAGNOSIS. The diagnosis can be suspected from the clinical course and the characteristic EEG. Confirmation requires demonstration of an elevated antibody titer against rubeola, usually associated with elevated gamma globulin concentrations, in the cerebrospinal fluid. The cerebrospinal fluid is otherwise normal. The plasma rubeola antibody titer is also markedly elevated.

A similar progressive disorder of the nervous system may occur in children who were born with rubella embryopathy (chronic rubella panencephalitis).

MANAGEMENT. Some patients have improved or stabilized after several 6-week treatments of intraventricular α-interferon, starting at 105 U/m^2 body surface area/day combined with oral isoprinosine, 100 mg/kg/day. Courses may be repeated up to six times at 2- to 6-month intervals (Anlar et al, 1997).

Other Disorders of Gray Matter

Ceroid Lipofuscinosis

Several neurodegenerative disorders characterized by dementia and blindness are now considered to be forms of ceroid lipofuscinosis. When these disorders were first described, different eponymic designations were used, depending on the age at onset (Table 5-11). The common pathological feature is the accumulation of autofluorescent lipopigments, ceroid and lipofuscin within the brain, retina, and some visceral tissues. All of the neuronal lipofuscinoses are transmitted by autosomal recessive inheritance except for one adult form. The early-infantile form was described in the previous section. The early and late juvenile disorders are allelic. The early infantile, late infantile, and juvenile forms map to different chromosomes.

Late Infantile Neuronal-Ceroid Lipofuscinois (Jansky-Bielschowsky Disease)

CLINICAL FEATURES. Visual failure begins between 2 and 3 years and progresses slowly. The onset of seizures and dementia is at 2 to 4 years. The seizures are myoclonic, akinetic, and tonic-clonic and are usually refractory to anticonvulsant drugs. Severe ataxia develops, owing in part to seizures and in part to motor system deterioration. Myoclonus, involuntary movements, and dementia follow. Dementia sometimes precedes the first seizure.

Ophthalmoscopic findings are abnormal before visual symptoms occur. They include attenuation of vessels, early optic atrophy, and pigmentary degeneration of the macula. The loss of motor, mental, and visual function is relentlessly progressive, and within months the child is in a chronic vegetative state. Death is usually between 10 and 15 years.

DIAGNOSIS. Antemortem and prenatal diagnosis is accomplished by screening CLN2 protease activity in blood, followed by gene analysis when protease activity is diminished (Berry-Kravis et al, 2000).

MANAGEMENT. Seizures are difficult to control but may respond in part to a combination of valproate, clonazepam, and phenobarbital (see Chapter 1). No treatment is available for the underlying metabolic error.

Early-Juvenile Ceroid-Lipofuscinosis (Batten)

CLINICAL FEATURES. Onset of visual failure is between 4 and 5 years, and the onset of seizures and dementia is between 5 and 9 years. Loss of ambulation occurs during the second decade (Lauronen et al, 1999). Myoclonus is prominent. Death occurs between 10 and 20 years.

DIAGNOSIS. Macular degeneration and pigmentary aggregation are seen on ophthalmoscopic examination. Curvilinear bodies are seen in skin and rectal tissue.

MANAGEMENT. Treatment is the same as for the late-infantile form.

Late Juvenile Ceroid-Lipofuscinosis (Spielmeyer-Vogt Disease)

CLINICAL FEATURES. The mean age at onset of the juvenile disease is 6 years, with a range from 4 to 9 years. Decreasing visual acuity is the most prominent feature. Time to blindness is shorter than in the early-juvenile form. Ophthalmoscopic examination shows attenuation of retinal vessels, a patchy retinal atrophy that resembles retinitis pigmentosa, mild optic atrophy, and a granular discoloration of the macula that may have a bull's-eye appearance with a dull red spot in the center.

The dementia is characterized by declining school performance and behavioral disturbances. Delusions and hallucinations are common. Blindness and dementia are the only symptoms for many years. Late in the course, speech becomes slurred and Parkinson-like rigidity develops. Myoclonic jerks and tonic-clonic seizures begin some years after onset but are not usually severe. Death usually occurs within 15 years of onset.

DIAGNOSIS. Antemortem diagnosis is reasonably certain because of the characteristic retinal

Table 5-11
The Neuronal Ceroid Lipofuscinoses

	Infantile	Late-Infantile	Early-Juvenile	Late-Juvenile
Other Names	Santavuori-Haltia disease	Jansky-Bielschowsky disease	Batten or Spielmeyer-Vogt disease	Batten or Spielmeyer-Vogt disease
Age of Onset	6–12 months	2–3 years	4–10 years	8–12 years
Chrosome Location	1p (CLN1)	11p15.5 (CLN2)	16p12.1 (CLN3)	16p12.1 (CLN3)

changes and is confirmed by skin and conjunctival biopsy. Fingerprint bodies are present in the cytoplasm of several cell types. The electroretinogram shows depression or absence of retinal potentials early in the course. Leukocytes in the peripheral blood are frequently abnormal. Translucent vacuoles are present in lymphocytes, and azurophilic granules occur in neutrophils.

MANAGEMENT. Treatment is not available for the underlying metabolic defect. Seizures usually respond to standard anticonvulsant drugs.

Heller Syndrome

Heller syndrome was originally described as a progressive dementia of childhood affecting males and females between the ages of 1 and 4 years. The early-onset female cases are now believed to be Rett syndrome.

CLINICAL FEATURES. Heller syndrome probably has a male predominance. Affected children develop normally up to at least 30 months of age. Dementia progresses for 1 to 3 years and results in profound mental retardation with marked autistic features but no effect on motor skills.

DIAGNOSIS. The diagnosis is based on clinical symptoms. The syndrome is differentiated from Rett syndrome by the age at onset, male predominance, and lack of motor disturbances; and from infantile autism by the age at onset. All other causes of progressive dementia of childhood must be excluded (Table 5-4).

MANAGEMENT. Treatment is supportive.

Huntington Disease

Huntington disease (HD) is a chronic degenerative disease of the nervous system transmitted by autosomal dominant inheritance. The HD gene maps to chromosome 4p16.3 and codes for a protein known as *huntingtin*. Its function is unknown. The gene contains an expanded trinucleotide (CAG) repeat sequence. The normal number of repeats is less than 29. Adult-onset HD patients usually have more than 35 repeats, while juvenile-onset patients often have 50 or more (Andrew et al, 1997).

CLINICAL FEATURES. The age of onset is usually between 35 and 55 but may be as early as 2 years. Approximately 10% of affected children show symptoms before 20 years of age and 5% before 14 years of age. When HD begins in childhood, the father is the affected parent in 83% of cases and may be asymptomatic when the child is born. Extrachromosomal organelles,

such as mitochondria, are inherited exclusively from the mother and may delay the expression of the gene when the mother is the affected individual.

The initial features are usually progressive dementia and behavioral disturbances. Declining school performance often brings the child to medical attention. Rigidity, with loss of facial expression and associative movements, is more common than choreoathetosis and hyperkinesis in early-onset cases. Cerebellar dysfunction occurs in approximately 20% of cases and can be a major cause of disability. Ocular motor apraxia may also be present (see Chapter 15). Seizures, which are rare in adult-onset cases, are present in 50% of affected children. The course in childhood is relentlessly progressive, and the average duration from onset to death is 8 years.

DIAGNOSIS. Reliable molecular testing is available to determine the size of the expanded CAG repeat.

MANAGEMENT. Rigidity may be temporarily relieved with levodopa, bromocriptine, and amantadine. Neuroleptics are useful for behavioral control, but treatment is not available for the dementia.

Mitochondrial Encephalomyopathies

The mitochondrial encephalomyopathies are a diverse group of disorders with defects of oxidative metabolism. Three such disorders are described in the section on progressive encephalopathies of infancy. Later-onset mitochondrial disorders are characterized by progressive external ophthalmoplegia or myopathy. However, a late-onset form of poliodystrophy and a syndrome of myoclonic epilepsy associated with ragged-red fibers in skeletal muscle cause childhood dementia as the initial feature. Genetic transmission is by maternal inheritance.

Late-Onset Poliodystrophy

CLINICAL FEATURES. The clinical features are similar to those of progressive infantile poliodystrophy except that the onset of dementia is delayed until 6 years of age or later. The dementia may be preceded by years of intermittent vomiting, lethargy, and headaches. Generalized tonic-clonic seizures can precede the onset of dementia or at least bring the child, who is already showing poor school performance, to medical attention. The subsequent course is variable and probably depends on the underlying defect in mitochondrial metabolism. In many children a myopathy develops; others have spasticity and blindness.

DIAGNOSIS. Definitive diagnosis can be established only by postmortem examination. However, an elevated blood lactate concentration should suggest disturbed pyruvate utilization and prompt investigation of mitochondrial enzymes in liver and skeletal muscle. A carbohydrate load in the form of an oral glucose tolerance test may raise the blood lactate concentration to two or three times normal and worsen symptoms.

When myopathy is present in addition to dementia, muscle biopsy usually demonstrates ragged-red fibers (see Figure 8-3).

MANAGEMENT. Treatment is supportive.

Myoclonic Epilepsy and Ragged-Red Fibers

Myoclonic epilepsy and ragged-red Fibers (MERRF) is caused by point mutations in mitochondrial DNA (mtDNA). The phenotype can be produced by mutation in more than one mitochondrial gene. The severity of the clinical phenotype is proportional to the amount of mutant mtDNA.

CLINICAL FEATURES. Clinical heterogeneity is common even among members of the same family and ranges from severe central nervous system dysfunction to myopathy. Onset may be anytime during childhood or up until the fourth decade. An insidious decline in school performance is often the initial feature, but generalized tonic-clonic seizures or myoclonus may be the symptoms that first prompt medical consultation. The seizures may be induced by flickering light or watching television. Brief myoclonic twitching develops, often induced by action (action myoclonus), which may interfere with hand movement and posture. Ataxia is a constant feature as the disease progresses, and this may be due to action myoclonus rather than cerebellar dysfunction. Some patients have hearing loss, short stature, and endocrine dysfunction.

Neurological deterioration is progressive and may include spasticity, sensory loss, and central hypoventilation. Clinical evidence of myopathy is not always present.

DIAGNOSIS. Blood concentrations of pyruvate and lactate may be elevated. EEG shows slowing of the background rhythms and a photoconvulsive response. Ragged-red fibers are seen on muscle biopsy (see Figure 8-3).

MANAGEMENT. Anticonvulsant therapy may provide seizure control early in the course but often fails as the disease progresses. Glucose

loads should be avoided. Treatment is not available for the underlying defect.

Xeroderma Pigmentosum

Xeroderma pigmentosum (XP) is a group of uncommon neurocutaneous disorders characterized by susceptibility to sun-induced skin disorders and progressive neurological deterioration. XP is inherited as an autosomal recessive trait. Several different gene mutations have been associated with these disorders. In the United States, the most common form is termed XPAC and the gene has been mapped to chromosome 9q34.

CLINICAL FEATURES. A photosensitive dermatitis develops during the first year, and skin cancer may develop as well. Progressive psychomotor retardation and poor head growth leading to microcephaly are noted after age 3. Sensorineural hearing loss and spinocerebellar degeneration may develop after age 7. Approximately one third of patients are short in stature and some have a phenotype suggesting Cockayne syndrome, which is a separate genetic error (see Chapter 7) but also involves defective DNA repair (Broughton et al, 1995).

DIAGNOSIS. The diagnosis is suggested by the typical skin rash and neurological deterioration in both the central and peripheral nervous systems, and is confirmed by showing abnormal DNA repair in cultured fibroblasts.

MANAGEMENT. Treatment is not available. Radiation must be avoided.

Other Diseases of White Matter

Adrenoleukodystrophy

Adrenoleukodystrophy is a progressive demyelination of the central nervous system associated with adrenal cortical failure. It is transmitted by X-linked inheritance. Affected children have an impaired ability to oxidize very-long-chain fatty acids, especially hexacosanoic acid, because of deficiency of a peroxisomal acyl coenzyme A (CoA) synthetase. Very-long-chain fatty acids accumulate in tissues and plasma. Many cases previously designated as *Schilder disease* were probably the juvenile form of adrenoleukodystrophy.

Four phenotypes may coexist in the same family. The cerebral form accounts for approximately 56% of cases and is discussed in this section; a slowly progressive adrenomyeloneuropathy accounts for 25% of cases (see Chapter 12), and the remainder have only Addison disease or are asymptomatic.

CLINICAL FEATURES. The onset of the cerebral form is usually between 5 and 10 years of age but can be delayed until adolescence or adult life. The first symptoms are usually an alteration in behavior ranging from a withdrawn state to aggressive outbursts. Poor school performance follows invariably and may lead parents to seek psychological services. Neurological deterioration is then relentlessly progressive and includes disturbances of gait and coordination, loss of vision and hearing, and ultimate deterioration to a vegetative state. Seizures are a late manifestation. The average interval from onset to a vegetative state or death is 3 years.

DIAGNOSIS. The level of very-long-chain fatty acids in plasma is elevated in males of all ages, even in those who are asymptomatic, and in 85% of female carriers. Molecular-based diagnosis is available but is used primarily for genetic counseling.

T_2-weighted MRI shows high signal intensity in the periventricular white matter even in asymptomatic individuals. Adrenal insufficiency may be shown in most asymptomatic children by a subnormal response to stimulation by adrenocorticotropic hormone.

MANAGEMENT. Assessment of adrenal function and corticosteroid replacement therapy can be lifesaving but have no effect on nervous system involvement. Bone marrow transplantation is an option for boys and adolescents who are in the early clinical stages and have MRI evidence of brain involvement. Dietary therapy has no established benefit.

Cerebrotendinous Xanthomatosis

Cerebrotendinous xanthomatosis is a rare disorder transmitted as an autosomal recessive trait. It is caused by mutations in the sterol 27-hydroxylase gene located on the distal portion of chromosome 2q. Enzyme deficiency causes an absence of chenodeoxycholic acid in the bile and a marked increase of cholestanol in plasma. Sterols are stored in all tissues, but especially the central nervous system.

CLINICAL FEATURES. Dementia begins in early childhood but is insidious in its progression so that affected children seem mildly retarded rather than actively deteriorating. By age 15, cataracts are present and tendinous xanthomas begin to form. They are small at first and may go unnoticed until adult life. Progressive spasticity and ataxia develop during adolescence, and the patient becomes incapacitated in early adult life. A demyelinating neuropathy may be present as

well. Speech and swallowing are impaired, and death occurs from brainstem dysfunction or myocardial infarction.

DIAGNOSIS. The triad of cataracts, tendon xanthomas, and progressive neurological deterioration establishes the diagnosis, but all three features are not expressed completely until late in the course. Biochemical screening should be carried out in every child with cataracts or Achilles tendon xanthoma. The diagnosis is established by showing increased concentrations of cholestanol in plasma or xanthomas. MRI shows progressive cerebral atrophy and demyelination.

MANAGEMENT. Daily administration of 750 mg of chenodeoxycholic acid lowers blood cholestanol and improves nerve conduction velocities. Tendon xanthomas also resolve.

References

Andrew SE, Goldberg YP, Hayden MR. Rethinking genotype and phenotype correlations in polyglutamine expansion disorders. *Hum Mol Genet* 1997;6:2005–2010.

Anlar B, Yalaz K, Oktem F, et al. Long-term follow-up of patients with subacute sclerosing panencephalitis treated with intraventricular alpha-interferon. *Neurology* 1997;48:526–528.

Berry-Kravis E, Sleat DE, Sohar I, et al. Prenatal testing for late infantile neuronal ceroid lipofuscinosis. *Ann Neurol* 2000;47:254–257.

Brady RO. Therapy for the sphingolipidoses. *Arch Neurol* 1998;55:1055–1056.

Broughton BC, Thompson AF, Harcourt SA, et al. Molecular and cellular analysis of the DNA repair defect in a patient in xeroderma pigmentosum complementation group D who has the clinical features of xeroderma pigmentosum and Cockayne syndrome. *Am J Hum Genet* 1995;56:167–174.

Clifton-Bligh RJ, Wentworth JM, Heinz P, et al. Mutation of the gene encoding human TTF-2 associated with thyroid agenesis, cleft palate and choanal atresia. *Nature Genet* 1998;19:399–401.

DeLong GR, Heinz ER. The clinical syndrome of early-life bilateral hippocampal sclerosis. *Ann Neurol* 1997;42:11–17.

DiMauro S, De Vivo DC. Genetic heterogeneity in Leigh syndrome. *Ann Neurol* 1996;40:5–7.

Friedman JM, Birch PH. Type 1 neurofibromatosis: A descriptive analysis of the disorder in 1,728 patients. *Am J Med Genet* 1997;70:138–143.

Garbern J, Cambi F, Shy M, et al. The molecular pathogenesis of Pelizaeus-Merzbacher disease. *Arch Neurol* 1999;56:1210–1214.

Harding BN, Alsanjari N, Smith SJ, et al. Progressive neuronal degeneration of children with liver disease (Alpers' disease) presenting in young adults. *J Neurol Neurosurg Psychiatry* 1995;58:320–325.

Krivit W, Shapiro EG, Perters C, et al. Hematopoietic stem-cell transplantation in globoid-cell leukodystrophy. *N Engl J Med* 1998;338:1119–1126.

Lauronen L, Munroe PB, Jarvela I, et al. Delayed and protracted phenotypes of compound heterozygous juvenile neuronal ceroid lipofuscinosis. *Neurology* 1999; 52:360–365.

Luzuriaga K, Bryson Y, Krogstad P, et al. Combination treatment with zidovudine, didanosine, and nevirapine in infants with human immunodeficiency virus type 1 infection. *N Engl J Med* 1997;336:1343–1349.

Morris AAM, Leonard JV, Brown GK, et al. Deficiency of respiratory chain complex I is a common cause of Leigh disease. *Ann Neurol* 1996;40:25–30.

NIH Technology Assessment Panel on Gaucher Disease. Gaucher disease: Current issues in diagnosis and management. *JAMA* 1996;275:548–553.

North KN, Riccardi V, Samango-Sprouse C, et al. Cognitive function and academic performance in neurofibromatosis 1: Consensus statement from the NF1 cognitive disorders task force. *Neurology* 1997;48:1121–1127.

Online Mendelian Inheritance in Man, OMIM (TM). Baltimore: Johns Hopkins University. MIM number 31270. April 30, 1999.

Patterson MC. (Updated 25 January 2000). Niemann-Pick Disease, Type C. In GeneClinics: Medical Genetics Knowledge Base [database online]. University of Washington, Seattle. Available at http://www.geneclinics.org/profiles/npc. Accessed February 2000.

Pratt VM, Naidu S, Dlouhy SR, et al. A novel mutation in exon 3 of the proteolipid protein gene in Pelizaeus-Merzbacher disease. *Neurology* 1995;45:394–395.

Rapin I. Autism. *N Engl J Med* 1997;337:97–104.

Risser WL, Hwang L-Y. Problems in the current case definitions of congenital syphilis. *J Pediatr* 1996;129:499–505.

Roach ES, Gomez MR, Northrup H. Tuberous sclerosis complex consensus conference: Revised clinical diagnostic criteria. *J Child Neurol* 1998;13:624–628.

Roizen N, Swisher CN, Stein MA, et al. Neurological and developmental outcome in treated congenital toxoplasmosis. *Pediatrics* 1995;95:11–20.

Schuelke M, Smeitink J, Mariman E, et al. Mutant NDUFV1 subunit of mitochondrial complex I causes leukodystrophy and myoclonic epilepsy. *Nature Genet* 1999; 21:260–261.

Stibler H, Stephani U, Kutsch U. Carbohydrate-deficient glycoprotein syndrome—A fourth subtype. *Neuropediatrics* 1995;26:235–237.

Syvänen A-C, Järvalä I, Paunto T, et al. DNA diagnosis and identification of carriers of infantile and juvenile neuronal ceroid lipofuscinosis. *Neuropediatrics* 1997; 28:63–66.

Tarleton J, Saul RA. (Updated 10 June 1998) Fragile X Syndrome. In: GeneClinics: Medical Genetics Knowledge Base. [database online] University of Washington, Seattle. Available at http://www.geneclinics.org/profiles/pws. Accessed 15 January 2000.

Traeger EC, Rapin I. The clinical course of Canavan disease. *Pediatr Neurol* 1998;18:207–212.

Tumer Z, Horn N. Menkes disease: Recent advances and new aspects. *J Med Genet* 1997;34:265–274.

Väisänen M-L, Haataja R, Leisti J. Decrease in the CGG_n trinucleotide repeat mutation of the fragile X syndrome to normal size range during paternal transmission. *Am J Hum Genet* 1996;59:540–546.

Voznyi YV, Keulemans JLM, Mancini GMS, et al. A new simple enzyme assay for pre- and postnatal diagnosis of infantile neuronal ceroid lipofuscinosis (INCL) and its variants. *J Med Genet* 1999;36:471–474.

Wappner R, Cho S, Kronmal RA, et al. Management of phenylketonuria for optimal outcome: A review of guidelines for phenylketonuria management and a report of surveys of parents, patients, and clinic directors. *Pediatrics* 1999;104:e68.

Weiner DM, Ewalt DE, Roach ES, Hensle TW. The tuberous sclerosis complex: A comprehensive review. *J Am College Surg* 1998;187:548–561.

Welch GN, Loscalzo J. Homocysteine and atherothrombosis. *N Engl J Med* 1998;338:1042–1050.

Wraith JE. The mucopolysaccharidoses: A clinical review and guide to management. *Arch Dis Child* 1995; 72:263–267.

Chapter 6
The Hypotonic Infant

Definitions

Tone is the resistance of muscle to stretch. Two kinds of tone are measured clinically: phasic and postural. *Phasic tone* is a rapid contraction in response to a high-intensity stretch. It is examined by testing the tendon reflexes. When a hammer strikes the patellar tendon, the quadriceps muscle is stretched and the spindle apparatus, sensing the stretch, sends an impulse through the sensory nerve to the spinal cord. This information is transmitted to the alpha motor neuron, and the quadriceps muscle contracts (the monosynaptic reflex). *Postural tone* is the prolonged contraction of antigravity muscles in response to the low-intensity stretch of gravity. When postural tone is depressed, the trunk and limbs cannot be maintained against gravity and the infant is hypotonic.

The maintenance of normal tone requires intact central and peripheral nervous systems. Not surprisingly, hypotonia is a common symptom of neurological dysfunction and is encountered in diseases of the brain, spinal cord, nerves, and muscles (Table 6-1). One anterior horn cell and all the muscle fibers that it innervates make up a *motor unit*. A primary disorder of the anterior horn cell body is a *neuronopathy*, a primary disorder of the axon or its myelin covering is a *neuropathy*, and a primary disorder of the muscle fiber is a *myopathy*. In infancy and childhood, diseases of the brain are far more common than diseases of the motor unit. The term *cerebral hypotonia* is used to encompass all causes of postural hypotonia caused by a cerebral disease or defect.

The Appearance of Hypotonia

When lying supine, all hypotonic infants look much the same, regardless of the underlying cause or location of the abnormality within the nervous system. Spontaneous movement is lacking, the legs are fully abducted with the lateral surface of the thighs against the examining table, and the arms lie either extended at the sides of the body or flexed at the elbow with the hands beside the head. Pectus excavatum is present when the infant has long-standing weakness in the muscles of the chest wall. Infants who lie motionless eventually develop flattening of the occiput and loss of hair on the portion of the scalp that is in constant contact with the crib sheet. When the infant is placed in a sitting posture, the head falls forward, the shoulders droop, and the limbs hang limply.

Newborns who are hypotonic in utero may be born with dislocation of the hips, arthrogryposis, or both. Hip dislocation is a common feature of intrauterine hypotonia because the formation of a normal hip joint requires the forceful contraction of muscles to pull the head of the femur into the acetabulum. Arthrogryposis varies in severity from clubfoot, the most common manifestation, to symmetric flexion deformities of all limb joints. Joint contractures are believed to be a nonspecific consequence of intrauterine immobilization. However, among the several disorders that equally decrease fetal movement, some commonly produce arthrogryposis and others never do. The differential diagnosis of arthrogryposis is summarized in Table 6-2. As a rule, newborns with

Table **6-1**
Differential Diagnosis of Infantile Hypotonia (Gene Location)

Cerebral Hypotonia
"Benign" congenital hypotonia
Chromosome disorders
   Prader-Willi syndrome (15q11–13)
   Trisomy
Chronic nonprogressive encephalopathy
   Cerebral malformation
   Perinatal distress
   Postnatal disorders
Peroxisomal disorders
   Cerebrohepatorenal syndrome (Zellweger syndrome)
   Neonatal adrenoleukodystrophy
Other genetic defects
   Familial dysautonomia
   Oculocerebrorenal syndrome (Lowe syndrome)
Other metabolic defects
   Acid maltase deficiency (see "Metabolic Myopathies")
   Infantile GM_1 gangliosidosis (see Chapter 5)

Spinal Cord Disorders
Hypoxic-ischemia myelopathy
Injuries

Spinal Muscular Atrophies
Acute infantile
   Autosomal dominant
   Autosomal recessive (5q11–13)
   Cytochrome-c-oxidase deficiency
   X-linked
Chronic infantile
   Autosomal dominant
   Autosomal recessive (5q11–13)
   Congenital cervical spinal muscular atrophy
   Infantile neuronal degeneration
   Neurogenic arthrogryposis

Polyneuropathies
Congenital hypomyelinating neuropathy
Giant axonal neuropathy (see Chapter 7)
Hereditary motor-sensory neuropathies (see Chapter 7)

Disorders of Neuromuscular Transmission
Familial infantile myasthenia
Infantile botulism
Transitory myasthenia gravis

Fiber-Type Disproportion Myopathies
Central core disease (19q13)
Congenital fiber-type disproportion myopathy
   (translocation 10p11:17q25)
Myotubular (centronuclear) myopathy
   Acute (Xq28)
   Chronic
Nemaline (rod) myopathy
   Autosomal dominant (1q21–23)
   Autosomal recessive (2q)

Metabolic Myopathies
Acid maltase deficiency (17q23)
Cytochrome-c-oxidase deficiency
Phosphofructokinase deficiency (12q13.3)
Phosphorylase deficiency (11q13)

Muscular Dystrophies
Bethlem myopathy (see Chapter 7)
Congenital dystrophinopathy (see Chapter 7)
Congenital muscular dystrophy
   Merosin deficiency primary [6q2]
   Merosin deficiency secondary [9q31-33]
   Merosin positive [1p36-p35]
Congenital myotonic dystrophy [19q13]

Table **6-2**
Differential Diagnosis of Arthrogryposis

Cerebral malformations
Cerebrohepatorenal syndrome
Chromosomal disorders
Fetal, nonnervous system causes
Motor unit disorders
   Congenital benign spinal muscular atrophy
   Congenital cervical spinal muscular atrophy
   Congenital fiber-type disproportion myopathy
   Congenital hypomyelinating neuropathy
   Congenital muscular dystrophy
   Genetic myasthenic syndromes
   Infantile neuronal degeneration
   Myotonic dystrophy
   Neurogenic arthrogryposis
   Phosphofructokinase deficiency
   Transitory neonatal myasthenia
Nonfetal causes

arthrogryposis who require respiratory assistance do not survive extubation unless the underlying disorder is myasthenia. The tone of infants who appear hypotonic at rest can be further evaluated by the traction response, by vertical suspension, and by horizontal suspension.

The Traction Response

The traction response is the most sensitive measure of postural tone and can be tested in premature newborns within an isolette. Grasping the hands and pulling the infant to a sitting position initiates the response. In a normal infant the head lifts from the surface immediately with the body. When the sitting position is attained, the head is held erect in the midline. During traction the examiner should feel the infant pulling back against traction and observe flexion at the elbow, knee, and ankle. The traction response cannot be elicited in premature newborns of less than 33 weeks' gestation. After 33 weeks, the neck flexors show increasing success in lifting the head. At term only minimal head lag is present; when the sitting posture is attained, the head may continue to lag or may become erect momentarily and then fall forward. The presence of more than minimal head lag and of failure to counter traction by flexion of the limbs in the term newborn is abnormal and indicates hypotonia.

Vertical Suspension

To perform vertical suspension, the examiner places both hands in the infant's axillae and, without grasping the thorax, lifts straight up. The muscles of the shoulders should be strong enough to press down against the examiner's hands and allow the infant to suspend vertically without falling through. While the infant is in vertical suspension, the head is held erect in the midline and the legs are kept flexed at the knee, hip, and ankle. When a hypotonic infant is suspended vertically, the head falls forward, the legs dangle, and the infant may slip through the examiner's hands because of weakness in the shoulder muscles.

Horizontal Suspension

When suspended horizontally, a normal infant keeps the head erect, maintains the back straight, and flexes the elbow, hip, knee, and ankle joints. A healthy full-term newborn makes intermittent efforts to maintain the head erect, the back straight, and the limbs flexed against gravity. Hypotonic newborns and infants drape over the examiner's hands, with the head and legs hanging limply.

Approach to Diagnosis

The first step in diagnosis is to determine whether the disease is sited in the brain, spine, or motor unit. More than one site may be involved (Table 6-3). The brain and the peripheral nerves are concomitantly involved in some lysosomal and mitochondrial disorders. Both brain and skeletal muscles are abnormal in infants with acid maltase deficiency and neonatal myotonic dystrophy. Newborns with severe hypoxic-ischemic encephalopathy may have hypoxic injury to the spinal cord as well. Several motor unit disorders produce sufficient hypotonia at

Table 6-3
Combined Cerebral and Motor Unit Hypotonia

Acid maltase deficiency
Familial dysautonomia
Giant axonal neuropathy
Hypoxic-ischemic encephalomyopathy
Infantile neuronal degeneration
Lipid storage diseases
Mitochondrial (respiratory chain) disorders
Neonatal myotonic dystrophy
Perinatal asphyxia secondary to motor unit disease

birth to impair respiration and cause perinatal asphyxia (Table 6-4). Such infants may then have cerebral hypotonia as well. Newborns with spinal cord injuries are frequently the product of long, difficult deliveries in which brachial plexus injuries and hypoxic-ischemic encephalopathy are concomitant problems.

Clues to the Diagnosis of Cerebral Hypotonia

Cerebral hypotonia in newborns usually does not pose diagnostic difficulty and can be identified by the history and physical examination. Many clues to the diagnosis of cerebral hypotonia exist (Table 6-5), but most important is the presence of other abnormal brain functions: decreased consciousness and seizures. Cerebral malformation is the likely explanation for hypotonia in an infant with dysmorphic features or with malformations in other organs.

A tightly fisted hand in which the thumb is constantly enclosed by the other fingers and does not open spontaneously (*fisting*), and adduction of the thigh so that the legs are crossed when the infant is suspended vertically (*scissoring*), are considered precursors of spasticity and indicate cerebral dysfunction. Postural reflexes may be elicited in newborns and infants with cerebral

Table 6-4
Motor Unit Disorders with Perinatal Respiratory Distress

Acute infantile spinal muscular atrophy
Congenital hypomyelinating neuropathy
Congenital myotonic dystrophy
Familial infantile myasthenia
Neurogenic arthrogryposis
X-linked myotubular myopathy

Table 6-5
Clues to Cerebral Hypotonia

Abnormalities of other brain functions
Dysmorphic features
Fisting of the hands
Malformations of other organs
Movement through postural reflexes
Normal or brisk tendon reflexes
Scissoring on vertical suspension

---

hypotonia even when spontaneous movement is lacking. In some acute encephalopathies, and especially in metabolic disorders, the Moro reflex may be exaggerated. The tonic neck reflex is an important indicator of cerebral abnormality if the responses are excessive and obligatory and persist beyond 6 months of age. When hemispheric damage is severe but the brainstem is intact, turning the head produces full extension of both ipsilateral limbs and tight flexion on the contralateral side. An obligatory reflex is one in which these postures are maintained as long as the head is kept rotated. Tendon reflexes are generally normal or brisk, and clonus may be present.

Clues to Motor Unit Disorders

Disorders of the motor unit are not associated with malformations of other organs except for joint deformities and the maldevelopment of bony structures. The face sometimes looks dysmorphic when facial muscles are weak or when the jaw is underdeveloped.

Tendon reflexes are absent or depressed. Loss of tendon reflexes that is out of proportion to weakness is more likely caused by neuropathy than myopathy, whereas diminished reflexes that are consistent with the degree of weakness are more often caused by myopathy than neuropathy (Table 6-6). Muscle atrophy suggests motor unit disease but does not exclude the possibility of cerebral hypotonia. Failure of growth and even atrophy can be considerable in brain-damaged infants. The combination of atrophy and fasciculations is strong evidence of denervation. However, the observation of fasciculations in newborns and infants is often restricted to the tongue, and distinguishing fasciculations from normal random movements of an infant's tongue is difficult unless atrophy is present.

Postural reflexes, such as the tonic neck and Moro reflex, cannot be superimposed on weak muscles. The motor unit is the final common pathway of tone; limbs that will not move voluntarily cannot be moved reflexively.

Cerebral Hypotonia

Hypotonia is a feature of almost every cerebral disorder in newborns and infants. This section does not deal with conditions in which the major symptoms are states of decreased consciousness, seizures, and progressive psychomotor retardation. Rather, the discussion focuses on conditions in which hypotonia is sufficiently prominent that the examining physician may consider the possibility of motor unit disease.

Benign Congenital Hypotonia

The term *benign congenital hypotonia* is retrospective and refers to infants who are hypotonic at birth or shortly thereafter and later have normal tone. It encompasses many different pathological processes that affect the brain, the motor unit, or both. The majority of affected children have cerebral hypotonia. An increased incidence of mental retardation, learning disabilities, and other sequelae of cerebral abnormality are evident later in life, despite the recovery of normal muscle tone.

Chromosome Disorders

Despite considerable syndrome diversity, common characteristics of autosomal chromosome aberrations in the newborn are dysmorphic features of the hands and face and profound hypotonia (see Table 5-4). For this reason, chromosome studies are indicated for any hypotonic newborn with dysmorphic features of the hands and face, with or without other organ malformation (Table 6-7).

Prader-Willi Syndrome

The Prader-Willi syndrome is characterized by hypotonia, hypogonadism, mental retardation,

---

Table 6-6
Clues to Motor Unit Disorders

Absent or depressed tendon reflexes
Failure of movement on postural reflexes
Fasciculations
Muscle atrophy
No abnormalities of other organs

Table 6-7
Hypotonia and Dysmorphic Features

Cerebral dysgenesis
Cerebrohepatorenal syndrome
Congenital myotonic dystrophy
Chromosomal aberrations
Fiber-type disproportion myopathies
Neonatal adrenoleukodystrophy
Prader-Willi syndrome

short stature, and obesity. Approximately 70% of children with this syndrome have an interstitial deletion of the proximal long arm of chromosome 15(q11-13). Most patients, who do not have a deletion, have the syndrome on the basis of maternal disomy (both chromosomes 15 are from the mother). Paternal disomy of chromosome 15 causes Angelman syndrome.

CLINICAL FEATURES. Decreased fetal activity is reported in 75% of pregnancies and is associated with a 10% incidence of congenital hip dislocation and a 6% incidence of clubfoot. At birth the hypotonia is profound, and tendon reflexes are absent or greatly depressed. Feeding problems are invariable, and prolonged nasogastric tube feeding is common (Table 6-8). Cryptorchidism is present in 84% and hypogenitalism in 100%. However, some newborns lack the associated features and only show hypotonia (Miller et al, 1999).

Both hypotonia and feeding difficulty persist until 8 to 11 months of age and are later replaced by relatively normal muscle tone and insatiable hunger. Developmental milestones are delayed, and mental retardation is a constant feature. Minor abnormalities that become more obvious during infancy include a narrow bifrontal diameter of the skull, strabismus, almond-shaped eyes, enamel hypoplasia, and small hands and

Table 6-8
Difficulty of Feeding in the Alert Newborn

Congenital myotonic dystrophy
Familial dysautonomia
Genetic myasthenic syndromes
Hypoplasia of bulbar motor nuclei (see Chapter 17)
Infantile neuronal degeneration
Myophosphorylase deficiency
Neurogenic arthrogryposis
Prader-Willi syndrome
Transitory neonatal myasthenia

feet. Obesity is the rule during childhood. The combination of obesity and minor abnormalities of the face and limbs produces a resemblance among children with this syndrome.

DIAGNOSIS. Chromosome analysis with special reference to chromosome 15 is indicated in newborns with the triad of hypotonia, difficulty feeding, and cryptorchidism. Other studies are not helpful, and without chromosome analysis the diagnosis is delayed until obesity develops.

MANAGEMENT. Dietary supervision is needed to control obesity. No specific treatment is available.

Chronic Nonprogressive Encephalopathy

Cerebral dysgenesis may be due to known or unknown noxious environmental agents, chromosomal disorders, or genetic defects. In the absence of an acute encephalopathy, hypotonia may be the only symptom at birth or during early infancy. Hypotonia is usually worse at birth and gets better with time. Cerebral dysgenesis should be suspected when hypotonia is coupled with malformations in other organs or abnormalities in head size and shape. Magnetic resonance imaging (MRI) of the head is advisable when cerebral malformation is suspected. The identification of a cerebral malformation provides useful information not only for prognosis but also on the feasibility of aggressive therapy to correct malformations in other organs.

Brain injuries occur in the perinatal period and, less commonly, throughout infancy as a result of anoxia, hemorrhage, infection, and trauma. The sudden onset of hypotonia in a previously well newborn or infant, with or without signs of encephalopathy, should always suggest a cerebral cause. The premature newborn who shows a decline in spontaneous movement and tone may have an intraventricular hemorrhage. Hypotonia is an early feature of meningitis in full-term and premature newborns. Tendon reflexes may be diminished or absent during the acute phase.

Genetic Disorders

Familial Dysautonomia

Familial dysautonomia, the *Riley-Day syndrome*, was originally described as a genetic disorder transmitted by autosomal recessive inheritance in Ashkenazi Jews. The abnormal gene maps to chromosome 9q31-q33. Similar clinical syndromes also occur in non-Jewish infants; these are often sporadic, and the mode of inheritance is not clear.

CLINICAL FEATURES. In the newborn the important clinical features are meconium aspiration, poor or no sucking reflex, and hypotonia. Hypotonia is caused by disturbances in the brain, the dorsal root ganglia, and the peripheral nerves. Tendon reflexes are hypoactive or absent. The feeding difficulty is unusual and provides a clue to the diagnosis. Sucking and swallowing are normal separately but cannot be coordinated for effective feeding. Other clinical features that may be noted either in the newborn or later in infancy are pallor, temperature instability, absence of fungiform papillae of the tongue, diarrhea, abdominal distention, poor weight gain, lethargy, episodes of irritability, absence of corneal reflexes, labile blood pressure, and failure to produce overflow tears.

DIAGNOSIS. Ophthalmological examination is useful to detect the signs of postganglionic parasympathetic denervation: supersensitivity of the pupil, shown by a positive miotic response to 0.1% pilocarpine or 2.5% methacholine, corneal insensitivity, and absence of tears.

MANAGEMENT. Treatment is directed at symptoms. Bethanechol (Urecholine), 1 to 2 mg/kg/day orally, is thought to be helpful. Its use is based on the observation that injections of acetylcholine produce transitory relief of some symptoms. Longevity has increased because of improved treatment of symptoms.

Oculocerebrorenal Syndrome (Lowe Syndrome)

Oculocerebrorenal syndrome is transmitted by X-linked recessive inheritance (Xq26.1). Partial expression in the form of minor lenticular opacities is seen in female carriers (Lin et al, 1999).

CLINICAL FEATURES. The important features at birth are hypotonia and hyporeflexia, sometimes associated with congenital cataracts and glaucoma. The differential diagnosis of cataracts in newborns and infants is listed in Table 16-2. Features that appear later in infancy are mental retardation and a progressive disorder of the renal tubules resulting in metabolic acidosis, proteinuria, aminoaciduria, and defective acidification of the urine. Many infants die after failing to thrive. Others have mild symptoms, including growth retardation, borderline intellectual function, mild renal disturbances, and late-onset cataract formation. Life expectancy is normal in the milder cases.

DIAGNOSIS. Diagnosis depends on recognition of the clinical constellation. MRI shows diffuse and irregular foci of increased signal consistent with demyelination.

MANAGEMENT. Most patients require alkinization therapy, and many benefit from supplements of potassium, phosphate, calcium, and carnitine.

Peroxisomal Disorders

Peroxisomes are subcellular organelles that participate in the biosynthesis of ether phospholipids and bile acids; the oxidation of very-long-chain fatty acids (VLCFA), prostaglandins, and unsaturated long-chain fatty acids; and the catabolism of phytanate, pipecolate, and glycolate. Hydrogen peroxide is generated in the course of several oxidation reactions and catabolized by the enzyme catalase.

The infantile syndromes of peroxisomal dysfunction are all disorders of peroxisomal biogenesis; the intrinsic protein membrane can be identified, but all matrix enzymes are missing. The prototype is *cerebrohepatorenal (Zellweger) syndrome. Neonatal adrenoleukodystrophy* and *infantile Refsum disease* (see Chapter 16) are milder variants. Infantile hypotonia is a prominent feature of disorders of peroxisomal biogenesis, and one mild form resembles infantile spinal muscular atrophy (Baumgartner et al, 1998).

The Zellweger phenotype can be caused by mutations in several different genes. One maps to chromosome 2p15, with a second possible site at chromosome 7q21-q22. It is inherited as an autosomal recessive trait.

CLINICAL FEATURES. Affected newborns are poorly responsive and have severe hypotonia, arthrogryposis, and dysmorphic features. The arthrogryposis is characterized by limited extension of the fingers (camptodactyly) and flexion deformities of the knee and ankle. Sucking and crying are weak, and tendon reflexes are diminished or absent. Characteristic craniofacial abnormalities include a pear-shaped head owing to a high forehead and an unusual fullness of the cheeks, widened sutures, micrognathia, a high-arched palate, flattening of the bridge of the nose, and hypertelorism. Organ abnormalities include biliary cirrhosis, polycystic kidneys, retinal degeneration, and cerebral malformations secondary to abnormalities of neuronal migration.

Seizures usually begin shortly after birth but may begin anytime during infancy. They are difficult to control. Death from aspiration, gastrointestinal bleeding, or liver failure usually occurs within 6 months and almost always within 1 year.

DIAGNOSIS. VLCFA plasma concentrations are increased, levels of plasmalogens in red blood cell membranes are reduced, and the rate of synthesis of plasmalogens in cultured skin fibroblasts is reduced. Pipecolic acid levels are increased in plasma and urine, and excessive amounts of bile acid intermediates also are excreted in urine.

MANAGEMENT. Treatment is symptomatic, anticonvulsants for seizures and vitamin K for bleeding disorders.

Other Metabolic Defects

Infantile hypotonia is rarely the only manifestation of inborn errors of metabolism. Acid maltase deficiency causes a severe myopathy and is discussed with other metabolic myopathies. Hypotonia may be the only initial feature of generalized GM_1 gangliosidosis (Chapter 5).

Spinal Cord Disorders

Hypoxic-Ischemic Myelopathy

Hypoxic-ischemic encephalopathy is an expected outcome in severe perinatal asphyxia (see Chapter 1). Affected newborns are hypotonic and areflexic. These features have been attributed exclusively to the cerebral injury but also may be caused by spinal cord dysfunction. Concurrent ischemic necrosis of gray matter occurs in the spinal cord as well as in the brain. The spinal cord component is often found on postmortem examination but may also be shown in nonfatal cases by electromyography (EMG).

Spinal Cord Injury

Only in the newborn does spinal cord injury enter the differential diagnosis of hypotonia. Injuries to the cervical spinal cord occur almost exclusively during vaginal delivery; approximately 75% are associated with breech presentation and 25% with cephalic presentation. Because the injuries are always associated with a difficult and prolonged delivery, decreased consciousness is common and hypotonia may be falsely attributed to asphyxia or cerebral trauma. However, the presence of impaired sphincter function and loss of sensation below the midchest should suggest myelopathy.

Injuries in Breech Presentation

Traction injuries to the lower cervical and upper thoracic regions of the cord occur almost exclusively when the angle of extension of the fetal head exceeds 90%. Indeed, the risk of spinal cord injury to a fetus in breech position whose head is hyperextended is greater than 70%. In such cases, delivery should always be by cesarean section. The tractional forces applied to the extended head are sufficient not only to stretch the cord but also to herniate the brainstem through the foramen magnum. In addition, the hyperextended position compromises the vertebral arteries as they enter the skull.

The spectrum of pathological findings varies from edema of the cord without loss of anatomical continuity to massive hemorrhage (epidural, subdural, and intramedullary), which is most pronounced in the lower cervical and upper thoracic segments but may extend the entire length of the cord. Concurrent hemorrhage in the posterior fossa and laceration of the cerebellum may be present as well.

CLINICAL FEATURES. Mild tractional injuries, in which there is edema of the cord but not intraparenchymal hemorrhage or loss of anatomical continuity, produce few or no clinical features. The main feature is hypotonia, which may be falsely attributed to asphyxia.

Severe tractional injuries are accompanied by hemorrhage into the posterior fossa. Affected newborns are unconscious and atonic at birth. They have flaccid quadriplegia with diaphragmatic breathing. Most do not survive the neonatal period. Injuries restricted to the low cervical and high thoracic segments produce near-normal strength in the biceps muscles and weakness of the triceps muscles. The result is flexion of the arms at the elbows and flaccid paraplegia. Spontaneous movement and tendon reflexes in the legs are absent, but foot withdrawal from pinprick may occur as a spinal reflex. The infant has a distended bladder and dribbling of urine. Sensory levels are difficult to measure but may be deduced by the absence of sweating below the injury.

DIAGNOSIS. Radiographs of the vertebrae show no abnormalities because bony displacement does not occur. MRI of the spine shows intraspinal edema and hemorrhage.

Unconscious newborns are generally thought to have intracerebral hemorrhage or asphyxia (see Chapter 2), and the diagnosis of spinal cord injury may not be considered until consciousness is regained and the typical motor deficits are observed. Even then, a neuromuscular disorder may be suspected. The disturbance in bladder function and the development of progressive spastic paraplegia should alert the physician to the correct diagnosis.

MANAGEMENT. The treatment of spinal cord traction injuries of the newborn is similar to the management of cord injuries in older children (see Chapter 12).

Injuries in Cephalic Presentation

Injuries in cephalic presentation are high cervical cord injuries caused by twisting of the neck during midforceps rotation when the trunk fails to rotate with the head. The risk is greatest when amniotic fluid is absent because of delay from the time of membrane rupture to the application of forceps. The spectrum of injury varies from intraparenchymal hemorrhage to complete transection. Transection usually occurs at the level of a fractured odontoid process, with atlantoaxial dislocation.

CLINICAL FEATURES. Newborns are flaccid and fail to breathe spontaneously. Those with milder injuries may have shallow, labored respirations, but all require assisted ventilation at birth. Most are unconscious at birth owing to edema in the brainstem. When consciousness is regained, eye movements, sucking, and the withdrawal reflex are the only movements observed. Tendon reflexes are at first absent but later become exaggerated if the child survives. The bladder becomes distended, and overflow incontinence occurs. Priapism may be present. Sensation is difficult to assess because the withdrawal reflex is present.

Death from sepsis or respiratory complications generally occurs in the first week. Occasionally children have survived for several years.

DIAGNOSIS. Most children with high cervical cord injuries are thought to have neuromuscular disorders, especially infantile spinal muscular atrophy, because the limbs are flaccid but the eye movements are normal. EMG of the limbs should exclude that possibility. Radiographs of the cervical vertebrae usually do not show abnormalities, but MRI shows marked thinning or disruption of the cord at the site of injury.

MANAGEMENT. Newborns with high cervical cord injuries are intubated and provided with respiratory assistance before the diagnosis is established. Further management of spinal cord transection is discussed in Chapter 12.

Motor Unit Disorders

Evaluation of Motor Unit Disorders

In the diagnosis of cerebral hypotonia in infants, the choice of laboratory tests varies considerably, depending on the disease entity (Table 6-9). This is not the case with motor unit hypotonia. A battery of tests is available that readily define the anatomy and cause of pathological processes affecting the motor unit. DNA-based testing is now commercially available for many disorders and should be used instead of muscle or nerve biopsy when appropriate.

Serum Creatine Kinase

Increased serum concentrations of creatine kinase (CK) reflect skeletal or cardiac muscle necrosis. Blood should be drawn for CK determination before the performance of EMG or muscle biopsy because either procedure transiently elevates the serum concentration of CK. Laboratory reference values for the normal serum concentration are usually based on those of nonambulatory patients. Normal values tend to be higher in an ambulatory population, especially after exercise. The total concentration of CK and its isoenzymes increases significantly with acidosis. Levels as high as 1,000 IU/L may be recorded in severely asphyxiated newborns, but even normal newborns have a higher than normal concentration during the first 24 hours postpartum. A normal CK level in a hypotonic infant is strong evidence against a rapidly progressive myopathy, but it does not exclude fiber-type disproportion myopathies and some metabolic myopathies from the diagnosis. Conversely, a mild elevation in the CK concentration is sometimes encountered in rapidly progressive spinal muscular atrophies.

Table 6-9
Evaluation of Motor Unit Disorders

DNA-based testing
Edrophonium chloride (Tensilon test)
Electrodiagnosis
   Electromyography
   Nerve conduction studies
   Repetitive stimulation
Muscle biopsy
Nerve biopsy
Serum creatine kinase

Electrodiagnosis

EMG is extremely useful in the diagnosis of infantile hypotonia when an experienced physician performs the study. It enables the prediction of the final diagnosis in most infants younger than 3 months of age with hypotonia of motor unit origin. Hypotonic infants with normal EMG findings rarely show abnormalities on muscle biopsy. The needle portion of the study helps to distinguish myopathic from neuropathic processes. Myopathies are generally characterized by the appearance of brief, small-amplitude, polyphasic potentials (BSAPPs). Neuropathies are characterized by the presence of denervation potentials at rest (fibrillations, fasciculations, sharp waves) and motor unit potentials that are large, prolonged, and polyphasic. Studies of nerve conduction velocity are useful in distinguishing axonal from demyelinating neuropathies; demyelinating neuropathies cause greater slowing of conduction velocity. Repetitive nerve stimulation studies demonstrate disturbances in neuromuscular transmission.

Muscle Biopsy

Muscle biopsy should not be undertaken unless the tissue can be processed by histochemical techniques. The muscle selected for biopsy should be weak but still able to contract. When weakness is symmetric, one side is studied by EMG and the other is reserved for biopsy. Histochemical analysis is essential for the complete evaluation of muscle histology because special techniques are needed to demonstrate fiber types, muscle proteins, and storage materials. Human skeletal muscle can be arbitrarily divided into two fiber types on the basis of the intensity of the reaction to myosin adenosine triphosphatase (ATPase) at pH 9.4. Type I fibers react weakly to ATPase, are characterized by oxidative metabolism and serve a tonic function. Type II fibers react intensely to ATPase, utilize glycolytic metabolism and serve a phasic function. Type I and II fibers are generally equal in number and randomly distributed in each fascicle. Disorders may be characterized by abnormalities in fiber type number, fiber type size, or both.

The structural proteins of muscle are described and illustrated in Chapter 7. Merosin is the main protein associated with congenital muscular dystrophy. The important storage materials identified in skeletal muscle are glycogen and lipid. In most storage disorders, vacuoles are present in the fibers that contain the abnormal material. The vacuoles are seen with light microscopy, and the specific material is identified by its histochemical reaction.

Nerve Biopsy

Sural nerve biopsy is rarely needed in the diagnosis of infantile hypotonia and should be done only if sural neuropathy has been shown by electrodiagnosis. Its main use is in the diagnosis of hypomyelinating neuropathies.

The Tensilon Test

Edrophonium chloride (Tensilon) is a rapidly acting anticholinesterase that temporarily reverses weakness in patients with myasthenia. Ptosis and oculomotor paresis are the only functions that are reliably tested. Rare patients are supersensitive to edrophonium chloride and may stop breathing because of depolarization of endplates or an abnormal vagal response. Equipment for mechanical ventilation should always be available when the test is performed. In newborns, a subcutaneous injection of 0.15 mg/kg produces a response within 10 minutes. In infants, the drug is given intravenously at a dose of 0.2 mg/kg and reverses weakness within 1 minute.

Spinal Muscular Atrophies

The spinal muscular atrophies (SMA) are genetic disorders in which anterior horn cells in the spinal cord and motor nuclei of the brainstem are progressively lost. The mechanism is probably a defect in programmed cell death, wherein the deletion of cells, a normal process during gestation, continues after birth. The onset of weakness may be any age from birth to adult life. Some are marked by a generalized distribution of weakness, and others affect specific muscle groups. Those with onset in infancy usually cause generalized weakness and hypotonia. Infantile spinal muscular atrophy is one of the more common motor unit disorders causing infantile hypotonia.

Autosomal Recessive Forms

Two clinical syndromes of SMA, transmitted by autosomal recessive inheritance, are distinguished. One is an acute fulminating form that begins at birth or within the first 6 months (SMA I), and the other is a more chronic form that usually begins after 3 to 6 months of age (SMA II). SMA II is described in Chapter 7. Both types are associated with homozygous deletions of exons 7 and 8 in the survival motor neuron (SMN) gene on chromosome 5q13. Defects in exon 5 of the neuronal apoptosis inhibitory protein (NAIP) gene are found in 67% of infants with SMA type I and in 42% of children with SMA types II and III (see Chapter 7). The role of the NAIP gene is unknown, but associated defects may modify the phenotype (Stewart et al, 1998).

The overlap in clinical features between the three types is considerable, and two different clinical phenotypes can occur in a single family. The course among siblings is almost always the same, but both SMA I and SMA II sometimes occur among siblings and is then attributed to a larger deletion in the more affected child that also affects the NAIP gene (Parano et al, 1996). The age at onset does not consistently predict the degree of eventual disability, and the outcome should not be predicted at the time of initial diagnosis.

CLINICAL FEATURES. The age at onset is birth to 6 months. Reduced fetal movement may be reported when neuronal degeneration begins in utero. Affected newborns have generalized weakness involving proximal more than distal muscles, hypotonia, and areflexia. Newborns who are hypotonic in utero and weak at birth may have difficulty adapting to extrauterine life and experience postnatal asphyxia and encephalopathy. Most breathe adequately at first and appear alert despite the generalized weakness because facial expression is relatively well preserved and extraocular movement is normal. Some newborns have paradoxical respiration because intercostal paralysis and thoracic collapse occur before diaphragmatic movement is impaired, while others have diaphragmatic paralysis as an initial feature. Despite intrauterine hypotonia, arthrogryposis is not present. Neurogenic arthrogryposis may be a distinct entity and is described separately in this chapter.

When weakness begins in infancy, the decline in strength can be sudden or decremental. At times, the child seems to improve because of normal cerebral development, but the progression of weakness is relentless. Atrophy and fasciculations may be observed in the tongue. After the gag reflex is lost, feeding becomes difficult and death results from aspiration and pneumonia. When weakness is present at birth, death usually occurs by 6 months of age, but the course is variable when symptoms develop after 3 months of age. Some infants will attain sitting balance but will not walk. *Survival time should not be predicted.*

DIAGNOSIS. The diagnosis is readily established by showing the gene abnormality on chromosome 5q13. The serum concentration of CK is usually normal but may be mildly elevated in infants with rapidly progressive weakness. EMG studies show fibrillations and fasciculations at rest, and the mean amplitude of motor unit potentials is increased. Motor nerve conduction velocities may be slowed but are usually normal.

Muscle biopsy is unnecessary because of the commercial availability of DNA-based testing. The pathological findings in skeletal muscle are characteristic. Routine histological stains show groups of small fibers adjacent to groups of normal-sized or hypertrophied fibers. When the myosin ATPase reaction is applied, all hypertrophied fibers are type I, whereas medium-sized and small fibers are a mixture of types I and II (Figure 6-1). The normal random arrangement of fiber types is replaced by type grouping, a sign of reinnervation in which large numbers of fibers of the same type are contiguous. Some biopsy specimens show uniform small fibers of both types.

MANAGEMENT. Treatment is supportive. Prenatal diagnosis can be accomplished by DNA analysis of chorion villus biopsies.

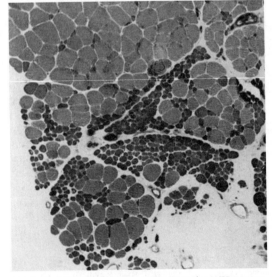

Figure 6-1. Infantile spinal muscular atrophy (ATPase reaction). The normal checkerboard pattern is lost. Groups of large type I fibers (*light shade*) are adjacent to groups of small type II fibers (*dark shade*).

Other Genetic Forms

A rare X-linked form of SMA has clinical features that are indistinguishable from those of SMA I. A second X-linked form, with linkage to markers in the region of chromosome Xp11.3-q11.2, has arthrogryposis as the initial feature. Hypotonia, areflexia, chest deformities, and facial dysmorphic features are associated. Life expectancy is variable.

A dominantly inherited SMA that affects only the legs occurs in newborns. The main features are joint deformities and nonprogressive weakness.

Cytochrome-*c*-Oxidase Deficiency

A boy with a marked SMA presented with hypotonia, severe axial and limb weakness, and normal bulbar muscle strength (Rubio-Gozalbo et al, 1999). He died at the age of 5 months from respiratory failure. Electrodiagnosis revealed positive sharp waves and fibrillation potentials with normal motor nerve conduction velocities. Muscle biopsy showed a preponderance of type I fibers, with atrophy of both fiber types. Cytochrome-*c*-oxidase (COX) activity was absent from all but intrafusal muscle fibers, and the activity was reduced in cultured skin fibroblasts. Western blot analysis showed decreased levels of all COX subunits. Analysis of mitochondrial DNA and the SMN gene was unrevealing.

Congenital Cervical Spinal Muscular Atrophy

This is a rare sporadic disorder characterized by severe weakness and wasting confined to the arms. Contractures of the shoulder, elbow, and wrist joints are present at birth. The legs are normal. Postnatal progression of weakness does not occur. Central nervous system function is normal. This cervical distribution of weakness is more commonly seen as a progressive disorder with onset in adolescence (see Chapter 7).

Infantile Neuronal Degeneration

This autosomal recessive disorder is caused by deficiency of α-N-acetylgalactosaminidase (Keulemans et al, 1996). The typical features of infantile spinal muscular atrophy are combined with degenerative changes in the cerebellum, thalamus, and peripheral sensory nerves.

CLINICAL FEATURES. All infants have hypotonia and areflexia, and some have arthrogryposis as well. The hypotonia is primarily caused by denervation but probably has a cerebral component. Half of the affected children have symptoms at birth and the remainder during infancy. Dyspnea, a weak cry, and difficulty feeding are prominent features in the newborns. All are dead within 5 months. The symptoms are the same when the onset is delayed until early infancy, and death occurs after age 2 years.

DIAGNOSIS. Infantile neuronal degeneration can be differentiated from infantile spinal muscular atrophy by electrophysiological studies. Motor nerve conduction velocities are slow, and sensory nerve responses are absent or reduced. Sialoglycopeptides are excreted in the urine.

MANAGEMENT. Treatment is not available.

Neurogenic Arthrogryposis

The term *neurogenic arthrogryposis* was originally used to denote the association of arthrogryposis with infantile spinal muscular atrophy. Transmission occurs by autosomal recessive inheritance in some families (Shohat et al, 1997) and by X-linked inheritance in others. Some individuals with autosomal recessive inheritance have deletions in the SMN gene. I am aware of two sets of identical twins in which one twin was born with neurogenic arthrogryposis and the other remained normal. This suggests that some sporadic cases may have nongenetic causes.

Families in whom neurogenic arthrogryposis is transmitted as an X-linked trait tend to have clinical or pathological features that distinguish them from others. Arthrogryposis may not occur in every affected family member, weakness or joint deformity may be limited to the legs or arms, and progression is minimal.

CLINICAL FEATURES. In neurogenic arthrogryposis the most active phase of disease occurs in utero. Severely affected newborns have respiratory and feeding difficulties, and some die of aspiration. The less severely affected ones survive and have little or no progression of their weakness. Indeed, the respiratory and feeding difficulties lessen with time. Contractures are present in both proximal and distal joints. Micrognathia and a high-arched palate may be associated features, and a pattern of facial anomalies suggesting trisomy 18 is present in some newborns. Newborns with respiratory distress at birth may not have a fatal course. Limb weakness may be minimal, and long intervals of stability occur.

DIAGNOSIS. The diagnosis is suspected in newborns with arthrogryposis with normal serum concentrations of CK and EMG findings compatible with a neuropathic process. Muscle histological examination reveals the typical pattern of denervation and reinnervation. Cranial MRI to look for cerebral malformations should be done in children with microcephaly.

MANAGEMENT. The joint deformities may respond to physical therapy, and an intensive program of rehabilitation should be initiated as soon after birth as possible.

Polyneuropathies

Polyneuropathies are uncommon in childhood and are even less common during infancy. Table 6-10 lists the polyneuropathies with onset in infancy. They are divided into those that primarily affect the myelin (demyelinating) or the axon (axonal). In newborns and infants, the term *demyelinating* also refers to disorders in which myelin has failed to form (*hypomyelinating*). Only with congenital hypomyelinating neuropathy is infantile hypotonia the initial feature. The others are more likely to start as progressive gait disturbance or psychomotor retardation. A complete discussion of the clinical approach to neuropathy is given in Chapter 7.

Table 6-10
Polyneuropathies with Possible Onset in Infancy

Axonal
Familial dysautonomia
Hereditary motor-sensory neuropathy type II (see Chapter 7)
Idiopathic with encephalopathy (see Chapter 7)
Infantile neuronal degeneration
Subacute necrotizing encephalopathy (see Chapters 5 and 10)

Demyelinating
Acute inflammatory demyelinating polyneuropathy (Guillain-Barré syndrome) (see Chapter 7)
Chronic inflammatory demyelinating polyneuropathy (see Chapter 7)
Congenital hypomyelinating neuropathy
Globoid cell leukodystrophy (see Chapter 5)
Hereditary motor-sensory neuropathy type I (see Chapter 7)
Hereditary motor-sensory neuropathy type III (see Chapter 7)
Metachromatic leukodystrophy (see Chapter 5)

Congenital Hypomyelinating Neuropathy

The term *congenital hypomyelinating neuropathy* encompasses several disorders with similar clinical and pathological features. Sporadic occurrence is the rule, but autosomal recessive inheritance is suggested by reports of disease in cousins and in siblings of both sexes (Tyson et al, 1997) (see Chapter 7).

CLINICAL FEATURES. The clinical features are indistinguishable from those of acute infantile spinal muscular atrophy. Arthrogryposis may be present. Newborns have progressive flaccid weakness and atrophy of the skeletal muscles, a bulbar palsy that spares extraocular motility, and areflexia. Respiratory insufficiency causes death during infancy.

Some children are not identified as abnormal until they fail to meet motor milestones. Examination shows diffuse weakness, distal atrophy, and areflexia. Weakness progresses slowly and is not life-threatening during childhood. Sensation remains intact.

DIAGNOSIS. The serum concentration of CK is normal, EMG findings are consistent with denervation, and motor nerve conduction velocities are usually less than 10 m/sec. The protein concentration of the cerebrospinal fluid is markedly elevated in almost every case. Screening for mutations in the peripheral myelin protein gene and the P zero myelin gene is essential to separate the genetic causes of this syndrome from those of chronic demyelinating inflammatory demyelinating polyneuropathies.

MANAGEMENT. Some infants with hypomyelinating neuropathies respond to treatment with oral prednisone. I have treated one newborn, who became normal, both clinically and electrophysiologically, by 1 year of age but relapsed several times later in childhood and then responded to prednisone and to intravenous immunoglobulin. Such children may have a connatal form of chronic inflammatory demyelinating neuropathy (see Chapter 7). Whatever the mechanism, every affected child should be given a course of oral prednisone, 2 mg/kg/day. Those who respond become stronger within 4 weeks of starting therapy. Following the initial response, the children should be maintained on alternate-day therapy, 0.5 mg/kg, for at least 1 year.

Disorders of Neuromuscular Transmission

Infantile Botulism

Human botulism ordinarily results from eating food contaminated by preformed exotoxin of the organism *Clostridium botulinum.* The exotoxin prevents the release of acetylcholine, causing a cholinergic blockade of skeletal muscle and end organs innervated by autonomic nerves. Infantile botulism is an age-limited disorder in which *C. botulinum* is ingested, colonizes the intestinal tract, and produces toxin in situ. Dietary contamination with honey or corn syrup accounts for almost 20% of cases, but in most the source is not defined (Cherington, 1998).

CLINICAL FEATURES. The clinical spectrum of infantile botulism includes asymptomatic carriers of organisms, mild hypotonia and failure to thrive, severe, progressive, life-threatening paralysis, and sudden infant death. Infected infants are between 2 and 26 weeks of age and usually live in a dusty environment adjacent to construction or agricultural soil disruption. The incidence is mainly between March and October. A prodromal syndrome of constipation and poor feeding is often reported. Progressive bulbar and skeletal muscle weakness and loss of tendon reflexes develop 4 to 5 days later. Typical features on examination include diffuse hypotonia, ptosis, dysphagia, weak cry, and dilated pupils that react sluggishly to light.

Infantile botulism is a self-limited disease generally lasting for 2 to 6 weeks. Recovery is complete, but relapse occurs in as many as 5% of babies.

DIAGNOSIS. The syndrome suggests postinfectious polyradiculoneuropathy (Guillain-Barré syndrome), infantile spinal muscular atrophy, or generalized myasthenia gravis. Clinical differentiation of infantile botulism from Guillain-Barré syndrome is difficult, and some reported cases of Guillain-Barré syndrome during infancy might actually have been infantile botulism. Infantile botulism differs from infantile spinal muscular atrophy by the early appearance of facial and pharyngeal weakness, the presence of ptosis and dilated pupils, and the occurrence of severe constipation. Infants with generalized myasthenia do not have dilated pupils, absent reflexes, or severe constipation.

Electrophysiological studies provide the first clue to the diagnosis. Repetitive stimulation between 20 and 50 Hz reverses the presynaptic block and produces an incremental increase in the size of the motor unit potentials in 90% of cases. The EMG shows short-duration, low-amplitude motor unit potentials. The diagnosis is confirmed by the isolation of organisms from the stool.

MANAGEMENT. The use of antitoxin and antibiotics does not influence the course of the disease.

Indeed, gentamicin, an agent that produces presynaptic neuromuscular blockade, may worsen the condition. Intensive care is necessary throughout the period of profound hypotonia, and many infants require ventilator support. Sudden apnea and death are a constant danger.

Familial Infantile Myasthenia

Several genetic defects causing myasthenic syndromes have been identified (Table 6-11). All are transmitted by autosomal recessive inheritance except for the slow channel syndrome, which is transmitted as an autosomal dominant trait (see Chapter 7). All genetic myasthenic syndromes are seronegative for antibodies that bind the acetylcholine receptor (AChR). The congenital myasthenia syndromes are classified on the basis of their genetic and clinical features (Middleton, 1996).

Few laboratories are able to determine the site of abnormality or the responsible gene. Therefore clinicians recognize two clinical syndromes: familial infantile myasthenia with prominent respiratory and feeding difficulty at birth, and congenital myasthenia with predominantly ocular findings (see Chapter 15). Familial infantile myasthenia can be caused by a presynaptic defect in acetylcholine resynthesis and packaging or by several postsynaptic defects involving the kinetics of the AChR or congenital endplate acetylcholinesterase deficiency.

CLINICAL FEATURES. Respiratory insufficiency and feeding difficulty may be present at birth. Many affected newborns require mechanical ventilation. Ptosis and generalized weakness either are present at birth or develop during infancy. Arthrogryposis may also be present. Although facial and skeletal muscles are weak,

---

Table 6-11
Genetic Myasthenic Syndromes

Presynaptic Defects
Defect in acetylcholine resynthesis or mobilization
Paucity of synaptic vesicles and reduced quantal release

Postsynaptic Defects
Endplate acetylcholinesterase deficiency
Kinetic abnormalities of the receptor without primary
    acetylcholine receptor (AChR) deficiency
    Abnormal interaction of acetylcholine and receptor
    High conductance and fast closure of the acetylcholine
      receptor channel
    Slow channel syndrome
Primary AChR deficiency

extraocular motility is usually normal. Within weeks the infants become stronger and no longer need mechanical ventilation. However, episodes of weakness and life-threatening apnea occur repeatedly throughout infancy and childhood, sometimes even into adult life.

DIAGNOSIS. The diagnosis is established by the intravenous or subcutaneous injection of edrophonium chloride, 0.15 mg/kg. The weakness and the respiratory distress are reversed almost immediately after intravenous injection and within 10 minutes of subcutaneous injection. Further confirmation can be accomplished by showing a decrement in the amplitude of successive motor unit potentials with repetitive nerve stimulation at low frequency. Identification of the precise defect requires special laboratory techniques.

MANAGEMENT. Long-term treatment with neostigmine or pyridostigmine is needed to prevent sudden episodes of apnea at the time of intercurrent illness. The weakness in some children responds to a combination of pyridostigmine and diaminopyridine (DAP). DAP is not commercially available in the United States but can be obtained on a compassionate use basis for individual patients. Information on the process can be obtained from Jacobus Pharmaceutical Company, Inc., Princeton, NJ, fax no. 609-799-1176. Thymectomy and immunosuppressive therapy are not beneficial.

Transitory Neonatal Myasthenia

A transitory myasthenic syndrome is observed in 10% to 20% of newborns of myasthenic mothers. The syndrome is believed to be due to the passive transfer of antibody directed against fetal AChR from the myasthenic mother to her normal fetus (Gardnerova et al, 1997). Fetal AChR is structurally different from adult AChR. The severity of symptoms in the newborn correlates with the ratio of fetal to adult AChR antibodies in the mother but not with the severity or duration of weakness in the mother.

CLINICAL FEATURES. Difficulty feeding and generalized hypotonia are the major clinical features. Affected children are eager to feed, but the ability to suck fatigues quickly and nutrition is inadequate. Symptoms usually arise within hours of birth but can be delayed until the third day. Some newborns have had intrauterine hypotonia and are born with arthrogryposis. Weakness of cry and lack of facial expression is present in 50%, but only 15% have limitation of extraocular movement and ptosis. Respira-

tory insufficiency is uncommon. Weakness becomes progressively worse in the first few days and then improves. The mean duration of symptoms is 18 days, with a range of 5 days to 2 months. Recovery is complete, and transitory neonatal myasthenia does not develop into myasthenia gravis later in life.

DIAGNOSIS. The diagnosis of transitory neonatal myasthenia is accomplished by showing high serum concentrations of AChR binding antibody in the newborn and temporary reversal of weakness by the subcutaneous or intravenous injection of edrophonium chloride, 0.15 mg/kg.

MANAGEMENT. Newborns with severe generalized weakness and respiratory distress should be treated with plasma exchange. For those who are less impaired, an intramuscular injection of 0.1% neostigmine methylsulfate before feeding sufficiently improves sucking and swallowing to allow adequate nutrition. The dose is progressively reduced as symptoms remit. Neostigmine may also be administered through a nasogastric tube at a dose 10 times the parenteral level.

Congenital Myopathies

Congenital myopathies are developmental disorders of skeletal muscle. The main clinical feature is infantile hypotonia. Diagnosis is established only by muscle biopsy. The common histological feature is that type I fibers are greater in number, but smaller in size, than type II fibers (Figure 6-2). Many infants with hypotonia and type I fiber predominance are later shown to have a cerebral abnormality; cerebellar aplasia is particularly common.

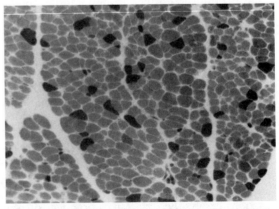

Figure 6-2. Fiber-type disproportion myopathy (ATPase reaction). Type I fibers (*light shade*) are more numerous than type II fibers (*dark shade*). Type II fibers are generally larger in diameter than type I fibers.

The term *congenital fiber-type disproportion myopathy* (CFTD) is used to describe newborns with hypotonia, and sometimes arthrogryposis, whose muscle biopsy specimens show type I predominance as the only histological abnormality. The biopsy specimens in some infants have not only a type I fiber predominance but also a unique histological feature for which their condition is named: central core disease, myotubular myopathy, and nemaline myopathy. Several other congenital myopathies, reported in one child or one family, are not discussed.

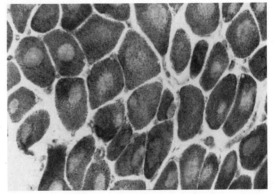

Figure 6-3. Central core disease (DPNH reaction). The center of every fiber has a central core that appears clear when oxidative enzyme reactions are applied.

Central Core Disease

Central core disease is a rare but distinct genetic entity transmitted by autosomal dominant inheritance. Mutations in the ryanodine receptor-1 gene (RYR1) on chromosome 19q13 are responsible for central core disease and malignant hyperthermia.

CLINICAL FEATURES. Mild hypotonia is noted immediately after birth or during infancy. Congenital dislocation of the hips is relatively common. Slowly progressive weakness begins after the age of 5 years. Weakness is greater in proximal than in distal limb muscles and is greater in the arms than in the legs. Tendon reflexes of weak muscles are depressed or absent. Extraocular motility, facial expression, and swallowing are normal. Some children become progressively weaker, have motor impairment, and develop kyphoscoliosis. In others, weakness remains mild and never causes disability.

All children with central core disease are at risk of malignant hyperthermia and should not be administered anesthetics without appropriate caution (see Chapter 8).

DIAGNOSIS. The serum concentration of CK is normal, and the EMG findings may be normal as well. More frequently the EMG suggests a myopathic process. Diagnosis depends on muscle biopsy. Sharply demarcated cores of closely packed myofibrils undergoing varying degrees of degeneration are present in the center of all type I fibers (Figure 6-3). Because of the tight packing of myofibrils, the cores are deficient in sarcoplasmic reticulum, glycogen, and mitochondria.

MANAGEMENT. Treatment is not available.

Congenital Fiber-Type Disproportion Myopathy

The congenital fiber-type disproportion (CFTD) myopathies are a heterogeneous group of diseases that have a similar pattern of muscle histology. The initial feature of all these diseases is infantile hypotonia. Both sexes are involved equally. Most cases are sporadic; some are clearly transmitted by autosomal dominant inheritance and others by autosomal recessive inheritance. One child with CFTD was biopsied again during infancy and found to have myotubular myopathy (Danon et al, 1997). Despite the label "congenital," an identical pattern of fiber-type disproportion may be present in patients who are asymptomatic at birth and first have weakness during childhood.

CLINICAL FEATURES. The severity of weakness in the newborn varies from mild hypotonia to respiratory insufficiency. Many had intrauterine hypotonia and show congenital hip dislocation, dysmorphic features, and joint contractures. Proximal muscles are weaker than distal muscles. Facial weakness, high-arched palate, ptosis, and disturbances of ocular motility may be present. When axial weakness is present in infancy, kyphoscoliosis often develops during childhood. Tendon reflexes are depressed or absent. Intellectual function is normal. Weakness is most severe during the first 2 years and then becomes relatively stable or progresses slowly.

DIAGNOSIS. The essential features seen in muscle specimens are type I fiber predominance and hypotrophy. Type I fibers are 15% smaller than type II fibers. Other laboratory studies are not helpful. The serum concentration of CK may be slightly elevated or normal, and the EMG may be consistent with a neuropathic process, a myopathic process, or both. Nerve conduction velocities are normal.

MANAGEMENT. Physical therapy should be initiated immediately, not only to relieve existing contractures but also to prevent new contractures from developing.

Myotubular (Centronuclear) Myopathy

Several clinical syndromes are included in the category of myotubular (centronuclear) myopathy. Some are clearly transmitted by X-linked inheritance, others by autosomal dominant inheritance, and still others by autosomal recessive inheritance. The autosomal dominant form has a later onset and a milder course. The common histological feature on muscle biopsy is an apparent arrest in the morphogenesis of the muscle fiber at the myotube stage.

Acute Myotubular Myopathy

The abnormal gene that causes acute myotubular myopathy has been mapped to the long arm of the X chromosome (Xq28) and has been designated MTM1. The protein encoded by the MTM1 gene is called *myotubularin* (OMIM, 1999).

CLINICAL FEATURES. The clinical features in the newborn are generalized hypotonia and respiratory distress. Decreased fetal movement during pregnancy, polyhydramnios, and fetal cardiac arrhythmias are common. Sucking, swallowing, and tendon reflexes are depressed or absent. Ptosis and ophthalmoplegia may be present. Repeated episodes of apnea, asphyxia, and pneumonia usually cause death during early infancy.

DIAGNOSIS. The serum concentration of CK is normal. The EMG may suggest a neuropathic process, a myopathic process, or both. Muscle biopsy shows type I fiber predominance and hypotrophy, the presence of many internal nuclei, and a central area of increased oxidative enzyme and decreased myosin ATPase activity.

MANAGEMENT. Treatment is not available.

Chronic Myotubular Myopathy

Chronic myotubular myopathy may be transmitted by either autosomal dominant or recessive inheritance.

CLINICAL FEATURES. In general, the recessive form starts later than the X-linked form and earlier than the dominant form. Some children with the disease have hypotonia at birth; others come to attention because of delayed motor development. Limb weakness may be predominantly proximal or distal. The axial and neck flexor muscles are weak as well. Ptosis, but not ophthalmoplegia, is sometimes present at birth. Infants have a slowly progressive ophthalmoplegia, loss of facial expression, continuing weakness of limb muscles, and loss of tendon reflexes. Many patients have seizures and mental deficiency.

DIAGNOSIS. The serum concentration of CK is normal, and EMG findings are abnormal but do not establish the diagnosis. Muscle biopsy is essential for diagnosis, and the histological features are identical to those of the acute form.

MANAGEMENT. Treatment is not available.

Nemaline (Rod) Myopathy

Nemaline myopathy can be transmitted by autosomal dominant or recessive inheritance. The dominant form is caused by mutations in the tropomyosin-3 gene on chromosome 1q22-23, and the much less common recessive form is caused by mutation in the gene encoding nebulin linked to chromosome 2q (North et al, 1997).

CLINICAL FEATURES. At least three different phenotypes are described in children. Two congenital types are transmitted by autosomal recessive inheritance: (1) a severe neonatal form that causes immediate respiratory insufficiency and neonatal death and (2) a milder form in which affected newborns often appear normal or are mildly hypotonic and attention is not sought until infancy, when achievement of motor milestones is delayed. This form tends to be slowly progressive, with greater weakness in proximal than distal muscles. Weakness of facial muscles causes a dysmorphic appearance in which the face appears long and narrow and the palate is high and arched. Axial weakness leads to scoliosis.

The childhood-onset form is transmitted by autosomal dominant inheritance. Onset of ankle weakness occurs late in the first or early in the second decade. The weakness is slowly progressive, and affected individuals may be wheelchair confined as adults.

DIAGNOSIS. The serum concentration of CK is either normal or only mildly elevated. EMG findings may be normal, and when abnormal they are not the basis for diagnosis. Muscle biopsy is essential for diagnosis. Within most children, if is not all, fibers are multiple small rod-like particles, thought to be derived from lateral expansion of the Z disk. The greatest concentration of particles is under the sarcolemma (Figure 6-4). Type I fiber predominance is a prominent feature.

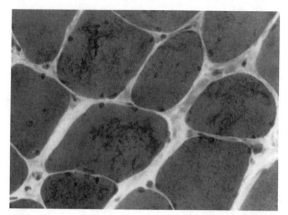

Figure 6-4. Nemaline (rod) myopathy (trichrome). A spectrum of fiber sizes is present. The small fibers are all type I and contain rod-like bodies in a subsarcolemmal position.

MANAGEMENT. Treatment is supportive. Parents who have the abnormal gene but are not weak may have rod bodies and fiber-type predominance in their muscles.

Muscular Dystrophies

Congenital Dystrophinopathy

Dystrophinopathies occasionally cause weakness at birth. In such cases, dystrophin is completely absent. Immunofluorescence reactions for all three domains of dystrophin should be done in newborns with the appearance of a congenital muscular dystrophy. See Chapter 7 for a complete discussion of dystrophinopathies.

Congenital Muscular Dystrophy

The congenital muscular dystrophies (CMD) are a group of myopathies characterized by hypotonia at birth or shortly thereafter, the early formation of multiple joint contractures, and diffuse muscle weakness and atrophy. They are broadly divided according to the absence or presence of merosin in muscle (Tomé, 1999). Merosin (laminin α2), located in the extracellular matrix, is the linking protein for the dystroglycan complex (see Figure 7-3). The merosin-deficient CMD are further divided into primary and secondary types. The secondary merosin deficiencies also have severe brain migrational disorders that cause mental retardation and seizures.

Merosin-Positive Congenital Muscular Dystrophy

The phenotype associated with merosin-positive CMD is not homogeneous. Transmission is by autosomal recessive inheritance with considerable genetic heterogeneity. One form, mapped to chromosome 1p36-p35, consistently shows early rigidity of the spine, scoliosis, and reduced vital capacity, as are found in the *rigid spine syndrome* (Flanigan et al, 2000). Another form, the *muscle-eye-brain syndrome,* maps to chromosome 1p34-p32 and clinically resembles the Walker-Warberg syndrome.

CLINICAL FEATURES. Approximately half of affected individuals are abnormal at birth because of some combination of hypotonia, poor ability to suck, and respiratory distress. Developmental motor milestones are almost always delayed. Limb-girdle weakness is the rule, generalized weakness may be present, and about half of the individuals have facial weakness. Joint deformities may be present at birth or develop during infancy in half of the patients.

DIAGNOSIS. The serum concentration of CK is mildly elevated, and muscle biopsy shows fiber necrosis and regeneration. Brain MRI is normal.

MANAGEMENT. Physical therapy is important to prevent and reduce contractures.

Primary Merosin-Deficient Congenital Muscular Dystrophy

The abnormal gene site for primary merosin-deficient CMD is chromosome 6q22-23 (Pegoraro et al, 1998). The phenotype associated with merosin deficiency is generally more severe than the phenotypes in which merosin is present.

CLINICAL FEATURES. Hypotonia, arthrogryposis, and respiratory insufficiency are severe at birth. The infant has generalized limb weakness, with proximal muscles affected earlier and more severely than distal muscles. Facial and neck weakness is common, but extraocular motility is normal. Tendon reflexes may be present or absent and are often difficult to test because of joint contractures. Contractures at birth may involve any joint, but torticollis and clubfoot are particularly common, and congenital dislocation of the hips is often an associated feature.

Muscles are not hypertrophied. Motor development is delayed because of weakness and contractures. The best motor achievement is the ability to sit unsupported. Intelligence is either normal or borderline subnormal. Chronic hypoventilation leading to respiratory failure is the usual cause of death.

DIAGNOSIS. The serum concentration of CK is high in the newborn and tends to decline with age. Asymptomatic siblings and parents may have elevated serum concentrations of CK.

EMG findings are consistent with a myopathic process. The muscle histological appearance is characteristic. Features include a variation in fiber size with occasional central nucleation, extensive fibrosis and proliferation of adipose tissue, fibers undergoing regeneration and degeneration, and thickening of the muscle spindle capsule. A mononuclear infiltrate surrounding muscle fibers is often present early in the course. Cases of "neonatal polymyositis" are now believed to be merosin-deficient CMD (Pegoraro et al, 1996).

Infants who are merosin deficient have an abnormal T_2 MRI signal in the cerebral white matter indicating hypomyelination mainly in the occipital horns. Structural disturbances of the occipital cortex may be associated (Philpot et al, 1999).

MANAGEMENT. Physical therapy is important to prevent further contractures. Antenatal diagnosis is not available.

Secondary Merosin Deficiency Myopathies

There are at least three disorders in which congenital muscular dystrophy coexists with involvement of the central nervous system: the *Walker-Warberg syndrome, Fukuyama congenital muscular dystrophy* (FCMD) in Japanese patients, and muscle-eye-brain disease in Finnish patients. The abnormal gene site for Walker-Warberg syndrome and FCMD is chromosome 9q31-33, and transmission is by autosomal recessive inheritance. Muscle-eye-brain disease does not link to chromosome 9q.

The major feature is a disturbance of cellular migration to the cortex between the fourth and fifth gestational months, resulting in polymicrogyria, lissencephaly, and heterotopia (Haltia et al, 1997). Other abnormalities may include fusion of the frontal lobes, hydrocephalus, periventricular cysts, optic nerve atrophy, hypoplasia of the pyramidal tracts, reduction in the number of anterior horn cells, and inflammation of the leptomeninges.

Merosin expression is reduced but not absent in the Walker-Warberg syndrome and FCMD and normal in the muscle-eye-brain disease (Wewer et al, 1995). An abnormal MRI T_2 signal in the centrum semiovale that resembles hypomyelination is a marker of abnormal merosin expression.

CLINICAL FEATURES. FCMD is the most common form of muscular dystrophy in Japan. A history of spontaneous abortion is recorded for 25% of mothers who have affected children.

Affected newborns are normal at birth but soon develop hypotonia, an expressionless face, a weak cry, and an ineffective suck. Weakness affects proximal more than distal limb muscles. Mild contractures of the elbow and knee joints may be present at birth or develop later. Tendon reflexes are usually absent. Pseudohypertrophy of the calves develops in half of cases.

Symptoms of cerebral involvement are present early in infancy. Febrile or nonfebrile generalized seizures are usually the first manifestation. Development is always globally delayed, and microcephaly is the rule. Weakness and atrophy are progressive and result in severe disability, cachexia, and death before 10 years of age.

The cerebral and muscle abnormalities of the Walker-Warberg syndrome are the same as those in FCMD. The major differences are the presence of ocular abnormalities and the occurrence in non-Japanese children. Ocular abnormalities include corneal clouding, cataracts, retinal dysplasia or detachment, and optic nerve hypoplasia.

DIAGNOSIS. The serum concentration of CK is generally elevated, and the EMG indicates a myopathy. Muscle biopsy specimens show excessive proliferation of adipose tissue and collagen out of proportion to the degree of fiber degeneration. Typical MRI abnormalities are dilatation of the cerebral ventricles and subarachnoid space and lucency of cortical white matter.

MANAGEMENT. Treatment is supportive.

Congenital Myotonic Dystrophy

Myotonic dystrophy is a multisystem disorder transmitted by autosomal dominant inheritance. Symptoms usually begin in the second decade (see Chapter 7). The disease is caused by an unstable DNA triplet in the DMPK gene (chromosome 19q13) that repeats 50 to several thousand times in successive generations; the number of repeats correlates with the severity of disease, but the phenotype should not be predicted by the repeat size alone (Gharehbaghi-Schnell et al, 1998). Repeat size changes from mother to child are greater than from father to child, and for this reason the mother is usually the affected parent when a child has CMD. A mother with repeats of 100 units has a 90% chance that her child will have repeats of 400 units or more.

The main features during pregnancy are reduced fetal movement and polyhydramnios. Fifty percent of babies are born prematurely. Labor may be prolonged because of inadequate uterine contraction, and forceps assistance is frequently needed. Severely affected newborns have inadequate diaphragmatic and intercostal muscle function and are incapable of spontaneous respiration. In the absence of prompt intubation and mechanical ventilation, many will die immediately after birth.

Prominent clinical features in the newborn include facial diplegia, in which the mouth is oddly shaped so that the upper lip forms an inverted V; generalized muscular hypotonia; joint deformities ranging from bilateral clubfoot to generalized arthrogryposis; and gastrointestinal dysfunction, including choking, regurgitation, aspiration, swallowing difficulties, and gastroparesis. Limb weakness in the newborn is more often proximal than distal. Tendon reflexes are usually absent in weak muscles. Myotonia, an abnormality in muscle relaxation after contraction, is not elicited by percussion and may not be demonstrable on EMG.

Neonatal mortality is 16%, a frequent cause of death being cardiomyopathy. Survivors usually gain strength and are usually able to walk; however, a progressive myopathy similar to the late-onset form occurs eventually. Severe mental retardation is the rule, and may result from a combination of early respiratory failure and a direct effect of the mutation on the brain (Ashizawa, 1998).

DIAGNOSIS. The diagnosis of congenital myotonic dystrophy in the newborn requires examination of the mother. She is likely to have many clinical features of the disease and myotonia on EMG. The diagnosis can be confirmed by showing DNA amplification on chromosome 19 in both mother and child. Nonsymptomatic family members at risk should be tested for the carrier state.

MANAGEMENT. The immediate treatment is intubation and mechanical ventilation. Fixed joints respond to physical therapy and casting. Gastroparesis may be alleviated by metoclopramide therapy.

Metabolic Myopathies

Acid Maltase Deficiency (Pompe Disease)

Acid maltase is a lysosomal enzyme, present in all tissues, that hydrolyzes maltose and other branches of glycogen to yield glucose. It has no function in maintaining blood glucose concentrations. Three distinct clinical forms of deficiency are recognized: infantile, childhood (see Chapter 7), and adult. All are transmitted by autosomal recessive inheritance. The defective gene is located on chromosome 17q25.

CLINICAL FEATURES. The infantile form may begin immediately after birth but usually appears during the second month. Profound generalized hypotonia without atrophy and congestive heart failure are the initial symptoms. Hypotonia is the result of glycogen storage in the brain, spinal cord, and skeletal muscles, causing mixed signs of cerebral and motor unit dysfunction: decreased awareness and depressed tendon reflexes. The mixed signs may be confusing, but the presence of cardiomegaly is almost diagnostic. The electrocardiogram shows abnormalities, including short PR intervals and high QRS complexes on all leads. Most patients die of cardiac failure by 1 year of age.

DIAGNOSIS. Diagnosis is established by muscle biopsy. Large vacuoles containing glycogen are observed in muscle fibers. The diagnosis is established by showing deficient acid maltase activity in fibroblasts or other tissues.

MANAGEMENT. A high-protein diet has been found helpful in childhood form of the disease but has not yet proved useful in the infantile form.

Cytochrome-c-Oxidase Deficiency

The electron transfer chain and oxidative phosphorylation are the principal sources of adenosine triphosphate (ATP) synthesis (see Chapter 8). Deficiencies of mitochondrial enzymes that comprise the electron transfer chain in skeletal muscle may cause hypotonia in newborns or infants and exercise intolerance in older children. Deficiency of COX causes several different neuromuscular and cerebral disorders in childhood. Deficiency can result from mutations in either nuclear or mitochondrial DNA. The deficiency resides in complex I in 33%, in complex IV in 28%, and in complexes I and IV in 28%. Deficiency of complex II and complex III accounts for 4% and 7% of cases, respectively (von Kleist-Retzow et al, 1998). Most cases are sporadic.

Both a fatal and a benign form of infantile COX deficiency are recognized. Early in their course these forms are indistinguishable, but in the benign form a spontaneous increase in COX activity associated with increased strength occurs during infancy.

CLINICAL FEATURES. Clinical features vary with the number of enzyme deficiencies, the percentage reduction in enzyme activity, and the presence of mitochondrial enzyme deficiencies in organs other than muscle. Profound generalized weakness, causing difficulty in feeding, early respiratory failure, and death; severe lactic acidosis; and the *De Toni-Fanconi-Debré syndrome* (glycosuria, proteinuria, phosphaturia, and generalized aminoaciduria) characterize the complete syndrome. Onset is anytime within the first 6 months. Ptosis, ophthalmoplegia, and macroglossia may be present. Newborns with multiple enzyme deficiencies in multiple organs die within 6 months.

DIAGNOSIS. A deficiency in respiratory chain enzymes should be suspected in any hypotonic infant with lactic acidosis. The serum concentration of CK is elevated, but EMG findings may be normal. Muscle biopsy reveals vacuoles, mainly in type I fibers, with abnormal glycogen and lipid accumulations. Mitochondria are large, increased in number, and abnormal in structure (ragged-red fibers).

MANAGEMENT. No effective treatment is available for infants with overwhelming disease caused by multiorgan enzyme deficiency. The fatal and benign forms of the deficiency should be distinguished by immunohistochemical findings, and supportive care should be provided for newborns with the transitory form.

Phosphofructokinase Deficiency

The usual manifestations of muscle phosphofructokinase deficiency are cramps on exercise and myoglobinuria (see Chapter 8). Symptoms usually begin in childhood, and patients are otherwise asymptomatic. A rare neonatal form of phosphofructokinase deficiency exists and is transmitted by autosomal recessive inheritance.

CLINICAL FEATURES. The neonatal form is characterized by hypotonia, weakness, respiratory deficiency, and joint deformities. The tendon reflexes are diminished or absent. Cerebral and corneal abnormalities may be present. Death occurs during infancy or early childhood.

DIAGNOSIS. The serum concentration of CK is normal. The EMG, at least late in the disease, is consistent with a myopathic process. Muscle biopsy is critical for diagnosis. Light microscopy shows only nonspecific myopathy, but electron microscopy shows an abnormal accumulation of subsarcolemmal and intramyofibrillary glycogen. Large cytoplasmic vacuoles, as in acid maltase deficiency, are not present. Phosphofructokinase activity is absent in skeletal muscle but present in red blood cells and fibroblasts.

MANAGEMENT. Treatment is not available.

Phosphorylase Deficiency

Myophosphorylase deficiency (McArdle disease) is characterized by exercise intolerance in young adults and progressive myopathy in middle life (see Chapter 8). A rare neonatal form of variable severity has been recognized. It is reported in siblings and is probably transmitted, like the older onset forms, by autosomal recessive inheritance. Indeed, the enzyme deficiency appears identical at all ages, and the reason for clinical heterogeneity is not understood.

CLINICAL FEATURES. Newborns with myophosphorylase deficiency have difficulty with sucking and swallowing immediately postpartum or in the early neonatal period. In some, weakness is so profound that it produces immediate respiratory insufficiency. In others, weakness is progressive over several months or years. The child appears alert and has normal cranial nerve function. The tongue and heart are not affected. Tendon reflexes are depressed or absent.

DIAGNOSIS. The serum concentration of CK is elevated, and the EMG findings are abnormal, with features of both neuropathy and myopathy. Muscle biopsy is diagnostic. Fibers vary in size from atrophic to normal and contain peripheral vacuoles that react intensely for glycogen. The glycogen concentration of muscle is greatly elevated, and phosphorylase activity cannot be detected.

MANAGEMENT. A high-protein diet is useful in older patients with phosphorylase deficiency but has not yet been tried in newborns.

References

Ashizawa T. Myotonic dystrophy as a brain disorder. *Arch Neurol* 1998;55:291–293.

Baumgartner MR, Verhoeven NM, Jacobs C, et al. Defective peroxisome biogenesis with a neuromuscular disorder resembling Werdnig-Hoffmann disease. *Neurology* 1998;51:1427–1432.

Cherington M. Clinical spectrum of botulism. *Muscle Nerve* 1998;21:701–710.

Danon MJ, Giometti CS, Manaligod JR, et al. Sequential muscle biopsy changes in a case of congenital myopathy. *Muscle Nerve* 1997;20:561–569.

Flanigan KM, Kerr L, Bromberg MB. Congenital muscular dystrophy with rigid spine syndrome: A clinical, pathological, radiological, and genetic study. *Ann Neurol* 2000;47:152–161.

Gardnerova M, Eymard B, Morel E, et al. The fetal/adult acetylcholine receptor antibody ratio in mothers with myasthenia gravis as a marker for transfer of the disease to the newborn. *Neurology* 1997;48:50–54.

Gharehbaghi-Schnell EB, Finsterer J, Korschineck I, et al. Genotype-phenotype correlation in myotonic dystrophy. *Clin Genet* 1998;53:20–26.

Haltia M, Leivo I, Somer H, et al. Muscle-eye-brain disease: A neuropathological study. *Ann Neurol* 1997;41: 173–180.

Keulemans JLM, Reuser AJJ, Kroos MA, et al. Human alpha-*N*-acetylgalactosaminidase (alpha-NAGA) deficiency: New mutations and the paradox between genotype and phenotype. *J Med Genet* 1996;33:458–464.

Lin T, Lewis RA, Nussbaum RL. Molecular confirmation of carriers for Lowe syndrome. *Ophthalmology* 1999; 106:119–122.

Middleton LT. Congenital myasthenic syndromes: Report of the 34th ENMC International Workshop. *Neuromusc Disord* 1996;6:133–136.

Miller SP, Riley P, Shevell MI. The neonatal presentation of Prader-Willi syndrome revisited. *J Pediatr* 1999;134: 226–228.

North KN, Laing NG, Wallgren-Pettersson C, et al. Nemaline myopathy: Current concepts. *J Med Genet* 1997; 34:705–713.

Online Mendelian Inheritance in Man (OMIM).™ Johns Hopkins University, Baltimore MD. MIM Number: 310400: November 11, 1999.

Parano E, Pavone L, Falsaperla R, et al. Molecular basis of phenotypic heterogeneity in siblings with spinal muscular atrophy. *Ann Neurol* 1996;40:247–251.

Pegoraro E, Mancias P, Swerdlow SH, et al. Congenital muscular dystrophy with primary laminin α2 (merosin) deficiency presenting as inflammatory myopathy. *Ann Neurol* 1996;40:782–791.

Pegoraro E, Marks H, Garcia CA, et al. Laminin α2 muscular dystrophy: Genotype/phenotype studies of 22 patients. *Neurology* 1998;51:101–110.

Philpot J, Cowan F, Pennock J, et al. Merosin-deficient muscular dystrophy: The spectrum of brain involvement on magnetic resonance imaging. *Neuromusc Disord* 1999; 9:81–85.

Rubio-Gozalbo MD, Smeitink JAM, Ruitenbeek W, et al. Spinal muscular atrophy-like picture, cardiomyopathy, and cytochrome-*c*-oxidase deficiency. *Neurology* 1999; 52:383–386.

Shohat M, Lotan R, Magal N, et al. A gene for arthrogryposis multiplex congenita neuropathic type is linked to D5S394 on chromosome 5qter *Am J Hum Genet* 1997;61:1139–1143.

Stewart H, Wallace A, McGaughran J, et al. Molecular diagnosis of spinal muscular atrophy. *Arch Dis Child* 1998;78:531–535.

Tomé FMS. The saga of congenital muscular dystrophy. *Neuropediatrics* 1999;30:55–65.

Tyson J, Ellis D, Fairbrother U, et al. Hereditary demyelinating neuropathy of infancy: A genetically complex syndrome. *Brain* 1997;120:47–63.

von Kleist-Retzow JC, Cormier-Daire V, de Lonlay P, et al. A high rate (20%–30%) of parental consanguinity in cytochrome-oxidase deficiency. *Am J Hum Genet* 1998; 63:428–435.

Wewer UM, Durkin ME, Zhang X, et al. Laminin 2 chain and adhalin deficiency in the skeletal muscle of Walker-Warburg syndrome (cerebro-ocular dysplasia-muscular dystrophy). *Neurology* 1995;45:2099–2101.

Chapter 7
Flaccid Limb Weakness in Childhood

MOST CHILDREN WITH acute or chronic flaccid limb weakness have a disorder of the motor unit. Flaccid leg weakness may be the initial feature of disturbances in the lumbosacral region, but other symptoms of spinal cord dysfunction are usually present. Table 12-1 should also be consulted when considering the differential diagnosis of flaccid leg weakness without arm impairment. Cerebral disorders may cause flaccid weakness, but dementia (see Chapter 5) or seizures (see Chapter 1) are usually concomitant features.

Clinical Features of Neuromuscular Disease

Weakness is decreased strength, as measured by the force of a maximal contraction. Fatigue is inability to maintain a less than maximal contraction, as measured by exercise tolerance. Weak muscles are always more easily fatigued than normal muscles, but fatigue may occur in the absence of weakness. Conditions in which strength is normal at rest but fatigue or cramps occur on exercise are discussed in Chapter 8.

The Initial Complaint

Limb weakness in children is almost always noted first in the legs and then in the arms (Table 7-1). This is because many neuromuscular disorders affect the legs before the arms and symptoms of mild leg weakness are more obvious than mild arm weakness because walking is impaired. Delayed development of motor skills is often an initial complaint or a prominent feature in the history of children with neuromuscular disorders. Marginal motor delay in a child whose other developmental skills are normal is often overlooked as part of the spectrum of normal development. Older children with neuromuscular disorders are frequently referred for neurological examination because they are unable to keep up with peers or because they tire easily.

An abnormal gait can be the initial symptom of either proximal or distal leg weakness. With proximal weakness, the pelvis is not stabilized and waddles from side to side as the child walks. Running is especially difficult and accentuates the hip waddle. Descending stairs is particularly difficult in children with quadriceps weakness; the knee must be kept locked and stiff. Difficulty with ascending stairs suggests hip extensor weakness. Rising from the floor or a deep chair is difficult, and the hands are used to push off.

Stumbling is an early complaint when there is distal leg weakness, especially weakness of the evertors and dorsiflexors of the foot. Falling is first noted when the child walks on uneven surfaces. The child is thought to be clumsy, but

Table 7-1
Symptoms of Neuromuscular Disease

Abnormal gait
  Steppage
  Toe walking
  Waddling
Easy fatigability
Frequent falls
Slow motor development
Specific disability
  Arm elevation
  Climbing stairs
  Hand grip
  Rising from floor

after a while parents realize that the child is "tripping on nothing at all." Repeated ankle spraining occurs because of lateral instability. Children with foot drop tend to lift the knee high in the air so that the foot will clear the ground. The weak foot then comes down with a slapping motion (steppage gait).

Toe walking is commonly encountered in Duchenne muscular dystrophy because the pelvis is thrust forward to shift the center of gravity and the gastrocnemius muscle is stronger than the peroneal muscles. Toe walking is seen also in upper motor neuron disorders that cause spasticity and in children who have tight heel cords but no identifiable neurological disease. Muscular dystrophy is usually associated with hyporeflexia and spasticity with hyperreflexia. However, the ankle tendon reflex may be difficult to elicit when the tendon is tight for any reason.

Adolescents, but usually not children, with weakness complain of specific disabilities. A young woman with proximal weakness may have difficulty keeping her arms elevated to groom her hair or rotating the shoulder to get into and out of garments that have a zipper or hook in the back. Weakness of hand muscles is often brought to attention because of difficulty with handwriting. Adolescents may notice difficulty in unscrewing jar tops or working with tools. Teachers report to parents when children are slower than classmates in climbing stairs, getting up from the floor, and skipping and jumping. Parents may report a specific complaint to the physician, but more often they say that the child's problem is an inability to keep up with peers.

A child whose limbs are weak also may have weakness in the muscles of the head and neck. Specific questions should be asked about double vision, drooping eyelids, difficulty chewing and swallowing, change of facial expression and strength (whistling, sucking, chewing, blowing), and the clarity and tone of speech. Weakness of neck muscles is frequently noticed when the child is a passenger in a car that suddenly accelerates or decelerates. The neck muscles are unable to stabilize the head, which snaps backward or forward.

Physical Findings

The examination begins by watching the child sit, stand, and walk. A normal child sitting cross-legged on the floor can rise to a standing position in a single movement without using the hands.

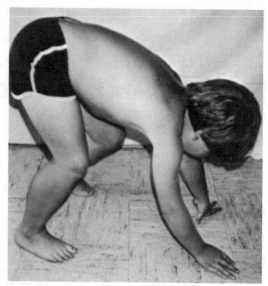

Figure 7-1. Gower sign. The child rises from the floor by pushing off with the hands to overcome proximal pelvic weakness.

This remarkable feat is lost sometime after age 15 in most children; and then rising from a low stool can be used to test proximal leg strength. The child with weak pelvic muscles uses the hands for assistance (Figure 7-1), and with progressive weakness the hands are used to climb up the legs (Gower sign).

After normal gait is observed, the child is asked to walk first on the toes and then on the heels (Table 7-2). Inability to walk on the toes indicates gastrocnemius muscle weakness, and inability to walk on the heels indicates weakness of the anterior compartment muscles.

Push-ups are a quick test of strength in almost all arm muscles. Most normal children can do

Table 7-2
Signs of Neuromuscular Disease

Observation
Atrophy and hypertrophy
Fasciculations
Functional ability

Palpation
Muscle texture
Tenderness

Examination
Joint contractures
Myotonia
Strength
Tendon reflexes

at least one push-up. The child is then asked to touch the tip of the shoulder blade with the ipsilateral thumb. This is an impossible task when the rhomboids are weak.

Finally, face and eye movements are tested. The best test of facial strength is to blow out the cheeks and hold air against compression. Normally the lips are smooth. Wrinkling of the perioral tissues and failure to hold air indicate facial weakness. During this period of observation and again during muscle strength testing, the physician should look for atrophy or hypertrophy. Wasting of muscles in the shoulder is easily seen because bony prominences stand out even further. Wasting of hand muscles causes flattening of the thenar and hypothenar eminences. Wasting of the quadriceps muscles causes a tapering appearance of the thigh that is exaggerated when the patient is asked to tense the thigh by straightening the knee. Atrophy of the anterior tibial and peroneal muscles gives the anterior border of the tibia a sharp appearance, and atrophy of the gastrocnemius muscle diminishes the normal contour of the calf.

Loss of tendon reflexes occurs early in denervation, especially when sensory nerves are involved, but tends to parallel the degree of weakness in myopathy. Tendon reflexes are usually normal even during times of weakness in patients with myasthenia gravis and may be normal between episodes of recurrent weakness in those with metabolic myopathies. Myotonia, a disturbance in muscle relaxation following contraction, is described in the section on myotonic dystrophy.

Progressive Proximal Weakness

Progressive proximal weakness in childhood is most often due to myopathy, usually a muscular dystrophy (Table 7-3). Juvenile spinal muscular atrophy is the only chronic denervating disease in which weakness is more proximal than distal. It is readily distinguished from myopathic disorders by electromyography (EMG) and muscle biopsy. Limb-girdle myasthenia is rare but is an important consideration because specific treatment is available (Table 7-4).

Spinal Muscular Atrophies

Autosomal Recessive Type

Three subtypes of spinal muscular atrophy (SMA) are distinguished by age at onset. The

---

Table 7-3
Progressive Proximal Weakness [Gene Location]

Spinal Cord Disorders (see Chapter 12)

Juvenile Spinal Muscular Atrophies
Autosomal dominant
Autosomal recessive [5q11-13]
GM$_2$ gangliosidosis (hexosaminidase A deficiency) [15q23-24]

Myasthenic Syndromes
Acquired limb-girdle myasthenia
Slow-channel syndrome

Myopathies
Muscular dystrophies
  Bethlem myopathy [21q]
  Duchenne/Becker dystrophy [Xp21.2]
  Facioscapulohumeral syndrome [4q35]
  Limb-girdle dystrophy [2p13-16, 4q12, 5q33-34, 13q12, 15q, 17q21]
  Severe childhood autosomal recessive muscular dystrophy
Inclusion body myopathy (autosomal dominant form)
Inflammatory myopathies
  Dermatomyositis
  Polymyositis
Metabolic myopathies
  Acid maltase deficiency [17q23]
  Carnitine deficiency
  Debrancher enzyme deficiency (see Chapter 8)
  Lipid storage myopathies
  Mitochondrial myopathies (see Chapter 8)
  Myophosphorylase deficiency (see Chapter 8)
Endocrine myopathies
  Adrenal cortex
  Parathyroid
  Thyroid

---

severe type (SMA I) always begins during infancy (see Chapter 6), the intermediate type (SMA II) may begin during infancy or early childhood, and the juvenile type (SMA III) begins after 18 months. The later-onset forms of SMA were initially thought to be genetically distinct from infantile SMA. However, despite considerable phenotypic heterogeneity, most cases of infantile and juvenile spinal muscular atrophy are caused by allelic defects on chromosome 5q11-13, the locus of the motor neuron survival gene (SMN).

An intermediate form of juvenile SMA with onset between 3 and 18 months months of age that is unrelated to the SMN region on chromosome 5q may exist (Nevo et al, 1996). Cases transmitted by autosomal dominant inheritance are rare and genetically distinct from those transmitted by autosomal recessive inheritance. CLINICAL FEATURES. In SMA II, fetal movements are normal and the child is normal at

Table 7-4
Distinguishing Features in Proximal Weakness

	Neuronopathy	Myopathy	Myasthenia
Tendon reflexes	Absent	Depressed or absent	Normal
Electromyography	Fasciculations; denervation potentials; high-amplitude polyphasic motor potentials	Brief, small-amplitude polyphasic motor units	Normal
Nerve conduction	Normal or mildly slow	Normal	Abnormal repetitive stimulation
Creatine kinase concentration	Normal or mildly elevated	Elevated	Normal
Muscle biopsy	Group atrophy, group typing	Fiber necrosis, fatty replacement, excessive collagen	Normal

birth. The initial feature of SMA II is delayed motor development. As a rule, affected children achieve sitting balance, do not stand unsupported, and are wheelchair confined. A fine hand tremor is often present. Contractures of the hips and knees and scoliosis eventually develop. Some of those affected die in childhood because of respiratory failure, but most survive into adult life.

An unusual form of SMA II is one that begins with head drop followed by generalized weakness and respiratory insufficiency. This variant causes death by 3 years of age.

The initial feature of SMA III is gait instability caused by proximal weakness. As in SMA II, a fine action tremor is common. Disease progression is very slow, sometimes in a stepwise fashion, and often seems arrested. Weakness may progress either to the distal muscles of the legs or to the proximal muscles of the arms. The hands are affected last. Facial muscles may be weak, but extraocular motility is always spared. Reflexes are uniformly reduced or absent. The sensory examination is normal. Cases with ophthalmoplegia are probably genetically distinct.

Some children have more profound weakness of the arms than of the legs and are likely to have facial weakness as well. Within a family, some children may have predominant leg weakness, whereas their siblings may have predominant arm weakness.

DIAGNOSIS. The diagnosis is established by showing the gene abnormality on chromosome 5. EMG and muscle biopsy are not needed if genetic analysis shows the appropriate mutation. The findings on both tests are similar to those described for SMA I in Chapter 6. The serum concentration of creatine kinase (CK) may be two to four times the upper limit of normal, and the increase in concentration correlates directly with the duration of illness.

MANAGEMENT. Proper management of spinal muscular atrophy in children increases longevity and decreases disability. The goals are to maintain function and prevent contractures. Children who quickly take to a wheelchair develop disuse atrophy. Dietary counseling is usually needed to prevent obesity, which only increases the strain on weak muscles. The prevention of contractures usually requires range of motion exercise and the early use of splints, especially at night. Families need genetic counseling.

Autosomal Dominant Type

The gene for the autosomal dominant type does not link to chromosome 5. A juvenile-onset type and an adult-onset type were thought to be genetically distinct but are now regarded as variable phenotypes. The onset of weakness is before age 10 years in most children, but some have mild joint contractures at birth. A new dominant mutation would be difficult to distinguish from the autosomal recessive form.

CLINICAL FEATURES. The pattern of weakness in the autosomal dominant type is somewhat more generalized than in the autosomal recessive type, but proximal muscles are still affected more severely than distal muscles. The weakness is slowly progressive and may stabilize after adolescence. Most patients walk and function well into middle and late adult life. Bulbar weakness is unusual and mild when present. Extraocular muscles are not affected. Tendon reflexes are depressed or absent in weak muscles. Joint contractures are uncommon.

DIAGNOSIS. The serum concentration of CK is normal or only mildly elevated. The EMG is the basis for diagnosis, as in the autosomal recessive type.

MANAGEMENT. Treatment for the dominant type is the same as for the recessive type. Genetic counseling should stress the complete penetrance of the phenotype. Antenatal diagnosis is not available. When the family has no history of spinal muscular atrophy, genetic counseling is difficult, but autosomal dominant inheritance should be considered if the onset is after 3 years of age.

GM$_2$ Gangliosidosis

The typical clinical expression of *hexosaminidase-A deficiency* is *Tay-Sachs disease* (see Chapter 5). Several phenotypic variants of the enzyme deficiency with onset throughout childhood and adult life are described. All are transmitted by autosomal recessive inheritance. The initial features of the juvenile-onset type mimic those of juvenile SMA (Navon et al, 1997).

CLINICAL FEATURES. Weakness, wasting, and cramps of the proximal leg muscles begin after infancy and frequently not until adolescence. These are followed by distal leg weakness, proximal and distal arm weakness, and tremor. Symptoms of cerebral degeneration (personality change, intermittent psychosis, dementia) become evident after motor neuron dysfunction is established.

Examination shows a mixture of upper and lower motor neuron signs. The macula is usually normal and the cranial nerves are intact, with the exception of atrophy and fasciculations in the tongue. Fasciculations also may be present in the limbs. Tendon reflexes are absent or exaggerated, depending on the relative severity of upper and lower motor neuron dysfunction. Plantar responses are sometimes extensor and sometimes flexor. Tremor, but not dysmetria, is present in the outstretched arms, and sensation is intact.

Some children never develop cerebral symptoms and have only motor neuron disease; some adults have only dementia and psychosis. The course is variable and compatible with prolonged survival.

DIAGNOSIS. The serum concentration of CK is normal or only mildly elevated. Motor and sensory nerve conduction velocities are normal, but needle EMG shows neuropathic motor units. The diagnosis is established by showing a severe deficiency or absence of hexosaminidase-A activity in leukocytes or cultured fibroblasts.

MANAGEMENT. No treatment is available. Heterozygote detection is possible because enzyme activity is partially deficient. Prenatal diagnosis is available.

Myasthenic Syndromes

Proximal weakness and sometimes wasting may occur in acquired immune-mediated myasthenia and in a genetic myasthenic syndrome.

Limb-Girdle Myasthenia

Immune-mediated myasthenia gravis that begins as progressive proximal weakness of the limbs and spares ocular motility is called *limb-girdle myasthenia*.

CLINICAL FEATURES. Onset is after 10 years of age, and girls are more often affected than boys. Weakness does not fluctuate with exercise. Muscles of facial expression may be affected, but other bulbar function is spared. Tendon reflexes are usually present but may be hypoactive. The clinical features suggest limb-girdle dystrophy or polymyositis.

DIAGNOSIS. Limb-girdle myasthenia should be suspected in every child with proximal weakness and preserved tendon reflexes. Repetitive nerve stimulation shows a decremental response, and the serum concentration of antibodies that bind the acetylcholine receptor is increased.

Families with limb-girdle myasthenia affecting two or more siblings have not been reported in recent years. Some of these families may have had the slow-channel syndrome or another genetic myasthenia.

MANAGEMENT. The treatment is the same as for other forms of antibody-positive myasthenia (see Chapter 15).

Slow-Channel Syndrome

The slow-channel syndrome is an inherited disorder of the ion channel of the skeletal muscle acetylcholine receptor (Gomez et al, 1996). It is transmitted by autosomal dominant inheritance. Some individuals have EMG evidence of disease without clinical symptoms.

CLINICAL FEATURES. No symptoms are present at birth. Onset is usually during infancy but can be delayed until adult life. Weakness of the cervical and scapular muscles is often the initial feature. Other common features are exercise intolerance, ophthalmoparesis, and muscle atrophy. Ptosis, bulbar dysfunction, and leg weakness are unusual. The syndrome progresses

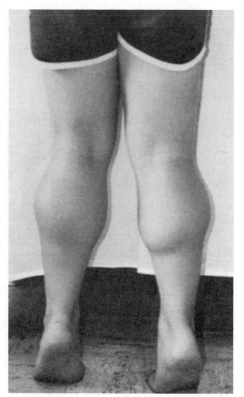

Figure 7-2. Enlarged calf muscles in DMD. Enlarged calves may be seen in other neuromuscular disorders.

slowly, and many patients do not come to medical attention until after the first decade.

DIAGNOSIS. Weakness does not respond either to injection or to oral administration of anticholinesterase medication. Two patients were hypersensitive to edrophonium (Tensilon) and responded with muscarinic side effects. Repetitive nerve stimulation at a rate of three stimuli per second causes an abnormal decremental response, and single-nerve stimulation causes a repetitive muscle potential. Muscle biopsy shows type I fiber predominance. Group atrophy, tubular aggregates, and an abnormal endplate configuration are present in some specimens.

MANAGEMENT. Cholinesterase inhibitors, thymectomy, and immunosuppression are not effective. Quinidine sulfate may improve strength (Harper and Engel, 1998).

Muscular Dystrophies

The dystrophies are a group of genetic myopathies that are usually caused by defects in structural proteins (Figure 7-2). Enzyme deficiencies, such as acid maltase deficiency, are not classified

as dystrophies. The abnormal gene and its product are known for most dystrophies.

Bethlem Myopathy

Bethlem myopathy is a slowly progressive limb-girdle muscular dystrophy transmitted by autosomal dominant inheritance. The abnormal gene has been linked to the collagen type VI gene located on chromosome 21 (Jöbsis et al, 1999).

CLINICAL FEATURES. The onset of contractures or weakness is always in the first 2 years. Diminished fetal movements and congenital hypotonia may be present. The usual initial features are congenital flexion contractures of the elbows, ankles, and interphalangeal joints of the last four fingers, but the spine is spared. The contractures are at first mild and unrecognized by parents. Mild proximal weakness and delayed motor development are common. Both the contractures and the weakness progress slowly and produce disability in middle life but do not shorten the life span. Tendon reflexes are normal or depressed. Cardiomyopathy does not occur.

DIAGNOSIS. The serum concentration of CK is normal or slightly elevated, EMG usually shows myopathy, and muscle biopsy shows a nonspecific myopathy.

MANAGEMENT. Physical therapy for contractures is the main treatment.

Duchenne and Becker Muscular Dystrophies

Duchenne muscular dystrophy (DMD) and Becker muscular dystrophy (BMD) are variable phenotypic expressions of a gene defect at the Xp21 site. Several different phenotypes are associated with abnormalities at the Xp21 site (Table 7-5). The abnormal gene product in both DMD and BMD is a reduced muscle content of the structural protein dystrophin. In DMD the

---

Table 7-5
Phenotypes Associated with the Xp21 Gene Site

Becker muscular dystrophy
Dilated cardiomyopathy without skeletal muscle weakness
Duchenne muscular dystrophy
Familial X-linked myalgia and cramps (see Chapter 8)
McLeod syndrome (elevated serum creatine kinase concentration, acanthocytosis, and absence of Kell antigen)
Mental retardation and elevated serum creatine kinase
Quadriceps myopathy

dystrophin content is less than 3% of normal, and in BMD the dystrophin content is 3% to 20% of normal. DMD has a worldwide distribution, with a mean incidence of 1 per 3,500 male births. The traditional phenotypic difference between the two dystrophies is that BMD has a later age of onset (after age 5), unassisted ambulation after age 15, and survival into adult life. However, a spectrum of intermediate phenotypes exists.

Quadriceps myopathy is characterized by slowly progressive weakness of the quadriceps muscle, calf enlargement, and an elevated serum concentration of CK. Another syndrome of dystrophin deficiency consists of mental retardation and an elevated concentration of serum CK without muscle weakness (North et al, 1996).

CLINICAL FEATURES. The initial feature in most boys with DMD is a gait disturbance; onset is always before age 5 and is often before age 3. Toe walking and frequent falling are typical complaints. A history of delayed achievement of motor milestones is often recalled in retrospect. Early symptoms are insidious and likely to be dismissed by both parents and physicians. Children may not be brought to medical attention until proximal weakness is sufficiently severe to cause difficulty in rising from the floor and an obvious waddling gait. At this stage, mild proximal weakness is present in the pelvic muscles and the Gower sign is present. The calf muscles are often large (Figure 7-3). The ankle tendon is shortened, and the heels do not quite touch the floor. Tendon reflexes may still be present at the ankle and knee but are difficult to obtain.

The decline in motor strength is linear throughout childhood. Motor function usually appears static between the ages of 3 and 6 years because of cerebral maturation. Most children maintain their ability to walk and climb stairs until 8 years of age. Between ages 3 and 8, the child shows progressive contractures of the ankle tendons and the iliotibial bands, increased lordosis, a more pronounced waddling gait, and increased toe walking. Gait is more precarious, and the child falls more often. Tendon reflexes at the knees and ankles are lost, and proximal weakness develops in the arms.

The range of intelligence scores in boys with DMD is shifted downward. While most of these boys function in the normal range, the percentage of those with learning disabilities and mental retardation is increased.

Considerable variability of expression occurs even within the DMD phenotype. On average, functional ability declines rapidly after 8 years of age because of increasing muscle weakness and contractures. By 9 years of age, some children require a wheelchair, but most can remain ambulatory until age 12 and may continue to stand in braces until age 16.

Scoliosis occurs in some boys and is not caused by early use of a wheelchair. Deterioration of vital capacity to less than 20% of normal leads to symptoms of nocturnal hypoventilation. The child awakens frequently and is afraid to sleep.

The immediate cause of death is usually a combination respiratory insufficiency and cardiomyopathy. In some patients with chronic hypoxia, intercurrent infection or aspiration causes respiratory arrest.

DIAGNOSIS. Before 5 years of age the serum concentration of CK is 10 times the upper limit of

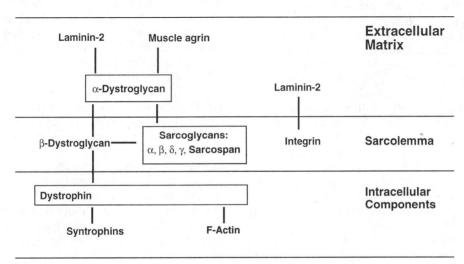

Figure 7-3. The structural proteins of muscle fibers.

normal. The concentration then declines with age at an approximate rate of 20% per year.

Mutation analysis is the standard for diagnosis, carrier detection, and fetal diagnosis. Intragenic deletions can be identified in 60% of affected boys and duplications in another 6%. Dystrophin analysis of muscle is useful to distinguish DMD from BMD.

MANAGEMENT. Although DMD is not curable, it is treatable. Prednisone, 0.75 mg/kg/day, increases strength and function. Treatment goals are to maintain function, prevent contractures, and provide psychological support not only for the child but also for the family. Every effort should be made to keep children standing and walking as long as possible. This is best accomplished by passive stretching exercises to prevent contractures, use of a lightweight plastic ankle-foot orthosis to maintain the foot in a neutral position during sleep, and use of long-leg braces when walking becomes precarious. Scoliosis cannot be prevented or reversed by external appliances; only surgery is effective to straighten the spine.

Facioscapulohumeral Syndrome

Progressive facioscapulohumeral (FSH) weakness is generally classified as a muscular dystrophy. However, patients with genetic FSH weakness may have histological evidence of myopathy, neuropathy, and inflammation. Therefore, the term *facioscapulohumeral syndrome* is used to designate this entity that, although predominantly a dystrophy, has elements of denervation.

The FSH syndrome is associated with a deletion at chromosome 4q35 (Ricci et al, 1999). The size of the deletion correlates with the severity of disease. Considerable interfamily and intrafamily heterogeneity exists. A family history may not be elicited because affected family members are unaware that they have a problem.

CLINICAL FEATURES. Weakness usually begins in the second decade. Initial involvement is often in the shoulder girdle, with subsequent spread to the humeral muscles. *The deltoid is always spared.* Facial weakness is present but often overlooked until late in the course. The progression of weakness is insidious, and diagnosis is often delayed. Late in the course, leg muscles may be involved. Anterior tibial weakness is most prominent, but proximal weakness may occur as well.

The course of FSH syndrome is variable. Many patients do not become disabled, and

their life expectancy is normal. Others are confined to a wheelchair in adult life. In the infantile form, progression is always rapid and disability is always severe (see Chapter 17).

Deafness and retinal vascular abnormalities are part of the phenotype. The most severe manifestations are retinal telangiectasia, exudation, and detachment (*Coates disease*).

DIAGNOSIS. The serum concentration of CK can be normal or increased to five times normal. The EMG may show denervation potentials, myopathic motor units, or both. Histological changes are minimal in many limb muscles and are never diagnostic. Occasional fibers are myopathic, some appear denervated, and inflammatory cells may be present. Definitive diagnosis is now accomplished by gene deletion studies.

MANAGEMENT. No treatment for the weakness is available. The retina should be carefully examined for Coates disease. Retinal telangiectasia can be treated by coagulation to prevent blindness.

Limb-Girdle Muscular Dystrophies

The term *limb-girdle muscular dystrophies* (LGMD) is used to describe progressive proximal muscle weakness. LGMD transmitted by X-linked inheritance are discussed in the section on DMD and BMD. Four forms of LGMD are transmitted by autosomal dominant inheritance. One with onset in adult life is not discussed here, the second is Bethlem myopathy, the third is associated with a severe cardiac conduction disturbances (van der Kooi et al, 1996), and the fourth is an inclusion body myopathy (discussed later in this chapter). Autosomal recessive types may begin in childhood or adult life and are distinguished by the location of the abnormal gene and in some cases by the abnormal gene product (Table 7-6). Many are caused by deficiencies in the dystrophin-associated glycoprotein complex called the *sarcoglycan* (Duggan et al, 1997). Some of the phenotypes are similar to DMD and explain most cases of affected females with a DMD phenotype (see the later section on Severe Childhood Autosomal Recessive Muscular Dystrophy).

CLINICAL FEATURES. Patients with slowly progressive symmetric proximal weakness, with or without facial involvement, and diminished or absent tendon reflexes should be considered to have LGMD if other specific entities can be excluded. Either the pelvic or the shoulder girdle muscles can be affected first.

Table 7-6
Autosomal Recessive Limb-Girdle Muscular Dystrophies

LGMD	Location	Gene Product	Clinical Features
LGMD-2A	15q	Calpain 3	Onset at 8–15 years, progression variable
LGMD-2B	2p13-16	Dysferlin	Onset at adolescence, mild weakness; gene site is the same as for Miyoshi myopathy
LGMD-2C	13q12	Sarcoglycan	Duchenne-like, severe childhood autosomal recessive muscular dystrophy (SCARMD1)
LGMD-2D	17q21	α Sarcoglycan (adhalin)	Duchenne-like, severe childhood autosomal recessive muscular dystrophy (SCARMD2)
LGMD-2E	4q12	β Sarcoglycan	Phenotype between Duchenne and Becker muscular dystrophies
LGMD-2F	5q33-34	Sarcoglycan	Slowly progressive, growth retardation

DIAGNOSIS. The most common problem in differential diagnosis is to distinguish LGMD from BMD; indeed, many males in whom LGMD is diagnosed will prove to have BMD when dystrophin is measured. The distinction between these dystrophies is important for accurate genetic counseling. In addition to DMD and BMD, conditions to be considered in the differential diagnosis include juvenile spinal muscular atrophy, glycogen storage myopathies, endocrine myopathies, and polymyositis.

The serum concentration of CK is elevated, and the EMG findings are consistent with a myopathy. Muscle histological findings vary with the stage of disease. The earliest changes are variation in fiber size and an increase in internal nuclei. Later, fiber splitting and an uneven distribution of mitochondria produce a moth-eaten appearance when histochemical reagents for oxidative enzymes are applied. Both fiber types are affected equally.

MANAGEMENT. The treatment goals in LGMD are the same as those for DMD. The only difference is that contractures are not as serious a problem.

Severe Childhood Autosomal Recessive Muscular Dystrophy

Severe childhood autosomal recessive muscular dystrophy (SCARMD) can be caused by deficiency of any of the subunits of the sarcoglycan complex of proteins associated with dystrophin (see Table 7-6). Sarcoglycan complex defects account for 11% of children with Duchenne phenotypes.

CLINICAL FEATURES. Both sexes are affected equally. The clinical features are identical to those described for the dystrophinopathies.

DIAGNOSIS. SCARMD should be suspected in all girls with a Duchenne phenotype and in boys who appear to have DMD but show normal dystrophin content in muscle. Immunohistochemical reagents can be applied to muscle sections to show the absence or presence of the sarcoglycan components. Mutation analysis is becoming available for diagnosis.

MANAGEMENT. Management is the same as for DMD.

Inflammatory Myopathies

The inflammatory myopathies are a heterogeneous group of disorders whose causes are infectious, immune-mediated, or both. A progressive proximal myopathy occurs in adults, but not in children, with acquired immune deficiency syndrome (AIDS). However, the concentration of serum CK is elevated in children with AIDS treated with zidovudine. Acute infectious myositis is described in the section on acute generalized weakness. The conditions discussed in this section are considered idiopathic.

Dermatomyositis

Dermatomyositis is a systemic angiopathy in which vascular occlusion and infarction account for all pathological changes observed in muscle, connective tissue, skin, gastrointestinal tract, and small nerves. More than 30% of adults with dermatomyositis have an underlying malignancy, but cancer is not a factor before the age of 16. The childhood form of dermatomyositis is a relatively homogeneous disease.

CLINICAL FEATURES. Peak incidence is generally between the ages of 5 and 10 years, but an onset as early as 4 months has been reported. The initial features may be insidious or fulminating. An insidious onset is characterized by fever, fatigue, and anorexia in the absence of rash or weakness. These symptoms may persist for weeks or months and suggest an underlying infection. Dermatitis precedes myositis in most children. The characteristic rash is marked by an erythematous discoloration and edema of the upper eyelids that spread to involve the entire periorbital and malar regions. Erythema and edema of the extensor surfaces overlying the joints of the knuckles, elbows, and knees develop later. With time the skin appears atrophic and scaly.

The myopathy is characterized by proximal weakness, stiffness, and pain. Weakness becomes generalized, and flexion contractures develop rapidly and cause joint deformities. Tendon reflexes become increasingly difficult to obtain and finally disappear.

Calcinosis of subcutaneous tissue, especially under discolored areas of skin, occurs in 60% of children. When severe, it produces an armor-like appearance, termed *calcinosis universalis,* on radiographs. In some children stiffness is the main initial feature, and skin and muscle symptoms are only minor.

In the past, gastrointestinal tract infarction was a leading cause of death. The mortality rate has fallen to less than 5% with modern treatment.

DIAGNOSIS. The combination of fever, rash, myalgia, and weakness is compelling evidence for the diagnosis of dermatomyositis. The serum concentration of CK is usually elevated early in the course. During the time of active myositis, the resting EMG shows increased insertional activity, fibrillations, and positive sharp waves; muscle contraction produces brief, small-amplitude polyphasic potentials. The diagnostic feature on muscle biopsy is perifascicular atrophy (Figure 7-4). Capillary necrosis usually starts at the periphery of the muscle fascicle and causes ischemia in the adjacent muscle fibers. The most profound atrophy occurs in fascicular borders that face large connective tissue septae. Type I and type II fibers are affected equally.

MANAGEMENT. The inflammatory process is thought to be active for approximately 2 years. Corticosteroids may suppress the inflammatory response and provide symptomatic relief but do not cure the underlying disease. The best results are obtained when corticosteroids are started early in high doses and are maintained for long periods of time.

Prednisone is initiated at 2 mg/kg/day, not to exceed 100 mg/day. The response follows a predictable pattern. Temperature returns to normal within 48 hours. The serum CK concentration returns to normal by the second week,

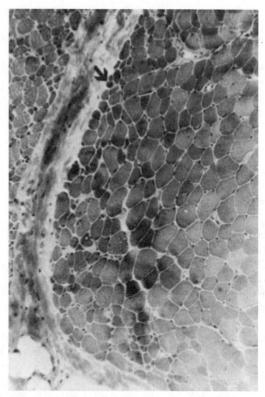

Figure 7-4. Perifascicular atrophy in childhood dermatomyositis (trichrome stain). The muscle fibers at the edge of each fascicle are atrophied (*arrow*).

and muscle strength increases simultaneously. When these events occur, prednisone should be given on alternate days in the same dosage to reduce the frequency and severity of corticosteroid-induced side effects. Alternate-day or every-day therapy is equally effective if the doses are large and the treatment is maintained. As muscle strength increases, the original dosage of alternate-day prednisone is tapered by 10% per month for 5 months. Further reductions are then made at a rate of 5% per month. For most children the alternate-day maintenance dosage needed for normal muscle strength and a normal serum CK concentration is 25% of the starting dosage. The response of the skin rash to prednisone is variable; in some children the rash heals completely, but most will have some permanent scarring from the disease.

Although most children show a dramatic improvement and seem normal within 3 months, prednisone must be continued for a full 2 years. If treatment is discontinued prematurely, relapse is invariable. Calcinosis and contractures are more likely to develop in children treated intermittently. Corticosteroids also are useful in the treatment of calcinosis universalis. In addition to prednisone, a well-structured program of physical therapy is needed to prevent contractures.

Eighty percent of children with dermatomyositis have a favorable outcome if high-dose prednisone is started within 4 months of the onset of symptoms. Children who do not respond immediately to high-dose prednisone should be started on oral methotrexate, 10 to 20 mg/m^2, given twice weekly. Regular monitoring of liver function and the white blood cell count is required.

Plasmapheresis or courses of intravenous immunoglobulin may be used in children whose condition is refractory to corticosteroids or to reduce the dosage when adverse side effects limit therapy (Sansome and Dubowitz, 1995).

Once the disease becomes inactive, reactivation is unlikely. However, late progression or recurrence may occur and should be treated with an additional 1-year course of corticosteroids.

Polymyositis

Polymyositis without evidence of other target organ involvement is uncommon before puberty. Children with systemic lupus erythematosus may have myalgia and arthralgia as early symptoms, but generally they do not have muscle weakness at onset. Skin, joint, and systemic manifestations are usually well established before the onset of myopathy. Polymyositis in children is similar to the disorder in adult life except that malignancy is not usually a causative factor.

CLINICAL FEATURES. Polymyositis begins as a symmetric proximal weakness that develops insidiously and progresses to a moderate handicap within weeks to months. The patient may have prolonged periods of stability or even remission that suggest the diagnosis of LGMD because of the slow progress. Tendon reflexes are present early in the course but become hypoactive as muscle bulk is lost. Cardiorespiratory complications are less common in childhood than in adult polymyositis.

DIAGNOSIS. The serum CK concentration is not always increased, but EMG almost always shows both myopathic and neuropathic features. Muscle biopsy may show several different patterns of abnormality, and perivascular inflammation may not be present. Instead, features of myopathy, denervation, or both are observed.

MANAGEMENT. The same treatment schedule suggested for childhood dermatomyositis should be used for children with polymyositis.

Unfortunately, the response to corticosteroids is far less predictable in polymyositis than in dermatomyositis. Children who do not respond to corticosteroids should be treated with methotrexate. Plasmapheresis and intravenous immunoglobulins are reasonable alternatives when other remedies fail.

Metabolic Myopathies

Acid Maltase Deficiency

The initial features of acid maltase deficiency may occur in infancy, childhood, or adult life. The enzyme defect is the same regardless of the age of onset, and different ages of onset may occur within the same family. Why the age at onset varies so widely is unknown. The speed of progression is variable, but the severity of cardiorespiratory involvement correlates with the amount of residual enzyme activity. The abnormal gene is on chromosome 17 and is transmitted by autosomal recessive inheritance.

CLINICAL FEATURES. Infants with acid maltase deficiency have glycogen storage in both skeletal and cardiac muscles. Death occurs from cardiac failure during infancy (see Chapter 6).

In the childhood form, only skeletal muscle is involved and the main clinical feature is slowly progressive proximal limb weakness. Tendon reflexes are hypoactive or unobtainable. Some children have mild hypertrophy of the calves simulating DMD. The weakness is steadily progressive and leads to disability and respiratory insufficiency by 20 years of age. A late age at onset predicts a more benign course.

DIAGNOSIS. The diagnosis of acid maltase deficiency is established by showing glycogen storage in muscle fibers and the absence of acid maltase in muscle or fibroblasts.

MANAGEMENT. Treatment is not available.

Other Carbohydrate Myopathies

Slowly progressive proximal weakness is sometimes the initial features of McArdle disease and debrancher enzyme deficiency. Both disorders must at least be considered in the differential diagnosis. The initial symptom of these disorders is usually exercise intolerance, and for this reason they are discussed in Chapter 8.

Muscle Carnitine Deficiency

Carnitine is an essential cofactor in the transfer of long-chain fatty acids across the inner mitochondrial membrane and modulates the ratio of acyl to acylcoenzyme A. Its deficiency causes a failure in the production of energy for metabolism and the storage of triglycerides. It occurs (1) in newborns receiving total parenteral alimentation, (2) in several systemic disorders, (3) as the result of several genetic disorders of organic acid metabolism, (4) in children treated with valproate, (5) and as a primary genetic defect that causes deficiency of the cellular carnitine transporter.

The primary genetic defect, on chromosome 5, is transmitted by autosomal recessive inheritance (Shoji et al, 1998). The clinical features may be restricted to skeletal muscle or may include systemic symptoms resembling those of Reye syndrome (see Chapter 2).

CLINICAL FEATURES. The main clinical feature of muscle carnitine deficiency is the childhood onset of slowly progressive proximal weakness, affecting the legs before and more severely than the arms. Sudden exacerbations or a fluctuating course are superimposed. Occasionally patients have recurrent attacks of myoglobinuria and cardiomyopathy. The cardiomyopathy is usually asymptomatic but is recognized on electrocardiography (ECG) and echocardiography.

DIAGNOSIS. The serum concentration of CK is elevated. EMG findings are nonspecific. Muscle biopsy specimens show a vacuolar myopathy with lipid storage mainly in type I fibers. The biochemical measurement of carnitine, both free and total, is needed to establish the diagnosis.

MANAGEMENT. Dietary therapy with L-carnitine is usually effective. Diarrhea is the major side effect. The usual dosage is 100 mg/kg/day in three or four divided doses.

Other Lipid Myopathies

Children with progressive proximal weakness associated with lipid storage in muscle and normal carnitine content usually have a disturbance of mitochondrial fatty acid oxidation. These disorders are genetically heterogeneous and difficult to distinguish from other mitochondrial myopathies.

CLINICAL FEATURES. Progressive proximal weakness begins anytime from early childhood to adolescence. The legs are affected first and then the arms. Exercise intolerance is noted, and in some cases the ingestion of fatty foods leads to nausea and vomiting. The pattern and progression of weakness may simulate those of DMD even to the presence of calf hypertrophy.

Limb weakness is steadily progressive, and cardiomyopathy may develop.

DIAGNOSIS. The serum concentration of CK is markedly elevated. EMG findings are abnormal and are consistent with a myopathic process. Muscle biopsy is critical to diagnosis. Type I muscle fibers contain fatty droplets. Carnitine and carnitine palmitoyl transferase levels are normal.

MANAGEMENT. Patients with fat intolerance may show improvement on a diet free of long-chain fatty acids.

Endocrine Myopathies

Progressive proximal limb weakness may occur in children with hyperthyroidism, hypothyroidism, hyperparathyroidism, hypoparathyroidism, hyperadrenalism, and hypoadrenalism.

CLINICAL FEATURES. Systemic features of endocrine disease usually predate the onset of weakness. However, weakness may be the initial feature in primary or secondary hypoparathyroidism and in thyroid disorders. Weakness is much more prominent in the legs than in the arms. Tendon reflexes, even in weak muscles, are normal or diminished but generally are not absent.

DIAGNOSIS. The serum concentration of CK is typically normal. EMG is not useful for diagnosis. Many endocrinopathies produce both neuropathy and myopathy. In Cushing disease and in hyperparathyroidism, muscle histological studies show type II fiber atrophy. Other endocrinopathies show nonspecific myopathic changes that vary with the severity of disease.

MANAGEMENT. Treating the underlying endocrinopathy corrects the weakness.

Progressive Distal Weakness

Neuropathy is the most common cause of progressive distal weakness (Table 7-7). Among the slowly progressive neuropathies of childhood, hereditary disorders are far more common than acquired disorders. The only common acquired neuropathy is acute inflammatory demyelinating polyradiculoneuropathy (Guillain-Barré syndrome), in which weakness evolves rapidly.

Diagnosis in Neuropathy and Neuronopathy

The initial feature of neuropathy in children is progressive symmetric distal weakness affecting

Table 7-7
Progressive Distal Weakness
[Gene Location]

Spinal Cord Disorders (see Chapter 12)

Motor Neuron Diseases
Juvenile amyotrophic lateral sclerosis [2q33, 9q34, 15q12]
Spinal muscular atrophies
    Autosomal dominant forms [7p]
    Autosomal recessive forms
    Nonfamilial Asian (see Chapter 13)

Neuropathies
Hereditary motor sensory neuropathies
    Charcot-Marie-Tooth disease (see Table 7-9)
    Familial amyloid neuropathy (see Chapter 9)
    Giant axonal neuropathy [16q24]
    Other genetic neuropathies
    Other lipid neuropathies
    Pyruvate dehydrogenase deficiency (see Chapter 10)
    Refsum disease
    Sulfatide lipidoses: metachromatic leukodystrophy
Neuropathies with systemic diseases
    Drug-induced
    Systemic vasculitis
    Toxins
    Uremia
Idiopathic neuropathy
    Chronic axonal neuropathy
    Chronic demyelinating neuropathy

Myopathies
Autosomal dominant childhood myopathy [17p11]
Autosomal dominant infantile myopathy
Autosomal recessive distal (Miyoshi) myopathy [2p12-14]
Inclusion body myopathies
Myotonic dystrophy [19q13]

Scapulo (humeral) Peroneal Syndrome
Emery-Dreifuss muscular dystrophy type 1 [Xq28]
Emery-Dreifuss muscular dystrophy type 2 [1q21.2-q21.3]
Scapuloperoneal myopathy [12q13.3-q15]
Scapuloperoneal neuronopathy [12q24.1-q24.31]

the legs and then the arms. When sensation is disturbed, dysesthesias consisting of tingling, "pins and needles," or a burning sensation in the feet are felt. Dysesthesias usually occur in acquired but not in hereditary neuropathies. The progression of weakness and sensory loss are in a distal to proximal direction (glove and stocking distribution). Tendon reflexes are lost early, especially when sensory fibers are affected.

An important first step in diagnosis is to determine the primary site of the disorder: cell body (anterior horn cell), nerve axon, or myelin. This is accomplished by electrodiagnosis (Table 7-8). In primary disorders of the cell body (neuronopathy), fibrillations and fasciculations are seen in resting muscle. With voluntary contraction the number of motor unit potentials is reduced but the amplitude is normal or increased

because of collateral reinnervation. Motor conduction nerve velocity is normal or only slightly diminished, and the amplitude of sensory action potentials is normal. In axonopathies the EMG shows fibrillations at rest and a reduced number of motor unit potentials that are normal or increased in amplitude. High-amplitude potentials may be polyphasic. Motor nerve conduction velocity is normal or mildly reduced, and the amplitude of sensory action potentials may also be reduced. Demyelinating neuropathies are characterized by marked slowing of motor conduction velocity and reduced amplitude of sensory evoked potentials. EMG findings may be normal early in the course.

Juvenile Amyotrophic Lateral Sclerosis

Autosomal recessive forms map to chromosomes 2q33 and 15q12. The autosomal dominant form maps to chromosome 9q34 (Rabin et al, 1999).

CLINICAL FEATURES. Age at onset is after 12 years, and progression is slow. The clinical features are some combination of spastic paraplegia and wasting of the hands or peroneal atrophy. Bulbar and pseudobulbar palsy are present in the recessive forms but not in the dominant form.

DIAGNOSIS. Diagnosis depends on the family history and the clinical features.

MANAGEMENT. Only supportive therapy is available.

Spinal Muscular Atrophy

The distal form of SMA is genetically heterogeneous. Sometimes the disease is segmental (*juvenile progressive segmental SMA*) and affects only the hands or the feet. The trait may be transmitted by autosomal dominant or recessive inheritance. The dominant form maps to chromosome 7p (Ellsworth et al, 1999) and may be allelic to the axonal form of Charcot-Marie-Tooth disease.

CLINICAL FEATURES. These disorders usually begin with weakness and wasting in the anterior compartment of the legs associated with pes cavus deformities of the feet. Tendon reflexes may be preserved. In some families with dominantly inherited disease, the weakness begins in the plantar flexors, causing inability to stand on the toes. In other families, weakness and wasting are more prominent in the hands, especially the thenar muscles and first dorsal interossei.

Table 7-8
Electrodiagnosis in Neuropathy

	Neuronopathy	Axonal	Demyelinating
Fasciculations	+++	+++	+
Denervation potentials	+++	+++	+
Reduced number of motor units	+++	+++	0
High-amplitude potentials	+++	+++	0
Slow motor velocity	0	+	+++
Reduced sensory potentials	0	+	+++

0, absent; +, rare; +++, common.

In the severe autosomal recessive form, weakness progresses to involve the proximal muscles of the legs and sometimes the hands. Weakness in the arms varies among families but shows concordance within an individual family. Approximately 25% of patients have scoliosis. Calf atrophy or hypertrophy may be present, even among members of the same family.

Juvenile segmental SMA is primarily a disorder of teenage males, probably transmitted by autosomal recessive inheritance. Atrophy of the hands, often asymmetric, progresses for 2 to 4 years and sometimes involves the forearms. Fasciculations and cramps are common. The atrophy usually arrests, but may progress to involve the legs and can be associated with hyperreflexia. Progressive atrophy with hyperreflexia in the legs suggests a link between juvenile segmental SMA and familial amyotrophic lateral sclerosis.

DIAGNOSIS. Electrodiagnosis is critical to distinguish these disorders from peripheral neuropathies. Motor nerve conduction velocity is normal despite total denervation of the small muscles of the foot. Sensory evoked potentials are also normal. The serum concentration of CK is usually normal but may be mildly elevated. Muscle biopsy specimens show nonspecific changes of denervation, and the sural nerve is normal.

MANAGEMENT. Hand and foot braces may help to prolong function.

Charcot-Marie-Tooth Disease

The terms *Charcot-Marie-Tooth* (CMT) *disease* and *hereditary motor and sensory neuropathy* (HMSN) are interchangeable (Byrd, 1999). Each encompasses several genetic neuropathies that are further subdivided on the basis of mo-

lecular and linkage findings (Table 7-9). The typical patient has progressive distal weakness, mild to moderate sensory loss, depressed or tendon reflexes, and high-arched feet.

Charcot-Marie-Tooth 1 (CMT1): Demyelinating Type

CMT1 (HMSN-I) is an autosomal dominant form of demyelinating neuropathy. It consists of cases with DNA duplications on chromosome 17p (CMT1A) and cases in which the abnormal gene is mapped to chromosome 1q (CMT1B). The 17p11 duplication accounts for more than 95% of cases and causes trisomic expression of the peripheral myelin protein, PMP-22 (Birouk et al, 1997). Deletion in the 17p11 region with monosomic expression of PMP-22 causes *hereditary polyneuropathy with liability to pressure palsies* (see Chapter 13).

CLINICAL FEATURES. The subtypes are clinically indistinguishable and are designated solely on the basis of molecular findings. CMT1B tends to be more disabling than CMT1A and has proximal as well as distal weakness. CMT1C is identical to CMT1A.

CMT1 is not usually a severe disorder in childhood. The main early features are pes cavus, weakness of the peroneal muscles, and diminished reactivity of the ankle tendon reflex. With time the anterior tibial as well as the peroneal muscles become weak, producing foot drop. The calf muscles become weak in some families but may hypertrophy in some families with the 17p duplication. Eventually, usually after 20 years of age, weakness spreads to the proximal muscles of the legs and hands. Scoliosis is unusual. Cramps with exercise are present in weak muscles. Position sense becomes im-

Table 7-9
Charcot-Marie-Tooth Disease

Disease	Inheritance	Gene	Locus	Gene Product
CMT1A	AD	PMP-22	17p11	Peripheral myelin protein
CMT1B	AD	MPZ	1q22-q23	Glycoprotein P0
CMT1C	AD	?	?	?
CMT2A	AD	?	1p36-p35	?
CMT2B	AD	?	3q13-q22	?
CMT2C	AD	?	?	?
CMT2D	AD	?	7p14	?
CMT4A	AR	?	8q13-q21	?
CMT4B	AR	?	11q23	?
CMT4C	AR	?	5q23-33	?
CMT4D	AR	?	8q24	?
CMT4E	AR	EGR2	10q21	?
CMTX	XLD	GJB1	Xq13-21	Connexin 32

EGR2, early growth response 2 gene; GJB1, gap junction beta-1 protein; MPZ, myelin protein zero; PMP-22, peripheral myelin protein-22.

paired in the fingers and toes. Dysesthesias are never a problem.

Peripheral nerves are enlarged in adults but not in children. The enlargement is caused by repeated episodes of demyelination and remyelination.

DIAGNOSIS. Diagnosis relies on characteristic clinical findings and a family history of the disease. Motor nerve conduction velocities are less than 50% of normal in affected individuals. The cerebrospinal fluid protein content is usually normal in children but may be elevated in adults. A DNA-based test is available for CMT1A that detects more than 95% of cases. Persons with CMT1A have three copies of the PMP-22 gene.

MANAGEMENT. No specific treatment is available, but proper foot care may minimize discomfort and maximize function. Shoes should be roomy and soft to prevent rubbing against bony prominences. Footwear that is molded to the shape of the foot is especially useful. When foot drop is present, a lightweight plastic ankle-foot orthosis that fits into the patient's own shoe not only lifts the foot but also prevents turning and injury of the ankle.

Charcot-Marie-Tooth 2 (CMT2): Neuronal Type

CMT2 is transmitted by autosomal dominant inheritance and clinically resembles CMT1, except that the nerve conduction velocity is either normal or mildly abnormal. Four subtypes are recognized (Table 7-9).

CLINICAL FEATURES. The peak period at onset of CMT2A and CMT2B is during the second decade. Distal weakness begins in the legs and can be asymmetric. The hands are affected later. Tendon reflexes are absent at the ankle in CMT2A but are preserved in CMT2B (Elliot et al, 1997). Tendon reflexes may be preserved at the knee and elbow in both forms. Most children with CMT2A have mild distal sensory loss. Sensory loss is more prominent in CMT2B. Progression of symptoms is slow, and disability does not occur until middle adult life.

CMT2C is different from the other types because of prominent vocal cord and respiratory (intercostal and diaphragmatic) muscle paralysis. The onset is insidious and difficult to date precisely. The initial symptom may be hoarseness or frequent tripping, but neonatal respiratory disturbance also occurs. The course is one of progressive peroneal atrophy with minimal sensory deficit. CMT2D includes prominent weakness and atrophy of the hands.

DIAGNOSIS. The cerebrospinal fluid protein content is normal, as is the serum concentration of CK. Because the pathological process is primarily axonal rather than demyelinating, motor nerve conduction velocities are either normal or only mildly slowed (60% or more of normal). The EMG shows a denervation pattern in affected muscles. DNA-based testing is not available.

MANAGEMENT. Management is the same as for CMT1.

Charcot-Marie-Tooth 3 (CMT3): Dejerine-Sottas Syndrome

CMT3 (HMSN III) was originally described as a severe demyelinating neuropathy of infancy and childhood associated with very slow nerve conduction velocity, elevated cerebrospinal fluid protein, marked clinical weakness, and hypertrophic nerves with onion bulb formation. Patients with CMT3 are now known to be heterozygous for point mutations in either the PMP-22 gene, which causes CMT1A; or the Po myelin gene, which causes CMT1B or various types of CMT4; or the EGR2 gene, which causes CMT4E. Therefore, CMT3 is now reclassified as CMT1A, CMT1B, or CMT4.

Charcot-Marie-Tooth 4 (CMT4)

CMT4 comprises several different disorders that are characterized by progressive motor and sensory neuropathy and autosomal recessive inheritance. None of the genes for the CMT4 subtypes has been identified. The subcategories are based on clinical characteristics, ethnic background, and genetic linkage assignments.

CLINICAL FEATURES. Affected people have the typical CMT phenotype. CMT4A occurs in Tunisia. Distal muscle weakness develops in the second year, and proximal muscles are involved by age 10. Associated findings include mild sensory loss, absent tendon reflexes, skeletal deformities, and scoliosis.

CMT4B occurs in Italian families and causes progressive distal and proximal weakness of the legs between 2 and 3 years. Pes cavus is common, and facial weakness may develop. Most persons are wheelchair bound by age 20 and dead by the fourth or fifth decade.

CMT4C occurs in North Africa and Western Europe, especially among Arab populations. Affected individuals have a motor and sensory neuropathy in the legs, often associated with pes cavus foot deformity and a progressive scoliosis.

CMT4D occurs in Bulgarian gypsies and has the distinguishing characteristic of sensory neural deafness, with onset in the third decade.

CMT4E is associated with mutations in the EGR2 gene. One recessive and two dominant mutations have been reported. The clinical picture is either that of a congenital hypomyelinating neuropathy (see Chapter 6) or a CMT1 phenotype (Warner et al, 1999).

DIAGNOSIS. All members of the CMT4 group are demyelinating neuropathies with normal protein concentrations in the spinal fluid. Nerve conduction velocities are slow (15–17 m/sec). No specific clinical or genetic test is available.

MANAGEMENT. The treatment plan is similar to that for other CMTs.

Charcot-Marie-Tooth X (CMTX)

CMTX is inherited in an X-linked dominant pattern and is associated with mutations in the connexin 32 genes.

CLINICAL FEATURES. Affected males have a moderate to severe peripheral neuropathy that tends to be more severe than that seen in CMT1A. Females have a mild neuropathy or are asymptomatic. Symptoms develop in males during the first decade. The initial physical findings are depressed or absent tendon reflexes and foot drop. Mild to moderate sensory loss in the feet and hearing loss may be associated.

DIAGNOSIS. CMTX is detected by a DNA-based test of the connexin 32 gene. The test detects 100% of cases and is commercially available.

MANAGEMENT. The treatment plan is similar to that for other CMTs.

Other Genetic Neuropathies

Giant Axonal Neuropathy

Giant axonal neuropathy is a rare disorder transmitted by autosomal recessive inheritance. The gene maps to chromosome 16q24. The underlying defect is one of generalized intermediate filament organization, with neurofilaments predominantly affected. Central and peripheral axons are both affected.

CLINICAL FEATURES. Males and females are affected equally, and many are from consanguineous marriages. Affected children are pale and thin and have a chronic polyneuropathy accompanied by kinky pale hair. Gait impairment usually begins by 3 years of age but can appear later. Symmetric distal atrophy of leg muscles is a constant early feature. Vibratory and proprioceptive sensations in the legs are profoundly impaired, and tendon reflexes are decreased or absent. Central involvement may result in cerebellar dysfunction, dementia, optic atrophy, and cranial neuropathies.

DIAGNOSIS. Sural nerve biopsy shows enlarged axons filled with disrupted neurofilaments that are surrounded by a thin or fragmented myelin sheath. Large myelinated nerve fibers are mainly affected. Magnetic resonance imaging (MRI) of the brain may show increased signal intensity of the white matter.

MANAGEMENT. No specific treatment is available.

Refsum Disease

Refsum disease is an inborn error of phytanic acid metabolism caused by mutations in the gene encoding phytanoyl-CoA hydroxylase (Mihalik et al, 1997). The gene locus is chromosome 10pter–p11.2. The disease is inherited as an autosomal recessive trait.

CLINICAL FEATURES. The initial symptoms are insidious and difficult to date. Age at onset varies from the first to the third decade. The main features are retinitis pigmentosa, chronic or recurrent polyneuropathy, and cerebellar ataxia. Retinitis pigmentosa is a constant finding and is indispensable for diagnosis. Night blindness is often the first symptom. The neuropathy is hypertrophic, symmetric, and distal, affecting both motor and sensory fibers. Vibration and position sense are more diminished than pain and temperature. Tendon reflexes become progressively hyporesponsive and are finally lost. The ataxia may be of cerebellar origin; nystagmus and intention tremor are sometimes present, but could be caused by sensory neuropathy. Other symptoms include progressive loss of hearing, cataracts, cardiomyopathy, ichthyosis, and pes cavus.

The course is variable; there may be steady progression, long periods of stability, or remissions and exacerbations. Sudden death may occur from cardiac arrhythmia caused by cardiomyopathy.

DIAGNOSIS. The serum phytanic acid concentration is markedly increased. Enzyme activity can be measured in cultured fibroblasts.

MANAGEMENT. Phytanic acid is not produced endogenously and must be derived completely from the diet. Exacerbations of disease correlate well with the blood level of phytanic acid. Treatment involves a combination of diet and plasma exchange. Treatment should be started as soon as the diagnosis is suspected and continued for life. This has proved successful in preventing progression of symptoms and in reversing symptoms already present.

Sulfatide Lipidosis: Metachromatic Leukodystrophy

Metachromatic leukodystrophy is an inherited disorder of myelin metabolism caused by deficient activity of the enzyme arylsulfatase A. The gene defect is transmitted by autosomal recessive inheritance. Infantile, juvenile, and adult forms are recognized. Only the late infantile form is discussed in this section.

CLINICAL FEATURES. After a period of normal development, gait disturbances develop, usually before 2 years of age but sometimes not until age 4. Initial features may be spasticity, ataxia, or distal weakness of the feet with loss of the ankle tendon reflex. Progressive weakness of all limbs results in generalized hypotonia and hyporeflexia. Weakness, dementia, and optic atrophy are progressive. Death occurs within several years of onset.

DIAGNOSIS. The protein content of the cerebrospinal fluid is elevated, and motor nerve conduction velocities are reduced at the time of initial leg weakness. Subcortical demyelination with a posterior predominance of white matter abnormalities is seen on MRI. The diagnosis is established by showing the absence of arylsulfatase A in white blood cells. Prenatal diagnosis is possible by analysis of arylsulfatase A in amniocytes.

MANAGEMENT. Bone marrow transplantation early in the course of disease may slow its progress.

Other Lipid Disorders

Peripheral neuropathy occurs in globoid cell leukodystrophy (Krabbe disease), but it is not as prominent a feature as in metachromatic leukodystrophy. The usual initial features are psychomotor retardation and irritability rather than flaccid weakness (see Chapter 5). Tendon reflexes may be absent or hyperactive, and motor nerve conduction velocity is reduced in half of the cases. The cerebrospinal fluid protein concentration is always elevated.

Cockayne syndrome is characterized by progeria, small stature, ataxia, retinitis pigmentosa, deafness, and mental retardation (see Chapter 16). A primary segmental demyelinating neuropathy is present in 10% to 20% of cases but is not an initial symptom. The main features are hyporeflexia and reduced motor nerve conduction velocity. Other disorders of lipid metabolism in which demyelinating neuropathy is present, but not an important feature, include Niemann-Pick disease, Gaucher disease, and Farber disease.

Neuropathies with Systemic Disease

Drug-Induced Neuropathy

Several drugs that are used widely in children, such as phenytoin, can cause neuropathy. Such neuropathies are usually subclinical, detected only by electrodiagnosis or because of loss of the ankle tendon reflex. Drugs that commonly produce clinical evidence of motor and sensory neuropathy are isoniazid, nitrofurantoin, vincristine, and zidovudine.

Isoniazid

CLINICAL FEATURES. The initial symptoms are numbness and paresthesias of the fingers and toes. If treatment is continued, superficial sensation is diminished in a glove-and-stocking pattern. Distal limb weakness follows and is associated with tenderness of the muscles and burning dysesthesias. The ankle tendon reflex is diminished or absent.

DIAGNOSIS. Isoniazid neuropathy should be suspected whenever a neuropathy develops in a child taking the drug.

MANAGEMENT. Isoniazid interferes with pyridoxine metabolism and produces neuropathy by causing a pyridoxine deficiency state. The administration of pyridoxine along with isoniazid prevents neuropathy without interfering with antituberculous activity. The longer the symptoms are allowed to progress, the longer the time until recovery. Although pyridoxine can prevent the development of neuropathy, it has little effect on the speed of recovery once neuropathy is established.

Nitrofurantoin

CLINICAL FEATURES. Nitrofurantoin neuropathy most often occurs in patients with impaired renal function. A high blood concentration of nitrofurantoin causes an axonal neuropathy. The initial features are usually paresthesias, followed within a few days or weeks by glove-and-stocking sensory loss and weakness of distal muscles. Pure motor neuropathy is occasionally present.

DIAGNOSIS. Nitrofurantoin neuropathy should be suspected in any child who has neuropathy and is taking the drug. It may be difficult to distinguish from uremic neuropathy.

MANAGEMENT. Recovery is usually complete when the drug is stopped. Occasional patients have developed complete paralysis and death despite discontinuation of nitrofurantoin.

Vincristine

CLINICAL FEATURES. Neuropathy is an expected complication of vincristine therapy. The ankle tendon reflex is lost first; later, other tendon reflexes become less reactive and may be lost. The first symptoms are paresthesias, often starting in the fingers rather than the feet and pro-gressing to mild loss of superficial sensation but not position sense. Weakness follows sensory loss and is evidenced by clumsiness in the hands and cramps in the feet. Distal muscles are affected more than proximal muscles and extensors more than flexors. Weakness may progress rapidly, with loss of ambulation in a few weeks. The initial weakness may be asymmetric and suggests mononeuropathy multiplex.

DIAGNOSIS. Electrodiagnostic features are consistent with axonal neuropathy; fibrillations and fasciculations are seen on the EMG, but motor nerve conduction velocity is normal.

MANAGEMENT. The neuropathy is dose related, and usually the patient recovers 1 to 3 months after the drug is discontinued.

Toxins

Several heavy metals, inorganic chemicals, and insecticides produce polyneuropathies in children. In adults, heavy metal poisoning is generally caused by industrial exposure, agricultural exposure, or attempted homicide. Small children who have a single accidental ingestion are more likely to have acute symptoms of systemic disease or central nervous system dysfunction than a slowly progressive neuropathy. Sometimes, progressive distal weakness is an early sign in older children addicted to sniffing glue or gasoline. Even in these cases, symptoms of central nervous system dysfunction are usually present.

Uremia

Some degree of neuropathy occurs at some time or in many children undergoing long-term periodic hemodialysis. Uremic neuropathy is more common in males than in females, but the reason for the gender bias is unknown.

CLINICAL FEATURES. The earliest symptoms may be muscle cramps in the hands and feet, burning feet or restless legs, and loss of the ankle tendon reflex. After the initial sensory symptoms, the disorder progresses to a severe distal, symmetric, mixed motor, and sensory polyneuropathy affecting the legs more than the arms. The rate of progression is variable and may be fulminating or may evolve over several months.

A pure motor neuropathy develops in some children with uremia. Symptoms begin after hemodialysis is started. The rapid progression of distal weakness in all limbs does not respond to dialysis but may be reversed by renal transplantation.

DIAGNOSIS. Uremia causes an axonal neuropathy, but chronic renal failure causes segmental demyelination that is out of proportion to axonal changes. Therefore motor nerve conduction velocity measurements are useful to monitor the severity of neuropathy. Slow conduction velocities are present even before clinical symptoms occur. Reduced creatine clearance correlates with slowing of the conduction velocity.

MANAGEMENT. Early neuropathy can be reversed by dialysis. Patients with severe neuropathy rarely recover fully despite adequate treatment.

Vasculitis and Vasculopathy

Polyneuropathy and mononeuropathy multiplex are relatively common neurological complications of vasculitis in adults but not in children. Children with lupus erythematosus are generally sicker than adults, but peripheral neuropathy is neither an initial nor a prominent feature of their disease. Motor and sensory neuropathies occur in children with chronic juvenile rheumatoid arthritis.

Idiopathic Axonal Neuropathy

CLINICAL FEATURES. Most axonal neuropathies are either hereditary or toxic. Glue sniffing is an example of a toxic cause. Some children have a progressive axonal neuropathy for which no cause can be determined. Progressive weakness of the feet, with or without sensory impairment, is often the initial feature. A hereditary basis can sometimes be established by electrodiagnostic studies in parents and siblings.

DIAGNOSIS. The EMG shows fibrillations and fasciculations, but motor nerve conduction velocity is normal or only mildly delayed. The protein content of the cerebrospinal fluid is normal.

MANAGEMENT. Children with idiopathic axonal neuropathies usually have a slowly progressive weakness that does not respond to corticosteroids. However, occasional patients do respond, and a 2-month trial of prednisone is indicated in patients with subacute progression of disease. These responsive cases may be variants of chronic inflammatory demyelinating neuropathy, in which both axonal involvement and demyelination are present.

Myopathies

Hereditary Distal Myopathies

Three clinical forms of hereditary distal myopathy are described in children. Two are dominant

traits and one is recessive. One of the dominant forms occurs in infancy and the other in childhood or later. Welander distal myopathy has an adult onset and is not discussed here. The recessive form begins during adolescence or later and is linked to chromosome 2p12-14.

Autosomal Dominant Infantile-Onset Distal Myopathy

CLINICAL FEATURES. Hereditary distal myopathy with onset in infancy begins anytime during the first 2 years. The first signs are foot drop and weakness in the hand extensor muscles. Little or no progression occurs throughout the remainder of childhood. Some children have pseudohypertrophy of the calves, scoliosis, or pes cavus.

DIAGNOSIS. The serum CK concentration is usually normal, but EMG shows brief, small-amplitude polyphasic potentials, occasional fibrillations, and myotonia. Muscle biopsy specimens show fiber-type disproportion in which type I fibers are more numerous but smaller than type II fibers.

MANAGEMENT. Braces for foot drop are needed.

Autosomal Dominant Childhood-Onset Distal Myopathy

This is the clinical phenotype that most resembles Gower's distal myopathy (Laing et al, 1995). The gene site is on chromosome 14 and may be allelic to Welander distal myopathy.

CLINICAL FEATURES. Age at onset is after 4 years and may be delayed to the third decade. The initial weakness is in the toe and ankle extensors and the neck flexors. Weakness of the finger extensors develops years later, with relative sparing of the finger flexors and intrinsic hand muscles. Some proximal limb muscles are mildly affected late in life, but walking is usually preserved.

DIAGNOSIS. EMG findings are consistent with a myopathic process. Muscle biopsy specimens show variation in fiber size, nuclear clumps, moth-eaten type I fibers, and small-angulated type II fibers. The serum concentration of CK is one to three times the upper limit of normal.

MANAGEMENT. Treatment is not usually needed.

Autosomal Recessive Distal (Miyoshi) Myopathy

This disorder is allelic to type 2B LGMD2B. Both are caused by mutation in the gene encoding the skeletal muscle protein dysferlin, and both phenotypes may occur in the same family

(Matsuda et al, 1999). The abnormal gene site is on chromosome 2p13.3-p13.1.

CLINICAL FEATURES. Onset of weakness is between 15 and 25 years of age. Weakness and atrophy in the calf muscles are the initial features, with relative sparing of the anterior compartment. The ankle jerk reflex is lost, but other tendon reflexes are normal. Slowly progressive weakness is the rule, with eventual involvement of the proximal leg muscles and then the arms. Ambulation is usually preserved (Linssen et al, 1997).

DIAGNOSIS. The peculiar pattern of calf atrophy is almost diagnostic. The serum CK concentration is at least five times the upper limit of normal; this distinguishes Miyoshi myopathy from the other distal myopathies. EMG findings are consistent with a myopathy, and muscle biopsy shows a chronic active myopathy without vacuoles.

MANAGEMENT. Most patients are not greatly impaired and do not require assistive devices.

Inclusion Body Myopathies

This group of disorders is defined by the presence of vacuolar degeneration of muscle fibers, accompanied by intrafiber clusters of paired helical filaments (Askansas and Engel, 1998). When inflammation is an associated feature, the condition is called *inclusion body myositis;* when inflammation is lacking, the condition is called *inclusion body myopathy.* In general, inclusion body myositis is a sporadic disorder with onset after age 30 years, whereas inclusion body myopathy is hereditary and may begin in childhood.

Inclusion body myopathy may be inherited as either an autosomal dominant or an autosomal recessive trait. One autosomal recessive form maps to chromosome 9.

CLINICAL FEATURES. The autosomal recessive form with linkage to chromosome 9 occurs among several ethnic groups in the Middle East and in Japan. The main feature is leg weakness, more distal than proximal, that always spares the quadriceps. Onset is after age 10 years. A second recessive form found in in French Canadians, not linked to chromosome 9, does not spare the quadriceps.

The age at onset of the autosomal dominant form is in adolescence. Painless weakness occurs first in the proximal muscles of the pelvis. The progression of weakness is slow. The biceps and triceps muscles are affected next, but the interval between leg and arm weakness may be as long

as 10 years. Facial weakness may occur. Dysphagia, fatigue, myalgia, and paresthesias may occur later in the course. Tendon reflexes are either reduced or absent. This form of inclusion body myopathy should be considered in cases of autosomal dominant LGMD.

DIAGNOSIS. The serum concentration of CK is normal or only mildly elevated. EMG shows abnormal spontaneous electrical activity: increased insertion activity and fibrillations. Short-duration motor units and polyphasic potentials are the rule, but long-duration motor units are also observed. Motor and sensory conduction velocities are normal unless a concomitant neuropathy is present.

Light microscopy characteristically shows muscle fibers with single or multiple vacuoles rimmed with basophilic material. Electron microscopy is needed to show the filamentous inclusions, usually adjacent to vacuoles.

MANAGEMENT. The weakness does not respond to corticosteroid or immunosuppressive therapy.

Myotonic Dystrophy

Myotonic dystrophy is a multisystem disorder transmitted by autosomal dominant inheritance with variable penetrance. An unstable DNA region on chromosome 19 that can amplify 50 to several thousand times causes the disease. Amplification increases in successive generations and correlates with more severe disease. A neonatal form, which occurs in children born to mothers with myotonic dystrophy, is described in Chapter 6.

CLINICAL FEATURES. The onset of symptoms is usually during adolescence or later. The major features are myotonia (a disturbance in muscle relaxation after contraction), weakness in the face and distal portion of the limbs, cataracts, frontal baldness, and multiple endocrinopathies. The pattern of muscle atrophy in the face is so stereotyped that all patients with the disease have a similar facies. The face is long and thin because of wasting of the temporal and masseter muscles, and the neck is thin because of atrophy of the sternocleidomastoid muscles. The eyelids and corners of the mouth droop and the lower part of the face sags, producing the appearance of sadness.

Although medical treatment is rarely sought before adolescence, myotonia is usually present in childhood and can be detected by EMG, if not by clinical examination. Myotonia is demonstrated by percussion of muscle, usually the thenar eminence, which dimples and remains dimpled at the site of percussion. In addition, the thumb abducts and remains in that position for several seconds. The physician can also detect myotonia by shaking hands with the patient, who has difficulty letting go and releases the grip in part by flexing the wrist to force the finger flexors to open.

Some patients have little or no evidence of muscle weakness, only cataracts, frontal baldness, or endocrine disturbances. However, when muscle weakness is present before age 20, it is likely to be relentlessly progressive, causing severe distal weakness in the hands and feet by adult life. Smooth and cardiac muscle involvement may be present and is characterized by disturbed gastrointestinal motility. Endocrine disturbances include testicular atrophy, infertility in women, hyperinsulinism, adrenal atrophy, and disturbances in growth hormone secretion.

DIAGNOSIS. The diagnosis of myotonic dystrophy is usually based on clinical features and a family history. EMG studies show myotonia (the appearance of motor unit potentials that wax and wane in amplitude and frequency), myopathic potentials, and involvement of peripheral large-diameter motor and sensory fibers. Muscle biopsy is not needed to confirm the diagnosis. Studies to show the presence and number of trinucleotide repeats are commercially available and are the best method to detect asymptomatic individuals and for prenatal diagnosis.

MANAGEMENT. Myotonia frequently responds to drugs that stabilize membranes: mexiletine is probably the most effective; procainamide, phenytoin, and carbamazepine are also useful. However, it is weakness, not myotonia, that disables the patient. Braces for foot drop are usually required as the disease progresses.

Scapulo (Humeral) Peroneal Syndromes

Progressive weakness and atrophy affecting the proximal muscles of the arms and the distal muscles of the legs may result from neuronopathy or myopathy. Some patients with dominantly inherited scapulo (humeral) peroneal syndromes are a variant phenotype of FSH syndrome, whereas others do not show linkage to the FSH locus on chromosome 4q35. One family with mainly myopathic weakness has shown linkage to chromosome 12 (Wilhelmsen et al, 1996).

Emery-Dreifuss Muscular Dystrophy Type 1 (EDMD1)

EDMD1 is transmitted by X-linked recessive inheritance. The abnormal gene product is *emerin*.

CLINICAL FEATURES. The onset of symptoms is between 5 and 15 years of age. The earliest feature of the disease is the development of contractures in the flexors of the elbows, the ankle tendon, and the extensors of the hand. This is followed by muscle weakness and wasting in the biceps and triceps muscles and then in the deltoid and other shoulder muscles. The peroneal muscles are severely affected. Calf hypertrophy does not occur. The progression of symptoms is slow, and the condition usually stabilizes by 20 years of age. In some patients, however, weakness progresses into adult life and ambulation is eventually lost.

All patients develop a cardiomyopathy that leads to permanent atrial paralysis. Bradycardia and syncope may precede muscle weakness or be delayed until the third decade. The earliest symptom is pathological fatigue on minor activity. A permanent pacemaker must be placed at the first sign of cardiac involvement. Sudden death is common.

Female heterozygotes develop a cardiomyopathy late in life and also require a pacemaker. They do no develop skeletal muscle weakness.

DIAGNOSIS. Neither EMG nor muscle biopsy is diagnostic. The diagnosis is established either by demonstrating the genetic defect or by emerin staining of skin biopsy specimens (Mora et al, 1997).

MANAGEMENT. Treatment is available for the muscle weakness, but cardiac arrhythmia should be treated early by implantation of a permanent pacemaker.

Emery-Dreifuss Muscular Dystrophy Type 2 (EDMD2)

EDMD2 is transmitted by autosomal dominant inheritance. The gene locus, on chromosome 1, contains the gene for lamin A/C (Bonne et al, 1999). The phenotype is the same as for EDMD1.

Scapuloperoneal Myopathy

This is a dominantly inherited disorder with usual onset in adult life. The phenotype is similar to that of facioscapulohumeral dystrophy except that the face is not usually involved. The abnormal gene is on chromosome 12 and therefore is different from that of FSH dystrophy.

Scapuloperoneal Neuronopathy

A dominantly inherited neuronopathic scapuloperoneal syndrome with increasing severity in successive generations has been described in a French Canadian family (Isozumi et al, 1996). This family validates the hypothesis that congenital absence of muscle groups and progressive spinal muscular atrophy is a continuum of disturbed programmed cell death.

CLINICAL FEATURES. Males are generally affected more severely than females. The phenotypic expression varies from congenital absence of muscle groups (congenital laryngeal abductor palsy, Möbius syndrome, clubfoot) to progressive neurogenic atrophy. Congenital absence of muscles may be noted at birth without progression of weakness, or scapuloperoneal weakness may develop during the first two decades. In later generations, weakness progresses to severe disability that causes loss of ambulation, hand weakness, and laryngeal paralysis requiring tracheotomy by adolescence.

DIAGNOSIS. The concentration of serum CK is normal. EMG shows denervation potentials with normal conduction velocity, and muscle biopsy findings are consistent with chronic denervation atrophy.

MANAGEMENT. Treatment is not available.

Acute Generalized Weakness

The sudden onset or rapid evolution of generalized flaccid weakness, in the absence of symptoms of encephalopathy, is always due to disorders of the motor unit. Among the disorders listed in Table 7-10, acute inflammatory demyelinating polyradiculoneuropathy (Guillain-Barré syndrome) is by far the most common.

The combination of acute weakness and rhabdomyolysis, as evidenced by myoglobinuria, indicates that muscle is degenerating rapidly. This may occur in some disorders of carbohydrate and fatty acid metabolism (see Chapter 8), after intense and unusual exercise, in some cases of infectious and idiopathic polymyositis, and in intoxication with alcohol and cocaine. Death from renal failure is a possible outcome in patients with rhabdomyolysis.

Infectious Disease

Acute Infectious Myositis

Acute myositis in children most often follows influenza or other respiratory infections (Mackay et al, 1999). Boys are affected more often than girls.

CLINICAL FEATURES. Ordinarily, prodromal respiratory symptoms persist for 3 to 8 days before

---

Table 7-10
Acute Generalized Weakness
[Gene Location]

Infectious Disorders
Acute infectious myositis
Acute inflammatory polyradiculoneuropathy
    (Guillain-Barré syndrome)
Acute axonal neuropathies
Chronic inflammatory polyradiculoneuropathy (CIDP)
Enterovirus infections

Metabolic Disorders
Acute intermittent porphyria (see Chapter 9)
Hereditary tyrosinemia (see Chapter 9)

Neuromuscular Blockade
Botulism
Corticosteroid induced quadriplegia
Tick paralysis

Intensive Care Unit Weakness

Periodic Paralysis
Andersen syndrome
Familial hypokalemic (FPPI) [1q31-32]
Familial hyperkalemic (FPPII) [17q23-25]
Familial normokalemic (FPPIII)

---

the onset of severe symmetric muscle pain and weakness, which may cause severe disability within 24 hours. Pain and tenderness are most severe in the calf muscles. Tendon reflexes are present.

DIAGNOSIS. The serum concentration of CK is elevated, usually more than 10 times the upper limit of normal.

MANAGEMENT. Spontaneous resolution of the myositis occurs almost immediately. Bed rest is required for 2 to 7 days until pain subsides, after which the patient recovers completely.

Acute Inflammatory Demyelinating Polyradiculoneuropathy (AIDP)

AIDP, more commonly called *Guillain-Barré syndrome* (GBS), is an acute monophasic demyelinating neuropathy in which abnormal immune responses are directed against peripheral nerves. More than half of patients describe an antecedent viral infection. Respiratory tract infections are more common than gastrointestinal infections (Paradiso et al, 1999). Enteritis caused by specific strains of *Campylobacter jejuni* is more often the inciting disease in the acute axonal form of GBS than in the demyelinating form.

CLINICAL FEATURES. The natural history of AIDP in children is substantially the same as in adults. The clinical features are so stereotyped that the diagnosis is usually established without laboratory confirmation. This is especially important because the characteristic laboratory features may not be present at the onset of clinical symptoms. The two essential features are progressive motor weakness involving more than one limb and areflexia. Weakness is frequently preceded by insidious sensory symptoms that are usually ignored. These consist of fleeting dysesthesias and muscle tenderness in limbs that are soon to become paralytic. Weakness progresses rapidly, and approximately 50% of patients will reach a nadir by 2 weeks, 80% by 3 weeks, and the rest by 4 weeks. The weakness may be ascending or descending but is relatively symmetric qualitatively, if not quantitatively. Tendon reflexes are absent in all weak muscles and can be absent even before the muscle is weak. Bilateral facial weakness occurs in as many as one half of cases. Autonomic dysfunction (arrhythmia, labile blood pressure, and gastrointestinal dysfunction) is commonly associated, and a syndrome of acute autonomic dysfunction without paralysis may be a variant.

Recovery of function usually begins 2 to 4 weeks after progression stops. In children recovery is almost always complete. The prognosis is best when recovery begins early. Respiratory paralysis is unusual, but if respiratory function can be supported during the critical time of profound paralysis, complete recovery is expected. **Diagnosis.** Examination of the cerebrospinal fluid was once critical in distinguishing GBS from acute poliomyelitis. In the absence of poliomyelitis, cerebrospinal fluid examination is less important. A physician first sees most children during the second week of symptoms. At that time, the concentration of protein may be normal or elevated and the number of mononuclear leukocytes per cubic millimeter may be 10 or fewer.

Electrophysiological studies are more important for diagnosis, especially to distinguish AIDP from acute axonal neuropathy. AIDP has a better prognosis than acute axonal neuropathy. **Management.** Respiratory function must be carefully monitored. Intubation is needed if vital capacity falls rapidly to less than 50% of normal. Adequate control of respiration should prevent death from the disorder. Corticosteroids are not helpful because, although they may produce some initial improvement, they tend to prolong the course. Children too weak to walk without assistance recover more quickly after plasma exchange or the use of intravenous immune globulin.

Acute Motor Axonal Neuropathy (AMAN)

The axonal form of GBS occurs more often in rural and economically deprived populations than does AIDP and often follows enteritis (Paradiso et al, 1999).

Clinical Features. The clinical features are indistinguishable from the AIDP except that sensation is not usually affected. Maximal weakness, symmetric quadriparesis, and respiratory failure usually occur in 1 week. Tendon reflexes are absent early in the course. Distal atrophy occurs. Recovery is slow, and the mean time to ambulation is 5 months.

Diagnosis. The cerebrospinal fluid cell count is normal, but the protein concentration is increased after 1 or 2 weeks. Electrophysiological studies are consistent with an axonopathy rather than a demyelinating neuropathy, and sensory nerve action potentials are normal.

Management. Respiratory support is often needed. Specific treatment is not available, but most children recover spontaneously.

Chronic Inflammatory Demyelinating Polyradiculoneuropathy

Acquired demyelinating neuropathies occur in both an acute and a chronic form. The acute form is called *Guillain-Barré syndrome* (GBS) and is described in the section that follows (Table 7-10). The chronic form is called *chronic inflammatory demyelinating polyradiculoneuropathy* (CIDP). The acute and chronic forms may be difficult to distinguish from each other at the onset of symptoms but are identified by their subsequent course.

CIDP, like GBS, is generally believed to be immune-mediated. However, although a clear relationship exists between GBS and a preceding infection, the provocative stimulus for CIDP is unknown (Simmons et al, 1997a).

Clinical Features. CIDP affects adults more often than children, but a similar syndrome may be present even at birth (see Chapter 6). The usual initial features are weakness and paresthesias in the distal portions of the limbs causing a gait disturbance. Cranial neuropathies are unusual. Mandatory criteria for diagnosis are (1) progressive or relapsing motor and sensory dysfunction of more than one limb, of a peripheral nerve nature, developing over at least 2 months, and (2) areflexia or hyporeflexia, usually affecting all four limbs. The course is monophasic in a quarter of children and has a relapsing course in the remainder (Nevo et al, 1996). Three-quarters have residual weakness.

DIAGNOSIS. Exclusionary criteria in establishing the diagnosis of CIDP are a family history of a similar disorder, a pure sensory neuropathy, other organ involvement, or abnormal storage of material in nerves. The protein content of the cerebrospinal fluid is always greater than 0.45 g/L, and a small number of mononuclear cells may be present. Motor nerve conduction velocity is less than 70% of the lower limit of normal in at least two nerves. Sural nerve biopsy shows features of demyelination. Cellular infiltration of the nerve is uncommon, and evidence of vasculitis excludes the diagnosis of CIDP.

Acquired demyelinating neuropathies in children can be differentiated from familial demyelinating neuropathies by electrodiagnosis. Acquired neuropathies show a multifocal disturbance of conduction velocity, whereas in hereditary disorders conduction is uniformly slowed throughout the length of the nerve.

MANAGEMENT. The ideal management of patients with CIDP is not established. Chronic use of prednisone, intravenous immune globulin (IVIG), or plasma exchange is effective (Simmons et al, 1997b). As a rule, long-term corticosteroid use is needed, and relapse may follow discontinuation of therapy. The outcome is more favorable in children than in adults.

Enterovirus Infections

Poliovirus, coxsackievirus, and the echovirus group are small RNA viruses that inhabit the intestinal tract of humans. They are neurotropic and produce paralytic disease by destroying the motor neurons of the brainstem and spinal cord. Of this group, poliovirus causes the most severe and devastating disease. Coxsackievirus and echoviruses are more likely to cause aseptic meningitis, although they can cause an acute paralytic syndrome similar to that of poliomyelitis.

CLINICAL FEATURES. Enterovirus infections occur in epidemics during the spring and summer. The most common syndrome associated with poliovirus infection is a brief illness characterized by fever, malaise, and gastrointestinal symptoms. Aseptic meningitis occurs in more severe cases. The extreme situation is paralytic poliomyelitis. It begins with fever, sore throat, and malaise lasting for 1 to 2 days. After a brief period of apparent well-being, fever recurs in association with headache, vomiting, and signs of meningeal irritation. Pain in the limbs or over the spine is an antecedent symptom of limb pa-

ralysis. Flaccid muscle weakness develops rapidly thereafter. The pattern of muscle weakness varies, but it is generally asymmetric. One arm or leg is affected more than other limbs.

Bulbar polio may occur with or without spinal cord disease and is life-threatening. Affected children have prolonged episodes of apnea and require respiratory assistance. Several motor cranial nerves may be involved as well, but the extraocular muscles are spared.

The introduction of inactivated poliomyelitis vaccine in 1954, followed by the use of live-attenuated vaccine in 1960, has abolished the disease in the Western hemisphere and Europe. Nearly all recently reported cases are vaccine related. Vaccine-associated poliomyelitis should not be a future problem, as inactivated polio vaccine has replaced the live-attenuated vaccine.

DIAGNOSIS. The diagnosis can be suspected from clinical findings and confirmed by isolation and viral typing from stool and nasopharyngeal specimens. The cerebrospinal fluid initially shows a polymorphonuclear reaction, with the cell count ranging from 50/mm^3 to 200/mm^3. After 1 week, lymphocytes predominate; after 2 to 3 weeks, the total cell count decreases. The protein content is elevated early and remains elevated for several months.

MANAGEMENT. Treatment is supportive.

Neuromuscular Blockade

A fulminating form of myasthenia gravis in which generalized weakness progresses to respiratory distress within 12 to 18 hours has been described in infants. Bulbar and limb paralysis are present. No recent reports have been published, and earlier cases may have been infantile botulism (see Chapter 6).

Children treated for prolonged periods with neuromuscular blocking agents for assisted ventilation may remain in a flaccid state for days or weeks after the drug is discontinued. This is especially true in newborns receiving several drugs that block the neuromuscular junction.

Botulism

Clostridium botulinum produces a toxin that interferes with the release of acetylcholine at the neuromuscular junction. An infantile form of botulism is described in Chapter 6, but most cases occur after infancy in people who eat food, usually preserved at home, contaminated with the organism.

CLINICAL FEATURES. The first symptoms are blurred vision, diplopia, dizziness, dysarthria, and dysphagia, which have their onset 12 to 36 hours after the ingestion of toxin. Some patients have only bulbar signs; in others, flaccid paralysis develops in all limbs. Patients with generalized weakness always have ophthalmoplegia, but the pupillary response is usually spared. Tendon reflexes may be present or absent.

DIAGNOSIS. Repetitive supermaximal nerve stimulation at a rate of 20 to 50 stimuli per second produces an incremental response characteristic of a presynaptic defect. The electrical abnormality evolves with time and may not be demonstrable in all limbs on any given day.

MANAGEMENT. Botulism can be fatal because of respiratory depression. Treatment relies primarily on supportive care, which is similar to the management of GBS. Antitoxin does not influence the course of the disease.

Corticosteroid-Induced Quadriplegia

The administration of high-dose intravenous corticosteroids, especially in combination with a neuromuscular blocking agent, may cause acute generalized weakness (Rich et al, 1996).

CLINICAL FEATURES. Most patients with this syndrome receive corticosteroids to treat asthma. The onset of weakness is 4 to 14 days after treatment is started. The weakness is usually diffuse at onset but may be limited to proximal or distal muscles. Tendon reflexes are usually preserved. Complete recovery is the rule.

DIAGNOSIS. The serum CK concentration may be normal or elevated. EMG shows brief, small-amplitude polyphasic potentials, and the muscle is electrically inexcitable to direct stimulation.

MANAGEMENT. Respiratory assistance may be needed. Cessation of the offending drugs usually ends the disorder and allows the patient to recover spontaneously.

Tick Paralysis

In North America, the female tick of the species *Dermacentor andersoni* and *D. variabiis* elaborates a salivary gland toxin that induces paralysis. The mechanism of paralysis may be similar to that of botulinum toxin (Grattan-Smith et al, 1997).

CLINICAL FEATURES. Affected children are usually less than 5 years of age. The clinical syndrome is similar to GBS, except that ocular motor palsies and pupillary abnormalities are common. A severe generalized flaccid weakness, usually first affecting the legs, develops rapidly and is sometimes associated with bifacial palsy. Respiratory paralysis requiring assisted ventilation is common. Tendon reflexes are usually absent or greatly depressed. Dysesthesias may be present at the onset of weakness, but loss of sensation cannot be shown on examination.

DIAGNOSIS. The cerebrospinal fluid protein concentration is normal. Nerve conduction study results may be normal or may show mild slowing of motor nerve conduction velocities. The amplitude of the compound muscle action potentials is often decreased. High rates of repetitive stimulation may show a normal result or an abnormal incremental response.

MANAGEMENT. Strength returns quickly once the North American tick is removed. However, the tick may be hard to find, because it is frequently hidden in body hair. In contrast, paralysis may worsen over 1 to 2 days after removal of the Australian tick before improvement begins.

Intensive Care Unit Weakness

Prolonged muscle weakness may occur in people with severe illness requiring intensive care. Formerly, many such cases were treated with neuromuscular blocking agents and corticosteroids and represent examples of the "corticosteroid-induced quadriplegia" described above. Others, who were treated with corticosteroids but not neuromuscular blocking agents develop a corticosteroid myopathy with an increased blood concentrations of CK and histological evidence of myofiber necrosis (Hansen et al, 1997).

A third group develops an intensive care quadriplegia in the absence of treatment with neuromuscular blocking agents or corticosteroids (Showalter and Engel, 1997). These cases are associated with the depletion of myosin from muscle. Muscle biopsy is needed to distinguish the several types of prolonged weakness that may occur in people with severe illness requiring intensive care.

Periodic Paralyses

The periodic paralyses are usually classified in relation to serum potassium: hyperkalemic, hypokalemic, or normokalemic. In addition, periodic paralysis may be primary (genetic) or secondary. Secondary hypokalemic periodic paralysis is caused by urinary or gastrointestinal loss of potassium. Urinary loss accompanies primary hyperaldosteronism, licorice intoxication, amphotericin B therapy, and several renal tubular defects. Gastrointestinal loss most often occurs with severe chronic diarrhea, prolonged gastrointestinal intubation and vomiting, and a draining gastrointestinal fistula. Either urinary or gastrointestinal loss, or both, may occur in children with anorexia nervosa who overuse diuretics or induce vomiting. Hypokalemic periodic paralysis is also seen with thyrotoxicosis, especially in Asians. Secondary hyperkalemic periodic paralysis is associated with renal or adrenal insufficiency.

Familial Hypokalemic Periodic Paralysis

Familial hypokalemic periodic paralysis (FPPI) is transmitted by autosomal dominant inheritance with decreased penetrance in women. FPPI results from mutations in the gene encoding the muscle dihydropyridine (DHP)-sensitive calcium channel alpha-1 subunit that maps to chromosome 1q31–32.

CLINICAL FEATURES. The onset of symptoms occurs before 16 years of age in 60% of cases and by 20 years of age in the remainder. Attacks of paralysis are at first infrequent but then may occur several times a week. Factors that trigger an attack include rest after exercise (therefore many attacks occur early in the morning), a large meal with high carbohydrate content, emotional or physical stress, alcohol ingestion, and exposure to cold. Before and during the attack the patient may have excessive thirst and oliguria. The weakness begins with a sensation of aching in the proximal muscles. Sometimes only the proximal muscles are affected; at other times there is complete paralysis so that the patient cannot even raise the head. Facial muscles are rarely affected, and extraocular motility is always normal. Respiratory distress does not occur. When the weakness is most extreme, the muscles feel swollen and the tendon reflexes are absent. Most attacks last for 6 to 12 hours and some for the whole day. Strength recovers rapidly, but after several attacks residual weakness may be present.

DIAGNOSIS. During the attack, the serum potassium concentration may fall to l.5 mEq/L (1.5 mmol/L) and ECG changes occur, including bradycardia, flattening of T waves, and prolongation of the PR and QT intervals. The muscle is electrically silent and not excitable. Attacks can be provoked by the oral administration of glucose, 2 g/kg, with 10 to 20 units of crystalline insulin given subcutaneously. The serum potassium concentration falls, and an attack of paralysis is initiated within 2 to 3 hours.

MANAGEMENT. Acute attacks in patients with good renal function are treated by repeated oral doses of potassium. In adolescents 5 to 10 g is used. Smaller amounts should be considered for younger children. Daily use of carbonic anhydrase inhibitors is beneficial in many families to prevent attacks (Tawil et al, 2000).

Familial Hyperkalemic Periodic Paralysis

Familial hyperkalemic periodic paralysis (FPPII) is transmitted by autosomal dominant inheritance and occurs with equal frequency in both sexes. It is caused by a defect of the gene encoding the sodium channel on chromosome 17q23–25 (Hudson et al, 1995). Myotonia of the eyelids, face, and hands is sometimes an associated symptom, and such cases are referred to as *paramyotonia congenita.*

CLINICAL FEATURES. The onset of weakness is in early childhood and sometimes in infancy. As in hypokalemic periodic paralysis, resting after exercise may provoke attacks. However, only moderate exercise is required. Weakness begins with a sensation of heaviness in the back and leg muscles. Sometimes the patient can delay the paralysis by walking or moving about. In infants and small children, the attacks are characterized by an episode of floppiness in which the child lies around and cannot move. In older children and adults, both mild and severe attacks may occur. Mild attacks last for less than an hour and do not produce complete paralysis. More than one mild attack may occur in a day. Severe attacks are similar to the complete flaccid paralysis seen in hypokalemic periodic paralysis and may last for several hours. Residual weakness may persist after several severe attacks.

DIAGNOSIS. Myotonia in patients with hyperkalemic periodic paralysis is mild and may occur only on exposure to cold. Laying a towel soaked in ice water over the patient's eyes for a few minutes elicits the myotonia. After the towel is removed, the patient is asked to look up briefly and then to look down quickly. When the eyelids are myotonic, the lids cannot come down quickly and a rim of sclera is exposed.

During attacks the serum concentration of potassium increases but may not increase sufficiently to be abnormal. When the potassium concentration is high, ECG changes are consistent with hyperkalemia. The oral administration of potassium chloride just after exercise in the fasting state provokes an attack. During the attack the muscles are electrically silent.

MANAGEMENT. Acute attacks seldom require treatment because they are brief. Daily use of carbonic anhydrase inhibitors is beneficial to prevent attacks. The mechanism by which these drugs are effective in preventing attacks of both hyperkalemic and hypokalemic periodic paralysis is unknown.

Familial Normokalemic Periodic Paralysis

Several families have experienced an autosomal dominant inherited periodic paralysis in which no alteration in the serum concentration of potassium could be detected (FPPIII). These cases may represent hyperkalemic periodic paralysis in which the flux of potassium into the serum was insufficient to be detected.

Andersen Potassium-Sensitive Cardiodysrhythmic Periodic Paralysis (Andersen Syndrome)

Andersen syndrome is a distinct channelopathy affecting both skeletal and cardiac muscles (Canun, 1999). The genetic defect does not involve the α-subunit of the skeletal muscle's sodium channel and the cardiac muscle potassium channel responsible for most long Q-T intervals.

CLINICAL FEATURES. The main features are dysmorphic features, periodic paralysis, and a prolonged Q-T interval. The dysmorphic features include a broad nose, low-set ears, a small mandible, and syndactyly. The periodic paralysis may be associated with hyperkalemia, hypokalemia, or normokalemia. The prolonged Q-T interval may be the only feature in some individuals. The initial feature may be an arrhythmia, especially ventricular tachycardia, or attacks of paralysis.

DIAGNOSIS. The diagnosis should be suspected in any dysmorphic child with a prolonged Q-T interval or a periodic paralysis.

MANAGEMENT. The arrhythmias associated with prolonged Q-T interval are life-threatening and must be treated. Affected members with periodic paralysis are responsive to oral potassium.

References

Askansas V, Engel WK. Sporadic inclusion-body myositis and hereditary inclusion-body myopathies. Diseases of oxidative stress and aging? *Arch Neurol* 1998;55:915–920.

Birouk N, Gouider R, Guern EL, et al. Charcot-Marie-Tooth disease type 1A with 17p11.2 duplication. *Brain* 1997;120:813–823.

Bonne G, Di Barletta MR, Varnous S, et al. Mutations in the gene encoding lamin A/C cause autosomal dominant Emery-Dreifuss muscular dystrophy. *Nature Genet* 1999;21:285–288.

Byrd TD. (Updated 31 August 1999) Charcot-Marie-Tooth Hereditary Neuropathy Overview. In: GeneClinics: Medical Genetic Knowledge Base [database online]. University of Washington, Seattle. Available at http://www.geneclinics.org/profiles/pws. Accessed 1 January 2000.

Canun S, Perez N, Beirana LG. Andersen syndrome autosomal dominant in three generations. *Am J Med Genet* 1999;85:147–156.

Duggan DJ, Gorospe JR, Fanin M, et al. Mutations in the sarcoglycan genes in patients with myopathy. *N Engl J Med* 1997;336:618–624.

Elliot JL, Kwon JM, Goodfellow PJ, et al. Hereditary motor and sensory neuropathy IIB: Clinical and electrodiagnostic characteristics. *Neurology* 1997;48:23–28.

Ellsworth RE, Ionasescu V, Searby C, et al. The CMT2D locus: Refined genetic position and construction of a bacterial clone-based physical map. *Genome Res* 1999;9:568–574.

Gomez CM, Maselli R, Gammack J. A β-subunit mutation in the acetylcholine receptor channel gate causes severe slow-channel syndrome. *Ann Neurol* 1996;39:712–723.

Grattan-Smith PJ, Morris JG, et al. Clinical and neurophysiological features of tick paralysis. *Brain* 1997;120:1975–1987.

Hanson P, Dive A, Brucher J-M, et al. Acute corticosteroid myopathy in intensive care patients. *Muscle Nerve* 1997;20:1371–1380.

Harper CM, Engel AG. Quinidine sulfate therapy for the slow-channel congenital myasthenic syndrome. *Ann Neurol* 1998;43:480–484.

Hudson AJ, Ebers GC, Bulman DE. The skeletal muscle sodium and chloride channel diseases. *Brain* 1995;118:547–563.

Isozumi K, DeLong R, Kaplan J, et al. Linkage of scapuloperoneal spinal muscular atrophy to chromosome 12q24.1-q24.31. *Hum Mol Genet* 1996;5:1377–1382.

Jöbsis GJ, Boers JM, Barth PG, et al. Bethlem myopathy: A slowly progressive congenital muscular dystrophy. *Brain* 1999;122:649–655.

Laing NG, Laing BA, Meredith C, et al. Autosomal dominant distal myopathy: Linkage to chromosome 14. *Am J Hum Genet* 1995;56:422–427.

Linssen WH, Notermans NC, Van der Graaf Y, et al. Miyoshi-type distal muscular dystrophy. Clinical spectrum in 24 Dutch patients. *Brain* 1997;120:1989–1996.

Mackay MT, Kornberg AJ, Shield LK, et al. Benign acute childhood myositis. Laboratory and clinical features. *Neurology* 1999;53:2127–2131.

Matsuda C, Aoki M, Hayashi YK, et al. Dysferlin is a surface-associated protein that is absent in Miyoshi myopathy. *Neurology* 1999;53:1119–1122.

Mihalik SJ, Morrell JC, Kim D, et al. Identification of PAHX, a Refsum disease gene. *Nature Genet* 1997;17:185–189.

Mora M, Cartegni L, Di Blasi C, et al. X-linked Emery-Dreifuss muscular dystrophy can be diagnosed from skin biopsy or blood sample. *Ann Neurol* 1997;42:249–253.

Navon R, Khosravi R, Melki J, et al. Juvenile-onset spinal muscular atrophy caused by compound heterozygosity for mutations in the HEXA gene. *Ann Neurol* 1997;41:631–638.

Nevo Y, Pestronk A, Kornberg AM, et al. Childhood chronic inflammatory demyelinating neuropathies: Clinical course and long-term follow-up. *Neurology* 1996;47:98–102.

North KN, Miller G, Iannaccone ST, et al. Cognitive dysfunction as the major presenting feature of Becker's muscular dystrophy. *Neurology* 1996:461–465.

Paradiso G, Tripoli J, Galicchio S, et al. Epidemiological, clinical, and electrodiagnostic findings in childhood Guillain-Barré syndrome: A reappraisal. *Ann Neurol* 1999;46:701–707.

Rabin BA, Griffin JW, Crain BJ, et al. Autosomal dominant juvenile amyotrophic lateral sclerosis. *Brain* 1999;122: 1539–1550.

Ricci E, Galluzzi G, Deidda G, et al. Progress in the molecular diagnosis of facioscapulohumeral muscular dystrophy and correlation between the number of KpnI repeats at the 4q35 locus and clinical phenotype. *Ann Neurol* 1999;45:751–757.

Rich MM, Teener JW, Raps EC, et al. Muscle is electrically inexcitable in acute quadriplegic myopathy. *Neurology* 1996;46:731–736.

Sansome A, Dubowitz V. Intravenous immunoglobulin in juvenile dermatomyositis—four year review of nine cases. *Arch Dis Child* 1995;72:25–28.

Shoji Y, Koizumi A, Kayo T, et al. Evidence for linkage of human primary systemic carnitine deficiency with D5S436: A novel gene locus on chromosome 5q. *Am J Hum Genet* 1998;63:101–108.

Showalter CJ, Engel AE. Acute quadriplegic myopathy: Analysis of myosin isoforms and evidence for calpain-mediated proteolysis. *Muscle Nerve* 1997;20:316–322.

Simmons Z, Wald JJ, Albers JW. Chronic inflammatory polyradiculoneuropathy in children: I. Presentation, electrodiagnostic studies, and initial clinical course, with comparison to adults. *Muscle Nerve* 1997a;20:1008–1015.

Simmons Z, Wald JJ, Albers JW. Chronic inflammatory polyradiculoneuropathy in children: II. Long-term follow-up, with comparison to adults. *Muscle Nerve* 1997b;20:1569–1575.

Tawil R, McDermott MP, Brown R Jr, et al. Randomized trials of dichlorphenamide in the periodic paralyses. *Ann Neurol* 2000;47:46–53.

Tawil R, Myers GJ, Weiffenbach B, et al. Scapuloperoneal syndromes. Absence of linkage to the 4q35 FSHD locus. *Arch Neurol* 1995;52:1069–1072.

van der Kooi AJ, Ledderhof TM, de Voogt WG, et al. A newly recognized autosomal dominant limb girdle muscular dystrophy with cardiac involvement. *Ann Neurol* 1996;39:636–642.

Warner LE, Svaren J, Milbrandt J, et al. Functional consequences of mutations in the early growth response 2 gene (EGR2) correlate with severity of human myelinopathies. *Hum Mol Gen* 1999;8:1245–1251.

Wilhelmsen KC, Blake DM, Lynch T, et al. Chromosome 12-linked autosomal dominant scapuloperoneal muscular dystrophy. *Ann Neurol* 1996;39:507–520.

Chapter 8
Cramps, Muscle Stiffness, and Exercise Intolerance

A **CRAMP IS** an involuntary painful contraction of a muscle or part of a muscle. Cramps can occur in normal children during and after vigorous exercise and after excessive loss of fluid or electrolytes. Such cramps are characterized on electromyography (EMG) by the repetitive firing of normal motor unit potentials. Stretching the muscle relieves the cramp. Muscle that is partially denervated is particularly susceptible to cramping not only during exercise but also during sleep. Night cramps may awaken patients with neuronopathies, neuropathies, or root compression. Cramps during exercise occur also in patients with several different disorders of muscle energy metabolism. These cramps differ from other cramps in that they are not detected by electrodiagnostic examination.

Muscle stiffness and spasms are sometimes called cramps by patients but are actually prolonged contractions of several muscles that are able to impose postures. Such contractions may or may not be painful. When painful, they lack the explosive character of cramps. Prolonged contractions occur when muscles fail to relax (myotonia) or when motor unit activity is continuous (Table 8-1). Prolonged, painless muscle contractions occur also in dystonia and in other movement disorders (see Chapter 14).

Many normal children, especially preadolescent boys, complain of pain in their legs at night and sometimes during the day, especially after a period of increased activity. These pains are not true cramps. The muscle is not in spasm, the pain is diffuse and aching in quality, and the discomfort lasts for an hour or longer. Stretching the muscle does not relieve the pain. This is not a symptom of neuromuscular disease and, for want of better understanding, is usually referred to as *growing pains*. Symptoms are relieved by mild analgesics or heat.

Table 8-1
Diseases with Abnormal Muscle Activity

Continuous Motor Unit Activity
Neuromyotonia
Paroxysmal ataxia and myokymia (see Chapter 10)
Schwartz-Jampel syndrome
Stiff man syndrome
Thyrotoxicosis

Cramps-Fasciculation Syndrome

Myotonia
Myotonia congenita
Myotonia fluctuans

Systemic Disorders
Hypoadrenalism
Hypocalcemia (tetany)
Strychnine poisoning
Hypothyroidism
Uremia

Exercise intolerance is a relative term for an inability to maintain exercise at an expected level. The causes of exercise intolerance considered in this chapter are fatigue and muscle pain. Fatigue is a normal consequence of exercise and occurs in everyone at some level of activity. In general, weak children become fatigued more quickly than children who have normal strength. Many children with exercise intolerance and cramps, but no permanent weakness, have a defect in an enzyme needed to produce energy for muscular contraction (Table 8-2). Several such inborn errors of metabolism have been defined, and others are yet to be defined. Even when the full spectrum of biochemical tests is available, the metabolic defect cannot be identified in some children in whom cramps develop

Table 8-2
Diseases with Decreased Muscle Energy

Defects of Carbohydrate Utilization
Lactate dehydrogenase deficiency
Myophosphorylase deficiency
Phosphofructokinase deficiency
Phosphoglycerate kinase deficiency
Phosphoglycerate mutase deficiency

Defects of Fatty Acid Oxidation
Carnitine palmitoyl transferase 2 deficiency
Very-long-chain acyl coenzyme A dehydrogenase
    deficiency

Mitochondrial (Respiratory Chain) Myopathies

Myoadenylate Deaminase Deficiency

Table 8-3
Electromyography in Muscle Stiffness

Normal Between Cramps*
Brody myopathy
Defects of carbohydrate metabolism
Defects of lipid metabolism
Mitochondrial myopathies
Myoadenylate deaminase deficiency
Rippling muscle disease
Tubular aggregates

Silent Cramps
Brody disease
Defects of carbohydrate metabolism
Rippling muscle disease
Tubular aggregates

Continuous Motor Activity
Neuromyotonia
Schwartz-Jampel syndrome
Stiff man syndrome

Myotonia
Myotonia congenita
Myotonic dystrophy
Schwartz-Jampel syndrome

Myopathy
Emery-Dreifuss muscular dystrophy
Rigid spine syndrome
X-linked myalgia

* Or may be myopathic.

after exercise and who have clear-cut evidence of muscle disease.

Myasthenia gravis is a disorder characterized by exercise intolerance, but it is not covered in this chapter because the usual initial symptoms are either isolated cranial nerve disturbances (see Chapter 15) or limb weakness (see Chapters 6 and 7).

Conditions that produce some combination of cramps and exercise intolerance can be divided into three groups: diseases with abnormal muscle activity, diseases with decreased energy for muscle contraction, and myopathies. As a rule, the first and third groups are symptomatic at all times, whereas the second group is symptomatic only with exercise. The first group requires EMG for diagnosis.

EMG should be the initial diagnostic test in patients with muscle stiffness that is not due to spasticity or rigidity. It usually leads to the correct diagnosis (Table 8-3).

Abnormal Muscle Activity

Continuous Motor Unit Activity

Continuous motor unit activity (CMUA) is caused by the uncontrolled release of acetylcholine (ACh) packets at the neuromuscular junction. The EMG features of CMUA are repetitive muscle action potentials in response to a single nerve stimulus; high-frequency bursts of motor unit potentials of normal morphology that start and stop abruptly; and rhythmically firing doublets, triplets, and multiplets. During long bursts the potentials decline in amplitude. This activity is difficult to distinguish from normal voluntary

activity. CMUA is seen in a heterogeneous group of disorders characterized clinically by some combination of muscular pain, fasciculations, myokymia, contractures, and cramps (Table 8-4).

Disorders with CMUA can be subdivided into syndromes in which the primary defect is believed to be within the spinal cord (stiff man syndrome) and those in which the primary defect is believed to be within the peripheral nerve

Table 8-4
Abnormal Muscle Activity

Fasciculations: Spontaneous, random twitching of a group of muscle fibers
Fibrillation: Spontaneous contraction of a single muscle fiber, not visible through the skin
Myotonia: Disturbance in muscle relaxation following voluntary contraction or percussion
Myokymia: Repetitive fasciculations causing a quivering or undulating twitch
Neuromyotonia: Continuous muscle activity characterized by muscle rippling, muscle stiffness, and myotonia

(neuromyotonia). Neuromyotonia is also called *Isaac syndrome*. These disorders may be sporadic or familial in occurrence. When familial, they are usually transmitted by autosomal dominant inheritance.

Neuromyotonia

The primary abnormality in neuromyotonia is in the nerve or the nerve terminal. Most childhood cases are sporadic in occurrence, but some are transmitted by autosomal dominant inheritance. An autoimmune process directed against the potassium channel may account for some sporadic cases (Shillito et al, 1995).

CLINICAL FEATURES. The clinical triad includes involuntary muscle twitching (fasciculations or myokymia), muscle cramps or stiffness, and myotonia. Excessive sweating is frequently associated with the muscle stiffness. The age at onset is anytime from birth to adult life.

The initial features are muscle twitching and cramps brought on by exercise. Later these symptoms occur also at rest and even during sleep. The cramps may affect only distal muscles, causing painful posturing of the hands and feet. As a rule, the legs are affected more severely than the arms. These disorders are not progressive and do not lead to permanent disability. Attacks of cramping become less frequent and less severe with age.

In some children, cramps and fasciculations are not as prominent as stiffness, which causes abnormal limb posturing associated frequently with excessive sweating. The legs are more often affected than the arms, and the symptoms suggest dystonia (see Chapter 14). Limb posturing may begin in one foot and remain asymmetric for months. Most cases are sporadic.

Muscle mass, muscle strength, and tendon reflexes are normal. Fasciculations are sporadic and are seen only after prolonged observation.

DIAGNOSIS. Some adult-onset cases are associated with malignancy, but this is never the case in children. Muscle fibers fire repetitively at a rate of 100–300 Hz, either continuously or in recurring bursts, producing a pinging sound. The discharge continues during sleep and persists after procaine block of the nerve. The intramuscular nerve twigs are the probable sites of the activity (Torbergsen et al, 1996).

MANAGEMENT. Carbamazepine and phenytoin, at usual anticonvulsant doses, are both effective in reducing or abolishing symptoms.

Schwartz-Jampel Syndrome

The Schwartz-Jampel syndrome (SJS) is a hereditary disorder, probably transmitted by autosomal recessive inheritance. It is characterized by short stature, skeletal abnormalities, and persistent muscular contraction and hypertrophy.

Giedion et al. (1997) found that some children had mild skeletal changes that may be secondary to CMUA (SJS-1), while others had primary bone dysplasia with CMUA (SJS-2). The first group shows linkage to chromosome 1p36.1-p34, while the second group does not.

CLINICAL FEATURES. SJS-1 corresponds to the original description of Schwartz and Jampel. Bone deformities are not prominent at birth. CMUA of the face is the main feature producing a characteristic triad that includes narrowing of the palpebral fissures (blepharophimosis), pursing of the mouth, and puckering of the chin. Striking or even blowing on the eyelids induces blepharospasm. CMUA in the limbs produces stiffness of gait and exercise intolerance. Motor development during the first year is slow, but intelligence is normal.

SJS-2 has prominent bone deformities at birth that suggest the Morquio syndrome (osteochondrodystrophy). Neonatal mortality is high.

DIAGNOSIS. EMG shows CMUA. Initial reports suggested incorrectly that the abnormal activity seen on the EMG and expressed clinically was myotonia. Myotonia may be present, but CMUA is responsible for the facial and limb symptoms. The serum concentration of creatine kinase (CK) can be mildly elevated. The histological appearance of the muscle is usually normal but may show variation in fiber size and an increased number of central nuclei.

MANAGEMENT. Muscle stiffness is diminished by phenytoin or carbamazepine. Early treatment with relief of muscle stiffness reduces the severity of subsequent muscle deformity.

Stiff Man (Stiff Person) Syndrome

Stiff man syndrome is a sporadic condition of adult life that may be immune-mediated (Kissel and Elble, 1998). It is rare in children. A genetic form of stiff man syndrome, transmitted by autosomal dominant inheritance, was described in infants but is now considered to be startle disease (hyperekplexia). Startle disease is described in Chapter 1 because the main features in children and adults are paroxysmal, but the initial symptom in newborns is stiffness. It is not stiff man syndrome.

CLINICAL FEATURES. Following an initial period of aching and tightness in the truncal muscles, involuntary painful spasms occur without spinal deformity. Abdominal wall rigidity and contraction of thoracolumbar paraspinal muscles cause a hyperlordosis that is characteristic of the disease. The spasms are triggered by startle and by emotional upset and are relieved by sleep. Limb and bulbar muscles are not involved (Barker et al, 1998). Tendon reflexes are active or hyperactive, and no evidence of muscle atrophy is found.

DIAGNOSIS. Individuals with stiff man syndrome and their relatives have an increased incidence of several organ-specific autoimmune disorders, especially insulin-dependent diabetes and hypothyroidism. Serum antibodies against glutamic acid decarboxylase and pancreatic islet cells are present in 60% of patients.

MANAGEMENT. Diazepam and baclofen are the mainstays of treatment but provide only partial symptomatic relief of the spasms. Prednisone, plasma exchange, and intravenous immunoglobulin may be useful in patients with evidence of antibodies against glutamic acid decarboxylase or pancreatic islet cells.

Myotonia Congenita

Myotonia congenita is a genetic disorder characterized by muscle stiffness and hypertrophy. Weakness is not prominent, but muscle function may be impaired by stiffness. The disease can be transmitted as either an autosomal dominant (Thomsen disease) or autosomal recessive (Becker disease) trait. Many cases are sporadic and cannot be classified genetically. In general, the autosomal recessive form has a later onset and more severe myotonia than the dominant form. Mild weakness may occur in the recessive form. However, the overlap of clinical features is considerable, and the clinical features alone cannot determine the pattern of genetic transmission. Both are associated with abnormalities in the chloride channel, the gene for which is located on chromosome 7q35 (Barchi, 1998).

CLINICAL FEATURES. Clinical features are stereotyped. After rest, muscles are stiff and difficult to move. With activity the stiffness disappears and movement may be normal. One of my patients played Little League baseball and could not sit while he was waiting to bat for fear that he would be unable to get up. The onset is usually dated to infancy. In the recessive form, the myotonia causes generalized muscle hypertrophy, which gives the infant a Herculean appearance. The tongue, face, and jaw muscles are sometimes involved. Stiffness is painless and is exacerbated by exposure to cold. Percussion myotonia is present. Muscle mass, strength, and tendon reflexes are normal.

DIAGNOSIS. EMG establishes the diagnosis. Repetitive discharges at rates of 20 to 80 cycles/sec are recorded when the needle is first inserted into the muscle and again on voluntary contraction. Two types of discharges are seen: a biphasic spike potential of less than 5 ms and a positive wave of less than 50 ms. The amplitude and frequency of potentials wax and wane, producing a characteristic sound. No evidence of dystrophy is demonstrated. The serum concentration of CK is normal. Muscle biopsy specimens in patients with either the dominant or the recessive form do not contain type IIb fibers.

MANAGEMENT. Myotonia does not always require treatment but sometimes can be relieved by phenytoin or carbamazepine at ordinary anticonvulsant doses. Mexiletine is probably the more effective drug and has become my first choice.

Myotonia Fluctuans

Myotonia fluctuans is a disorder of the muscle sodium channel on chromosome 17q23-25 (Hudson et al, 1995). It is transmitted by autosomal dominant inheritance, and its clinical features are similar to those of myotonia congenita.

CLINICAL FEATURES. The onset of stiffness is usually in the second decade and is made worse by exercise or by potassium ingestion. Myotonia affects the extraocular muscles as well as the trunk and limbs. The severity of myotonia fluctuates on a day-by-day basis. "Warming up" usually relieves symptoms, but exercise may also worsen symptoms. A bad day may follow a day of exercise or potassium ingestion, but neither precipitant causes immediate worsening of myotonia. Cooling does not trigger or worsen myotonia.

DIAGNOSIS. EMG shows myotonia, and muscle biopsy is normal. DNA analysis shows a mutation in the gene for the sodium channel subunit.

MANAGEMENT. Daily use of mexilitine or acetazolamide may be effective to relieve the stiffness.

Systemic Disorders

Hypoadrenalism

A small percentage of patients with Addison disease complain of cramps and pain in truncal muscles. At times, paroxysmal cramps occur in the lower torso and legs and cause the patient to double up in pain. The symptoms are relieved by hormone replacement.

Hypocalcemia and Hypomagnesemia

Tetany caused by dietary deficiency of calcium is rare in modern times, except in newborns fed cow's milk. Hypocalcemic tetany is more likely to result from hypothyroidism or hyperventilation-induced alkalosis.

The initial symptom of tetany is tingling around the mouth and in the hands and feet. With time, the tingling increases in intensity and becomes generalized. This is followed by spasms in the muscles of the face, hands, and feet. The hands assume a typical posture in which the fingers are extended, the wrist is flexed, and the thumb is abducted. Fasciculations and laryngeal spasm may be present. Percussion of the facial nerve, either just anterior to the ear or over the cheek, produces contraction of the muscles innervated by that branch of the nerve.

A similar syndrome is encountered with magnesium deficiency. In addition to the tetany, encephalopathy occurs. Restoring the proper concentration of serum electrolytes relieves the cramps associated with hypocalcemia and hypomagnesemia.

Strychnine Poisoning

Strychnine is sometimes used as an adulterant in cocaine because it is a white, odorless powder that is readily available as rat poison. It is a competitive antagonist of glycine, a central nervous system inhibitory neurotransmitter. The clinical features of poisoning are apprehension, nausea, muscle twitching, extensor spasm, opisthotonos, and seizures. Excessive muscle contraction causes myoglobinuria and lactic acidosis. Intravenous diazepam reduces spasms and can prevent death.

Thyroid Disease

Muscle aches, cramps, and stiffness are the initial features in up to half of patients with hypothyroidism. Stiffness is worse in the morning, especially on cold days, and is probably caused by slowing of both muscular contraction and relaxation. This is different from myotonia, in which only relaxation is affected. Indeed, the stiffness of hypothyroidism is made worse by activity and may be painful, whereas myotonia is relieved by activity and is painless. The slow-

ing of muscular contraction and relaxation is sometimes demonstrated when tendon reflexes are tested. The response tends to "hang up."

Percussion of a muscle produces a localized knot of contraction called *myoedema*. This localized contraction lasts for up to 1 minute before slowly returning to normal.

Myokymia, CMUA of the face, tongue, and limbs, and muscle cramps develop occasionally in patients with thyrotoxicosis. Restoring the euthyroid state reverses all of the neuromuscular symptoms of hypothyroidism and hyperthyroidism.

Uremia

Uremia is a known cause of polyneuropathy (see Chapter 7). However, 50% of patients complain of nocturnal leg cramps and flexion cramps of the hands even before clinical evidence of polyneuropathy is present. Excessive use of diuretics may be the triggering factor. Muscle cramps occur also in approximately one third of patients undergoing hemodialysis. Monitoring with EMG during dialysis documents a buildup of spontaneous discharges, which after several hours, usually toward the end of dialysis treatment, culminate in repetitive high-voltage discharges associated with clinical cramps. Because standard dialysis fluid is slightly hypotonic, many nephrologists have attempted to treat the cramps by administering hypertonic solutions. Either sodium chloride or glucose solutions relieve cramps in most patients. The cramps apparently result from either extracellular volume contraction or hypo-osmolarity. Similar cramps occur in children with severe diarrhea or vomiting.

Decreased Muscle Energy

Three sources for replenishing adenosine triphosphate (ATP) during exercise are available: the phosphorylation of adenosine diphosphate (ADP) to ATP by phosphocreatine (PCr) within the exercising muscles; glycogen and lipids within the exercising muscles; and glucose and triglycerides brought to the exercising muscles by the blood. A fourth and less efficient source is derived from ADP via an alternate pathway using adenylate kinase and deaminase. PCr stores are the main source from which ATP is replenished during intense activity of short duration. During the first 30 seconds of intense endurance exercise, PCr is decreased by 35% and muscle glycogen stores are reduced by 25%. Exercise lasting longer than 30 seconds is associated with the mobilization of substantial amounts of carbohydrate and lipid.

The glucose required to sustain a single powerful contraction can be provided by the breakdown of muscle glycogen (glycogenolysis) and the anaerobic metabolism of glucose to pyruvate (glycolysis) (Figure 8-1). Anaerobic glycolysis is an inefficient mechanism for producing energy and is not satisfactory for endurance exercise. Endurance requires that pyruvate generated in muscle by glycolysis be metabolized aerobically in the mitochondria. Oxidative metabolism provides high levels of energy for every molecule of glucose metabolized (Figure 8-1).

The central compound of oxidative metabolism in mitochondria is acetylcoenzyme A (acetyl-CoA). Acetyl-CoA is derived from pyruvate, from fatty acids, and from amino acids. When exercise is prolonged, fatty acids become an important substrate to maintain muscular contraction. Acetyl-CoA is oxidized through the Krebs cycle and releases hydrogen ions that reduce nicotinamide adenine dinucleotide (NAD). These reduced compounds then enter a sequence of oxidation-reduction steps in the respiratory chain that liberate energy. Energy is stored as ATP. This process of liberating and storing energy is called *oxidation-phosphorylation coupling*. The production of energy for muscular contraction is therefore impaired by disorders that prevent the delivery of glucose or fatty acids, the oxidation process in the mitochondria, or the creation of ATP.

Clinical Features of Decreased Muscle Energy

Exercise intolerance is the invariable result of any disturbance in the biochemical pathways that support muscle contraction. The common symptom is fatigue. Other symptoms are myalgia and cramps. Muscle pain the day after strenuous exercise is expected after unaccustomed exercise. Muscle pain develops during exercise when the mechanisms to supply energy for contraction are impaired.

The *ischemic exercise test* had been the first step in the diagnosis of muscle energy disorders, but it has become less important with the ease of tissue diagnosis by muscle biopsy and the commercial availability of methods for measuring enzyme activity in fibroblasts. I have stopped using the test. It is almost impossible to get a child to cooperate sufficiently to do the test properly.

Defects of Carbohydrate Utilization

Myophosphorylase Deficiency (McArdle Disease)

Myophosphorylase is encoded by a gene on chromosome 11q13. It exists in two forms: phosphorylase a is the active form and phosphorylase b is the inactive form. Phosphorylase b kinase is the enzyme that converts the inactive form to the active form. It is in turn activated by a protein kinase. Deficiencies of either enzyme result in exercise intolerance.

Myophosphorylase deficiency is transmitted by autosomal recessive inheritance. The gene is encoded on chromosome 11q13. Reports of autosomal dominant inheritance may represent manifesting heterozygotes. Phosphorylase activity is deficient only in muscle; the first step of glycogenolysis is prevented, and muscle glycogen is unavailable to produce glucose for energy. Liver phosphorylase concentrations are normal, and hypoglycemia does not occur.

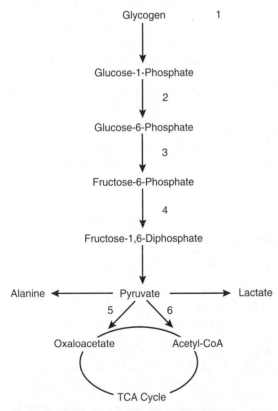

Figure 8-1. Glycogen metabolism. 1. Myophosphorylase, initiates glycogen breakdown; 2. Phosphoglucomutase; 3. Phosphoglucose isomerase; 4. Phosphofructokinase; 5. Pyruvate carboxylase; 6. Pyruvate dehydrogenase complex.

CLINICAL FEATURES. The severity of symptoms varies with the percentage of enzyme activity. Children with only mild deficiency states have few or no symptoms until adolescence. Aching becomes increasingly prominent and then, after an episode of vigorous exercise, severe cramps are noted in the exercised muscles. Myoglobinuria is sometimes present. The pain can last for hours. Thereafter, exercise leads to repeated bouts of cramps that cause a decline in the overall level of activity. Pain begins soon after vigorous exercise is initiated, and myoglobinuria is noted several hours later. Some patients exercise through the pain by slowing down just before the time of fatigue. Once that point is passed, exercise may continue unimpeded. This is probably due to an increase in cardiac output, the use of blood glucose and free fatty acids as a substrate for muscle metabolism, and the recruitment of more motor units.

Examination is generally unrevealing. Muscle mass and strength and the tendon reflexes are usually normal. Weakness is detected only in adult patients, and even then the tendon reflexes are normal.

Myophosphorylase deficiency can also be manifested as slowly progressive proximal weakness that begins during childhood or adult life. Affected individuals may never complain of cramps on exercise or of myoglobinuria. Tendon reflexes are preserved until late in the course of disease.

DIAGNOSIS. EMG examination is usually normal. The serum concentration of CK is elevated, and myoglobin may appear in the urine coincidentally with the cramps.

Salient features of muscle biopsy specimens are histochemical evidence of subsarcolemmal blebs containing glycogen and the absence of phosphorylase. Muscle fiber degeneration and regeneration are present immediately after an episode of cramps and myoglobinuria. Definitive diagnosis requires the biochemical demonstration of decreased myophosphorylase activity.

MANAGEMENT. Creatine supplementation may increase muscle function (Vorgerd et al, 2000). Patients usually learn to live with their disorder by controlling their level of exercise.

Other Disorders of Glucose Utilization

A syndrome identical to myophosphorylase deficiency—cramps on exercise and myoglobinuria—has also been described in four other enzyme deficiencies associated with the anaerobic

glycolysis of carbohydrates (see Figure 8-1). They are muscle phosphofructokinase (PFK) deficiency, muscle phosphoglycerate kinase deficiency, muscle phosphoglycerate mutase deficiency, and lactate dehydrogenase deficiency. All are transmitted by autosomal recessive inheritance except phosphoglycerate kinase deficiency, which is an X-linked trait. PFK deficiency is the most common member of this group and has also been described as a cause of infantile hypotonia (see Chapter 6). Attacks may be associated with nausea, vomiting, and muscle pain. The mutase deficiency occurs mainly in Afro-Americans.

Muscle biopsy results show subsarcolemmal collections of glycogen, but the histochemical reaction for phosphorylase is normal. These disorders are correctly identified by biochemical analysis.

Defects of Long-Chain Fatty Acid Metabolism

Long-chain fatty acids are the principal lipid oxidized to produce acetyl-CoA.

Carnitine Palmitoyl Transferase 2 Deficiency

The mitochondrial oxidation of fatty acids is the main source of energy for muscles during prolonged exercise and during fasting. The carnitine palmitoyl transferase (CPT) enzyme system is essential for the transfer of fatty acids across the mitochondrial membrane. This system includes CPT-1 in the outer mitochondrial membrane and CPT-2 and carnitine-acylcarnitine translocase in the inner mitochondrial membrane.

CPT-2 deficiency is transmitted as an autosomal recessive trait (gene locus 1p32) and has three main phenotypes. The most severe phenotype is a fatal nonketotic-hypoglycemic encephalopathy of infants, and the less severe phenotypes are characterized by exercise intolerance in children and recurrent myoglobinuria in adults. CPT-2 deficiency is the most common metabolic disorder of skeletal muscle. The phenotypic variations in the muscle diseases caused by CPT-2 deficiency probably relate to the type of molecular defect, and to superimposed environmental factors, such as prolonged fasting, exercise, cold exposure, and intercurrent illness.

CLINICAL FEATURES. The features of CPT-2 deficiency usually begin between the ages of 15 and 25. No difficulty is experienced in performing even heavy exercise of short duration. However, pain, tenderness, and swelling of muscles develop after sustained aerobic exercise. Severe muscle cramps, as in myophosphorylase deficiency, do not occur. Associated with the pain may be actual muscle injury characterized by an increased serum concentration of CK and myoglobinuria. Muscle injury may also accompany periods of prolonged fasting, especially in patients on low-carbohydrate, high-fat diets.

In the interval between attacks, results of muscle examination, serum concentration of CK, and EMG are usually normal. People with CPT-2 deficiency are at risk for malignant hyperthermia.

DIAGNOSIS. The diagnosis is suggested by the clinical features and established by measuring the concentration of CPT-2 in muscle. Muscle histology is usually normal between attacks.

MANAGEMENT. Frequent carbohydrate feedings and the avoidance of prolonged aerobic activity minimize muscle destruction.

Very-Long-Chain Acyl Coenzyme A Dehydrogenase Deficiency

The chain length of their preferred substrates describes four mitochondrial acyl CoA dehydrogenases: short (SCAD), medium (MCAD), long (LCAD), and very long (VLCAD). The first three are located in the mitochondrial matrix, and deficiency causes recurrent coma (see Chapter 2). VLCAD is bound to the inner mitochondrial membrane, and deficiency causes exercise-induced myoglobinuria (Straussberg et al, 1997).

CLINICAL FEATURES. Onset is usually in the second decade but can be as early as 4 years. Pain and myoglobinuria occur during or following prolonged exercise or fasting. Weakness may be profound. Carbohydrate ingestion before or during exercise reduces the intensity of pain. Examination between attacks is normal.

DIAGNOSIS. The serum CK concentration is slightly elevated between attacks and increased further at the time of myoglobinuria. EMG is consistent with myopathy, and muscle biopsy shows lipid storage in type I fibers. Plasma free fatty acids but not ketones increase during a 24-hour fast, suggesting impaired ketogenesis.

MANAGEMENT. Frequent small carbohydrate feeds, dietary fat restriction, and carnitine supplementation reduce the frequency of attacks.

Mitochondrial (Respiratory Chain) Myopathies

The respiratory chain, located in the inner mitochondrial membrane, consists of five protein complexes: complex I (NADH–coenzyme Q reductase); complex II (succinate–coenzyme Q reductase); complex III (reduced coenzyme Q–cytochrome-*c* reductase); complex IV (cytochrome *c* oxidase); and complex V (ATP synthase) (Figure 8-2).

Coenzyme Q is a shuttle between complexes I and II and complex III. A defect of coenzyme Q has been recorded in only one newborn with seizures, abnormal ocular movements, and lactic acidosis.

The clinical syndromes associated with mitochondrial disorders are continually expanding and revised. The organs affected are those highly dependent on aerobic metabolism: nervous system, skeletal muscle, heart, and kidney (Table 8-5). Exercise intolerance, either alone or in combination with symptoms of other organ failure, is a common feature of mitochondrial disorders. Although several clinical syndromes have been defined, they do not correspond exactly with any one of the respiratory complexes (Table 8-6).

CLINICAL FEATURES. The age at which mitochondrial myopathies begin ranges from birth to adult life but is before 20 in most patients. Half of patients have ptosis or ophthalmoplegia, one fourth have exertional complaints in the limbs, and one fourth have cerebral dysfunction. With time, considerable overlap occurs among the three groups. Seventy-five percent eventually have ophthalmoplegia, and 50% have exertional complaints. Pigmentary retinopathy occurs in 33% and neuropathy in 25%.

Exercise intolerance usually develops by 10 years of age. With ordinary activity, active muscles become tight, weak, and painful. Cramps and myoglobinuria are unusual but may occur. Nausea, headache, and breathlessness are sometimes associated features. During these episodes

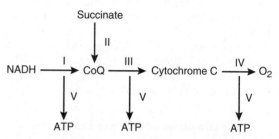

Figure 8-2. Respiratory complexes. complex I (NADH-coenzyme Q reductase); complex II (succinate-coenzyme Q reductase); complex III (reduced coenzyme Q-cytochrome *c* reductase); complex IV (cytochrome *c* oxidase); complex V (ATP synthase).

Table 8-5
Clinical Features of Mitochondrial Disease

Nervous System
Ataxia
Central apnea
Deafness
Dementia
Hypotonia
Mental retardation
Neuropathy
Ophthalmoplegia
Optic atrophy
Retinitis pigmentosa

Heart
Cardiomyopathy
Conduction defects

Kidney
Aminoaciduria
Hyperphosphaturia

Skeletal Muscle
Exercise intolerance
Myopathy

Table 8-6
Mitochondrial Disorders

Complex I (NADH-Coenzyme Q Reductase)
Congenital lactic acidosis, hypotonia, seizures, and apnea
Exercise intolerance and myalgia
Kearns-Sayre syndrome (see Chapter 15)
Metabolic encephalopathy, lactic acidosis, and stroke (see Chapter 11)
Progressive infantile poliodystrophy (see Chapter 5)
Subacute necrotizing encephalomyelopathy (see Chapter 5)

Complex II (Succinate-Coenzyme Q Reductase)
Encephalomyopathy (?)

Complex III (Coenzyme QH$_2$-Cytochrome *c* Reductase)
Cardiomyopathy
Kearns-Sayre syndrome (see Chapter 15)
Myopathy and exercise intolerance with or without progressive external ophthalmoplegia

Complex IV (Cytochrome *c* Oxidase)
Fatal neonatal hypotonia (see Chapter 6)
Menkes syndrome (see Chapter 5)
Myoclonus epilepsy and ragged red fibers
Progressive infantile poliodystrophy (see Chapter 5)
Subacute necrotizing encephalomyelopathy (see Chapter 5)
Transitory neonatal hypotonia (see Chapter 6)

Complex V (Adenosine Triphosphate Synthase)
Congenital myopathy
Neuropathy, retinopathy, ataxia, and dementia
Retinitis pigmentosa, ataxia, neuropathy, and dementia

the serum concentration of lactate and CK may increase. Generalized weakness with ptosis and ophthalmoplegia may follow prolonged periods of activity or fasting. Such symptoms may last for several days, but recovery is usually complete.

DIAGNOSIS. A mitochondrial myopathy should be considered in all children with exercise intolerance and ptosis or ophthalmoplegia. This combination of symptoms may also suggest myasthenia gravis. However, in myasthenia the ocular motor features fluctuate, while in mitochondrial myopathies they are constant.

Some children with mitochondrial myopathies have an increased concentration of serum lactate after exercise. An easy-to-perform test is the glucose-lactate tolerance test. During an ordinary oral glucose tolerance test, lactate and glucose determinations are made at the same time. In some children with mitochondrial disorders, lactic acidoses develops and glucose is slow to clear.

Muscle biopsy specimens show a clumping of the mitochondria, which become red when the Gomori trichrome stain is applied (Figure 8-3). These muscle cells are called *ragged-red fibers*. Commercial laboratories can identify several specific respiratory complex disturbances.

MANAGEMENT. Treatment with a "cocktail" that includes riboflavin, ubiquinone, vitamin C, menadione, and niacin is popular but has no established benefit.

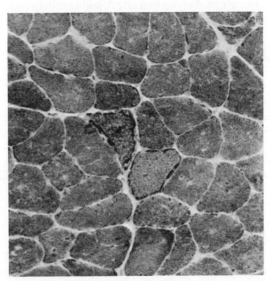

Figure 8-3. Ragged-red fibers (trichrome stain). The mitochondria are enlarged and stain intensely with hematoxylin.

Myoadenylate Deaminase Deficiency

The gene for the muscle form of adenosine monophosphate deaminase is encoded on chromosome 1p. Deficiency of myoadenylate deaminase is clearly a familial trait, and the mode of inheritance is probably autosomal recessive. The deficiency state has been shown in infants with hypotonia, in children with progressive myopathies and recurrent rhabdomyolysis, in children and adults with exercise intolerance, and in asymptomatic individuals. Establishing a cause-and-effect relationship between myoadenylate deaminase deficiency and exercise intolerance in any particular individual is often difficult because most people with the deficiency state are asymptomatic.

CLINICAL FEATURES. The typical history is one of intermittent muscle pain and weakness with exercise. The pain varies from a diffuse aching to a severe cramping type associated with muscle tenderness and swelling. Between attacks the children are normal. Symptoms last for 1 to 20 years, with a mean duration of less than 9 years.

DIAGNOSIS. During attacks the serum concentration of CK may be normal or markedly elevated. EMG and muscle histological studies are usually normal. The diagnosis is suggested by the forearm exercise test. Patients with myoadenylate deaminase deficiency fail to generate ammonia but show normal elevations of lactate. However, ammonia levels may fail to rise even in normal individuals, and enzyme analysis of muscle is required for diagnosis.

Obligate heterozygotes have a reduced concentration of myoadenylate deaminase in muscle but are capable of normal ammonia production and are asymptomatic.

MANAGEMENT. Treatment is not available.

Myopathic Stiffness and Cramps

This section deals with several conditions that cause muscle stiffness or cramps, or both, in which the primary abnormality is thought to be in skeletal muscle.

Brody Myopathy

The autosomal recessive, but not the autosomal dominant, form of Brody myopathy is caused by a mutation in the gene (16p12) that encodes the fast-twitch skeletal muscle calcium-activated ATPase in sarcoplasmic reticulum (Odermatt et al, 1997)

CLINICAL FEATURES. The main clinical feature is difficulty of relaxation after contraction. Myotonia is suspected but not supported by EMG. Symptoms of exercise-induced stiffness and cramping begin in the first decade and become progressively worse with age. Unlike myotonia, stiffness becomes worse rather than better with continued exercise. Exercise can be resumed after a period of rest. Muscle strength and tendon reflexes are normal.

DIAGNOSIS. Patients with Brody disease are thought to have myotonia, but the cramps are not shown on EMG, suggesting myophosphorylase deficiency. Muscle histology reveals type II atrophy. The diagnosis is established only by showing the biochemical defect.

MANAGEMENT. Dantrolene, which reduces the myofibrillar Ca^{2+} concentration by blocking Ca^{2+} release from the sarcoplasmic reticulum, provides symptomatic relief. Verapamil may also be useful.

Cramps and Tubular Aggregates

Tubular aggregates are abnormal double-walled structures that originate from the sarcoplasmic reticulum and are located in a subsarcolemmal position (Figure 8-4). They are found in muscle biopsy specimens from patients with a variety of neuromuscular disorders. In some families there is progressive myopathy, and in others there is only cramps or myalgia.

Sporadic Cases

CLINICAL FEATURES. Onset is usually in the second or third decade. Cramps may occur at rest or be induced by exercise. Thigh and calf muscles are usually affected and become swollen, stiff, and tender. Cramping occurs more often in cold weather and may also occur at night, interfering with sleep. Myalgia is present between cramps.

Episodic stiffness of the mouth and tongue interferes with speech. Cramps are not associated with myoglobinuria. Muscle mass, strength, and tendon reflexes are normal.

DIAGNOSIS. The serum concentration of CK is normal. EMG results are normal except that in some patients the cramps are electrically silent. Muscle histology results are the basis for a diagnosis. Light and electron microscopic examinations show tubular aggregates in type II fibers.

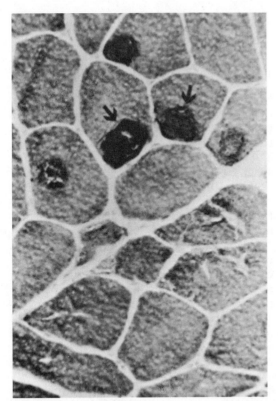

Figure 8-4. Tubular aggregates (ATPase reaction). Dark material is present beneath the sarcolemma in type I and type II fibers (*arrows*).

No evidence of glycogen or lipid storage is present.

MANAGEMENT. The cramps do not respond to medication.

Autosomal Dominant Cases

CLINICAL FEATURES. Muscle aches, cramps, and proximal weakness begin in the second decade. The cramps are exercise induced but also may occur at rest and during sleep. The legs are usually more severely affected than the arms, but the pattern of cramping varies from family to family. Weakness, when it occurs, is mild and progresses slowly.

DIAGNOSIS. The serum concentration of CK is moderately elevated. EMG results suggest a myopathic process in some families and a neuropathic process in others. Muscle biopsy may show tubular aggregates in type I and type II fibers. Type I fiber predominance and type II hypotrophy are present in some patients.

TREATMENT. No treatment is available for either the myopathy or the cramps.

Familial X-Linked Myalgia and Cramps

Familial X-linked myalgia and cramps is another phenotype associated with a decreased amount of skeletal muscle dystrophin, which is usually associated with Becker muscular dystrophy (see Chapter 7). Almost all cases are male (Samaha and Quinlan, 1996), except for one female who also had hypertrophy of the calves (Malapart et al, 1995). Half of the males and the one female showed a deletion in the dystrophin gene.

CLINICAL FEATURES. Symptoms begin in early childhood, frequently between 4 and 6 years of age. The boys first have cramps with exercise and then cramps at rest. Usually the limb muscles are affected, but chest pain may occur as well. The cramping continues throughout life but is not associated with atrophy or weakness. Tendon reflexes are normal.

DIAGNOSIS. Affected family members have elevated concentrations of serum CK, especially after exercise. The EMG and muscle biopsy are usually normal or show only mild, nonspecific changes. This disorder and the *McLeod phenotype* (acanthocytosis, elevated serum concentration of CK, and absence of the Kell antigen) may be allelic conditions. EMG and muscle biopsy show nonspecific myopathic changes. DNA analysis may be normal or may show a deletion either in the first third of the dystrophin gene or in exons 45–52.

MANAGEMENT. Phenytoin, carbamazepine, and nifedipine do not relieve the cramps. Exercise avoidance is the only way to avoid cramping.

Malignant Hyperthermia

Malignant hyperthermia (MH) is a disorder of calcium regulation in skeletal muscle. It is transmitted as an autosomal dominant trait. Susceptibility was first localized to chromosome 19q13.1 and the skeletal muscle ryanodine receptor. However, MH proved to be genetically heterogeneous, with additional loci on chromosomes 17q, 7q, and 3q. Several neuromuscular disorders, such as carnitine palmitoyl transferase deficiency 2, muscular dystrophy, and central core disease, are known to predispose to the syndrome. Attacks of muscular rigidity and necrosis in association with a rapid rise in body temperature are triggered by the administration of several inhalation anesthetics or by succinylcholine. Nonanesthetic triggers of rhabdomyolysis in susceptible persons include severe exercise in hot conditions, neuroleptic drugs, alcohol, and infections.

CLINICAL FEATURES. The first symptoms are tachycardia, tachypnea, muscle fasciculations, and increasing muscle tone. Body temperature rises dramatically, as much as 2° C per hour. All muscles become rigid, and a progressive and severe metabolic acidosis develops. Seizures and death may occur if the patient is not treated promptly.

DIAGNOSIS. The diagnosis is based on the response to anesthesia or succinylcholine. The serum concentration of CK rises to 10 times the upper limit of normal. No reliable test for identifying susceptible individuals is available.

MANAGEMENT. Treatment includes termination of anesthesia, body cooling, treatment of metabolic acidosis, and intravenous injection of dantrolene, 1 to 2 mg/kg, which may be repeated every 5 to 10 minutes up to a total dose of 10 mg/kg. When malignant hyperthermia is suspected, pretreatment with dantrolene before an anesthetic is used.

Neuroleptic Malignant Syndrome

Neuroleptic malignant syndrome, like MH, is a disorder of the skeletal muscle calcium channels.

CLINICAL FEATURES. Several neuroleptic agents may induce an idiosyncratic response characterized by muscle rigidity, hyperthermia, altered states of consciousness, and autonomic dysfunction in susceptible individuals. Phenothiazines, butyrophenones, and thioxanthenes have all been implicated. Persons of all ages have been affected, but young men predominantly. Symptoms develop over 1 to 3 days. The first symptoms are rigidity and akinesia, followed by fever, excessive sweating, urinary incontinence, and hypertension. Consciousness fluctuates, and the 20% mortality rate is due to respiratory failure.

DIAGNOSIS. The diagnosis is based primarily on clinical findings. The only helpful laboratory test results are an increased serum concentration of CK and a leukocytosis.

MANAGEMENT. The offending neuroleptic agent must be promptly withdrawn and general supportive care provided. Bromocriptine reverses the syndrome completely.

Rigid Spine Syndrome

Rigid spine syndrome encompasses a heterogeneous group of disorders. The phenotype has been associated with a merosin-positive congenital muscular dystrophy (see Chapter 6) and

with Emery-Dreifuss muscular dystrophy (see Chapter 7).

Rippling Muscle Disease

Several families are reported under different titles in which mechanical stimulation produces electrically silent contractions. The disorder is transmitted by autosomal dominant inheritance, and the responsible gene is localized to chromosome 1q in some families. It is a disorder of skeletal muscle calcium channels that is different from the defects causing MH and the neuroleptic malignant syndrome (Stephan and Hoffman, 1999).

CLINICAL FEATURES. The onset of symptoms is usually in the second decade. Muscle pain and cramps follow exercise and persist for several hours. Stiffness occurs during rest after the patient exercises or maintains posture for long periods. Percussion of muscles causes local swelling and a peculiar rippling movement that lasts for 10 to 20 seconds. Muscle hypertrophy develops. Muscle strength, tone, and coordination, as well as tendon reflexes, are normal.

DIAGNOSIS. The serum CK concentration is mildly elevated, and muscle biopsy findings are normal. EMG of the muscle swelling after percussion does not show any electrical activity.

MANAGEMENT. No treatment is available.

References

Barchi RL. Phenotype and genotype in the myotonic disorders. *Muscle Nerve* 1998;21:1119–1121.

Barker RA, Revesz T, Thom M, et al. Review of 23 patients affected by the stiff man syndrome: Clinical subdivision into stiff trunk (man) syndrome, stiff limb syndrome, and progressive encephalomyelitis with rigidity. *J Neurol Neurosurg Psychiatry* 1998;65:633–640.

Giedion A, Boltshauser E, Briner J, et al. Heterogeneity in Schwartz-Jampel chondrodystrophic myotonia. *Eur J Pediatr* 1997;156:214–223.

Hudson AJ, Ebers GC, Bulman DE. The skeletal muscle sodium and chloride channel diseases. *Brain* 1995;118:547–563.

Kissel JT, Elble RJ. Stiff-person syndrome. Stiff opposition to a simple explanation. *Neurology* 1998;51:11–14.

Malapart D, Recan D, Leturcq F, et al. Sporadic lower limb hypertrophy and exercise induced myalgia in a woman with dystrophin gene deletion. *J Neurol Neurosurg Psychiatry* 1995;59:552–554.

Odermatt A, Taschner PEM, Scherer SW, et al. Characterization of the gene encoding human sarcolipin (SLN), a proteolipid associated with SERCA1: Absence of structural mutations in five patients with Brody disease. *Genomics* 1997;45:541–553.

Stephan DA, Hoffman EP. Physical mapping of the rippling muscle disease locus. *Genomics* 1999;55:268–274.

Samaha FJ, Quinlan JG. Myalgia and cramps: Dystrophinopathy with wide-ranging laboratory findings. *J Child Neurol* 1996;11:21–24.

Shillito P, Molenaar PC, Vincent A, et al. Acquired neuromyotonia: Evidence for autoantibodies directed against K⁺ channels of peripheral nerves. *Ann Neurol* 1995;38: 714–722.

Straussberg R, Harel L, Varsano I, et al. Recurrent myoglobinuria as a presenting feature of very long chain acyl coenzyme A dehydrogenase deficiency. *Pediatrics* 1997; 93:894–896.

Torbergsen T, Stålberg E, Brautaset NJ. Generator sites for spontaneous activity in neuromyotonia. An EMG study. *Electroencephalogr Clin Neurophysiol* 1996;101: 69–78.

Vorgerd M, Grehl T, Jäger M, et al. Creatine therapy in myophosphorylace deficiency (McArdle disease). A placebo-controlled crossover trial. *Arch Neurol* 2000; 57:956–963.

Chapter 9
Sensory and Autonomic Disturbances

THIS CHAPTER DEALS primarily with sensory disturbances of the limbs and trunk. Autonomic dysfunction is often associated with sensory loss but sometimes occurs alone. Sensory disturbances of the face are considered in Chapter 17.

Sensory Symptoms

The important symptoms of disturbed sensation are pain, dysesthesias, and loss of sensibility. Peripheral neuropathy is the most common cause of disturbed sensation at any age. As a rule, hereditary neuropathies are more likely to cause loss of sensibility without discomfort, whereas acquired neuropathies are more likely to be painful. Discomfort is more likely than numbness to bring a patient to medical attention.

Nerve root pain generally follows the course of a dermatome and is ordinarily described as deep and aching. The pain is more proximal than distal and may be constant or intermittent. When intermittent, the pain may radiate in a dermatomal distribution. The most common cause of root pain in adults is sciatica associated with lumbar disk disease. Disk disease also occurs in adolescents, usually because of trauma. In children, root pain is more commonly caused by radiculitis. Examples of radiculitis are the migratory aching of a limb preceding paralysis in the Guillain-Barré syndrome (see Chapter 7) and the radiating pain in a C5 distribution that heralds an idiopathic brachial neuritis (see Chapter 13).

Polyneuropathy involving small nerve fibers causes dysesthetic pain. This pain differs from previously experienced discomfort and is described as pins and needles, tingling, or burning.

Table 9-1
Patterns of Sensory Loss

Pattern	Site
All limbs	Spinal cord or peripheral nerve
Both legs	Spinal cord or peripheral nerve
Glove-and-stocking	Peripheral nerve
Legs and trunk	Spinal cord
One arm	Plexus
One leg	Plexus or spinal cord
Unilateral arm and leg	Brain or spinal cord

It is often compared to the abnormal sensation felt when dental anesthesia is wearing off. The discomfort is superficial, distal, and usually symmetric. Dysesthetic pain is never a feature of hereditary neuropathies in children.

Loss of sensibility is the sole initial feature in children with sensory neuropathy. Diagnosis is often delayed because clumsiness is the initial feature and strength is normal, as are tests of cerebellar function. Tendon reflexes are absent. The combination of areflexia and clumsiness should suggest a sensory neuropathy.

The pattern of sensory loss as a guide to the anatomical site of abnormality is summarized in Table 9-1.

Brachial Neuritis

Three painful arm syndromes are acute idiopathic brachial neuritis (also called *neuralgic amyotrophy* or *brachial plexitis*), familial recurrent brachial neuritis, and complex regional pain syndrome (*reflex sympathetic dystrophy*). In the first two syndromes, transitory pain in the shoulder or arm is followed by muscle atrophy.

Monoplegia is the prominent feature (see Chapter 13). Although muscle atrophy also occurs in complex regional pain syndrome, pain is the prominent feature. This syndrome is discussed later in this chapter.

Complex Regional Pain Syndrome I

A working group of the International Association for the Study of Pain developed a new terminology (Rowbotham, 1998) that separates reflex sympathetic dystrophy (RSD) from causalgia. *Complex regional pain syndrome (CRPS) I* replaces the term RSD and is defined as "a pain syndrome that develops after an injury, is not limited to the distribution of a single peripheral nerve, and is disproportional to the inciting event." CRPS II requires demonstrable peripheral nerve injury and replaces the term *causalgia*.

CLINICAL FEATURES. The essential feature of CRPS I is sustained burning pain in a limb combined with vasomotor and pseudomotor dysfunction, leading to atrophic changes in skin, muscle, and bone following trauma. The mechanism remains a debated issue, and several different central and peripheral mechanisms probably produce the same result.

The mean age at onset in children is 11 years, and girls are affected more often than boys. CRPS I frequently follows trauma to one limb, with or without fracture. The trauma may be relatively minor, and the clinical syndrome is so unusual that many affected individuals are first labeled "hysterical" or "malingering." Time until onset after injury is usually within 1 or 2 months, but the average interval from injury to diagnosis is 1 year.

The first symptom is pain at the site of injury, which progresses either proximally or distally without regard for dermatomal distribution or anatomical landmarks. Generalized swelling and vasomotor disturbances of the limb follow in 80% of children. Pain is intense, described as burning or aching, and is out of proportion to the injury. It may be maximally severe at onset or may become progressively worse for 3 to 6 months. Movement or dependence exacerbates the pain, causing the arm to be held in a position of abduction and internal rotation, as if it is swaddled to the body. The hand becomes swollen and hyperesthetic and feels warmer than normal.

Children with CRPS I do better than adults. Reported outcomes vary widely, probably based on the standard of diagnosis. In my own experience, most begin recovering within 6 to 12 months. Long-term pain is unusual, as are the trophic changes of the skin and bones that often occur in adults. Recovery is usually complete, and recurrence is unusual.

DIAGNOSIS. The diagnosis is based on the clinical features and cannot be confirmed by laboratory tests. Because the syndrome follows accidental or surgical trauma, litigation is commonplace, and careful documentation of the examination is needed. One simple test is to immerse the affected limb in warm water. Wrinkling of the skin of the fingers or toes requires intact sympathetic innervation. The absence of wrinkling is evidence of a lesion in either the central or the peripheral sympathetic pathway. The other unaffected limb is used as a control.

MANAGEMENT. Most children can be managed with range of motion exercise and over-the-counter analgesics. Treatment of more severe syndromes, as occur in adults, includes the oral administration of guanethidine, anticonvulsants, gabapentin (Wheeler et al, 2000), prednisone with or without stellate ganglion blockade, and sympathectomy. No specific treatment modality is established as effective (Hooshmand and Hashmi, 1999).

Congenital Insensitivity (Indifference) to Pain

Most children with congenital insensitivity to pain have a hereditary sensory neuropathy. Specific tests for sensory neuropathy and complete postmortem examinations were not performed in many early reports of this condition. This section is restricted to those children and families with congenital insensitivity to pain in whom sensory neuropathy was excluded and a central defect was at fault. Mild mental retardation is often associated. Several affected children are siblings with consanguineous parents. Autosomal recessive inheritance is therefore suspected. The Lesch-Nyhan syndrome is a specific metabolic disorder characterized by self-mutilation (presumably because of indifference to pain) and mental retardation without evidence of sensory neuropathy (see Chapter 5).

CLINICAL FEATURES. Children with congenital insensitivity to pain come to medical attention when they begin to crawl or walk. Their parents recognize that injuries do not cause crying and that the children fail to learn the potential of injury from experience. The result is repeated bruising, fractures, ulcerations of the fingers and toes, and mutilation of the tongue. Sunburn and frostbite are common.

Examination shows absence of the corneal reflex and insensitivity to pain and temperature but relative preservation of touch and vibration sensations. Tendon reflexes are present, an important differential point from sensory neuropathy.

DIAGNOSIS. The results of electromyography (EMG), nerve conduction studies, and examination of the cerebrospinal fluid are normal.

MANAGEMENT. No treatment is available for the underlying insensitivity, but supportive care is needed for the repeated injuries. Life is shortened by injuries and recurrent infections.

Foramen Magnum Tumors

Extramedullary tumors in and around the foramen magnum are known for false localizing signs and for mimicking other disorders, especially syringomyelia and multiple sclerosis. In children, neurofibroma caused by neurofibromatosis is the only tumor found in this location.

CLINICAL FEATURES. The most common initial symptom is unilateral or bilateral dysesthesias of the fingers. Suboccipital or neck pain occurs as well. These symptoms are often ignored early in the course. Numbness and tingling usually begin in one hand and then migrate to the other. Dysesthesias in the feet are a late occurrence. Gait disturbances, incoordination of the hands, and bladder disturbances generally follow the sensory symptoms and are so alarming that they prompt medical consultation.

Many patients have café au lait spots, but few have evidence of subcutaneous neuromas. Weakness may be confined to one arm, one side, or both legs; 25% of patients have weakness in all limbs. Atrophy of the hands is uncommon. Sensory loss may involve only one segment or may have a "cape" distribution. Pain and temperature are usually diminished, and other sensory disturbances may be present. Tendon reflexes are brisk in the arms and legs. Patients with neurofibromatosis may have multiple neurofibromas causing segmental abnormalities in several levels of the spinal cord.

DIAGNOSIS. Magnetic resonance imaging (MRI) is the best method for showing abnormalities at the foramen magnum.

MANAGEMENT. Symptoms can be relieved completely by surgical excision of a neurofibroma of the C2 root.

Hereditary Metabolic Neuropathies

Acute Intermittent Porphyria

Acute intermittent porphyria is inherited as an autosomal dominant disorder that results from an error in pyrrole metabolism due to deficiency of porphobilinogen (PBG) deaminase. The gene location is 11q23.3. Individuals with similar degrees of enzyme deficiency may have considerable variation in phenotypic expression (Puy et al, 1997).

CLINICAL FEATURES. Approximately 90% of individuals with acute intermittent porphyria never have clinical symptoms. Those who do rarely have symptoms before puberty. Symptoms are periodic and occur at irregular intervals. The attacks are triggered by alterations in hormonal levels during a normal menstrual cycle or pregnancy and by exposure to certain drugs, especially barbiturates. The most common clinical feature of acute intermittent porphyria is an attack of severe abdominal pain, often associated with vomiting, constipation, or diarrhea. Tachycardia, hypertension, and fever may be associated. Pain in the limbs is common, and muscle weakness often develops. The weakness is a result of a motor neuropathy that causes greater weakness in proximal than distal muscles and in the arms more than the legs. Tendon reflexes are usually decreased and may be absent in weak muscles. Approximately half of the patients have symptoms of cerebral dysfunction; mental changes are particularly common, and seizures can sometimes occur. Chronic mental symptoms, such as depression and anxiety, sometimes continue even between attacks.

DIAGNOSIS. Acute intermittent porphyria should be suspected in people with acute or episodic neurological or psychiatric disturbances. Increased amounts of amino-levulinic acid and PBG are excreted during attacks, but levels may be normal between attacks. Definitive diagnosis requires measurment of PBG deaminase activity in erythrocytes. The risk of attacks correlates with the excretion of PBG in the urine when the patient is free of symptoms.

MANAGEMENT. The most important aspect of managing symptomatic disease is to prevent acute attacks. This is done in part by avoiding known precipitating factors. During an attack, patients frequently need to be hospitalized because of severe pain. Carbohydrates are believed to reduce porphyrin synthesis and should be administered intravenously daily at a dose of 300 to 500 g as a 10% dextrose solution.

Haem-arginate and cimetidine have been used for prophylactic therapy (Rogers, 1997).

Hereditary Tyrosinemia

Hereditary tyrosinemia type I, caused by deficiency of the enzyme fumarylacetoacetate hydrolase, is transmitted by autosomal recessive inheritance.

CLINICAL FEATURES. The major features are acute and chronic liver failure and a renal Fanconi syndrome. However, recurrent attacks of painful dysesthesias or paralysis are a prominent feature of the disease in half of children.

The attacks usually begin at 1 year of age and are preceded by an infection in half of the cases. Perhaps because of the child's age, the pain is poorly localized to the legs and lower abdomen. Associated with the pain is axial hypertonicity that ranges in severity from mild neck stiffness to opisthotonus. Generalized weakness occurs in 30% of attacks and may necessitate respiratory support. Less common features of attacks are seizures and self-mutilation. Between attacks, the child appears normal.

DIAGNOSIS. The diagnosis of hereditary tyrosinemia is based on showing an increased blood concentration of tyrosine and a deficiency of fumarylacetoacetate hydrolase. The crises are caused in part by an acute axonal neuropathy that can be shown by EMG studies. Succinylacetone, a metabolite of tyrosine, accumulates and inhibits porphyrin metabolism. Increased urinary excretion of gamma-aminolevulinic acid is present in both acute intermittent porphyria and hereditary tyrosinemia.

MANAGEMENT. Ninety percent of patients treated with the drug 2-(2-nitro-4-trifluoromethylbenzoyl)-1,3-cyclohexanedione (NTBC) have shown a favorable response (Holme and Lindstedt, 1998). Liver transplantation is the definitive treatment.

Hereditary Sensory and Autonomic Neuropathy

The classification of hereditary sensory and autonomic neuropathy (HSAN) attempts to syn-

---

Table 9-2
Disturbances of Sensation

Brachial Neuritis
Neuralgic amyotrophy (see Chapter 13)
Recurrent familial brachial neuropathy (see Chapter 13)

Complex Regional Pain Syndrome I (Reflex Sympathetic Dystrophy)

Congenital Insensitivity (Indifference) to Pain
Lesch-Nyhan syndrome
Mental retardation
With normal nervous system

Foramen Magnum Tumors

Hereditary Metabolic Neuropathies
Acute intermittent porphyria
Hereditary tyrosinemia

Hereditary Sensory and Autonomic Neuropathy (HSAN)
HSAN I (autosomal dominant)
HSAN II (autosomal recessive)
HSAN III (familial dysautonomia)
HSAN IV (with anhydrosis)
HSAN with spastic paraplegia

Lumbar Disk Herniation

Syringomyelia

Thalamic Syndromes

---

thesize information based on natural history, mode of inheritance, and electrophysiological characteristics. Table 9-2 provides a list of HSANs. Many of these phenotypes may be caused by several different genetic errors. In addition to the condition listed, several other disorders are described whose genetic status remains uncertain. Among these is *congenital sensory neuropathy with selective loss of small myelinated fibers*, classified as *HSAN V*, in which pain fibers are lost selectively.

Hereditary Sensory and Autonomic Neuropathy Type I

Hereditary sensory and autonomic neuropathy type I (HSAN I) appears in the literature under several names, most commonly *hereditary sensory radiculoneuropathy*. Transmission is by autosomal dominant inheritance. As with other dominantly inherited neuropathies, variable expression is the rule. Therefore, the history alone is insufficient to determine whether the parents are affected; physical examination and electrophysiological studies are required. HSAN type I has been mapped to chromosome 9q22.1-22.3.

CLINICAL FEATURES. Symptoms begin during the second decade or later. The major clinical features are lancinating pains in the legs and ulcerations of the feet. However, initial symptoms are usually insidious, and the precise onset is often difficult to date. A callus develops on the sole of the foot, usually in the skin overlying a weight-bearing bony prominence. The callus blackens, becomes necrotic, and breaks down into an ulcer that is difficult to heal. The ulcer is preceded by sensory loss, but often it is the ulcer, and not the sensory loss, that first brings the patient to medical attention. Although plantar ulcers are an important feature, they are not essential for diagnosis. Most patients with HSAN I do not have ulcers. When the proband has typical features of plantar ulcers and lancinating pain, other family members may have sensory loss in the feet, mild pes cavus or peroneal atrophy, and loss of the ankle tendon reflex.

Sensory loss in the feet is a constant feature, whereas sensory loss in the hands is variable. The hands are never affected as severely as the feet, and finger ulcers do not occur. The sensations of pain and temperature are lost before the sensations of touch and pressure. In some patients the dissociation of sensory loss is constant, whereas in others the dissociation is only a first stage before the development of global sensory loss. The ankle tendon reflex is absent, and the quadriceps tendon reflex may also be absent. Tendon reflexes in the arms are preserved.

Foot ulcers are caused by trauma to the insensitive skin of the feet. They occur more often and are more difficult to heal in boys than in girls, in individuals who wear ill-fitting shoes, and in individuals who are on their feet much of the day. Lancinating pain is a late occurrence. It comes as recurring attacks usually affecting a single arm or leg. Other limbs may be affected on subsequent days. The intensity of pain varies.

DIAGNOSIS. Autosomal dominant inheritance and sensory loss in the feet are essential for the diagnosis. The presence of plantar ulcers and lancinating pain is helpful but not critical for the diagnosis. HSAN I can be differentiated from familial amyloid polyneuropathy on clinical grounds. Urinary incontinence, impotence, and postural hypotension are frequent features of amyloidosis but do not occur in HSAN I.

Electrophysiological studies show slowing of sensory nerve conduction velocity and the absence sensory nerve action potentials. Sural nerve biopsy reveals a marked decrease or absence of myelinated fibers and a mild to moderate reduction of small myelinated fibers.

MANAGEMENT. No treatment is available for the neuropathy, but plantar ulcers can be prevented by good foot care. Tight shoes and activities that cause trauma to the feet should be avoided. Weight bearing must be discontinued at the first sign of a plantar ulcer. Much of the foot mutilation reported in previous years was due to secondary infection of the ulcers. Infection can be avoided by the use of warm soaks, elevation, and antibiotics.

Hereditary Sensory and Autonomic Neuropathy Type II

Hereditary sensory and autonomic neuropathy type II (HSAN II) probably includes several disorders transmitted by autosomal recessive inheritance. No chromosomal linkage has been identified. Some cases are relatively static, and others have a progressive course. Many of the cases are sporadic, instances of parental consanguinity have been reported, and siblings are affected in some families.

CLINICAL FEATURES. Symptoms probably begin during infancy and possibly at the time of birth. Infantile hypotonia is common (see Chapter 6). Unlike HSAN I, which affects primarily the feet, HSAN II involves the arms and legs equally, as well as the trunk and forehead. The result is a diffuse loss of all sensation; touch and pressure are probably affected earlier and to a greater extent than temperature and pain. Affected infants and children are constantly hurting themselves without a painful response and are sometimes believed to have congenital absence of pain. The absence of the protection that pain provides against injury results in ulcerations and infections of the fingers and toes, stress fractures, and injuries to long bones. Loss of deep sensibility causes injury and swelling of joints, and loss of touch makes simple tasks, such as tying shoes, manipulating small objects, and buttoning buttons, difficult if not impossible. Tendon reflexes are absent throughout. Sweating is diminished in all areas of decreased sensibility, but no other features of autonomic dysfunction are present.

HSAN II may be associated with impaired hearing, taste, and smell, with retinitis pigmentosa, or with the early onset of cataracts. It is not clear whether such cases represent separate genetic disorders or are part of the phenotypic spectrum of a single genetic disorder.

DIAGNOSIS. The diagnosis relies primarily on the history and examination. Absence of sensory nerve action potentials confirms that the congenital absence of pain is due to peripheral neuropathy and not to a cerebral abnormality. Motor nerve conduction velocities are normal, as are the morphological characteristics of motor unit potentials. Fibrillations are sometimes present. Sural nerve biopsy reveals an almost complete absence of myelinated fibers.

The boundary between HSAN II and HSAN IV (discussed later) is difficult to delineate. Mental retardation and anhydrosis are more prominent in HSAN IV than in HSAN II.

MANAGEMENT. No treatment is available for the neuropathy. However, parents must be vigilant for painless injuries. Discoloration of the skin and swelling of joints or limbs should raise the possibility of fracture. Children must be taught to avoid activities that might cause injury and to examine themselves for signs of superficial infection.

Hereditary Sensory and Autonomic Neuropathy Type III

Hereditary sensory and autonomic neuropathy type III (HSAN III) is ordinarily referred to as *familial dysautonomia* or the *Riley-Day syndrome*. This disorder is present at birth. Cardinal features are hypotonia, feeding difficulties, and poor control of autonomic function. Because neonatal hypotonia is prominent, the disorder is discussed in Chapter 6.

Hereditary Sensory and Autonomic Neuropathy Type IV

Hereditary sensory and autonomic neuropathy type IV (HSAN IV) is probably a heterogeneous group of disorders transmitted by autosomal recessive inheritance. The major features are congenital insensitivity to pain, anhidrosis, and mental retardation. All the clinical abnormalities are present at birth, and although complications of the pain-free state are a continuous problem, the underlying disease may not be progressive.

CLINICAL FEATURES. The initial symptoms are usually caused by anhidrosis rather than insensitivity to pain. Affected infants have repeated episodes of fever, sometimes associated with seizures. These episodes usually occur during the summer and are caused by the inability to sweat in response to exogenous heat. Sweat glands are present in the skin but lack sympathetic innervation. Most infants are hypotonic and areflexic. Developmental milestones are attained slowly, and by 2 or 3 years of age the child has had several self-inflicted injuries caused by pain insensitivity. Injuries may include ulcers of the fingers and toes, stress fractures, self-mutilation of the tongue, and Charcot joints.

Sensory examination shows widespread absence of pain and temperature sensation. Touch, vibration, and stereognosis are intact in some patients. Tendon reflexes are absent or hypoactive. The cranial nerves are intact and the corneal reflex and lacrimation are normal. Mild to moderate retardation is present in almost every case. Other features, present in some children, are blond hair and fair skin, Horner syndrome, and aplasia of dental enamel.

DIAGNOSIS. Familial dysautonomia (HSAN III) and HSAN IV have many features in common and are easily confused. However, insensitivity to pain is not prominent in HSAN III, and fungiform papillae of the tongue are present in HSAN IV. Anhidrotic ectodermal dysplasia is another hereditary disorder that shares many features with HSAN IV. Affected children also have unexplained fevers and abnormalities of tooth formation. However, children with ectodermal dysplasia are anhidrotic because sweat glands are absent. The nervous system is intact, and sensation to pain is present. Diagnosis of HSAN IV depends primarily on the clinical features but can be confirmed by demonstrating the absence of sensory evoked potentials, the absence of an axon reflex when histamine is injected into the skin, and the presence of sweat glands on skin biopsy specimens.

MANAGEMENT. No treatment is available for the underlying disease. However, constant vigilance is required to prevent injuries to the skin and bones with secondary infection.

Hereditary Sensory and Autonomic Neuropathy with Spastic Paraplegia

Most cases of hereditary sensory and autonomic neuropathy with spastic paraplegia have occurred in siblings, and autosomal recessive inheritance is suspected. Some patients with HSAN I or HSAN II have mild signs of corticospinal tract dysfunction, such as brisk reflexes and extensor plantar responses, but it is reasonable to consider these cases separately the present.

CLINICAL FEATURES. The initial clinical feature may be progressive sensory neuropathy or spasticity. Eventually, the sensory symptoms affect all modalities and cause disability. Children with early spasticity have a stiff-legged gait during infancy or early childhood and delayed motor milestones. Tendon reflexes in the legs are increased, plantar responses are extensor, and sphincter control may not be attained.

Relative insensitivity to pain is the initial feature of the sensory neuropathy. This is characterized by repeated episodes of injury, ulcerations of the fingers and toes, and fractures. Pain and temperature sensations are much more severely affected than are the sensations of touch and vibration. Intelligence is normal, and cranial nerves are unaffected. As the neuropathy becomes more profound, tendon reflexes, which initially were brisk, become depressed and are lost.

When the disease begins during infancy or early childhood, the course is relentlessly progressive and may lead to early death. Disease with onset in the second decade has a slower progression.

DIAGNOSIS. A diagnosis cannot be established during early stages of the disease when spastic paraplegia is present but neuropathy is not. The development of insensitivity to pain and ulcers of the feet and fingers are essential for the diagnosis. Nerve conduction studies show prolonged sensory latencies and reduced amplitude of action potentials. Motor conduction velocity may be normal. Sural nerve biopsy shows an axonopathy with a profound loss of myelinated fibers of all diameters and also of some unmyelinated fibers.

MANAGEMENT. No treatment for the underlying disease is available, but symptomatic care is needed to prevent injury to the hands and feet.

Lumbar Disk Herniation

Lumbar disk herniation in children is usually caused by trauma. Almost all cases occur after age 10; they are more common in boys than in girls and are frequently sports related. Because lumbar disk herniation is unusual in children, diagnosis may be delayed for months or years.

CLINICAL FEATURES. The initial features are pain and inability to function normally because of pain and inability to move the back. Straight leg raising and bending forward from the waist are impaired. Frequently the pain has been present for a long time because most children will accommodate to their disability. Sensation to pinprick may be diminished in the distribution of the L-5 and S-1 dermatome, and the ankle

tendon reflex is diminished or absent in more than half of patients.

DIAGNOSIS. Radiographs of the lumbosacral spine reveal minor congenital anomalies (hemivertebrae, sacralization of the lumbar spine) in an unusually large number of cases. The diagnosis is confirmed by MRI of the spine or by myelography.

MANAGEMENT. Bed rest provides immediate relief in most patients. The indication for surgical treatment is pain that persists and limits function in spite of adequate medical measures.

Syringomyelia

Syringomyelia is a generic term for a fluid-filled cavity within the substance of the spinal cord. The cavity varies in length and may extend into the brainstem. A cephalic extension is termed *syringobulbia*. The cavity, or *syrinx*, is centrally placed in the gray matter and may enlarge in all directions. The cervicothoracic region is a favorite site, but thoracolumbar syrinx also occurs, and occasionally a syrinx extends from the brainstem to the conus medullaris.

The mechanism of syrinx formation has been debated. Cavitation of the spinal cord sometimes follows trauma and infarction, but these are not important mechanisms of syringomyelia in children. In childhood, primary syringomyelia is generally regarded as either a congenital malformation or a cystic astrocytoma. In the past, a congenital cyst could be distinguished from astrocytoma only by postmortem examination. Astrocytomas of the spinal cord, like those of the cerebellum, may have large cysts with only a nubbin of solid tumor. The development of MRI has greatly enhanced antemortem diagnosis of cystic astrocytoma by showing small areas of increased signal intensity in one or more portions of the cyst. Cystic astrocytoma is more likely to produce symptoms during the first decade, whereas congenital syringomyelia becomes symptomatic in the second decade or later and is usually associated with the Chiari anomaly. Cystic astrocytoma of the spinal cord is considered further in Chapters 12 and 13; this section deals primarily with congenital syringomyelia.

CLINICAL FEATURES. The initial symptoms of syringomyelia depend on the cyst's location. Because the cavity is near the central canal, crossing fibers subserving pain and temperature are often affected first. When the syrinx is in the cervical area, pain and temperature are typically lost in a "cape" or "vest" distribution. However, early involvement is often unilateral or at least asymmetric and sometimes involves the fingers before the shoulders. Touch and pressure are ordinarily preserved until the cyst enlarges into the posterior columns or the dorsal root entry zone. Loss of pain sensibility in the hands often leads to injury, ulceration, and infection, as seen in hereditary sensory and autonomic neuropathies. Pain is prominent. Complaints include neck ache, headache, back pain, and radicular pain (Milhorat et al., 1996).

Scoliosis is common, and torticollis may be an initial sign in children with cervical cavities. As the cavity enlarges into the ventral horn, weakness and atrophy develop in the hands and may be associated with fasciculations; pressure on the lateral columns causes hyperreflexia and spasticity in the legs. Very long cavities may produce lower motor neuron signs in all four limbs. Sphincter control is sometimes impaired. The posterior columns are generally the last to be affected, so that vibration sense and touch are preserved until relatively late in the course. The progress of symptoms is extremely slow and insidious. The spinal cord accommodates well to the slowly developing pressure within. Thus, at the time a physician is consulted, a long history of minor neurological handicaps such as clumsiness or difficulty running may be elicited.

Bulbar signs are relatively uncommon and usually asymmetric. They include hemiatrophy of the tongue with deviation on protrusion, facial weakness, dysphasia, and dysarthria. The descending pathway of the trigeminal nerve is frequently affected, causing loss of pain and temperature sensations on the same side of the face as the facial weakness and tongue hemiatrophy. **DIAGNOSIS.** MRI is the diagnostic test of choice. It not only shows the cavity (Figure 9-1) and the Chiari malformation, but also the presence of small foci of glioma.

MANAGEMENT. Syrinxes occurring with hydrocephalus and communicating with the fourth ventricle do well following ventriculoperitoneal shunt. Syrinxes associated with Chiari I malformations collapse after shunting from the syrinx to the cerebellopontine angle, and noncommunicating syrinxes often collapse after excision of an extramedullary obstruction.

Thalamic Pain

The thalamic pain syndrome occurs almost exclusively in adults following infarction of the

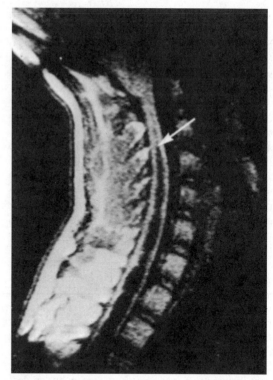

Figure 9-1. Cervical syringomyelia. MRI demonstrates a long cavity (*arrow*) beginning just below the foramen magnum.

thalamus. Similar symptoms sometimes occur in patients with thalamic glioma. The location of the lesion is usually the ventroposterolateral nucleus of the thalamus. Thalamic-type pain also occurs with lesions of the parietal lobe, medial lemniscus, and dorsolateral medulla (Mac-Gowan et al., 1997).

CLINICAL FEATURES. Touching the affected limb or part of the body produces intense discomfort described as "sharp," "crushing," or "burning." Suffering is considerable, and the quality of the pain is unfamiliar to the patient. Several different modes of stimulation, such as changes in ambient temperature, auditory stimulation, and even changes in emotional state, can accentuate the pain. Despite the severity of these dysesthesias, the affected limb is otherwise anesthetic to ordinary sensory testing.

DIAGNOSIS. The presence of thalamic pain should prompt imaging studies to determine the presence of tumor, infarction, or demyelinating disease.

MANAGEMENT. The combination of levodopa and a peripheral decarboxylase inhibitor may be helpful for relieving pain. If this does not prove satisfactory, some combination of analgesic and tranquilizing medication should be administered.

References

Holme E, Lindstedt S. Tyrosinaemia type I and NTBC (2-(2-nitro-4-trifluoromethylbenzoyl)-1,3-cyclohexanedione). *J Inherit Metab Dis* 1998;21:507–517.

Hooshmand H, Hashmi M. Complex regional pain syndrome (reflex sympathetic dystrophy syndrome): Diagnosis and therapy—A review of 824 patients. *Pain Digest* 1999;9:1–24.

MacGowan DGL, Janal MN, Clark WC, et al. Central poststroke pain and Wallenberg's lateral medullary infarction. Frequency, character, and determinants in 63 patients. *Neurology* 1997;49:120–125.

Milhorat TH, Kotzen RM, Mu HT, et al. Dysesthetic pain in patients with syringomyelia. *Neurosurgery* 1996;38:940–946.

Puy H, Deybach JC, Lamoril J, et al. Molecular epidemiology and diagnosis of PBG deaminase gene defects in acute intermittent porphyria. *Am J Hum Genet* 1997;60:1373–1383.

Rogers PD. Cimetidine in the treatment of acute intermittent porphyria. *Ann Pharmacother* 1997;31:365–367.

Rowbotham MC. Complex regional pain syndrome type I (reflex sympathetic dystrophy). More than a myth. *Neurology* 1998;51:4–5.

Wheeler DS, Vaux KK, Tam DA. Use of gabapentine in the treatment of childhood reflex sympathetic dystrophy. *Ped Neurol* 2000;22:220–231.

Chapter 10
Ataxia

THE TERM *ATAXIA* is used to denote disturbances in the fine control of posture and movement that are normally controlled by the cerebellum and its major input systems from the frontal lobes and the posterior columns of the spinal cord. The initial and most prominent feature is usually an abnormal gait. The ataxic gait is wide-based, lurching, and staggering, and it provokes disquiet in an observer for fear that the patient is in danger of falling. The same gait is seen in people who are attempting to walk in a vehicle that has several directions of motion at once, such as a railroad train.

When an abnormality occurs in the vermis of the cerebellum, the child cannot sit still but constantly moves the body to and fro and bobs the head (titubation). In contrast, disturbances of the cerebellar hemispheres cause a tendency to veer in the direction of the affected hemisphere, with dysmetria and hypotonia in the ipsilateral limbs. Bifrontal lobe disease may produce symptoms and signs that are indistinguishable from those of cerebellar disease.

Loss of sensory input to the cerebellum, because of peripheral nerve or posterior column disease, necessitates constant looking at the feet to know their location in space. The gait is also wide-based, but is not so much lurching as careful. The foot is raised high with each step and slaps down heavily on the ground. Station and gait are considerably worse with the eyes closed, and the patient may actually fall to the floor (Romberg sign). Sensory ataxia is more likely to cause difficulty with fine finger movements than with reaching for objects.

Other features of cerebellar disease are a characteristic speech that varies in volume and has an increased separation of syllables (scanning speech), hypotonia, limb and ocular dysmetria, and tremor.

The differential diagnosis of a child with acute ataxia or recurrent attacks of ataxia (Table 10-1) is quite different from that of a child with chronic static or progressive ataxia (Table

---

Table 10-1
Acute or Recurrent Ataxia

Brain Tumor

Conversion Reaction

Drug Ingestion

Encephalitis (Brainstem)

Genetic Disorders
Dominant recurrent ataxia
Episodic ataxia type 1
Episodic ataxia type 2
Hartnup disease
Maple syrup urine disease
Pyruvate dehydrogenase deficiency

Migraine
Basilar
Benign paroxysmal vertigo

Postinfectious-Immune
Acute postinfectious cerebellitis
Miller Fisher syndrome
Multiple sclerosis
Myoclonic encephalopathy and neuroblastoma

Pseudoataxia (Epileptic)

Trauma
Hematoma (see Chapter 2)
Postconcussion
Vertebrobasilar occlusion

Vascular Disorders
Cerebellar hemorrhage
Kawasaki disease

10-2). Therefore, these two presentations are discussed separately in the text. However, a slowly progressive ataxia may be noticed "acutely," and children with recurrent ataxia may never return to baseline after each attack and have a progressive ataxia superimposed on the acute attacks.

Acute or Recurrent Ataxia

The two most common causes of ataxia among children who were previously healthy and then suddenly have an ataxic gait are drug ingestion and acute postinfectious cerebellitis. Migraine, brainstem encephalitis, and an underlying neuroblastoma are the next considerations. Recurrent ataxia is uncommon and is usually caused by hereditary disorders; migraine is the most common cause, and disorders of pyruvate metabolism are second.

Table 10-2
Chronic or Progressive Ataxia

Brain Tumors
Cerebellar astrocytoma
Cerebellar hemangioblastoma (Von Hippel-Lindau disease)
Ependymoma
Medulloblastoma
Supratentorial tumors (see Chapter 4)

Congenital Malformations
Basilar impression
Cerebellar aplasias
Cerebellar hemisphere aplasia
Dandy-Walker malformation (see Chapter 18)
Vermal aplasia
Chiari malformation

Hereditary Ataxias
Autosomal dominant inheritance (see Table 10-3)
Autosomal recessive inheritance
  Abetalipoproteinemia
  Ataxia-telangiectasia
  Ataxia with diffuse central nervous system
    hypomyelination
  Ataxia with episodic dystonia
  Friedreich ataxia
  Hartnup disease
  Juvenile GM_2 gangliosidosis
  Juvenile sulfatide lipidoses
  Maple syrup urine disease
  Marinesco-Sjögren syndrome
  Pyruvate dehydrogenase deficiency
  Ramsay Hunt syndrome
  Refsum disease (HSMN IV) (see Chapter 7)
  Respiratory chain disorders (see Chapter 8)
X-linked inheritance
  Adrenoleukodystrophy (see Chapter 5)
  Leber optic neuropathy (see Chapter 16)
  With adult-onset dementia
  With deafness
  With deafness and loss of vision

Brain Tumor

Primary brain tumors ordinarily cause chronic progressive ataxia and are discussed later in this chapter. However, ataxia may be acute if the brain tumor bleeds or causes hydrocephalus. In addition, early clumsiness may be overlooked until it becomes severe enough to cause an obvious gait disturbance. For this reason, brain imaging is recommended for most children with acute cerebellar ataxia.

Conversion Reaction

CLINICAL FEATURES. Hysterical gait disturbances are common in children, especially girls between 10 and 15 years of age. Hysteria is involuntary, usually provides a secondary gain, and should be distinguished from malingering, which is a voluntary act. Hysterical gait disturbances are often extreme. The child appears to sit without difficulty but when brought to standing immediately begins to sway from the waist. A wide-based stance is not used to increase stability. Instead the child lurches, staggers, and otherwise travels across the room from object to object. The lurching maneuvers are often complex and require extraordinary balance. Strength, tone, sensation, and tendon reflexes are normal.

DIAGNOSIS. Hysterical gait disturbances are usually diagnosed by observation; laboratory tests are not ordinarily required to exclude other possibilities.

MANAGEMENT. Determination of the precipitating stress is important. Conversion may represent a true call for help in a desperate situation such as child abuse. Such cases require referral to a multispecialty team able to deal with the whole family.

Most children with hysterical gait disturbances are responding to a more immediate and less serious life stress. Symptoms can usually be treated by the use of suggestion and do not require psychiatric referral except when conversion is used repeatedly to handle stress.

Drug Ingestion

The incidence of accidental drug ingestion is highest between ages 1 and 4 years.

CLINICAL FEATURES. An overdose of most psychoactive drugs causes ataxia, disturbances in personality or sensorium, and sometimes seizures. Toxic doses of anticonvulsant drugs, especially phenytoin, may cause marked nystagmus and ataxia without an equivalent alteration in sensorium. Excessive use of antihistamines in the treatment of an infant or young child with allergy or an upper respiratory tract infection may cause ataxia. This is especially true in children with otitis media, who may have underlying unsteadiness because of middle-ear infection.

DIAGNOSIS. The parents or care providers of every child with acute ataxia should be carefully questioned concerning drugs intentionally administered to the child and other drugs accessible in the home. Specific inquiry concerning the use of anticonvulsant or psychoactive drugs by family members is mandatory. Urine should be screened for drug metabolites, and blood should be sent for analysis when a specific drug is suspected.

MANAGEMENT. Treatment depends on the specific drug ingested and its blood concentration. In most cases of ataxia caused by drug ingestion, the drug can be safely eliminated spontaneously if vital function is not compromised, if acid-base balance is not disturbed, and if liver and kidney function is normal. In life-threatening situations, dialysis may be necessary while vital function is supported in an intensive care unit.

Encephalitis (Brainstem)

Ataxia may be the initial feature of viral encephalitis affecting primarily the structures of the posterior fossa. Echoviruses, coxsackieviruses, adenoviruses, and *Coxiella burnetti* have been implicated as etiological agents (Sawaishi et al, 1999).

CLINICAL FEATURES. Cranial nerve dysfunction is often associated with the ataxia. Generalized encephalitis characterized by declining consciousness and seizures may develop later. Meningismus is sometimes present. The course is variable, and although most children recover completely, some are left with considerable neurological impairment. Those who have only ataxia and cranial nerve palsies, with no disturbance of neocortical function, tend to recover best. Such cases cannot be distinguished from the Miller Fisher syndrome on clinical grounds alone.

DIAGNOSIS. Diagnosis requires showing a cellular response, primarily mononuclear leukocytes, in the cerebrospinal fluid, with or without some elevation of the protein content. Prolonged interpeak latencies of the brainstem auditory evoked response are evidence of an abnormality within the brainstem parenchyma and not the peripheral sensory input system. The electroencephalogram (EEG) is usually normal in children with brainstem encephalitis who have a normal sensorium.

MANAGEMENT. No specific treatment is available for the viral infection.

Genetic Disorders

Dominant Recurrent Ataxias

At least two distinct genetic defects are recognized that cause episodic ataxia, episodic ataxia type 1 (EA-1) and episodic ataxia type 2 (EA-2). Both are the result of ion channel mutations. EA-1 is caused by mutations in a potassium channel gene and EA-2 by mutations in a voltage-dependent calcium channel (Bird, 1999).

Episodic Ataxia Type 1 (Paroxysmal Ataxia and Myokymia)

EA-1 is caused by a mutation of the potassium channel gene on chromosome 12p. It is probably related to the syndrome of paroxysmal choreoathetosis (see Chapter 1) (Lubbers et al, 1995). The additional feature of continuous motor unit activity (see Chapter 8) suggests a defect in membrane stability affecting the central and peripheral nervous systems.

CLINICAL FEATURES. The onset of attacks is usually between 5 and 7 years of age. The child has sudden awareness that an attack is to begin by the sensation of spreading limpness or stiffness lasting for a few seconds. Incoordination, trembling of the head or limbs, and blurry vision often follow. Some children feel warm and perspire. Some can continue standing or walking, but most sit down. Attacks usually last for less than 10 minutes but can be as long as 6 hours. They may begin spontaneously but are usually brought on by sudden and unexpected movement (kinesigenic). Startle and anxiety increase the potential for attacks. Myokymia of the hands is observed even between attacks.

DIAGNOSIS. The clinical diagnosis is based on the history of typical attacks and the family history. Electromyography (EMG) confirms the diagnosis by showing continuous motor unit activity, most often in the hands but also in the proximal arm muscles and sometimes in the face.

MANAGEMENT. Acetazolamide reduces the frequency of attacks or completely stops them in about half of patients. The effect is noted within a few days. Some patients respond to phenytoin or other anticonvulsants.

Episodic Ataxia Type 2 (Acetazolamide-Responsive Ataxia)

EA-2, one form of spinocerebellar ataxia (SCA6), and one type of familial hemiplegic migraine all represent allelic mutations in the same calcium channel gene on chromosome 19p. About half of patients have migraine headaches; some episodes may be typical of basilar migraine (Baloh et al, 1997).

CLINICAL FEATURES. Clinical heterogeneity is considerable despite genetic localization to the 19p site. The onset is generally during school age or adolescence. The child first becomes unsteady and is then unable to maintain posture because of vertigo and ataxia. Vomiting is frequent and severe. Jerk nystagmus, sometimes with a rotary component, is seen during attacks. One to three attacks may occur each month, with symptoms lasting for 1 hour to 1 day. Attacks become milder and less frequent with age. Slowly progressive truncal ataxia and nystagmus may persist between attacks. In some patients ataxia is the only symptom, others have only vertigo, and still others have only nystagmus. Most affected individuals are normal between attacks, but some are phenotypically indistinguishable from those with SCA6 (see discussion on Progressive Hereditary Ataxias later in this chapter).

DIAGNOSIS. Diagnosis is based on the clinical features and a family history of the disorder. Magnetic resonance imaging (MRI) may show selective atrophy of the cerebellar vermis. Basilar artery migraine and benign paroxysmal vertigo can be distinguished from dominant recurrent ataxia because in these conditions, older family members have migraine but do not have recurrent ataxia. Further, attacks of benign paroxysmal vertigo rarely last more than a few minutes.

MANAGEMENT. Daily oral acetazolamide prevents recurrence of attacks in almost every case. The mechanism of action is unknown. The dose is generally 125 mg twice a day in young children and 250 mg twice a day in older children. Flunarizine, 5 to 10 mg/day, may serve as an alternative therapy when acetazolamide is not tolerated. Anticonvulsant and antimigraine medications are without value.

Hartnup Disease

Hartnup disease is a rare disorder transmitted by autosomal recessive inheritance. The basic error is a defect of amino acid transport in kidney and small intestine. The result is aminoaciduria and the retention of amino acids in the small intestine. Tryptophan is converted to nonessential indole products instead of nicotinamide.

CLINICAL FEATURES. Affected children are normal at birth but may be slow in attaining developmental milestones. Most achieve only borderline intelligence; others are normal. Affected individuals are photosensitive and have a severe pellagra-like skin rash after exposure to sunlight. The rash is attributed to nicotinamide deficiency. Many patients have episodes of limb ataxia, sometimes associated with nystagmus. Mental changes, ranging from emotional instability to delirium, or states of decreased consciousness may occur. Tone is decreased, and the tendon reflexes are normal or exaggerated. The neurological disturbances are triggered by stress or intercurrent infection and may be due to the intestinal absorption of toxic amino acid breakdown products.

Most patients have both rash and neurological disturbances, but each can occur without the other. Symptoms progress over several days and last for a week to a month before recovery occurs.

DIAGNOSIS. The constant feature of Hartnup disease is aminoaciduria involving neutral monoaminomonocarboxylic amino acids. These include alanine, serine, threonine, asparagine, glutamine, valine, leucine, isoleucine, phenylalanine, tyrosine, tryptophan, histidine, and citrulline.

MANAGEMENT. The rash can be prevented by daily oral administration of nicotinamide, 50 to 300 mg. Nicotinamide (25 to 300 mg/day) supplementation may reverse the skin and neurological complications. A high-protein diet is also recommended to make up for the amino acid loss.

Maple Syrup Urine Disease (Intermittent)

Maple syrup urine disease is a disorder of branched-chain amino acid metabolism caused by deficiency of the enzyme branched-chain keto-acid dehydrogenase. The defect is transmitted by autosomal recessive inheritance. Three phenotypes are associated, depending on the percentage of enzyme deficiency. The *classic* form begins as seizures in the newborn (see Chapter 1), the *intermediate* form causes progressive mental retardation (see Chapter 5), and the *intermittent* form causes recurrent attacks of ataxia and encephalopathy.

CLINICAL FEATURES. Affected individuals are normal at birth. Between 5 months and 2 years, episodes of ataxia, irritability, and progressive lethargy are provoked by minor infections, surgery, or a diet that is rich in protein. The length of an attack is variable; most children recover spontaneously, but some die of severe metabolic acidosis. Psychomotor development remains normal in survivors.

DIAGNOSIS. The urine has a maple syrup odor during the attack, and the blood and urine have elevated concentrations of branched-chain amino acids and ketoacids. Between attacks the concentrations of branched-chain amino acids and ketoacids are normal in both blood and urine. The diagnosis is established by showing the enzyme deficiency in cultured fibroblasts.

MANAGEMENT. Children with intermittent maple syrup disease need a protein-restricted diet. Some have a thiamine-responsive enzyme defect, and 1 g of thiamine a day should be tried for acute attacks. If this is successful, a maintenance dose of 100 mg/day is recommended. The main objective during an acute attack is to reverse ketoacidosis. Protein should not be given. Peritoneal dialysis may be helpful in life-threatening situations.

Pyruvate Dehydrogenase Deficiency

The pyruvate dehydrogenase (PDH) complex is responsible for the oxidative decarboxylation of pyruvate to carbon dioxide and acetyl-coenzyme A (acetyl-CoA). Disorders of the complex are associated with several neurological conditions, including subacute necrotizing encephalomyelopathy (Leigh syndrome), mitochondrial myopathies, and lactic acidosis. The complex contains three main components that are termed E1, E2, and E3. E1 consists of two alpha subunits encoded on the X chromosome and two beta subunits. An X-linked form of PDH-E1 deficiency is characterized by episodes of intermittent ataxia and lactic acidosis. E1 deficiency is the most common form of PDH deficiency.

CLINICAL FEATURES. The clinical features range from severe neonatal lactic acidosis and death to episodic ataxia with lactic and pyruvic acidosis and spinocerebellar degeneration. Most patients show mild developmental delay during early childhood. Episodes of ataxia, dysarthria, and sometimes lethargy usually begin after 3 years of age. In more severely affected patients, episodes may begin during infancy and are associated with generalized weakness and states of decreased consciousness. Some attacks are spontaneous, but others are provoked by intercurrent infection, stress, or a high-carbohydrate meal. Attacks recur at irregular intervals and may last for periods ranging from 1 day to several weeks.

The severity of neurological dysfunction in any individual probably reflects the level of residual enzyme activity. Those with generalized weakness are also areflexic and have nystagmus or other disturbances in ocular motility. Ataxia is the predominant symptom. Intention tremor and dysarthria may be present. Hyperventilation is common and may be caused by metabolic acidosis. Patients with almost complete PDH deficiency die of lactic acidosis and central hypoventilation during infancy.

DIAGNOSIS. PDH deficiency should be suspected in children with lactic acidosis, hypotonia, progressive or episodic ataxia, the Leigh disease phenotype, and recurrent polyneuropathy. The pyruvic acid concentration is elevated, and the lactate-to-pyruvate ratio is low. The blood concentration of lactate may be elevated between attacks; lactate and pyruvate concentrations are always elevated during attacks. Some children have hyperalaninemia as well. The diagnosis may be further verified by an oral glucose tolerance test. When oral glucose is administered, hyperglycemia is prolonged and the blood concentration of lactate is elevated. The test may provoke clinical symptoms. The diagnosis is established by analysis of enzyme activity in cultured fibroblasts, leukocytes, or muscle.

MANAGEMENT. Patients are usually treated with thiamine (100 to 600 mg/day) and a high-fat (>55%), low-carbohydrate diet. Unfortunately, current treatments do not prevent disease progression in most patients. In addition, daily oral acetazolamide, 125 mg twice a day in small children and 250 mg twice a day in older children, may significantly abort the attacks. Biotin, carnitine, coenzyme Q10, and thiamine supplements have been used in several patients, but the value of vitamin supplementation has not been established.

Migraine

Basilar Migraine

The term *basilar (artery) migraine* is used to characterize recurrent attacks of brainstem or cerebellar dysfunction that occur as symptoms of a migraine attack. Girls are affected more often than boys. The peak incidence is during adolescence, but attacks may occur at any age.

Infant-onset cases are more likely to be manifested as benign paroxysmal vertigo.

CLINICAL FEATURES. Gait ataxia occurs in approximately 50% of patients. Other symptoms include visual loss, vertigo, tinnitus, alternating hemiparesis, and paresthesias of the fingers, toes, and corners of the mouth. An abrupt loss of consciousness, usually lasting for only a few minutes, may be reported. Cardiac arrhythmia and brainstem stroke are rare life-threatening complications. Neurological disturbances are usually followed by a severe, throbbing, occipital headache. Nausea and vomiting occur in less than one third of cases.

Children may have repeated basilar migraine attacks, but with time the episodes evolve into a pattern of classic migraine. Even during attacks of classic migraine, the patient may continue to complain of vertigo and even ataxia.

DIAGNOSIS. EEG should be done to distinguish basilar migraine from benign occipital epilepsy. The EEG shows occipital intermittent delta activity during and just after an attack in basilar migraine and occipital discharges in epilepsy.

MANAGEMENT. Basilar artery migraine is treated the same way as other forms of migraine (see Chapter 3). A prophylactic agent should be used when attacks are frequent.

Benign Paroxysmal Vertigo

Benign paroxysmal vertigo is primarily a disorder of infants and preschool children but may occur in older children.

CLINICAL FEATURES. Episodes are characterized by the sudden onset of vertigo. True cerebellar ataxia is not present, but vertigo is so profound that posture cannot be maintained. The child either lies motionless on the floor or indicates the need to be held by a parent. Consciousness is not altered, and headache is not reported. The predominant symptoms are pallor, nystagmus, and fright. Episodes last only for minutes and may recur at irregular intervals. Attacks decrease in frequency and stop completely. Migraine develops in 21% (Lindskog et al, 1999).

DIAGNOSIS. The diagnosis is primarily clinical, and laboratory tests are useful only to exclude other possibilities. A family history of migraine, though not necessarily paroxysmal vertigo, can be obtained in 40% of cases. Some parents indicate that they experience vertigo with their attacks of migraine. Only in rare cases does a parent have a history of benign paroxysmal vertigo.

MANAGEMENT. The attacks are so brief and harmless that treatment is seldom indicated.

Postinfectious/Immune Disorders

In many of the conditions discussed in this section, an altered immune state is blamed for cerebellar dysfunction and sometimes for other neurological deficits. Preceding viral infections are usually incriminated but are documented in only half of cases. Natural varicella infections and the varicella vaccine are recognized as definite preceding causes. No other vaccine has been linked to acute cerebellar ataxia.

Acute Cerebellar Ataxia

Acute cerebellar ataxia usually affects children between 2 and 7 years of age, but it may occur as late as 16 years. Males and females are affected equally, and the incidence among family members is not increased.

CLINICAL FEATURES. The onset is explosive. A previously healthy child awakens from a nap and cannot stand. *Ataxia is maximal at onset.* Some worsening may occur during the first hours, but a longer progression, or a waxing and waning course, makes the diagnosis unlikely. Ataxia varies from mild unsteadiness while walking to complete inability to stand or walk. Even when ataxia is severe, sensorium is clear and the child is otherwise normal. Tendon reflexes may be present or absent; their absence suggests the Miller Fisher syndrome. Nystagmus, when present, is usually mild. Chaotic movements of the eyes (opsoclonus) should suggest the myoclonic encephalopathy-neuroblastoma syndrome.

Symptoms may begin to remit after a few days, but recovery of normal gait takes 3 weeks to 5 months. Patients with pure ataxia of the trunk or limbs and only mild nystagmus are likely to recover completely. Marked nystagmus or opsoclonus (see the section on Myoclonic Encephalopathy/Neuroblastoma Syndrome later in this chapter), tremors of the head and trunk, or moderate irritability are likely to be followed by persistent neurological sequelae.

DIAGNOSIS. The diagnosis of acute postinfectious cerebellitis is one of exclusion. Every child should have drug screening, and most will have a brain imaging study. The necessity of imaging the brain in typical cases, especially those with varicella infection, is debatable. Lumbar puncture is indicated when encephalitis is suspected.

MANAGEMENT. Acute postinfectious cerebellitis is a self-limited disease. Treatment is not required.

Miller Fisher Syndrome

Miller Fisher syndrome is characterized by ataxia, ophthalmoplegia, and areflexia. A similar disorder with ataxia and areflexia but without ophthalmoplegia is called *acute ataxic neuropathy*. Some believe that Miller Fisher syndrome is a variant of Guillain-Barré syndrome; others believe that it is a form of brainstem encephalitis. In support of the hypothesis of a Guillain-Barré-like immune-mediated hypothesis is the finding that *Campylobacter jejuni* is a causative agent in both Miller Fisher syndrome and Guillain-Barré syndromes (Jacobs et al, 1995).

CLINICAL FEATURES. A viral illness precedes the neurological symptoms by 5 to 10 days in 50% of cases. Either ophthalmoparesis or ataxia may be the initial feature. Both are present early in the course. The initial ocular motor disturbance is paralysis of upgaze, followed by loss of lateral gaze and then downgaze. Recovery takes place in the reverse order. The Bell phenomenon may be preserved despite paralysis of voluntary upward gaze, suggesting the possibility of supranuclear palsy. Ptosis occurs but is less severe than the vertical gaze palsy.

Ataxia is more prominent in the limbs than in the trunk and, like the areflexia, is probably caused by decreased peripheral sensory input. Weakness of the limbs may be noted. Unilateral or bilateral facial weakness occurs in a significant minority of children. Recovery generally begins within 2 to 4 weeks after symptoms become maximal and is complete within 6 months.

DIAGNOSIS. The clinical distinction between the Miller Fisher syndrome and brainstem encephalitis can be difficult. Disturbances of sensorium, multiple cranial nerve palsies, an abnormal EEG, or prolongation of the interpeak latencies of the brainstem auditory evoked response should suggest brainstem encephalitis. The cerebrospinal fluid profile in Miller Fisher syndrome parallels that of Guillain-Barré syndrome. A cellular response is noted early in the course, and protein elevation occurs later.

MANAGEMENT. Corticosteroids, adrenocorticotropic hormone (ACTH), and plasmapheresis are not beneficial. The outcome in untreated children is excellent.

Multiple Sclerosis

Multiple sclerosis is usually a disease of young adults, but 3% to 5% of cases occur in children less than 6 years of age (Ruggieri et al, 1999). Whether the childhood forms of multiple sclerosis are etiologically distinct from the adult types is not established.

CLINICAL FEATURES. The female-to-male ratio varies from 1.5:3. Ataxia, concurrent with a febrile episode, is the most common initial feature in children, followed by encephalopathy, hemiparesis, or seizures. Intranuclear ophthalmoplegia, unilateral or bilateral, develops in one third of patients (see Chapter 15).

The clinical features that occur in multiple sclerosis are so variable that a single prototype cannot be provided. The essential feature is repeated episodes of demyelination in noncontiguous areas of the central nervous system. Each episode is characterized by the rapid development of focal neurological deficits that persist for weeks or months; afterward the child has partial or complete recovery. Recurrences are separated by months or years and are frequently associated with febrile illnesses. Lethargy, nausea, and vomiting sometimes accompany the attacks in children but rarely in adults.

The child is usually irritable and shows truncal and limb ataxia. Tendon reflexes are generally brisk throughout. The long-term outcome is unpredictable.

DIAGNOSIS. Multiple sclerosis may be suspected at the time of the first attack, but definitive diagnosis requires recurrence to establish a polyphasic course. Examination of the cerebrospinal fluid at the time of exacerbation shows fewer than 25 lymphocytes/mm^3, a normal or mildly elevated protein content, and sometimes the presence of oligoclonal bands.

MRI is the best technique to show demyelination (Figure 10-1), but the extent and severity of lesions may not correlate with the clinical syndrome. Visual evoked responses are useful to document prior or concurrent optic neuritis, and peroneal somatosensory evoked responses can be used to document myelitis.

MANAGEMENT. A short course of corticosteroids is recommended at the time of acute exacerbations. Methylprednisolone, 500 to 1,000 mg, depending on the age, is generally administered, then rapidly tapered and discontinued. Experience is not available in children with the drugs used to prevent relapses in adults.

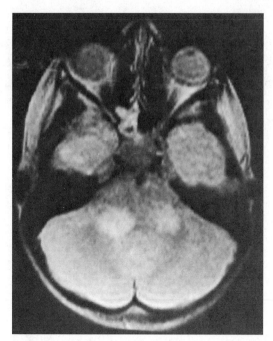

Figure 10-1. MRI in multiple sclerosis. Two areas of increased signal intensity are present in the cerebellum.

Myoclonic Encephalopathy/ Neuroblastoma Syndrome

Myoclonic encephalopathy is a syndrome characterized by chaotic eye movements (dancing eyes, opsoclonus), myoclonic ataxia, and encephalopathy. The pathophysiological mechanism is an altered immune state. It was generally thought either to occur as an idiopathic syndrome or to be secondary to an occult neuroblastoma. With improved imaging techniques, the percentage of cases in which neuroblastoma cannot be found is diminishing.

CLINICAL FEATURES. The mean age at onset is 18 months, with a range from 1 month to 4 years (Russo et al, 1997). Unlike acute postinfectious cerebellitis and Miller Fisher syndrome, in which neurological symptoms are fully expressed within 1 to 2 days, the evolution of symptoms in myoclonic encephalopathy may take a week or longer.

Either ataxia or chaotic eye movements may bring the child to medical attention. Almost half of affected children show personality change or irritability, suggesting the presence of a more diffuse encephalopathy. Some are described as having ataxia, but the imbalance is actually myoclonus, constant rapid muscular contractions that have an irregular occurrence and a widespread distribution (see Chapter 14). Opsoclonus is a disorder of ocular muscles that is similar to myoclonus. Spontaneous, conjugate, irregular jerking of the eyes in all directions is characteristic. The movements are most prominent with attempts to change fixation and are then associated with blinking or eyelid flutter. Opsoclonus persists even in sleep and becomes more severe with agitation.

DIAGNOSIS. The myoclonic encephalopathy syndrome can be diagnosed on clinical grounds, but laboratory investigation is required to determine the underlying cause. The presence of an occult neuroblastoma should be suspected in all children with recurrent ataxia or the myoclonic encephalopathy syndrome. Acute ataxia that progresses over several days or waxes and wanes is more likely to be caused by neuroblastoma than by postinfectious acute cerebellar ataxia.

The occult neuroblastoma is equally likely to be in the chest or the abdomen. In contrast, only 10% to 15% of neuroblastomas are in the chest when myoclonic encephalopathy is absent. The usual studies to detect neuroblastoma are MRI of the chest and abdomen (Figure 10-2), and measurement of the urinary excretion of homovanillic acid (HVA) and vanillylmandelic acid (VMA).

MANAGEMENT. Neuroblastoma, when located, should be removed. However, the long-term neurological outcome is the same whether or not a neuroblastoma is found. Partial or complete remission of the neurological symptoms may occur regardless of whether neuroblastoma is pres-

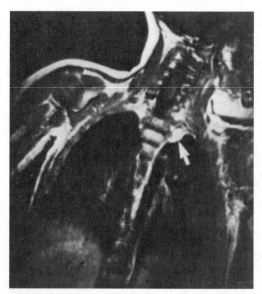

Figure 10-2. MRI demonstrates an apical neuroblastoma (*arrow*) in a child with normal radiographs and CT of the chest.

ent. In most patients the course is prolonged, with waxing and waning of neurological dysfunction. Either ACTH or oral corticosteroids provide partial or complete relief of symptoms in 80% of patients. Marked improvement usually occurs 1 to 4 weeks after initiation of therapy. Relapses occur when therapy is discontinued but may also occur while treatment is in progress. More than half of affected children are left with impaired motor and/or intellectual function.

Pseudoataxia (Epileptic)

CLINICAL FEATURES. Ataxia and other gait disturbances can be the only clinical features of seizure activity. Both limb and gait ataxia may be present, and the child's epilepsy may not have been previously recognized. If the child is already taking anticonvulsant drugs, the gait disturbance may be blamed on overdose. During the ataxic episode the child may appear inattentive or confused. Like other seizure manifestations, ataxia is sudden in onset and episodic.

DIAGNOSIS. The absence of nystagmus should suggest that ataxia is a seizure manifestation and is not caused by drug toxicity. The usual EEG findings concurrent with ataxia are prolonged, generalized, 2- to 3-Hz spike-wave complexes that have a frontal predominance. This is the typical EEG finding in the Lennox-Gastaut syndrome (see Chapter 1). Such discharges are ordinarily associated with myoclonic jerks or akinetic seizures. Either one occurring momentarily, but repeatedly, could interrupt smooth movement and produce ataxia.

MANAGEMENT. Pseudoataxia usually responds to anticonvulsant drugs. Clonazepam and valproate are most often used for slow spike-wave discharges (see Chapter 1).

Trauma

Mild head injuries are common in children and are an almost daily occurrence in toddlers. Recovery is always complete despite considerable parental concern. More serious head injuries, associated with loss of consciousness, seizures, and cerebral contusion, are less common but still account for several thousand deaths in children annually. Ataxia may follow head injuries, even mild injuries. In most of these cases the ataxia is part of the so-called postconcussion syndrome, in which imaging studies do not show any structural derangement of the nervous system. In others a cerebellar contusion or posterior fossa hematoma may be present (see Chapter 2).

Ataxia may also follow cervical injuries, especially during sports. These are usually caused by trauma to the vertebrobasilar artery.

Postconcussion Syndrome

CLINICAL FEATURES. Many adults complain of headache, dizziness, and mental changes following even a mild head injury. Some of these symptoms also occur after head injury in children and probably represent a transitory derangement of cerebral function caused by the trauma. Even mild head trauma can cause a cerebral axonopathy, which may explain the persistence of symptoms.

In infants and small children the most prominent postconcussive symptom is ataxia. This is not necessarily a typical cerebellar ataxia but may be only an unsteady gait. No limb dysmetria is present, and other neurological functions are normal.

In older children with postconcussive syndromes, headache and dizziness are as common as ataxia. The headache is usually described as low grade and constant. It is often an analgesic-rebound headache (see Chapter 3). Gait is less disturbed, possibly because an older child better compensates for dizziness, but the sensation of unsteadiness is still described.

DIAGNOSIS. The diagnosis is based on the clinical syndrome. Cranial computed tomography (CT) at the time of injury to exclude intracranial hemorrhage is normal but MRI may show foci of high signal intensity on T_2-weighted images, indicating axonal injury.

MANAGEMENT. Ataxia usually clears completely within 1 month and always within 6 months. Decreased activity during this time is recommended. Usually no further treatment is required.

Vertebrobasilar Occlusion

Trauma to the vertebrobasilar arteries may occur with chiropractic manipulation and sports injuries. The vertebral arteries are encased in bony canals from C2 to the foramen magnum. Sudden stretching of the arteries by hyperextension or hyperflexion of the neck causes endothelial injury and thrombosis.

CLINICAL FEATURES. Symptoms are noted within minutes or hours of injury. Vertigo, nausea, and vomiting are the initial symptoms of brainstem ischemia. Occipital headache may be present as well. Ataxia is due to incoordination of the limbs on one side. It may be maximal at onset or progress over several days.

Examination shows some combination of unilateral brainstem disturbances (diplopia, facial weakness) and ipsilateral cerebellar dysfunction.

DIAGNOSIS. CT or MRI shows a unilateral infarction in the cerebellar hemisphere. The lateral medulla may also be infarcted. The location of arterial thrombosis is visualized by arteriography.

MANAGEMENT. Many children recover completely in the months that follow injury. The value of anticoagulation has not been established.

Vascular Disorders

Cerebellar Hemorrhage

Spontaneous cerebellar hemorrhage in children, in the absence of a coagulopathy, is due to arteriovenous malformation, even though less than 10% of intracranial arteriovenous malformations in children are in the cerebellum. The two major features of cerebellar hemorrhage are ataxia and headache.

Kawasaki Disease

Kawasaki disease is a systemic vasculitis that occurs predominantly in infants and children.

CLINICAL FEATURES. Five of the following six criteria are required for diagnosis: fever, conjunctival congestion, reddening of the oropharynx and lips, indurative edema of the limbs, polymorphic exanthems, and lymphadenopathy. Arthralgia, carditis, and aseptic meningitis may be associated features. The disease is thought to be identical to childhood polyarteritis nodosa.

Multiple infarcts may occur in the brain. Acute ataxia, facial palsy, ocular motor palsies, and hemiplegia may occur. The prognosis is guarded, partly because of the neurological complications but mainly because of coronary artery disease.

DIAGNOSIS. Clinical features of multisystem disease are essential for diagnosis. Abnormal laboratory findings include an increased sedimentation rate, a positive test for C-reactive protein, and increased serum complement and globulin levels. Typical changes of arteritis are demonstrated by skin biopsy.

MANAGEMENT. Intravenous high-dose gammaglobulin is an effective method of treatment. Aspirin is usually recommended.

Chronic or Progressive Ataxia

Brain tumor is always an initial concern when progressive ataxia develops in previously normal children, especially if headache is present as well (see Table 10-2). Congenital abnormalities that cause ataxia are often associated with some degree of mental deficiency. The onset of symptoms may occur during infancy or be delayed until adult life. Friedreich ataxia is the most common hereditary form of progressive ataxia. The causes of chronic or progressive ataxia are usually easy to diagnose, and many are treatable. Failure to establish a diagnosis can have unfortunate consequences for the child.

Brain Tumors

Neuroectodermal tumor is the second most common malignancy of childhood and the most common solid tumor. Posterior fossa tumors are more common than supratentorial tumors between the ages of 1 and 8 years and account for approximately 50% of brain tumors in children of all ages. The four major tumors of the posterior fossa are cerebellar astrocytoma, brainstem glioma, ependymoma, and medulloblastoma. The initial feature of brainstem glioma is cranial nerve dysfunction and not ataxia (see Chapter 15). Although this discussion is limited to tumors of the posterior fossa, it is important to remember that supratentorial brain tumors may also cause ataxia. Approximately one quarter of children with supratentorial brain tumors have gait disturbances at the time of their first hospitalization, and many show signs of cerebellar dysfunction. Gait disturbances occur with equal frequency whether supratentorial tumors are in the midline or the hemispheres, whereas cerebellar signs are more common with midline tumors.

Cerebellar Astrocytoma

Cerebellar astrocytomas comprise 12% of brain tumors in children. The tumor usually grows slowly in the cerebellar hemisphere and consists of a large cyst with a mural nodule. It may be in the hemisphere, in the vermis, in both the hemisphere and vermis, or may occupy the fourth ventricle. Midline tumors are likely to be solid.

CLINICAL FEATURES. Both genders are affected equally. The peak incidence is at 5 to 9 years of age but may be as early as infancy. Headache is the most common initial complaint in school-age children, whereas unsteadiness of gait and vomiting are the initial symptoms in preschool children. Headache can be insidious and intermittent; typical morning headache and vomiting are rare. The first complaints of headache and nausea are usually attributed to a flu-like illness. Only when symptoms persist is the possibility of increased intracranial pressure considered. In infants and small children, symptoms of increased intracranial pressure are often relieved by the separation of cranial sutures. For this reason, gait disturbances without headache or vomiting are the common initial sign of cerebellar astrocytoma in infants.

Papilledema is present in most affected children at initial examination but is often absent in infants with separation of cranial sutures. Ataxia is present in three quarters, dysmetria in half, and nystagmus in only a quarter. Ataxia varies in severity from a wide-based, lurching gait to a subtle alteration of gait observed only with tandem walking or quick turning. It is caused in part by the cerebellar location of the tumor and in part by hydrocephalus. When the tumor is in the cerebellar hemisphere, ipsilateral or bilateral dysmetria may be present. Other neurological signs sometimes present in children with cerebellar astrocytoma are abducens palsy, multiple cranial nerve palsies, stiff neck, and head tilt.

DIAGNOSIS. MRI is the best imaging study for diagnosis.

MANAGEMENT. Children with life-threatening hydrocephalus should undergo a shunting procedure as the first step in treatment. The shunt relieves many of the symptoms and signs, including ataxia. Corticosteroids are sufficient to relieve pressure in many children with less severe hydrocephalus.

The 5-year survival rate after surgical removal approaches 95%. The mural nodule must be located and removed at surgery or the tumor may recur. The amount of tumor resected is difficult to determine at the time of resection, and postoperative imaging studies are used to improve upon the surgeon's estimate. The need for adjuvant radiotherapy is not established.

Deeper tumors that involve the floor of the fourth ventricle are rarely removed in toto. Local recurrence is common after partial resection. Repeat surgery may be curative in some cases, but postoperative radiation therapy appears to offer a better prognosis following partial resection. The overall disease-free survival rates following either surgery alone or surgery and ra-diotherapy are 92% at 5 years and 88% at 25 years. Chemotherapy is not currently recommended for low-grade cerebellar astrocytomas, regardless of the degree of surgical resection.

High-grade cerebellar astrocytoma (glioblastoma) is rare in children. More than 30% of childhood patients have dissemination of tumor through the neuraxis (spinal cord drop metastases). Examination of cerebrospinal fluid for cytological features and complete myelography are recommended following surgical resection in all patients with glioblastoma. If either result is abnormal, whole-axis radiation therapy is indicated.

Cerebellar Hemangioblastoma (Von Hippel-Lindau Disease)

Von Hippel-Lindau (VHL) disease is a multisystem disorder transmitted by autosomal dominant inheritance (Maher and Kaelin, 1997). The most prominent features are hemangioblastomas of the cerebellum and retina. All children with cerebellar hemangioblastomas have VHL disease. Among adults, 60% have isolated tumors and do not have the genetic defect. The expression of VHL disease is variable even within the same kindred. The most common features are cerebellar and retinal hemangioblastoma (59%), renal carcinoma (28%), and pheochromocytoma (7%).

CLINICAL FEATURES. Mean age at onset of cerebellar hemangioblastoma in VHL disease is 32 years; onset before 15 is unusual. The initial features are headache and ataxia. Retinal hemangioblastomas occur at a younger age and may cause visual impairment from hemorrhage as early as the first decade. They may be multiple and bilateral and appear on ophthalmoscopic examination as a dilated artery leading from the disk to a peripheral tumor with an engorged vein. Spinal hemangioblastomas are intramedullary in location and lead to syringomyelia. Pheochromocytomas are seen in 7% to 19% of patients and may be the only clinical manifestation.

DIAGNOSIS. The gene for VHL disease is a tumor-suppressor gene that maps to chromosome 3p25. Identification of the gene locus allows the identification of asymptomatic, affected family members who need annual examinations to look for treatable abnormalities. Such examinations should include indirect ophthalmoscopy and renal ultrasound, as well as gadolinium-enhanced MRI of the brain every 3 years.

The clinical diagnosis of VHL disease is based on the presence of any of the following: more than one hemangioblastoma of the central nervous system, an isolated hemangioblastoma associated with a visceral cyst or renal carcinoma, or any known manifestation with a family history of disease.

MANAGEMENT. Cryotherapy or photocoagulation of smaller retinal lesions can lead to complete tumor regression without visual loss. Cerebellar hemangioblastoma should be treated surgically and can often be totally extirpated.

Ependymoma

Posterior fossa ependymoma is derived from the cells that line the roof and floor of the fourth ventricle. These tumors can extend into both lateral recesses and grow out to the cerebellopontine angle. They account for 10% of primary brain tumors in children.

CLINICAL FEATURES. Eight percent of all childhood brain tumors are ependymomas. The peak incidence in children is from birth to 4 years. Both genders are affected equally. The clinical features evolve slowly and are often present for several months before consultation is sought. Symptoms of increased intracranial pressure are the first feature in 90% of children. Disturbances of gait and coordination, neck pain, or cranial nerve dysfunction are the initial features in the remainder. Half of affected children have ataxia, usually of the vermal type, and one third have nystagmus. Head tilt or neck stiffness is present in one third of children and indicates extension of tumor into the cervical canal.

Although steady deterioration is expected, some children have an intermittent course. Episodes of headache and vomiting, ataxia, and even nuchal rigidity lasting for days or weeks are followed by periods of well-being. These intermittent symptoms are caused by transitory obstruction of the fourth ventricle or aqueduct by the tumor acting in a ball-valve fashion.

DIAGNOSIS. MRI is better than CT at showing the tumor's location in the fourth ventricle and its extraventricular extensions. The ventricular system is almost always markedly dilated.

MANAGEMENT. The goals of surgical therapy are to relieve the hydrocephalus and to remove as much tumor as possible without damaging the fourth ventricle. Postoperative irradiation to the posterior fossa is indicated. Neuraxis radiation is not recommended unless leptomeningeal disease is recognized at diagnosis. Poor prognostic features include an age of less than 2 to 5 years

at diagnosis, brainstem invasion, and a radiation dose of less than 4,500 cGy.

Medulloblastoma

Medulloblastoma is a primitive neuroectodermal tumor (PNET) with the capacity to differentiate into neuronal and glial tissue. Most tumors are in the vermis or fourth ventricle, with or without extension into the cerebellar hemispheres. Approximately 10% are in the hemisphere alone.

CLINICAL FEATURES. Most series indicate a male-to-female ratio of 3:2. Ninety percent of cases have their onset during the first decade and the remainder during the second decade. Medulloblastoma is the most common primary brain tumor with onset during infancy.

The tumor grows rapidly, and the interval between onset of symptoms and medical consultation is generally brief; 2 weeks in 25% of cases and less than a month in 50%. Vomiting is an initial symptom in 58% of children, headache in 40%, an unsteady gait in 20%, and torticollis or stiff neck in 10%. The predominance of vomiting with or without headache as an early symptom is probably caused when the tumor irritates the floor of the fourth ventricle. Gait disturbances are more common in young children and are characterized by refusal to stand or walk rather than by ataxia.

Two thirds of children have papilledema at the time of initial examination. Truncal ataxia and limb ataxia are equally common, and both may be present. Only 22% of children have nystagmus. Tendon reflexes are hyperactive when hydrocephalus is present and hypoactive when the tumor is causing primarily cerebellar dysfunction.

DIAGNOSIS. Medulloblastoma is readily diagnosed with CT or MRI (Figure 10-3). The tumors are highly vascular and become enhanced when contrast medium is used.

MANAGEMENT. The prognosis for children with medulloblastoma is greatly improved by the combined use of surgical extirpation, radiation therapy, and chemotherapy. The role of surgery is to provide histological identification, debulk the tumor, and relieve obstruction of the fourth ventricle. Ventriculoperitoneal shunting may be needed to reduce intracranial pressure even before decompressive resection.

The overall 5-year survival rate is approximately 40%. Survival is better in children who have gross total tumor resection compared with partial resection or biopsy. Craniospinal radia-

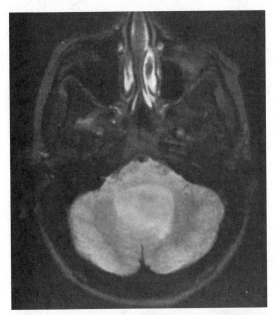

Figure 10-3. MRI of medulloblastoma. The tumor is seen as an enhancing mass in the vermis of the cerebellum.

tion increases survival better than local field radiation. Survival is significantly improved by the use of adjuvant chemotherapy.

Congenital Malformations

Basilar Impression

Basilar impression is a disorder of the craniovertebral junction in which the odontoid process is displaced posteriorly and compresses the spinal cord or brainstem.

CLINICAL FEATURES. The first symptoms are often head tilt, neck stiffness, and headache. The onset of symptoms is frequently precipitated by minor trauma to the head or neck. Examination shows ataxia, nystagmus, and hyperreflexia.

DIAGNOSIS. MRI is the best method to visualize the cervicomedullary junction and may also be useful to delineate an associated Chiari malformation or syringobulbia (Figure 10-4).

MANAGEMENT. Surgical decompression of the foramen magnum usually relieves symptoms.

Cerebellar Malformations

Congenital Hemisphere Hypoplasia

Congenital hypoplasia of the cerebellum can be unilateral or bilateral. Unilateral cerebellar hypoplasia is not associated with genetic disorders (Ramaekers et al, 1997). More than half of pa-

tients with bilateral disease have an identifiable genetic disorder transmitted by autosomal recessive inheritance. The common histological feature is the absence of granular cells, with relative preservation of Purkinje cells. In some hereditary forms, granular cell degeneration may continue postnatally and cause progressive cerebellar dysfunction during infancy.

CLINICAL FEATURES. Developmental delay and hypotonia are the first features suggesting a cerebral abnormality in the infant. Titubation of the head is a constant feature, and some combination of ataxia, dysmetria, and intention tremor is also noted. A jerky, coarse nystagmus is usually present. Tendon reflexes may be increased or diminished. Those with hyperactive reflexes probably have congenital abnormalities of the corticospinal tract in addition to cerebellar hypoplasia. Seizures occur in some hereditary and some sporadic cases. Other neurological signs and symptoms may be present, depending on associated malformations. Mental retardation is a constant feature but varies from mild to severe.

DIAGNOSIS. MRI is the study of choice (Figure 10-4). It shows not only the extent of cerebellar hypoplasia but also associated anomalies. The folial pattern of the cerebellum is prominent, and there is compensatory enlargement of the fourth ventricle, cisterna magna, and vallecula.

MANAGEMENT. No treatment is available.

Vermal Aplasia

Aplasia of the vermis is relatively common and often associated with other cerebral malformations. All or part of the vermis may be missing,

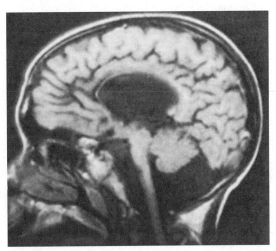

Figure 10-4. Aplasia of the cerebellum associated with thinning of the corpus callosum.

and when the vermis is incomplete, the caudal portion is usually lacking (Al Shahwan et al, 1995). Dominantly inherited aplasia of the anterior vermis is a rare condition.

CLINICAL FEATURES. Partial agenesis of the cerebellar vermis may be asymptomatic. Symptoms are nonprogressive and vary from only mild gait ataxia and upbeating nystagmus to severe ataxia.

Complete agenesis causes titubation of the head and truncal ataxia. Vermal agenesis is frequently associated with other cerebral malformations, producing a constellation of symptoms and signs referable to neurological dysfunction. Two such examples are the Dandy-Walker malformation (see Chapter 18) and the *Joubert syndrome.*

The clinical features of Joubert syndrome includes a characteristic facies, oculomotor apraxia, and hyperpnea intermixed with central apnea in the neonatal period (Maria et al, 1999). Cerebellar vermal agenesis is a constant feature of the Joubert syndrome, but several other cerebral malformations are usually present as well. More than one sibling in a family may be involved, but the parents are normal. All patients are mentally retarded, and some are microcephalic. Several affected children have died unexpectedly, possibly from respiratory failure.

DIAGNOSIS. MRI shows agenesis of the vermis of the cerebellum with enlargement of the cisterna magna. Other cerebral malformations, such as agenesis of the corpus callosum, may be observed as well.

MANAGEMENT. No treatment is available.

X-Linked Cerebellar Hypoplasia

One family with cerebellar hemispheric and vermal hypoplasia had a genetic defect that mapped to the short arm of the X chromosome (Illarioshkin et al, 1996). Developmental milestones are delayed, and affected males may also show some combination of nonprogressive ataxia, dysarthria, and external ophthalmoplegia. Intelligence is normal.

Chiari Malformation Type I

The type I Chiari malformation is a displacement of the cerebellar tonsils and posterior vermis of the cerebellum through the foramen magnum, compressing the spinomedullary junction. The type II Chiari malformation has an additional downward displacement of a dysplastic

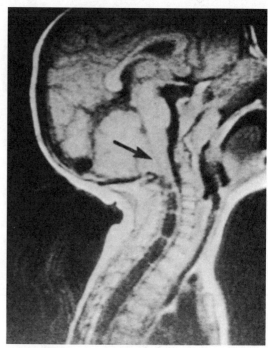

Figure 10-5. Chiari malformation. MRI shows displacement of the cerebellar tonsils (*arrow*) into the foramen magnum.

lower medulla and a lumbosacral meningomyelocele (see Chapter 12).

CLINICAL FEATURES. The onset of symptoms is frequently delayed until adolescence or adult life. Major clinical features are headache, head tilt, pain in the neck and shoulders, ataxia, and lower cranial nerve dysfunction. Physical signs vary among patients and may include weakness of the arms, hyperactive tendon reflexes in the legs, nystagmus, and ataxia. Chiari I is often an incidental finding on neuroimaging studies in children with headache.

DIAGNOSIS. MRI provides the best visualization of posterior fossa structures. The distortion of the cerebellum and the hindbrain is precisely identified (Figure 10-5).

MANAGEMENT. Surgical decompression of the foramen magnum to at least the C3 vertebra is recommended. More than half of patients are significantly improved by surgery.

Progressive Hereditary Ataxias

Autosomal Dominant Inheritance

Spinocerebellar Degenerations

A genotypic classification of the dominantly inherited ataxias has replaced the phenotypic classification that included Marie's ataxia, olivopontocerebellar atrophy (OPCA), and spino-cerebellar atrophies (SCA) (Bird, 1999). The progressive autosomal dominant ataxias with onset in childhood are listed in Table 10-3. The genetic abnormality is usually a trinucleotide repeat. SCA3 was originally described in Portuguese families from the Azores and is also called *Machado-Joseph Disease* (MJD).

CLINICAL FEATURES. The clinical features overlap, and they are best distinguished by genetic testing. Table 10-3 indicates a few distinguishing clinical features.

DIAGNOSIS. DNA-based genetic tests are available for the diagnosis of SCA1, SCA2, SCA3, SCA6, SCA7, and DRPLA.

MANAGEMENT. Treatment is symptomatic and, depending on the disease, may include anticonvulsants, muscle relaxants, and assistive devices.

Hypobetalipoproteinemia

CLINICAL FEATURES. Several different disorders are associated with hypocholesterolemia and reduced, but not absent, concentrations of apolipoprotein B and apolipoprotein A. Some patients with this lipid profile have no neurological symptoms; others have severe ataxia beginning in infancy. Malabsorption does not occur, but the infant fails to thrive and has progressive fatty cirrhosis of the liver. Severe hypotonia and absence of tendon reflexes are noted in the first months.

DIAGNOSIS. The diagnosis should be considered in children with unexplained progressive ataxia. The total serum lipid content is normal, but the concentration of triglycerides is increased. Total high- and low-density lipoprotein cholesterol concentrations are reduced, as are those of apolipoproteins.

MANAGEMENT. Administering 1,000 to 10,000 mg/day of DL-α-tocopherol prevents many of the complications of hypobetalipoproteinemia. Vitamins A and K also should be supplemented.

Autosomal Recessive Inheritance

Ataxia is a feature of many degenerative disorders but is a presenting or cardinal feature in the disorders discussed in this section.

Abetalipoproteinemia

Abetalipoproteinemia is caused by a molecular defect(s) in the gene for the microsomal triglyceride transfer protein (MTTP) at chromosome 4q22-q24. It is transmitted by autosomal recessive inheritance. Other terms for the disorder are *acanthocytosis* and the *Bassen-Kornzweig syndrome*. MMTP catalyzes the transport of triglyceride, cholesteryl ester, and phospholipid from phospholipid surfaces. The results are fat malabsorption and a progressive deficiency of vitamins A, E, and K.

CLINICAL FEATURES. Fat malabsorption is present from birth, and most newborns come to medical attention because of failure to thrive, vomiting, and large volumes of loose stool. The correct diagnosis may be made at that time.

Psychomotor development during infancy is delayed. A cerebellar ataxia develops in one

---

Table 10-3
Autosomal Dominant Cerebellar Ataxias: Clinical Characteristics

Disease	Average Onset (range in years)	Clinical Features (all include ataxia)
SCA1	4th decade (<10 to >60)	Pyramidal signs, peripheral neuropathy
SCA2	3rd–4th decade (<10 to >60)	Slow saccadic eye movement, peripheral neuropathy, decreased DTRs, dementia
SCA3	4th decade (10–70)	Pyramidal and extrapyramidal signs; lid retraction, nystagmus, decreased saccade velocity; amyotrophic fasciculations, sensory loss
SCA4	4th–5th decade (19–59)	Sensory axonal neuropathy
SCA5	3rd–4th decade (10–68)	Early onset, slow course
SCA7	3rd–4th decade (1/2–60)	Visual loss with retinopathy
SCA12	3rd (8–55)	Early tremor, late dementia
DRPLA	Rare (USA) 8–20 20% (Japan) 40–60s	Early onset correlates with shorter duration; chorea, seizures, dementia, myoclonus

ADCA, autosomal dominant cerebellar ataxias; DRPLA, dentatorubral-pallidoluysian atrophy; DTRs, deep tendon reflexes; EA, episodic ataxia; SCA, spinocerebellar ataxia.
Source: Adapted from Bird (1999).

third of children during the first decade and in almost every child by the end of the second decade. Tendon reflexes are usually lost by 5 years of age. Progressive limb ataxia is characterized by gait disturbances, dysmetria, and difficulty performing rapid alternating movements. Ataxia progresses until the third decade and then becomes stationary. Proprioceptive sensation is lost in the hands and feet, and pinprick and temperature sensations are mildly reduced. Sensory loss results from demyelination in the posterior columns of the spinal cord and the peripheral nerves.

Retinitis pigmentosa is an almost constant feature. The age at onset is variable but is usually during the first decade. The initial symptom is night blindness. Nystagmus is common and may be caused either by the cerebellar disturbance or by loss of central vision.

DIAGNOSIS. Severe anemia, with hemoglobin levels less than 8 g/dl (5 mmol/L), is common in young children but not in adults. The anemia may result from malabsorption and can be corrected with parenteral supplementation of iron or folate. Plasma cholesterol levels are less than 100 mg/dl (2.5 mmol/L), and triglyceride levels are less than 30 mg/dl (0.3 mmol/L). The diagnosis is confirmed by the absence of apolipoprotein B in plasma. Parents should be screened for apolipoprotein B as well. In abetalipoproteinemia the heterozygote is normal; if partial deficiency of apolipoprotein B is present, the diagnosis of familial hypobetalipoproteinemia is more likely.

MANAGEMENT. The neurological complications of abetalipoproteinemia are caused by chronic vitamin E deficiency. Dietary fat restriction and large oral doses of vitamin E (100 mg/kg/day) prevent the onset of symptoms or arrest their progression.

Ataxia Telangiectasia

Ataxia-telangiectasia (AT) primarily affects the nervous and immune systems. The gene associated with AT is a large gene located at chromosome 11q22-23, and more than 100 mutations have been discovered. The gene product is involved in cell-cycle progression and the checkpoint response to DNA damage. It is transmitted by autosomal recessive inheritance.

CLINICAL FEATURES. The principal feature is a progressive truncal ataxia that begins during the first year. In infants, choreoathetosis develops instead of, or in addition to, ataxia. The ataxia begins as clumsiness and progresses so slowly that cerebral palsy is often the erroneous diagnosis. Oculomotor apraxia is present in 90% of patients but may be mild at first and overlooked (see Chapter 15). Many children are said to have a dull or expressionless face. Intellectual development is normal at first but often lags with time. One third of children ultimately function in the mildly retarded range.

Telangiectasia usually develops after 2 years of age and sometimes as late as age 10. It first appears on the bulbar conjunctivae, giving the eyes a bloodshot appearance. Similar telangiectasia appears on the upper half of the ears, on the flexor surfaces of the limbs, and in a butterfly distribution on the face. Telangiectasia may be exacerbated by exposure to sun or by irritation or friction.

Recurrent sinopulmonary infection is one of the more serious features of the disease and reflects an underlying immunodeficiency. The synthesis of antibodies and certain immunoglobulin subclasses is disturbed because of disorders of B-cell and helper T-cell function. Serum and salivary IgA is absent in 70% to 80% of children, and IgE is absent or diminished in 80% to 90%. The IgM concentration may be elevated in compensation for the IgA deficiency. The thymus has an embryonic appearance, and the α-fetoprotein concentration is elevated in most patients.

Taken together, the many features of this disease suggest a generalized disorder of tissue differentiation and cellular repair. The result is an increased incidence of neoplasia, especially lymphoma and lymphocytic leukemia. Two thirds of patients are dead by 20 years of age. Infection is the most common cause of death, and neoplasia is second.

DIAGNOSIS. The diagnosis should be suspected in infants who have a combination of ataxia, chronic sinopulmonary infections, and oculomotor apraxia. As the child gets older, the addition of telangiectasia to the other clinical features makes the diagnosis a certainty. Complete studies of immunocompetence should be performed. Nearly all patients with AT have an elevated α-fetoprotein concentration, and approximately 80% have decreased serum IgA, IgE, or IgG. Especially characteristic is a selective deficiency of the IgG2 subclass. Some children with progressive childhood-onset ataxia and typical telangiectasia have normal serum α-fetoprotein and immunoglobulin levels.

The acanthocyte is an abnormal erythrocyte characterized by thorny projections from the cell surface that prevent normal rouleau formation and cause a very low erythrocyte sedimentation rate. Between 50% and 70% of peripheral erythrocytes undergo transformation to acanthocytes. Acanthocytes are also seen in association with other neurological disorders in which lipoproteins are normal (see the discussions of McLeod syndrome and neuroacanthocytosis).

MANAGEMENT. All infections must be treated vigorously. Intravenous antibiotics are sometimes required for what would otherwise be a trivial sinusitis in a normal child. Patients with AT are exquisitely sensitive to radiation, which produces cellular and chromosomal damage. Radiation may be a precipitant in the development of neoplasia. Therefore, despite the frequency of sinopulmonary infections, radiological studies must be minimized.

Ataxia with Diffuse Central Nervous System Demyelination

This disorder is apparently transmitted as an autosomal recessive trait because it occurs in male and female siblings (van der Knaap et al, 1997).

CLINICAL FEATURES. Development is normal during the first year. Some clumsiness may be noted during the second year, but the onset of progressive ataxia and diplegia is usually after age 2. The neurological deterioration is progressive, but episodes of progression may follow intercurrent illness. Dysarthria and seizures may occur, but cognitive function and ocular motility are relatively preserved. Optic atrophy may occur late in the course. Muscle tone is depressed, but tendon reflexes are exaggerated and the plantar response is extensor.

DIAGNOSIS. MRI shows progressive, diffuse, homogeneous hypodensity of the white matter. Lysosomal and peroxisomal enzyme concentrations are normal. No biochemical defect is identified.

MANAGEMENT. Treatment is supportive.

Friedreich Ataxia

Friedreich ataxia is the most common inherited ataxia. It is caused by an unstable triplet repeat of the *frataxin* gene on chromosome 9q13 (Pandolfo, 1999). The size of the triplet expansion correlates with an earlier age at onset and a more rapid progression.

CLINICAL FEATURES. Clinical criteria for diagnosis have become less important with the availability of molecular diagnosis. Heterozygotes are asymptomatic, and the presence of abnormal signs, such as pes cavus or scoliosis, in parents should suggest a dominantly inherited ataxia or Charcot-Marie-Tooth disease (Dürr et al, 1996).

The onset is usually between 2 and 16 years of age, but symptoms may begin earlier or later. The initial feature is ataxia or clumsiness of gait in 95% of cases and scoliosis in 5%. The course is one of steady deterioration; most patients are confined to a wheelchair within 20 years of onset. Dysarthria always develops. Disturbances of ocular motility occur in 32% of patients, deafness in 8%, and titubation of the head in 4%. Symptoms of cerebellar dysfunction are more severe and more common in the arms than in the legs. Finger-nose ataxia and difficulty in performing rapidly alternating movements develop in almost every patient. Only 28% of patients show the same symptoms in the legs, but spastic weakness is often present and may hide the cerebellar signs.

All tendon reflexes are absent in 75% of children. Absent tendon reflexes in the legs was thought to be an essential feature for diagnosis. It is now recognized that the abnormal gene location in children with Friedreich ataxia and retained reflexes maps to the same 9q location. Extensor plantar responses are present in 89%. Joint position sense and vibration sense are absent in the feet in 90% and in the hands in 27%. Light touch and pain sensations are impaired in less than 10% of patients.

Scoliosis develops in 79% and pes cavus in 55% of patients. The severity of the skeletal deformities varies and is usually mild. A hypertrophic cardiomyopathy characterized by dyspnea on exertion, palpitations, and angina develops in 40% of patients. Systolic ejection murmurs, heard best over the apex or left sternal edge, are relatively common.

Diabetes is present in 10% of patients and has its onset during the third decade. It tends to be severe, may be difficult to control with insulin, and significantly contributes to death from the disease.

DIAGNOSIS. The diagnosis is suggested by the clinical features and confirmed by molecular diagnosis. Motor nerve conduction velocities in the arms and legs are slightly slower than normal. In contrast, sensory action potentials are either absent or markedly reduced in amplitude. Spinal somatosensory evoked responses are usually absent.

Common changes on the electrocardiogram (ECG) are reduced amplitude of T waves and left or right ventricular hypertrophy. Arrhythmias and conduction defects are uncommon.

MANAGEMENT. The underlying disturbance is not curable, but symptomatic treatment is available. Severe scoliosis should be prevented by surgical stabilization. Regular ECG and chest radiographs to determine heart size are useful to monitor the development of cardiomyopathy. Chest pain on exertion responds to propranolol, and congestive heart failure responds to digitalis. Patients should be checked for diabetes and should be treated with insulin when necessary.

Juvenile GM₂ Gangliosidosis

All juvenile forms of both α- and β-hexosaminidase-A deficiency are transmitted by autosomal recessive inheritance. Some, like Tay-Sachs disease, are restricted to Ashkenazi Jews, whereas others occur in individuals of non-Jewish descent (see Chapter 5). In all of these conditions, GM₂ gangliosides are stored within the central nervous system.

CLINICAL FEATURES. A progressive ataxic syndrome occurs in patients with late-onset hexosaminidase-A deficiency. Age at onset is usually before 15 years. Affected children may be considered clumsy for several years before neurological deterioration is evident. Intention tremor, dysarthria, and limb and gait ataxia are prominent.

DIAGNOSIS. Any child with an apparent "spinocerebellar degeneration" may have juvenile GM₂ gangliosidosis. Diagnosis requires the measurement of α- and β-hexosaminidase activity in fibroblasts.

MANAGEMENT. No treatment is available.

Juvenile Sulfatide Lipidosis

Sulfatide lipidosis (metachromatic leukodystrophy) is a disorder of central and peripheral myelin metabolism usually caused by deficient activity of the enzyme arylsulfatase A. The defective gene is on chromosome 22q. The late infantile form is discussed in Chapters 5 and 7. The juvenile form is usually caused by arylsulfatase deficiency but may also be caused by saposin B deficiency.

CLINICAL FEATURES. Juvenile sulfatide lipidosis begins later and has a slower course than the late infantile disease. Onset is usually between 4 and 12 years. Initial symptoms are poor school performance, behavioral change, and a gait disturbance. These are followed by spasticity, progressive ataxia of the trunk and limbs, generalized tonic-clonic convulsions, and mental deterioration. Peripheral neuropathy is not a prominent clinical feature, but motor conduction velocities are usually prolonged late in the course. Protein concentration in the cerebrospinal fluid may be normal or only slightly elevated.

Progression is relatively rapid. Most children deteriorate into a vegetative state and die within 10 years. The time from onset to death ranges from 3 to 17 years and cannot be predicted by age at onset.

DIAGNOSIS. MRI shows widespread demyelination of the cerebral hemispheres. Patients with late-onset disease are often thought to have multiple sclerosis. Diagnosis requires the demonstration of reduced or absent arylsulfatase A in peripheral leukocytes. Those with reduced amounts should be tested for saposin B deficiency.

MANAGEMENT. Allogenic bone marrow transplantation is being tried on an experimental basis.

Marinesco-Sjögren Syndrome

Cerebellar ataxia, congenital cataracts, and mental retardation are the characteristic features of the Marinesco-Sjögren syndrome. This complex may have many causes. In some families, ragged-red fibers are seen on muscle biopsy, and exercise induces hyperlactemia suggesting a mitochondrial disorder. In other families, acute rhabdomyolysis with marked weakness follows a viral infection (Muller-Felber et al, 1998).

CLINICAL FEATURES. A constant feature is cataracts, which may be congenital or develop during infancy. The type of cataract varies and is not specific. Cerebellar dysfunction during infancy is characterized by dysarthria, nystagmus, and ataxia of the trunk and limbs. Strabismus and hypotonia are frequently present in childhood. Developmental delay is a constant feature but varies from mild to severe. Other features include short stature, delayed sexual development, pes valgus, and scoliosis.

Although the onset of symptoms is in infancy, the progress is slow or stationary. Ataxia leads to confinement in a wheelchair by the third or fourth decade, and the life span is significantly shortened.

DIAGNOSIS. Diagnosis of the Marinesco-Sjögren syndrome relies primarily on the triad of bilateral cataracts, progressive cerebellar ataxia, and mental retardation. The underlying biochemical defect is unknown, and laboratory tests are not helpful.

MANAGEMENT. Treatment is supportive.

Ramsay Hunt Syndrome

Ramsay Hunt syndrome, also termed *dyssynergia cerebellaris myoclonica,* is a progressive degeneration of the dentate nucleus and superior cerebellar peduncle characterized by myoclonus, cerebellar ataxia, and infrequent seizures in the absence of dementia. Many patients will prove to have mitochondrial encephalomyopathies (see Chapter 5). Sporadic occurrence is common. It is likely that this not a single entity, and the term is of questionable usefulness.

CLINICAL FEATURES. A general clinical picture can be delineated. The initial symptom is clumsiness, usually noted during the first decade, which evolves into progressive ataxia. Intention tremor and dysarthria may follow. Myoclonus usually begins in the second decade. It is present at rest but is made worse by attempted movement. Myoclonus may be so severe as to throw the patient to the floor. The combination of ataxia and myoclonus is severely disabling. Generalized tonic-clonic convulsions develop late in the course and are not a constant feature. Tendon reflexes are depressed, and scoliosis may be present.

DIAGNOSIS. The diagnosis of Ramsay Hunt syndrome is based on the combination of cerebellar ataxia and myoclonus. Variants with autosomal dominant inheritance, as well as other syndromes causing myoclonic epilepsy, must be considered (see Chapter 1). MRI may show atrophy of the pons, cerebellar peduncles, and cerebellum. EEG frequently shows epileptiform activity of the slow spike-wave type.

MANAGEMENT. Seizures usually respond to ordinary anticonvulsant drugs. Valproate is specifically useful in reducing the severity and frequency of myoclonus.

Sea-Blue Histiocytoses

Sea-blue histiocytoses are a heterogeneous group of neurovisceral storage diseases that includes Niemann-Pick disease. In many, the enzymatic error has not been established. Sea-blue histiocytes are large macrophages 20 to 60 μm in diameter with a single eccentric nucleus and a prominent nucleolus. Wright-Giemsa staining reveals blue or blue-green granules in the cytoplasm that contain ceroid, lipofuscin, and sphingomyelin. The histiocytes are present in the bone marrow, liver, and lymph glands.

CLINICAL FEATURES. The initial features may be hepatosplenomegaly or neurological deterioration. Onset of symptoms can be as early as 2 months of age, but more commonly occurs after 1 year and sometimes after 10 years of age. Ataxia and spasticity are prominent features. The initial progress of neurological dysfunction is so slow that the child is thought to have cerebral palsy. Involuntary movements and tremor may be present.

Neurological deterioration accelerates as the child gets older. Later symptoms include dementia, seizures, speech disturbances, and supranuclear ophthalmoplegia. Severe bulbar palsy leads to aspiration and death.

DIAGNOSIS. Sea-blue histiocytosis is a diagnosis of exclusion. When sea-blue histiocytes are present in the bone marrow or liver, an extensive search for a lysosomal enzyme defect must be made. Niemann-Pick disease type C should be especially suspected (see Chapter 5).

MANAGEMENT. No treatment is available. Liver transplantation was tried in one patient without success.

Other Metabolic Disorders

Hartnup disease and maple syrup urine disease were both described in the section on acute or recurrent ataxia. After an acute attack of these diseases, some patients never return to baseline but instead have chronic progressive ataxia. Such patients should be screened for metabolic disorders (Table 10-4). Refsum disease is an in-

---

Table 10-4
Metabolic Screening in Progressive Ataxias

Disease	Abnormality
Blood	
Abetalipoproteinemia	Lipoproteins, cholesterol
Adrenoleukodystrophy	Very-long-chain fatty acids
Ataxia-telangiectasia	IgA, IgE, α-fetoprotein
Hypobetalipoproteinemia	Lipoproteins, cholesterol
Mitochondrial disorders	Lactate, glucose-lactate tolerance
Sulfatide lipidoses	Arylsulfatase A
Urine	
Hartnup disease	Amino acids
Maple syrup urine disease	Amino acids
Fibroblasts	
Carnitine acetyltransferase deficiency	Carnitine acetyltransferase
GM_2 gangliosidosis	Hexosaminidase
Refsum disease	Phytanic acid
Bone Marrow	
Neurovisceral storage	Sea-blue histiocytes

born error of phytanic acid metabolism and is transmitted by autosomal recessive inheritance. The cardinal features are retinitis pigmentosa, chronic or recurrent polyneuropathy, and cerebellar ataxia. Affected individuals usually have either night blindness or neuropathy (see Chapter 7).

Disorders of pyruvate metabolism and the respiratory chain enzymes produce widespread disturbances in the nervous system and are described in Chapters 5, 7, and 8. The common features among the several disorders of mitochondrial metabolism include lactic acidosis, ataxia, hypotonia, ophthalmoplegia, mental retardation, and peripheral neuropathy. These disorders are suggested by a raised concentration of blood lactate or the production of lactic acidosis by administration of a standard glucose tolerance test. A deficiency of pyruvate dehydrogenase may produce acute, recurrent, or chronic ataxias and is discussed in the section on acute or recurrent ataxia. Respiratory chain disorders produce a combination of ataxia, dementia, myoclonus, and seizures.

X-Linked Inheritance

Ataxia may be the initial feature of the infantile form of adrenoleukodystrophy (see Chapter 5). The clinical features of adrenoleukodystrophy can mimic a spinocerebellar degeneration and should be considered in any family with only males affected. An X-linked ataxia associated with hypotonia, deafness, and loss of vision in early childhood occurs in some families. Other families have only ataxia and deafness. The abnormal gene site and gene product have not been established, and it is not possible to know if these are allelic or different disorders.

Ataxia with Dementia

CLINICAL FEATURES. Age at onset of ataxia with dementia is 2 to 3 years. The initial features are delayed developmental milestones, clumsiness, and intention tremor. Early school performance is acceptable. Progressive ataxia and spasticity develop in affected males during the second decade. Incoordination becomes progressively severe, leading to loss of ambulation. Progressive dementia begins in the third and fourth decades. Death usually occurs in the seventh decade.

Cerebellar, corticospinal, and intellectual functions are abnormal. Other neurological systems are intact.

DIAGNOSIS. CT or MRI shows cerebellar atrophy. No biochemical defect has been identified.

Adrenoleukodystrophy is a major consideration, and plasma concentrations of very-long-chain fatty acids should be determined.

MANAGEMENT. Treatment is supportive.

References

Al Shahwan SA, Bruyn GW, Al Deeb SM. Non-progressive familial congenital cerebellar hypoplasia. *J Neurol Sci* 1995;128:71–77.

Baloh RW, Yue Q, Furman J, et al. Familial episodic ataxia: Clinical heterogeneity in four families linked to chromosome 19. *Ann Neurol* 1997;41:8–16.

Bird TD. (Updated 25 October 1999) Ataxia Overview. In: GeneClinics: Medical Genetics Knowledge Base [database online]. University of Washington at Seattle. Available at http://www.geneclinics.org/profiles/pws. Accessed 30 December 1999.

Connolly AM, Dodson WE, Prensky AL, et al. Course and outcome of acute cerebellar ataxia. *Ann Neurol* 1994;35:673–679.

Dürr A, Cossee M, Agid Y, et al. Clinical and genetic abnormalities in patients with Friedreich's ataxia. *N Engl J Med* 1996;335:1169–1175.

Illarioshkin SN, Tanaka H, Markova ED, et al. X-linked nonprogressive congenital cerebellar hypoplasia: Clinical description and mapping to chromosome Xq. *Ann Neurol* 1996;40:75–83.

Jacobs BC, Endtz H, van der Meche FG, et al. Serum anti-GQ1b IgG antibodies recognize surface epitopes on *Campylobacter jejuni* from patients with Miller Fisher syndrome. *Ann Neurol* 1995;37:260–264.

Lindskog U, Ödkvist L, Noaksson L, et al. Benign paroxysmal vertigo in childhood: A long-term follow-up. *Headache* 1999;39:33–37.

Lubbers WJ, Brunt ERP, Scheffer H, et al. Hereditary myokymia and paroxysmal ataxia linked to chromosome 12 is responsive to acetazolamide. *J Neurol Neurosurg Psychiatry* 1995;59:400-405.

Maher ER, Kaelin WG Jr. von Hippel-Lindau disease. *Medicine* 1997;76:381–391.

Maria BL, Boltshauser E, Palmer SC, et al. Clinical features and revised diagnostic criteria in Joubert syndrome. *J Child Neurol* 1999;14:583–591.

Muller-Felber W, Zafiriou D, Scheck R, et al. Marinesco-Sjogren syndrome with rhabdomyolysis: A new subtype of the disease. *Neuropediatrics* 1998;29:97–101.

Pandolfo M. Molecular pathogenesis of Friedreich ataxia. *Arch Neurol* 1999;56:1201–1208.

Ramaekers VTh, Heimann G, Reul J, et al. Genetic disorders and cerebellar structural abnormalities in childhood. *Brain* 1997;120:1739–1751.

Ruggieri M, Polizzi A, Pavone L, et al. Multiple sclerosis in children less under 6 years of age. *Neurology* 1999;53:478–484.

Russo C, Cohen SL, Petruzzi J, et al. Long-term neurological outcome in children with opsoclonus-myoclonus associated with neuroblastoma: A report of the pediatric oncology group. *Med Pediatr Oncol* 1997;29:284–288.

Sawaishi Y, Takahashi I, Hirayama Y, et al. Acute cerebellitis caused by *Coxiella burnetti*. *Ann Neurol* 1999;45:124–127.

van der Knaap MS, Barth PG, Gabreëls FJM, et al. A new leukoencephalopathy with vanishing white matter. *Neurology* 1997;48:845–855.

Chapter 11
Hemiplegia

THE APPROACH TO children with hemiplegia must distinguish between acute hemiplegia, in which weakness develops within a few hours, and chronic progressive hemiplegia, in which weakness evolves over days, weeks, or months. The distinction between an acute and an insidious onset should be easy but can be problematic. In children with a slowly evolving hemiplegia, early weakness may be missed until an obvious level of functional disability is reached; then the hemiplegia seems new and acute.

An additional presentation of hemiplegia is found in infants who come to medical attention because they are slow in meeting motor milestones or are not using one hand. They have a static structural problem from birth (hemiplegic cerebral palsy), but the clinical features are not apparent until the child is old enough to use the affected limbs.

Magnetic resonance imaging (MRI) has become the diagnostic modality of choice for investigating all forms of hemiplegia, and is especially informative in hemiplegic cerebral palsy to show migrational defects that are also causing seizures. Magnetic resonance arteriography (MRA) is sufficiently informative to obviate the need for arteriography in most children.

Hemiplegic Cerebral Palsy

The term *hemiplegic cerebral palsy* comprises several pathological entities that result in limb weakness on one side of the body. In premature infants the most common cause is periventricular hemorrhagic infarction (see Chapter 4). In term infants the underlying causes are often cerebral malformations, cerebral infarction, and intracerebral hemorrhage. Imaging studies of the brain are useful to provide the family with a definitive diagnosis. This often relieves guilt and prevents litigation against the obstetrician.

Infants with hemiplegia from birth are often brought to evaluation because crawling or walking is delayed and attention is directed at the legs. An associated but seldom recognized feature is that hand dominance was established during the first year; *this is not normal*. Unilateral facial weakness is never associated, probably because bilateral corticobulbar innervation of the lower face persists until birth.

Infants with injury to the dominant hemisphere can develop normal speech in the nondominant hemisphere, but it is at the expense of visuoperceptual and spatial skills. Infants with hemiplegia and early-onset seizures are an exception; they show cognitive disturbances of verbal and nonverbal skills.

Congenital Malformations

Migrational defects comprise the majority of congenital malformations causing infantile hemiplegia (Figure 11-1). The affected hemisphere is often small and may show a unilateral perisylvian syndrome in which the sylvian fossa is widened (Sébire et al, 1996). A bilateral perisylvian syndrome with speech disturbances is described in Chapter 17. Seizures and mental retardation are often associated. As a rule, epilepsy is more common when infantile hemiplegia is caused by congenital malformations than by stroke.

Neonatal Infarction

Cerebral infarction from arterial occlusion occurs more often in full-term newborns than in

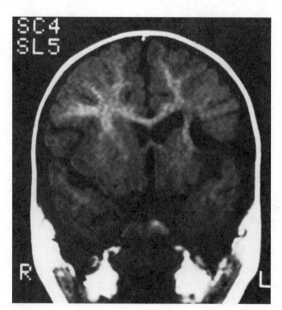

Figure 11-1. Schizencephaly. The rim of gray matter around the defect in the left hemisphere indicates that the abnormity is a schizencephaly rather than an infarction. The child's main abnormality was hemiplegia.

premature newborns. Three patterns of infarction are seen with MRI: (1) arterial border zone infarction is usually associated with resuscitation and probably is caused by hypotension; (2) multiartery infarction is less often associated with perinatal distress and may be caused by congenital heart disease, disseminated intravascular coagulation, and polycythemia; and (3) single-artery infarction can be caused by injury to the cervical portion of the carotid artery during a difficult delivery owing to either misapplication of obstetric forceps or hyperextension and rotation of the neck with stretching of the artery over the lateral portion of the upper cervical vertebrae. However, trauma is a rare associated event, and the cause of most single-artery infarctions, especially large infarctions in the frontal or parietal lobes, cannot be explained.

CLINICAL FEATURES. Newborns with large single-artery infarcts appear normal at birth but develop repetitive focal seizures during the first 4 days postpartum. Some recover fully, but most are left with a hemiparesis that spares the face.

DIAGNOSIS. MRI is necessary to show small infarcts, but large infarcts in the complete distribution of the middle cerebral artery can be detected by ultrasound. The size of the defect on MRI correlates directly with the probability of later hemiplegia (Mercuri et al, 1999). Follow-up imaging studies may show either unilateral enlargement of the lateral ventricle or porencephaly in

the distribution of the middle cerebral artery contralateral to the hemiparesis. Hemiatrophy of the pons contralateral to the abnormal hemisphere may be an associated feature.

Maternal use of cocaine during pregnancy can cause cerebral infarction and hemorrhage in the fetus. Cocaine can be detected in the newborn's urine during the first week postpartum. **MANAGEMENT.** Anticonvulsant drugs are usually effective for seizure control (see Chapter 1). Rehabilitative measures are the mainstay of therapy.

Neonatal Hemorrhage

Small unilateral parietal or temporal hemorrhages occur almost exclusively in term newborns and are not associated with either trauma or asphyxia. Larger hemorrhages into the temporal lobe sometimes result when excessive force is applied with obstetric forceps, but more often they are idiopathic. Intraventricular hemorrhage may be an associated feature.

CLINICAL FEATURES. Newborns with small hemorrhages are normal at birth and seem well until seizures begin, anytime during the first week. The symptoms of larger hemorrhages may be apneic spells, seizures, or both. Seizures may be focal or generalized, and hemiplegia or hypotonia is present on examination. Some infants recover completely, whereas others are left with hemiplegia and mental retardation.

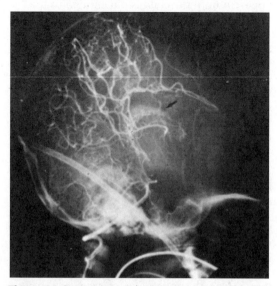

Figure 11-2. Moyamoya disease. Arteriography demonstrates occlusion of the carotid artery at the siphon and new anastomotic vessel formation (*arrow*).

DIAGNOSIS. Seizures and apneic spells usually prompt lumbar puncture to exclude the possibility of sepsis. The cerebrospinal fluid is grossly bloody. Computed tomography (CT) shows hemorrhage (Figure 11-2), and follow-up studies show focal encephalomalacia.

MANAGEMENT. Treatment is available for seizures but not for hemorrhage.

Acute Hemiplegia

The sudden onset of an acute, focal neurological deficit suggests either a vascular or an epileptic mechanism (Table 11-1). Infants and children who have acute hemiplegia can be divided almost equally into two groups according to whether or not the hemiplegia was preceded by epilepsia partialis continua. Both groups may have seizures on the paretic side after hemiplegia is established. Cerebral infarction, usually in the distribution of the middle cerebral artery, accounts for one quarter of cases in which seizures precede the hemiplegia and more than half of cases in which hemiplegia is the initial feature. Whatever the cause, the probability of a permanent motor deficit is almost 100% when the initial feature is epilepsia partialis continua and about 50% when it is not.

Alternating Hemiplegia

This is a rare and poorly understood clinical syndrome with hemiplegia as a cardinal feature (Rho and Chugani, 1998). Its nosological identity has been linked to migraine, epilepsy, and familial paroxysmal choreoathetosis. All cases are sporadic, with the exception of one family in whom chromosomal analysis showed a balanced reciprocal translocation in the patient, in all the affected living relatives, and in one unaffected sibling. In this family, the onset of attacks was before 18 months in all affected children except one child whose first attack was at age 3 years.

CLINICAL FEATURES. Onset is from birth to 54 months (mean, 8 months). The initial features are mild developmental delay and abnormal eye movements (Kramer et al, in press). Motor attacks may be hemiplegia, dystonia, or both. As a rule, young infants have more dystonic features and older children are more likely to have flaccid hemiplegia. Brief episodes of monocular or binocular nystagmus, lasting for 1 to 3 minutes, are often associated with both dystonic and hemiplegic attacks. Because the attacks have an abrupt onset, dystonia is often thought to be a seizure and hemiplegia a stroke. Most reports of epileptic seizures during infancy are probably dystonic attacks.

The duration of hemiplegia varies from minutes to days, and intensity waxes and wanes during a single episode. During long attacks, hemiplegia may shift from side to side or both sides may be affected. The arm is usually affected more than the leg, and walking may not be impaired. Hemiplegia disappears during sleep and reappears on awakening but not immediately.

Dystonic episodes may primarily affect the limbs on one side, causing hemidystonia, or affect the trunk, causing opisthotonic posturing. Some children scream during attacks as if in pain. Headache is sometimes reported at the onset of an attack but not afterward. Writhing movements that suggest choreoathetosis may be associated.

Mental retardation is recognized early in the course, and mental regression occurs with time. Stepwise neurological impairment occurs as well, as if recovery from individual attacks is incomplete.

DIAGNOSIS. Results of electroencephalography (EEG), cerebral arteriography, and MRI are normal. The diagnosis relies entirely on the clinical features.

MANAGEMENT. Anticonvulsant and antimigraine medications have consistently failed to prevent attacks or prevent progression. Flunarizine, a calcium channel-blocking agent, is recommended to reduce the frequency of attacks, but its efficacy is not established. Other calcium channel-blocking agents and anticonvulsant drugs have not been useful.

Alternating hemiplegia and dopa-responsive dystonia (see Chapter 14) share the feature of

---

Table 11-1
Differential Diagnosis of Acute Hemiplegia

Alternating hemiplegia
Asthmatic amyotrophy (see Chapter 13)
Cerebrovascular disease
Diabetes mellitus
Epilepsy
Hypoglycemia (see Chapter 2)
Kawasaki disease (see Chapter 10)
Migraine
Trauma
Tumor

episodic dystonia with diurnal variation, and levodopa-carbidopa should be tried in infants with attacks of dystonia.

Cerebrovascular Disease

The annual incidence of cerebral infarction in children after the newborn period is approximately 2.5 per 100,000. Half are ischemic and half are nontraumatic intracerebral and subarachnoid hemorrhages. The incidence rate is slightly higher in black than in white children. Approximately 25% of ischemic strokes in children are associated with a known risk factor (Table 11-2). The coexistence of multiple risk factors predicts a poor outcome (Lanthier et al, 2000).

Stroke is usually considered when a previously healthy child suddenly becomes hemiparetic or develops any focal neurological disturbance. Cranial CT or MRI confirms the diagnosis. Clinical features vary with the age of the child and the location of the stroke. Hemiplegia, either immediately or as a late sequela, is one of the more common features.

Infarction is identified on CT as an area of increased lucency that becomes enhanced with contrast material. As a rule, the lucency cannot be visualized in the first 24 hours after stroke. Cerebral infarction is often superficial, affecting both gray and white matter, and is in the distribution of a single artery. Multiple infarcts suggest either embolism or vasculitis. Small, deep lesions of the internal capsule are rare but can occur in infants.

The evaluation of a child with cerebral infarction is summarized in Table 11-3. The usual line of investigation includes tests for coagulopathies, vaculitis, and vasculopathies, a search for cardiac sources of emboli, and cerebral arteriography.

Intracerebral hemorrhage is readily identified as an area of increased density on a non–contrast-enhanced CT. It is frequently surrounded by edema and may produce a mass effect with shift of midline structures.

Arteriovenous Malformations

Supratentorial malformations may cause acute or chronic, progressive hemiplegia. Acute hemiplegia is usually caused by intraparenchymal hemorrhage. The major clinical features of hemorrhage into a hemisphere are loss of consciousness, seizures, and hemiplegia. Large hematomas shift midline structures and increase

Table 11-2
Causes of Stroke

Cerebrovascular Malformations
Arteriovenous malformation
Fibromuscular dysplasia
Hereditary hemorrhagic telangiectasia
Sturge-Weber syndrome

Coagulopathies/Hemoglobinopathies
Antiphospholipid antibodies/lupus anticoagulant
Congenital coagulation defects
Disseminated intravascular coagulation
Drug-induced thrombosis
Malignancy
Sickle cell anemia/disease
Thrombocytopenic purpura

Heart Disease
Arrhythmia
Atrial myxoma
Bacterial endocarditis
Cardiac catheterization
Cardiomyopathy
Cyanotic congenital defects
Mitral valve prolapse
Prosthetic heart valve
Rhabdomyoma
Rheumatic heart disease

Trauma
Arterial dissection
Blunt trauma to neck
Intraoral trauma
Vertebral manipulation

Vasculitis
Carotid infection
Drug abuse (amphetamines and cocaine)
Hemolytic-uremic syndrome (see Chapter 2)
Hypersensitivity vasculitis
Isolated angiitis
Kawasaki disease (see Chapter 10)
Meningitis (see Chapter 4)
Mixed connective tissue disease
Systemic lupus erythematosus
Takayasu arteritis
Varicella infection

Vasculopathies
Fabry disease
Homocystinuria (see Chapter 5)
Mitochondrial encephalopathy, lactic acidosis, and stroke (MELAS)
Moyamoya disease

intracranial pressure. Arteriovenous malformations are discussed fully in Chapter 4.

Brain Tumors

Acute hemiplegia from brain tumor is usually caused by hemorrhage into or around the tumor.

Table 11-3
Evaluation of Cerebral Infarction

Blood

Activated protein C resistance, antiphosphospholipid antibodies, apolipoproteins, cholesterol (high and low density), complete blood count, culture, erythrocyte sedimentation rate, factor V, free protein S, lactic acid, Leiden mutation, lupus anticoagulant, plasminogen, protein C, serum homocystine, and triglycerides	Bacterial endocarditis Homocystinuria Hypercoaguable state Hyperlipidemia Leukemia Lupus erythematosis MELAS Polycythemia Sickle cell anemia Vasculitis

Urine

Cocaine, urinalysis	Cocaine abuse Homocystinuria Nephritis Nephrosis

Heart

Echocardiography, electrocardiography	Bacterial endocarditis Congenital heart disease Mitral valve prolapse Rheumatic heart disease

Brain

Arteriography, magnetic resonance imaging	Arterial dissection Arterial thrombosis Arteriovenous malformation Fibromuscular hypoplasia Moyamoya disease Vasculitis

The underlying tumor may be hidden by the hemorrhage on CT and is better appreciated on MRI (see Chapter 4).

Carotid and Vertebral Artery Disorders

Cervical Infections

Unilateral and bilateral occlusions of the cervical portion of the internal carotid arteries may occur in children with a history of chronic tonsillitis and cervical lymphadenopathy. Whether this is cause and effect or coincidence is uncertain. It is speculated that tonsillitis produces carotid arteritis.

Unilateral cerebral infarction may occur in the course of cat-scratch disease (see Chapter 2) and mycoplasmal pneumonia. In both diseases, the presence of submandibular lymph node involvement is associated with arteritis of the adjacent carotid artery.

Necrotizing fasciitis is a serious cause of inflammatory arteritis with subsequent occlusion of one or both carotid arteries. The source of parapharyngeal space infection is usually chronic dental infection. Mixed aerobic and anaerobic organisms are isolated on culture.

CLINICAL FEATURES. The usual sequence in cervical arteritis is fever and neck tenderness followed by sudden hemiplegia. Bilateral hemiplegia may occur when both sides are infected.

DIAGNOSIS. The offending organism or organisms must be identified by culture of the throat or lymph node specimens. Carotid occlusion is identified by arteriography.

MANAGEMENT. Aggressive therapy with antibiotics, especially for necrotizing fasciitis, is indicated. The outcome is variable, and recovery may be partial or complete.

Fibromuscular Dysplasia

Fibromuscular dysplasia is an idiopathic segmental nonatheromatous disorder of the internal carotid artery. The cervical portion of the artery is most often affected.

CLINICAL FEATURES. Transitory ischemic attacks and stroke are the only clinical features. Fibromuscular dysplasia is primarily a disease of women over 50 years of age but can occur in children.

DIAGNOSIS. Arteriography shows an irregular contour of the internal carotid artery in the neck resembling a string of beads. Concomitant fibromuscular dysplasia of the renal arteries should be suspected if hypertension is present.

MANAGEMENT. The occlusion may be treated by operative transluminal balloon angioplasty or by carotid endarterectomy. The long-term prognosis in children is unknown.

Trauma to the Carotid Artery

Children may experience carotid thrombosis and dissection from seemingly trivial injuries sustained in child abuse (grabbing and shaking the neck) or during exercise and sports (Patel et al, 1995). The carotid artery also may be injured in the tonsillar fossa during a tonsillectomy or when a child falls with a blunt object (e.g., pencil, lollipop) in the mouth.

CLINICAL FEATURES. The onset of symptoms is usually delayed for several hours and sometimes days. The delay probably represents the time needed for thrombus to form within the artery.

Clinical features usually include hemiparesis, hemianesthesia, hemianopia, and aphasia when the dominant hemisphere is affected. Deficits may be transitory or permanent, but some recovery always occurs. Seizures are uncommon.

DIAGNOSIS. Carotid dissection and occlusion are safely visualized using MRA.

MANAGEMENT. Heparin is often recommended for the first week following thrombosis, but neither anticoagulation nor surgical repair has proven efficacy.

Trauma to the Vertebral Artery

Vertebral artery thrombosis or dissection may follow minor neck trauma, especially rapid neck rotation. The site of occlusion is usually at the C1-C2 level.

CLINICAL FEATURES. The usual features of vertebral artery injury are headache and brainstem dysfunction. Repeated episodes of hemiparesis associated with bitemporal throbbing headache and vomiting may occur and are readily misdiagnosed as basilar artery migraine. The outcome is relatively good, survival is the rule, and chronic neurological disability is unusual.

DIAGNOSIS. The clue to diagnosis is the presence of one or more areas of infarction on CT or MRI. This should raise the possibility of stroke and lead to arteriography. Occlusion of the basilar artery is then visualized.

MANAGEMENT. No treatment is proven to be effective, but aspirin prophylaxis is often recommended.

Cocaine Use

Cocaine is a potent vasoconstrictor that causes infarction in several organs. Stroke occurs mainly in young adults and may follow any route of administration but takes place more often when "crack" is smoked. The interval from administration to stroke is unknown in most cases but may be minutes to hours. Intracerebral hemorrhage and subarachnoid hemorrhage are more common than cerebral infarction and often occur in people with underlying aneurysms or arteriovenous malformations. Infarction is probably caused by vasospasm or vasculitis.

Heart Disease

Congenital Heart Disease

Cerebrovascular complications of congenital heart disease are most likely in children with cyanotic disorders. The usual complications are venous sinus thrombosis in infants and embolic arterial occlusion in children. Emboli may occur from valvular vegetations or bacterial endocarditis. In either case, the development of cerebral abscess is a major concern. Cerebral abscess of embolic origin is exceedingly uncommon in children younger than 2 years of age with congenital heart disease and occurs only as a complication of meningitis or surgery.

CLINICAL FEATURES. Venous thrombosis occurs most often in infants with cyanotic heart disease who are dehydrated and polycythemic. One or more sinuses may become occluded. Failure of venous drainage always increases intracranial pressure. Hemiparesis is a major clinical feature and may occur first on one side and then on the other when the sagittal sinus is obstructed. Seizures and decreased consciousness are almost always associated features. The mortality rate is high in infants with thrombosis of major venous sinuses, and most survivors have neurological morbidity.

Children with cyanotic heart disease are at risk for arterial embolism when vegetations are present within the heart or if a right-to-left shunt allows peripheral emboli to bypass the lungs and reach the brain. This can occur spontaneously or at the time of cardiac surgery. The potential for cerebral abscess formation increases in children with right-to-left shunt because decreased arterial oxygen saturation lowers cerebral resistance to infection.

The initial feature is sudden onset of hemiparesis associated with headache, seizures, and loss of consciousness. Seizures may at first be focal and recurrent but then become generalized.

DIAGNOSIS. MRI is the preferred procedure for the detection of venous thrombosis and emboli. A pattern of hemorrhagic infarction is seen adjacent to the site of venous thrombosis, and multiple areas of infarction are associated with embolization.

The CT appearance may be normal during the first 12 to 24 hours following embolization. By the next day, a low-intensity lesion can be observed with contrast enhancement. Although the sequence is consistent with a sterile embolus, the possibility of subsequent abscess formation must be considered. Enhanced CT or MRI should be repeated within 1 week to search for ring enhancement as a sign of abscess development.

MANAGEMENT. Treatment for venous thrombosis is primarily supportive and directed toward correcting dehydration and controlling increased intracranial pressure. Dexamethasone can be used to decrease cerebral volume, but osmotic diuretics are contraindicated and may cause further thrombosis. The infarction is usually hemorrhagic, and anticoagulants are contraindicated. Distinguishing a septic from a sterile thrombosis is impossible, and all infants should be treated with antibiotics.

Children with arterial emboli, but without evidence of hemorrhagic infarction, should undergo anticoagulation to prevent further embolization. If the infarction is associated with cerebral edema and a mass effect, dexamethasone should be administered as well. All such children should begin antibiotic therapy to prevent cerebral abscess formation. If an abscess does not form, antibiotics can be stopped after 1 week. If an abscess forms, therapy must be continued for 6 to 8 weeks.

Mitral Valve Prolapse

Mitral valve prolapse is a familial disorder present in 5% of children. It is almost always asymptomatic but is estimated to cause recurrent attacks of cerebral ischemia in 1 in every 6,000 cases each year. The attacks are attributed to sterile emboli from thrombus originating either from the prolapsing leaflet or at its junction with the atrial wall.

CLINICAL FEATURES. The initial feature is usually a transitory ischemic attack in the distribution of the carotid circulation producing partial or complete hemiparesis. Weakness usually clears within 24 hours, but recurrent episodes, not necessarily in the same arterial distribution, are the rule. Basilar insufficiency is less common and usually results in visual field defects. The interval between recurrences varies from weeks to years. Fewer than 20% of individuals are left with permanent neurological deficits.

DIAGNOSIS. Only 25% of patients have late systolic murmurs or a midsystolic click. In the remainder, a cardiac examination shows no abnormalities. Two-dimensional echocardiography is required to establish the diagnosis.

MANAGEMENT. No treatment is needed for asymptomatic children with auscultatory or electrocardiographic (ECG) abnormalities, nor is specific treatment available for a transient ischemic attack. However, once a child has suffered a transitory attack of ischemia, aspirin should be administered daily to reduce the likelihood of further thrombus formation in the heart.

Rheumatic Heart Disease

The frequency and severity of rheumatic fever and rheumatic heart disease in North America have been decreasing for several decades. Unfortunately, the incidence of acute rheumatic fever is now increasing. Rheumatic heart disease involves the mitral valve in 85% of patients, the aortic valve in 54%, and the tricuspid and pulmonary valves in less than 5%.

CLINICAL FEATURES. The main features of mitral valve disease are cardiac failure and arrhythmia. Aortic valve disease is often asymptomatic. Neurological complications are always due to bacterial endocarditis except in the immediate postoperative period, when embolization is the likely explanation. Symptoms are much the same as in congenital heart disease, except that cerebral abscess is less common.

DIAGNOSIS. Children are known to have rheumatic heart disease long before their first stroke. Multiple blood cultures may be needed to identify the organism and select the best drug for intravenous antibiotic therapy.

MANAGEMENT. Bacterial endocarditis must be treated vigorously with intravenous antibiotics.

Hypercoagulable States

A prethrombotic condition is present in 30% to 40% of children who experience an arterial ischemic stroke or sinovenous thrombosis (DeVeber et al, 1998; Bonduel et al, 1999). Inherited protein S and C deficiencies, defects of an anticoagulant (the *lupus anticoagulant*), and the *anticardiolipin antibody* are all important risk factors. Partial thrombosis of the sagittal sinus may also occur in young women taking oral contraceptives and during pregnancy.

CLINICAL FEATURES. The typical features of venous thrombosis are headache and obtundation caused by increased intracranial pressure, seizures, and successive hemiplegia on either side. An inherited hypercoaguable state should be suspected in children with recurrent venous thromboses, a family history of venous thrombosis, or thrombosis at an unusual site. Arterial thromboses usually cause ischemic stroke in the distribution of a single cerebral artery.

DIAGNOSIS. Venous thrombosis should be suspected when hemiplegia and increased intracranial pressure suddenly develop. The diagnosis of sagittal sinus thromboses is suggested when parasagittal hemorrhage or infarction is associated with a flow void in the sagittal sinus on MRI. Cerebral arteriography is the more definitive procedure. Laboratory studies are summarized in Table 11-3.

MANAGEMENT. Symptomatic treatment is directed at decreasing intracranial pressure and rehydrating the patient without increasing cerebral edema. Anticoagulant therapy is often required.

Ischemic Arterial Infarction

Capsular Stroke

Small, deep infarcts involving the internal capsule are usually seen in adults with hypertensive angiopathy. They also occur, but very rarely, in infants and young children. The onset of weakness is sudden and may occur during sleep or wakefulness.

CLINICAL FEATURES. The face and limbs are involved, and a typical hemiplegic posture and gait develop. Hypalgesia and decreased position sense are difficult to show in infants but can be seen in older children. Larger infarcts affecting the striatum and the internal capsule of the dominant hemisphere cause speech disturbances. At the onset of hemiplegia, the child is mute and lethargic. As speech returns, evidence of dysarthria and aphasia develops. Eventually speech becomes normal. Hemiplegia may clear completely in the following year, but some children have residual weakness of the hand.

DIAGNOSIS. MRI demonstrates capsular infarcts. A cause is rarely determined despite extensive study (see Table 11-3).

MANAGEMENT. A rehabilitative treatment program is recommended.

Cerebral Artery Infarction

Acute infantile hemiplegia may result from infarction in the distribution of the middle cerebral artery or one of its branches, the posterior cerebral artery, or the anterior cerebral artery.

CLINICAL FEATURES. Sudden hemiplegia is the typical initial feature. Hemianesthesia, hemianopia, and aphasia (with dominant hemisphere infarction) are present as well. Some children are lethargic at the onset of symptoms, but consciousness is seldom lost completely.

Epilepsia partialis continuans precedes hemiplegia in approximately one third of cases. When this is the case, permanent hemiplegia is a constant feature and epilepsy is common. When hemiplegia occurs without seizures, half of the patients recover completely and the remainder are left with partial paralysis.

DIAGNOSIS. Complete occlusion of the middle cerebral artery produces a large area of lucency on CT involving the cortex, underlying white matter, basal ganglia, and internal capsule. Occlusion of superficial branches of the middle cerebral artery produces a wedge-shaped area of lucency extending from the cortex into the subjacent white matter. Table 11-3 lists studies for hypercoaguable states.

MANAGEMENT. Seizures should be treated with anticonvulsant drugs (see Chapter 1). When seizures are intractable, hemispherectomy or commissurotomy should be considered (see the section an Epilepsy Surgery in Chapter 1).

Lipoprotein Disorders

Familial lipid and lipoprotein abnormalities may cause premature cerebrovascular disease in infants and children. These disorders are transmitted by autosomal dominant inheritance (Abram et al, 1996).

CLINICAL FEATURES. Ischemic episodes cause transitory or permanent hemiplegia, sometimes associated with hemianopia, hemianesthesia, and aphasia. The family has a history of cerebrovascular and coronary artery disease developing at an early age.

DIAGNOSIS. Most children have low plasma concentrations of high-density lipoprotein (HDL) cholesterol, others have high plasma concentrations of triglycerides, and some have both. The mechanism of arteriosclerosis is lipoprotein-mediated endothelial damage with secondary thrombus formation.

MANAGEMENT. Dietary treatment, lipid-lowering medications, and daily aspirin administration are indicated.

Mitochondrial Encephalopathy, Lactic Acidosis, and Stroke

Mitochondrial encephalopathy, lactic acidosis, and stroke (MELAS) is caused by mutations in the mitochondrial tRNA (Leu-UUR) gene (Smith et al, 1997).

CLINICAL FEATURES. Affected children are usually normal at birth. Onset during infancy is characterized by failure to thrive, growth retardation, and progressive deafness. The main neurological features in later-onset cases are recurrent attacks of prolonged migraine-like headaches and vomiting, seizures (myoclonic, focal, generalized) that often progress to status epilepticus, the sudden onset of focal neurological defects (hemiplegia, hemianopia, aphasia), and encephalopathy. Mental deterioration, when present, occurs anytime during childhood. Neurological abnormalities are initially intermittent and then become progressive, leading to coma and death.

DIAGNOSIS. MRI shows multifocal infarctions that do not conform to definite vascular territories. The initial infarctions are often in the occipital lobes; progressive disease affects the cerebral and cerebellar cortices, the basal ganglia, and the thalamus. The concentration of lactate in the blood and cerebrospinal fluid is elevated. Ragged-red fibers are noted on muscle biopsy (see Chapter 7). Genetic diagnosis is commercially available.

MANAGEMENT. Specific treatment is not available, but a cocktail of vitamins is often used.

Moyamoya Disease

Moyamoya disease is a chronic, progressive, noninflammatory vasculopathy. It results in a slowly progressive, bilateral occlusion of the internal carotid arteries starting at the carotid siphon. The basilar artery is sometimes occluded as well. Because the occlusion is slowly progressive, multiple anastomoses form between the internal and external carotid arteries. The result is a new vascular network at the base of the brain composed of collaterals from the anterior or posterior choroidal arteries, the basilar artery, and the meningeal arteries. On angiography, these telangiectasias produce a hazy appearance, like a puff of smoke, from which the Japanese word *moyamoya* is derived (Figure 11-2). The disorder is worldwide in distribution, with a female-to-male bias of 3 : 2.

CLINICAL FEATURES. The initial symptoms vary from recurrent headache to abrupt hemiparesis. Infants and young children tend to have an explosive onset characterized by the sudden development of complete hemiplegia affecting the face and limbs. The child is at least lethargic and sometimes comatose. When the child is sufficiently alert to be examined, hemianopia, hemianesthesia, and aphasia may be found. Some children have chorea of the face and all limbs that may be worse on one side. Recovery follows, but before it is complete, new episodes of focal neurological dysfunction occur on either the same or the opposite side. These episodes include hemiparesis, hemianesthesia, or aphasia, alone or in combination. The outcome is generally poor. Most children are left with chronic weakness on one or both sides, epilepsy, and mental retardation. Some have died.

Recurrent transient ischemic attacks are an alternative manifestation. These are characterized by episodic hemiparesis and dysesthesias lasting for minutes or hours. Consciousness is retained. Attacks are frequently triggered by hyperpnea or excitement and may recur daily. After 4 or 5 years, the attacks cease but the child may be left with residual deficits.

Repeated episodes of monoparesis or symptoms of subarachnoid hemorrhage are other possible features of moyamoya disease. Monoparesis generally occurs after infancy and subarachnoid hemorrhage after 16 years of age.

DIAGNOSIS. CT or MRI usually shows a large cerebral infarction caused by stenosis in the internal carotid artery. Definitive diagnosis requires arteriographic demonstration of bilateral stenosis in the distal internal carotid arteries and the development of collaterals in the basal ganglia and meninges. Studies should include a search for an underlying vasculopathy or coagulopathy.

MANAGEMENT. Treatment options depend on finding the underlying cause.

Sickle Cell Anemia

Sickle cell anemia is a genetic disorder of African-American children transmitted by autosomal recessive inheritance. Neurological complications occur in up to 25% of homozygotes and may occur at times of stress, such as surgery, in heterozygotes. The abnormal erythrocytes clog large and small vessels, decreasing total, hemispheric, or regional blood flow. Cerebral infarction usually occurs in the region of arterial border zones.

CLINICAL FEATURES. The major systemic features are jaundice, pallor, weakness, and fatigability from chronic hemolytic anemia. Half of homozygotes show symptoms by 1 year, and all have symptoms by 5 years of age.

Strokes occur at the time of a thrombotic, vaso-occlusive crisis. Such crises are frequently precipitated by dehydration or anoxia and are characterized by fever and pain in the abdomen and chest. Focal or generalized seizures are the initial neurological feature in 70% of patients. After the seizures have ended, hemiplegia and other focal neurological deficits are noted. Some recovery follows, but there is a tendency for recurrent strokes, epilepsy, and mental retardation. Strokes affecting both hemispheres produce a pseudobulbar palsy with brainstem dysfunction.

The worst case is a child who is in a coma and has meningismus. Such a case is usually caused by a diffuse decrease in cerebral blood flow associated with subarachnoid or intracerebral hemorrhage. The mortality rate is high.

DIAGNOSIS. The abnormal hemoglobin can be diagnosed at birth with acid agar gel electrophoresis or microcolumn chromatography. In most affected children, sickle cell anemia is diagnosed long before their first stroke. CT or MRI documents the extent of cerebral infarction and hemorrhage. After several such crises, cortical atrophy may be present. Cerebral arteriography should be avoided, because it offers little additional information and carries the risk of increasing ischemia.

MANAGEMENT. A vaso-occlusive crisis requires prompt hydration, oxygen administration, and transfusions of packed red blood cells. Hydration should not reach the point of increasing cerebral edema. Strokes can be prevented by a regimen of regular transfusions designed to keep the level of hemoglobin S below 30% (Adams et al, 1998).

Vasculopathies

Hypersensitivity Vasculitis

The term *hypersensitivity vasculitis* covers several disorders that have a known underlying cause (drugs, infection) and are characterized by purpura of the legs and venulitis. Neurological complications occur only in *Henoch-Schönlein purpura,* for which the cause is not established but is thought to be an antecedent infection.

CLINICAL FEATURES. The systemic features of Henoch-Schönlein purpura are fever, a purpuric rash on the extensor surfaces of the limbs, and abdominal pain with nausea and vomiting. Joint and renal disturbances may be present. Almost half of affected children have headache and abnormalities on EEG. Focal neurological deficits occur in one third of patients, with hemiplegia accounting for half of these cases. Hemiplegia may be preceded by a seizure and may be associated with hemianesthesia, hemianopia, and aphasia. These deficits may be permanent.

DIAGNOSIS. CT or MRI shows infarction, hemorrhage, or both.

MANAGEMENT. Corticosteroids are used to treat the underlying disease.

Isolated Angiitis of the Central Nervous System

Isolated angiitis of the central nervous system is an inflammation of small cerebral vessels. It is rare in children. The clinical features are recurrent headache, sometimes of a migrainous type, encephalopathy, and stroke. Arteriography shows multiple areas of irregular narrowing of the cerebral vessels. Corticosteroid therapy may be beneficial, but additional treatment with pulse cyclophosphamide is often required.

Systemic Lupus Erythematosus

Several collagen vascular disorders can cause neurological disturbances in adults, but systemic lupus erythematosus is the main cause in children. *Mixed connective tissue disease* is a rare cause of either large vessel occlusion or hemorrhage secondary to fibrinoid necrosis.

CLINICAL FEATURES. The clinical features of lupus in children are similar to those in adults except for a higher incidence of hepatosplenomegaly, chorea (see Chapter 14), nephritis, and avascular necrosis. Most children have fever, arthralgia, and skin rash at the time of diagnosis. Neurological features are present in one quarter of children at the time of diagnosis. Unlike systemic complaints, neurological disturbances are likely to progress or develop anew even after treatment is initiated. Neurological dysfunction develops in about one third of children sometime during the course of disease. Headache, seizures, cranial neuropathies, and mental disorders are common features. Hemiplegia usually follows a seizure and may be caused by cerebral infarction or hemorrhage.

Neurological episodes during treatment are often complications of immunosuppression, such as fungal meningitis, rather than primary complications of the underlying disease.

DIAGNOSIS. The diagnosis of lupus requires a compatible clinical syndrome and the detection of an abnormal titer of antinuclear antibody or anti-DNA antibody to native DNA. The presence of anticardiolipin antibodies is associated with hemolytic anemia and thrombotic events (Seaman et at, 1995). CT or MRI of the head is useful to determine the presence of hemorrhage or infarction. Results of cerebral arteriography may be normal.

MANAGEMENT. Large doses of corticosteroids are the mainstay of therapy, but the mortality is higher in children than in adults.

Takayasu Arteritis

Takayasu's disease primarily affects young women. Takayasu arteritis, a disorder of unknown cause, involves the aorta and its major branches.

CLINICAL FEATURES. Onset usually occurs between 15 and 20 years of age but may occur as early as infancy. Ninety percent of patients are female. The most common features are fever, weight loss, myalgias, arthralgia, hypertension, absent pulses, and vascular bruits. Stroke occurs in only 5% to 10% of patients and is usually characterized by focal seizures and sudden hemiplegia.

DIAGNOSIS. CT reveals a focal hypodense area, indicating infarction. Arteriography shows involvement of the ascending aorta and its major branches. Cardiac catheterization is necessary to define the full extent of arteritis. Some vessels have a beaded appearance; others terminate abruptly and have prestenotic dilatation.

MANAGEMENT. Corticosteroids are the treatment of choice. If the disease is left untreated, the mortality rate is 75%. Early diagnosis and treatment can lead to full recovery.

Diabetes Mellitus

Acute but transitory attacks of hemiparesis occur in children with insulin-dependent diabetes mellitus. Complicated migraine is a suggested mechanism, but the pathophysiology remains unknown.

CLINICAL FEATURES. Attacks frequently occur during sleep in a child with a respiratory illness. Hemiparesis is present on awakening; the face and arm are more affected than the leg. Sensation is intact, but aphasia is present if the dominant hemisphere is affected. Tendon reflexes may be depressed or brisk in the affected arm, and an extensor plantar response can usually be elicited. Headache is a constant feature and may be unilateral or generalized. Some patients are nauseated. The family does not have a history of migraine.

Attacks last for 3 to 24 hours, and recovery is complete. Recurrences are common.

DIAGNOSIS. Stroke is not a complication of juvenile insulin-dependent diabetes, except during episodes of ketoacidosis (see Chapter 2). Head CT in children with transitory hemiplegia does not show infarction.

MANAGEMENT. Although some children have further attacks, no way of preventing recurrences has been established. Prophylactic phenobarbital was useful in one child.

Epilepsy

Hemiparetic Seizures

Todd paralysis is a term used to describe hemiparesis that lasts for minutes or hours and follows a focal or generalized seizure. It most often occurs when seizures are prolonged or caused by an underlying structural abnormality. An ischemic mechanism has been suggested.

Hemiparesis may be a seizure manifestation as well as a postictal event. The seizures are called *hemiparetic* or *focal inhibitory* seizures. Todd paralysis may be difficult to distinguish from hemiparetic seizures, because it is not always clear whether a seizure preceded the hemiparesis or whether the hemiparesis is ictal or postictal.

CLINICAL FEATURES. The initial feature may be a brief focal seizure followed by flaccid hemiparesis or the abrupt onset of flaccid monoparesis or hemiparesis. Consciousness is not impaired, and the child seems well otherwise. The severity and distribution of weakness fluctuate, affecting one limb more than the other and sometimes the face. Tendon reflexes are normal in the hemiparetic limbs, but the plantar response may be extensor.

DIAGNOSIS. EEG shows recurrent spike-and-slow-wave discharges in the contralateral hemisphere. A radioisotope scan shows increased focal uptake in the affected hemisphere. Results of MRI, CT, and cerebral arteriography are normal.

MANAGEMENT. Seizures respond to standard anticonvulsant drugs (see Chapter 1).

Infections

Hemiplegia occurs during the course of bacterial meningitis, resulting from vasculitis or venous thromboses, and during the course of viral encephalitis, especially herpes simplex, resulting from parenchymal necrosis. In both bacterial and viral infections, hemiplegia is usually preceded by prolonged or repetitive focal seizures. Brain abscess may cause hemiplegia, but its evolution is usually slowly progressive rather than acute.

Varicella

Arterial ischemic strokes may occur during the course of varicella infection, and probably after varicella immunization, 1 week to several months after the appearance of rash (Sébire et al, 1999). The infarcts are small and located in the basal ganglia and internal capsule.

Migraine

Migraine is a hereditary disorder associated with, but not caused by, paroxysmal alterations in cerebral blood flow. Transitory neurological abnormalities may accompany the attack. These are caused by a primary neuronal disturbance rather than cerebral ischemia. However, cerebral infarction may occur in adolescents during a prolonged attack of classic migraine.

The occurrence of focal motor deficits, usually hemiplegia or ophthalmoplegia (see Chapter 15), during an occasional migraine attack is called *complicated migraine*. In some families, hemiplegic migraine is a familial trait.

Complicated Migraine

CLINICAL FEATURES. The family has a history of migraine, but other family members have not experienced hemiplegia during an attack. The evolution of symptoms is variable but usually includes scintillating or simple scotomas, unilateral dysesthesias of the hand and mouth, and unilateral weakness of the arm and face. The leg is usually spared. Occurring concurrently with hemiparesis is a throbbing frontotemporal headache contralateral to the affected hemisphere. Nausea and vomiting follow. The patient falls asleep and has usually recovered on awakening. Hemiparesis lasts for less than 24 hours.
DIAGNOSIS. Migraine is a clinical diagnosis that relies on a positive family history of the disorder. During an attack of hemiplegic migraine, an EEG focus of polymorphic delta activity is present in the hemisphere contralateral to the weakness. Neuroimaging studies are not indicated.
MANAGEMENT. The management of migraine is summarized in Chapter 3.

Familial Hemiplegic Migraine

Familial hemiplegic migraine differs from complicated migraine because other family members with migraine have had at least one hemiplegic attack. The trait is transmitted by autosomal dominant inheritance and one gene location is on chromosome 19p, allelic with the gene for hereditary paroxysmal cerebellar ataxia (Ahmed et al, 1996). The mechanism is a calcium channel disturbance. A second gene has been localized to chromosome 1 (Ducros et al, 1997).
CLINICAL FEATURES. Attacks are stereotyped, occur primarily in childhood or adolescence, may be precipitated by trivial head trauma, and rarely occur more often than once a year. The hemiplegia, although usually more severe in the face and arm, affects the leg too and always outlasts the headache. Hemianesthesia of the hemiplegic side is a prominent feature. Aphasia

occurs when the dominant hemisphere is affected. Confusion, stupor, or psychosis may be present during an attack. The psychosis includes both auditory and visual hallucinations, as well as delusions. Occasionally, patients have fever and a stiff neck.

Symptoms last for 2 or 3 days. When the attack is over, the neurological deficits usually resolve completely, but permanent sequelae are possible. A gaze-evoked nystagmus may persist between attacks (Elliott et al, 1996). Recurrent hemiplegic attacks may occur on either the same or the opposite side. Families with linkage to chromosome 1 may experience seizures during severe attacks.
DIAGNOSIS. A family history of hemiplegic migraine is essential for diagnosis.
MANAGEMENT. Acetazolamide is a useful prophylactic agent in several channelopathies and should be tried in children with familial hemiplegic migraine.

Trauma

Trauma accounts for half of all deaths in children. Approximately 10% of traumatic injuries in children are not accidental. Head injury is the leading cause of death from child abuse, and half of survivors are left with permanent neurological handicaps.

Epidural hematoma, subdural hematoma, cerebral laceration, and intracerebral hemorrhage can produce focal signs such as hemiplegia. However, brain swelling is such a prominent feature of even trivial head injury in children that diminished consciousness and seizures are the typical clinical features (see Chapter 2).

Tumors

The initial clinical feature of primary tumors of the cerebral hemispheres is more likely to be chronic progressive hemiplegia than acute hemiplegia. However, tumors may cause acute hemiplegia when they bleed or provoke seizures and must be considered in the evaluation of acute hemiplegia.

Chronic Progressive Hemiplegia

The important causes of chronic progressive hemiplegia are brain tumor, brain abscess, and arteriovenous malformations. The initial features of all three are often those of increased

Table 11-4
Progressive Hemiplegia

Arteriovenous malformation (see Chapter 4)
Brain abscess (see Chapter 4)
Cerebral hemisphere tumor (see Chapter 4)
Demyelinating diseases
    Adrenoleukodystrophy (see Chapter 5)
    Late-onset globoid leukodystrophy (see Chapter 5)
    Multiple sclerosis (see Chapter 10)
Sturge-Weber syndrome

intracranial pressure; they are discussed in Chapter 4. Progressive hemiplegia is sometimes an initial feature of demyelinating diseases, which are discussed in Chapters 5 and 10 (Table 11-4).

Sturge-Weber Syndrome

The Sturge-Weber syndrome (SWS) is a sporadic neurocutaneous disorder characterized by the association of a venous angioma of the pia mater with a port-wine stain of the face (Bodensteiner and Roach, 1999).

CLINICAL FEATURES. The cutaneous angioma is usually present at birth. It is flat and variable in size but usually involves the upper lid. The size of the cutaneous angioma does not predict the size of the intracranial angioma. It is unilateral in 70% of children and ipsilateral to the venous angioma of the pia. Even when the facial nevus is bilateral, the pial angioma is usually unilateral. The characteristic neurological and radiographic features of SWS may be present without the cutaneous angioma. Only 10% to 20% of children with a port-wine nevus of the forehead have a leptomeningeal angioma. Bilateral brain lesions occur in at least 15% of children.

Seizures occur in 80% of children with SWS. Onset is generally within the first year and the seizure type is usually focal motor, sometimes leading to partial or generalized status epilepticus (see Chapter 1). Eighty percent of children with SWS who have seizures in the first year will show developmental delay and mental retardation (Sujansky and Conradi, 1995).

Hemiplegia, contralateral to the facial angioma, occurs in up to 50% of children. It is often noted initially after a focal-onset seizure and progresses in severity after subsequent seizures. Transitory episodes of hemiplegia that cannot be related to clinical or EEG evidence of seizure activity may occur. Some episodes are associated with migraine-like headache, and others occur in the absence of other symptoms and may be caused by transitory ischemia. Glaucoma occurs in 71% of children with SWS, usually developing in the first decade.

DIAGNOSIS. The association of neurological abnormalities and a port-wine stain of the face should suggest SWS. The eyelid and the skin above the eye should be examined for angioma in any child with focal motor seizures. The pial angioma is best visualized by a contrast-enhanced MRI and only rarely by angiography.

MANAGEMENT. The seizures are often difficult to control with anticonvulsant medications. Hemispherectomy sometimes improves seizure control and may promote more normal intellectual development. Early hemispherectomy is recommended when seizure onset is in infancy. Corpus callosum section may be useful for patients with extensive disease.

References

Abram HS, Knepper LE, Warty VS, et al. Natural history, prognosis, and lipid abnormalities of idiopathic ischemic childhood stroke. *J Child Neurol* 1996;11:276–282.

Adams RJ, McKie VC, Hsu L, et al. Prevention of a first stroke by transfusions in children with sickle cell anemia and abnormal results on transcranial doppler ultrasonography. *N Engl J Med* 1998;339:5–11.

Ahmed MAS, Reid E, Cooke A, et al. Familial hemiplegic migraine in the west of Scotland: A clinical and genetic study of seven families. *J Neurol Neurosurg Psychiatry* 1996;61:616–620.

Bodensteiner J, Roach ES. Sturge-Weber Syndrome. Mt. Freedom, NJ: Sturge-Weber Foundation, 1999.

Bonduel M, Sciuccata G, Hepner M, et al. Prethrombotic disorders in children with arterial ischemic stroke and sinovenous thrombosis. *Arch Neurol* 1999;56:967–971.

DeVeber G, Monagle P, Chan A, et al. Prothrombotic disorders in infants and children with cerebral thromboembolism. *Arch Neurol* 1998;55:1539–1543.

Ducros A, Joutel A, Vahedi K, et al. Mapping of a second locus for familial hemiplegic migraine to 1q21-23 and evidence for further heterogeneity. *Ann Neurol* 1997;42:885–890.

Elliott MA, Peroutka SJ, Welch S, et al. Familial hemiplegic migraine, nystagmus, and cerebellar atrophy. *Ann Neurol* 1996;39:100-106.

Kramer U, Mikati MA, Zupanc ML, et al. Alternating hemiplegia of childhood: Clinical manifestations and long term outcome. *Neurology* in press.

Lanthier S, Carmant L, David M, et al. Stroke in children. The coexistence of multiple risk factors predicts poor outcome. *Neurology* 2000;54:371–378.

Mercuri E, Rutherford M, Cowan F, et al. Early prognostic indicators of outcome in infants with neonatal cerebral infarction: A clinical, electroencephalogram, and magnetic resonance imaging study. *Pediatrics* 1999;103:39–46.

Patel H, Smith RR, Garg BP. Spontaneous extracranial carotid artery dissection in children. *Pediatr Neurol* 1995;13:55–60.

Rho JM, Chugani HT. Alternating hemiplegia of childhood: Insights into its pathophysiology. *J Child Neurol* 1998; 13:39–45.

Seaman DE, Londino AV Jr, Kwoh CK, et al. Antiphospholipid antibodies in pediatric systemic lupus erythematosus. *Pediatrics* 1995;96:1040–1045.

Sébire G, Husson B, Dusser A, et al. Congenital unilateral perisylvian syndrome: Radiological basis and clinical correlations. *J Neurol Neurosurg Psychiatry* 1996; 61:52–56.

Sébire G, Meyer L, Chabrier S. Varicella as a risk factor for cerebral infarction in childhood: A case-control study. *Ann Neurol* 1999;45:679–680.

Smith ML, Hua XY, Marsden DL, et al. Diabetes and mitochondrial encephalopathy with lactic acidosis and stroke-like episodes (MELAS): Radiolabeled polymerase chain reaction is necessary for accurate detection of low percentages of mutation. *J Clin Endocrinol Metab* 1997;82:2826–2831.

Sujansky E, Conradi S. Sturge-Weber syndrome. Age of onset of seizures and glaucoma and the prognosis for affected children. *J Child Neurol* 1995;10:49–58.

White PH. Pediatric systemic lupus erythematosus and neonatal lupus. *Rheum Dis Clin North Am* 1994;20: 119–127.

Chapter 12
Paraplegia and Quadriplegia

THE TERM *PARAPLEGIA* is used in this text to denote partial or complete weakness of both legs, therefore obviating need for the term *paraparesis*. Many conditions described fully in this chapter are abnormalities of the spinal cord. The same spinal abnormality can cause paraplegia or quadriplegia, depending on the location of the injury. Therefore, the two are discussed together in this chapter. The term *quadriplegia* is used to denote partial or complete weakness of all limbs, and the term *quadriparesis* is not used.

Approach to Paraplegia

Weakness of both legs, without any involvement of the arms, suggests an abnormality of either the spinal cord or the peripheral nerves. Ordinarily, peripheral neuropathies are readily identified by the pattern of distal weakness and sensory loss, atrophy, and loss of tendon reflexes (see Chapters 7 and 9). In contrast, spinal paraplegia causes spasticity, exaggerated tendon reflexes, and a dermatomal level of sensory loss. Disturbances in the conus medullaris and cauda equina, especially congenital malformation, may produce a complex of signs in which spinal cord or peripheral nerve localization is difficult. Indeed, both may be involved. Spinal paraplegia may be asymmetric at first, and then the initial feature is monoplegia (see Chapter 13). When anatomical localization between the spinal cord and peripheral nerves is difficult, electromyography (EMG) and nerve conduction studies are useful in making the distinction.

Paraplegia is sometimes caused by cerebral abnormalities. In such a case, the child's arms as well as the legs are usually weak. However, leg weakness is so much greater than arm weakness that paraplegia is the chief complaint. It is important to remember that both the brain and the spinal cord may be abnormal and that the abnormalities can be in continuity (syringomyelia) or separated (Chiari malformation and myelomeningocele).

Spinal Paraplegia and Quadriplegia

The conditions that cause acute, chronic, or progressive spinal paraplegia are listed in Table 12-1. In the absence of trauma, spinal cord compression and myelitis are the main causes of an acute onset or rapidly progressive paraplegia. Spinal cord compression from any cause is a medical emergency requiring rapid diagnosis and therapy to avoid permanent paraplegia. Corticosteroids have the same dehydrating effect on the spinal cord as on the brain and provide transitory decompression before surgery.

Several techniques are available to visualize the spinal cord. Each has its place, and sometimes more than one technique must be used to achieve a comprehensive picture of the disease process. However, magnetic resonance imaging (MRI) is now the procedure of choice to visualize the spine. Computed tomography (CT) and radioisotope bone scanning are useful for visualizing the vertebral column, especially when osteomyelitis is suspected.

Symptoms and Signs

Clumsiness of gait, refusal to stand or walk, and loss of bladder or bowel control are the common complaints of spinal paraplegia. Clumsiness of gait is the usual feature of slowly progressive

Table 12-1
Spinal Paraplegia

Congenital Malformations
Arachnoid cyst
Arteriovenous malformations
Atlantoaxial dislocation
Caudal regression syndrome
Dysraphic states
  Chiari malformation
  Myelomeningocele
  Tethered spinal cord
Syringomyelia (see Chapter 9)

Familial Spastic Paraplegia
Autosomal dominant
Autosomal recessive
X-linked recessive

Infections
Asthmatic amyotrophy (see Chapter 13)
Diskitis
Epidural abscess
Herpes zoster myelitis
Polyradiculoneuropathy (see Chapter 7)
Tuberculous osteomyelitis

Lupus Myelopathy

Metabolic Disorders
Adrenomyeloneuropathy (adrenoleukodystrophy)
Argininemia
Krabbe disease

Neonatal Cord Infarction

Transverse Myelitis
Devic disease
Encephalomyelitis
Idiopathic

Trauma
Concussion
Epidural hematoma
Fracture dislocation
Neonatal cord trauma (see Chapter 6)

Tumors
Astrocytoma
Ependymoma
Ewing's sarcoma
Neuroblastoma

disorders. The decline in function can be sufficiently insidious to be overlooked for years. Refusal to stand or walk is a symptom of an acute process. When a young child refuses to support weight, the underlying cause may be weakness or pain. Sometimes both are present.

Scoliosis is a feature of many spinal cord disorders. It is seen with neural tube defects, spinal cord tumors, and several degenerative disorders. The presence of scoliosis, in females before puberty and in males of all ages, should strongly suggest either a spinal cord disorder or a neuromuscular disease (see Chapters 6 and 7).

Abnormalities in the skin overlying the spine, such as an abnormal tuft of hair, pigmentation, a sinus opening, or a mass, may indicate an underlying dysraphic state. Spina bifida is almost always an associated feature.

Foot deformities and especially stunted growth of a limb are malevolent signs of lower spinal cord dysfunction. The usual deformity is foreshortening of the foot, *pes cavus*. In such cases, disturbances of bladder control are often an associated feature.

Spinal myoclonus is often misdiagnosed as seizure activity or fasciculations. It is characterized by brief, irregular contractions of small groups of muscles and persists during sleep. Myoclonus is caused by irritation to pools of motor neurons and interneurons, usually by an intramedullary tumor or syrinx. The dermatomal distribution of the myoclonus localizes the site of irritation within the spinal cord.

Congenital Malformations

Some congenital malformations, such as caudal regression syndrome and myelomeningocele, are obvious at birth. Many others do not cause symptoms until adolescence or later. Congenital malformations must always be considered when progressive paraplegia appears in childhood.

Arachnoid Cysts

Arachnoid cysts of the spinal cord, like those of the brain (see Chapter 4), are usually asymptomatic and discovered incidentally on imaging studies. Familial cases should suggest neurofibromatosis type 2 (see Chapter 5).

CLINICAL FEATURES. Arachnoid cysts may be single or multiple and are usually thoracic. Symptomatic arachnoid cysts are unusual in childhood and are most often encountered in adolescents and young adults. The features are back or radicular pain and paraplegia. Symptoms are intensified when standing and intermittent upon changes in position. The pain tends to become more severe with time.

DIAGNOSIS. MRI is the diagnostic modality of choice. The cyst has the same MRI characteristics as cerebrospinal fluid.

MANAGEMENT. Shunting of the cyst is curative but should not be undertaken unless the cyst is known to be symptomatic. It is a common mistake to blame a subarachnoid cyst for symptoms that have another cause.

Arteriovenous Malformations

Arteriovenous malformations of the spinal cord are uncommon in childhood. The youngest known patient was 1 year old, and only 14% of childhood cases begin before age 5.

CLINICAL FEATURES. The progression of symptoms is usually insidious, and the time from onset to diagnosis may be several years. Subacute or chronic pain is the initial feature in one third of patients and subarachnoid hemorrhage in one quarter. Paraplegia is an early feature in only one third, but monoplegia or paraplegia is present in almost all children at the time of diagnosis. Most children have a slowly progressive spastic paraplegia and loss of bladder control.

When subarachnoid hemorrhage is the initial feature, the malformation is more likely to be in the cervical portion of the spinal cord. Blunt trauma to the spine may be a precipitating factor. The onset of paraplegia or quadriplegia is then acute and associated with back pain.

Back pain and episodic weakness that improve completely or in part may be initial features in some children, but impairment is progressive. This type of presentation is misleading, and diagnosis may be delayed for several years.

DIAGNOSIS. MRI is the first step in diagnosis. It distinguishes intramedullary from dural and extramedullary locations of the malformation and even allows recognition of thrombus formation. Arteriography is still necessary to demonstrate the intramedullary extent of the malformation and all of the feeding vessels.

MANAGEMENT. The potential approaches to therapy for intraspinal and intracranial malformations are similar (see Chapter 4).

Atlantoaxial Dislocation

The odontoid process is the major factor preventing dislocation of C1 onto C2. Aplasia of the odontoid process can occur alone or as part of Morquio syndrome, other mucopolysaccharidoses, Klippel-Feil syndrome, several types of genetic chondrodysplasia, and some chromosomal abnormalities (Crockard and Stevens, 1995). Asymptomatic atlantoaxial subluxation is thought to occur in 20% of children with Down syndrome as a result of congenital hypoplasia of the articulation of C1 and C2; symptomatic dislocation is much less common.

CLINICAL FEATURES. Congenital atlantoaxial dislocation produces an acute or slowly progressive quadriplegia that may begin anytime from the neonatal period to adult life. When the onset is in a newborn, the clinical features resemble an acute infantile spinal muscular atrophy (see Chapter 6). The infant has generalized hypotonia with preservation of facial expression and extraocular movement. The tendon reflexes are absent at first but then become hyperactive.

Dislocations during childhood frequently follow a fall or head injury. In such cases, symptoms may begin suddenly and include not only those of myelopathy but also those related to vertebral artery occlusion.

Morquio syndrome is primarily a disease of the skeleton, with only secondary abnormalities of the spinal cord. Beginning in the second year or thereafter, prominent ribs and sternum, knock-knees, progressive shortening of the neck, and dwarfism develop in affected children. The odontoid process is aplastic or absent. Acute, subacute, or chronic cervical myelopathy develops, sometimes precipitated by a fall. An insidious onset is characterized by loss of endurance, fainting attacks, and a "pins and needles" sensation in the arms.

The essential feature of the *Klippel-Feil syndrome* is a reduced number and abnormal fusion of cervical vertebrae. As in Morquio syndrome, the head appears to rest directly on the shoulders, the posterior hairline is low, and movement in all directions is limited. Elevation of the scapulae and deformity of the ribs (Sprengel deformity) are frequently present. Weakness and atrophy of the arm muscles and mirror movements of the hands are associated with the paraplegia. Associated abnormalities may be present in several different organ systems.

Symptomatic atlantoaxial dislocation in children with Down syndrome may occur anytime from infancy to the twenties. Females are affected more often than males. Symptoms include neck pain, torticollis, and an abnormal gait. Spinal cord compression is progressive and leads to quadriplegia and urinary incontinence.

DIAGNOSIS. Lateral radiographs of the cervical portion of the spine in extension and flexion may show atlantoaxial instability, but CT of the cervical vertebrae provides better documentation of the instability and of the spinal cord compression. When Morquio syndrome is suspected, the urine should be checked for keratan sulfate.

MANAGEMENT. Surgical stabilization of the atlantoaxial junction must be considered in any child with evidence of spinal cord compression. The choice of surgical procedure depends on the mechanism of compression.

Caudal Regression Syndrome

The term *caudal regression syndrome* covers several malformations of the caudal spine that range from sacral agenesis to *sirenomelia,* in which only one leg is present. The mechanism of caudal regression is poorly understood. Although the name implies that the cord was formed properly and then regressed, defects in neural tube closure and prosencephalization are often associated features. The risk of caudal regression is greater among infants of diabetic mothers. The clinical spectrum varies from absence of the lumbosacral spinal cord, resulting in small, paralyzed legs, to a single malformed leg associated with malformations of the rectum and genitourinary tract.

Chiari Malformation

The type I Chiari malformation is elongation of the cerebellar vermis with herniation of its caudal end through the foramen magnum. The type II malformation combines the cerebellar herniation with distortion and dysplasia of the medulla and occurs in more than 50% of children with lumbar myelomeningocele. The herniated portion may become ischemic and necrotic and can cause compression of the brainstem and upper cervical spinal cord.

CLINICAL FEATURES. Most Chiari I malformations are discovered as an incidental finding on MRI. *Do not assume that the malformation is the cause of the headache for which the MRI was ordered.* When symptomatic, the initial features are often insidious. Headache and neck pain are the first features in 38% of children and weakness in 56%. Eighty percent show motor deficits on examination, usually atrophy and hyporeflexia in the arms and spasticity and hyperreflexia in the legs. Sensory loss and scoliosis are each present in half of cases.

The type II malformation should be suspected in every child with myelomeningocele. In most cases, the cerebellar displacement is asymptomatic. Hydrocephalus may be caused by aqueductal stenosis or by an obstruction of the outflow of cerebrospinal fluid from the fourth ventricle due to herniation. Respiratory distress is the most important feature of the Chiari malformation and the usual cause of death. Rapid respirations, episodes of apnea, and Cheyne-Stokes respirations may occur. Other evidence of brainstem compression is poor feeding, vomiting, dysphagia, and paralysis of the tongue.

Sudden cardiorespiratory failure is the usual cause of death.

DIAGNOSIS. MRI is the best method to visualize the posterior fossa and cervical cord. CT may be helpful to further delineate bony abnormalities.

MANAGEMENT. Newborns with myelomeningocele and respiratory distress caused by the Chiari malformation are often treated with posterior fossa decompression (Bindal et al, 1995). Unfortunately, the results are not encouraging. Posterior fossa decompression is usually successful in relieving symptoms of cord compression in older children without myelomeningocele. Ventriculoperitoneal shunt may be required as well.

Myelomeningocele

Dysraphia comprises all defects in the closure of the neural tube and its coverings. Closure occurs during the third and fourth weeks of gestation. The mesoderm surrounding the neural tube gives rise to the dura, skull, and vertebrae but not to the skin. Therefore, defects in the final closure of the neural tube and its mesodermal case do not preclude the presence of a dermal covering.

Despite extensive epidemiological studies, the cause of myelomeningocele remains unknown. Causes are likely to be multifactorial, including both genetic and environmental factors. Because women who have previously had a child with dysraphia have an approximate 2% risk of recurrence, prenatal diagnosis can be offered to prevent repetition.

α-Fetoprotein is the principal plasma protein of the fetus and is present in amniotic fluid. When the fetus has a defect of the skin that allows the exudation of plasma proteins, the concentration of α-fetoprotein in the amniotic fluid increases. Prenatal diagnosis is possible in every case by the combination of measuring the maternal serum concentration of α-fetoprotein and performing an ultrasound examination of the fetus.

The incidence of dysraphic defects has been declining in the United States and the United Kingdom. This decline cannot be explained by antenatal screening alone and may be caused in part by changes in critical environmental factors.

Because the ingestion of folic acid supplements during early pregnancy reduces the incidence of neural tube defects, all women of childbearing age are advised to consume 0.4 mg of folic acid daily. Women with a prior history of delivering a child with a neural tube defect should take 4 mg/day of folic acid from at least 4 weeks before the conception through the first 3 months of pregnancy.

CLINICAL FEATURES. *Spina bifida cystica*, the protrusion of a cystic mass through the defect, is an obvious deformity of the newborn's spine. More than 90% are thoracolumbar. Among newborns with spina bifida cystica, the protruding sac is a meningocele without neural elements in 10% to 20% and is a myelomeningocele in the rest. Meningoceles tend to have a partial dermal covering and are often pedunculated, with a narrow base connecting the sac to the underlying spinal cord. Myelomeningoceles usually have a broad base, are poorly epithelialized, and ooze a combination of cerebrospinal fluid and serum. Remnants of the spinal cord are fused to the exposed portion of the dome.

In newborns with spina bifida cystica, it is important to determine the extent of neurological dysfunction caused by the myelopathy, the potential for the development of hydrocephalus, and the presence of other malformations in the nervous system and in other organs. When myelomeningocele is the only deformity, the newborn is alert and responsive and has no difficulty in feeding. Diminished consciousness or responsiveness and difficulty in feeding should suggest perinatal asphyxia or cerebral malformations such as hydrocephalus. Cyanosis, pallor, or dyspnea may be caused by associated malformations in the cardiovascular system. Multiple major defects are present in 27% of cases.

The spinal segments involved can be determined by locating the myelomeningocele with reference to the ribs and iliac crest. Several patterns of motor dysfunction may be observed, depending on the cyst's location. Motor dysfunction results from interruption of the corticospinal tracts and from dysgenesis of the segmental innervation. At birth the legs are flaccid and the hips are dislocated. Spastic paraplegia, a spastic bladder, and a level of sensory loss develop in infants with a thoracic lesion. Segmental withdrawal reflexes below the level of the lesion, which indicate the presence of an intact but isolated spinal cord segment below the cyst, are present in half of patients. Infants with deformities of the conus medullaris maintain a flaccid paraplegia, have lumbosacral sensory loss, lack a withdrawal response in the legs, and have a distended bladder with overflow incontinence.

Only 15% of newborns with myelomeningocele have clinical evidence of hydrocephalus at birth, but hydrocephalus can be detected in 60% of affected newborns by ultrasound. Hydro-cephalus eventually develops in 80%. The first clinical features of hydrocephalus often follow the repair of the myelomeningocele, but the two are not related. Aqueductal stenosis is the cause of hydrocephalus in three quarters of infants with myelomeningocele.

DIAGNOSIS. The diagnosis of spina bifida cystica is made by examination alone. EMG may be useful to clarify the distribution of segmental dysfunction. Cranial ultrasound should be performed on every newborn to look for hydrocephalus. MRI is useful to define malformations of the brain, especially the Chiari malformation (see Figure 10-5). This information may be needed in making therapeutic decisions. Even when hydrocephalus is not present at birth, ultrasound should be repeated in 2 to 4 weeks to evaluate ventricular size.

MANAGEMENT. Intrauterine surgery to close the back is an experimental procedure based on the hypotheses that exposure of the cord to amniotic fluid increases injury and increases hindbrain herniation (Tulipan et al, 1998). The usefulness of the procedure is not established.

The chance of surviving the first year is poor unless the back is closed shortly after birth. However, closure is not a surgical emergency and can be delayed for a week or longer without influencing the survival rate. Other factors associated with increased mortality are a high spinal location of the defect and clinical hydrocephalus at birth. The long-term outcome depends on the degree of mental retardation and the neurological deficit from the spinal defect.

Tethered Spinal Cord

The conus medullaris is sometimes anchored to the base of the vertebrae by a thickened filum terminale, a lipoma, a dermal sinus, or a diastematomyelia. Spina bifida occulta is usually an associated feature. As the child grows, the tether causes the spinal cord to stretch and the lumbosacral segments to become ischemic. The mitochondrial oxidative metabolism of neurons is impaired, and neurological dysfunction follows.

Dermal sinus is a midline opening of the skin usually marked by a tuft of hair or port-wine stain. It is caused by an abnormal invagination of ectoderm into the posterior closure site of the neural tube. Most sinuses terminate subcutaneously as a blind pouch or dermoid cyst. Others extend through a spina bifida to the developing neuraxis, at which point they attach to the dura or the spinal cord as a fibrous band or dermoid cyst. Such sinuses tether the spinal cord and may also serve as a route for bacteria from the skin to reach the subarachnoid space and cause meningitis.

Diastematomyelia consists of a bifid spinal cord (also called *diplomyelia*) that is normal in the cervical and upper thoracic regions and then divides into lateral halves (Figure 12-1). Two types of diastematomyelia occur with equal frequency. In one type, a dural sheath surrounds each half of the cord and the two halves are separated by a fibrous or bony septum. Once the cord separates, it never rejoins. In the other type, a single dural sheath surrounds both halves and a septum is not present. The two halves rejoin after one or two segments. Therefore, splitting of the spinal cord is not caused by the presence of a septum, but is instead a primary disturbance in the formation of luminal borders caused by faulty closure of the neural tube. It is usually associated with other dysraphic disturbances such as spina bifida occulta or cystica.

CLINICAL FEATURES. The initial features of a tethered spinal cord occur at any age from infancy to young adulthood. The clinical features vary with age. External signs of spinal dysraphism (tuft of hair, subcutaneous lipoma, dermal sinus) are present in more than half of patients, and spina bifida occulta or sacral deformity is present in almost 90%.

Infants and young children are most likely to show clumsiness of gait, stunted growth or deformity of one foot or leg, and disturbances in bladder function. These may occur alone or in combination. Consequently, the first specialist consulted may be an orthopedic surgeon, a urologist, a neurologist, or a neurosurgeon. The progression of symptoms and signs is insidious, and at first most children are believed to have a static problem. Children with only a clumsy gait or disturbances in urinary control tend to have normal or exaggerated tendon reflexes and an ex-

tensor plantar response. In some children, the ankle tendon reflex is diminished or absent on one or both sides. Children with foot deformity usually have pes cavus and stunted growth of the entire leg. The other leg may appear normal or have a milder deformity without a growth disturbance. The tendon reflexes in the deformed foot are more likely to be diminished than increased.

The initial feature of tethered spinal cord in older children and adolescents is either clumsiness of gait or scoliosis. Bilateral, but mild, foot deformities are sometimes present, and urinary incontinence and constipation may be reported. Tendon reflexes in the legs are usually exaggerated at the knees and ankles, and the plantar response is usually extensor.

DIAGNOSIS. EMG is not a useful screening procedure, as the results are almost always abnormal. Radiographs of the spine may show a spina bifida, but MRI is the appropriate diagnostic test and is particularly useful in the detection of lumbosacral lipoma. The essential feature of a tethered spinal cord is a low-lying conus medullaris. At 28 weeks' gestation, the tip of the conus is at the L3 vertebral level. It generally rises one level by 40 weeks' gestation. A conus that extends below the L2 to L3 interspace in children 5 years and older is always abnormal.

MANAGEMENT. Surgical relief of the tethering prevents further deterioration of neurological function. Improvement of preexisting deficits is accomplished in up to 50% of children (Cornette et al, 1998).

Familial Spastic Paraplegia

Familial spastic paraplegia is a heterogeneous group of genetic disorders in which the prominent clinical feature is progressive spastic paraplegia. Some families have pure spastic paraple-

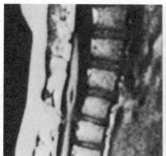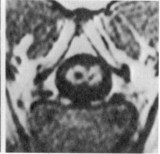

Figure 12-1. Diplomyelia. MRI shows two cords with two central canals. An enlarged segment with a cystic center is seen on longitudinal section.

gia, while others have clinical evidence of degeneration in the posterior columns or cerebellar pathways. Familial spastic paraplegia is transmitted by autosomal dominant inheritance in 70% of cases and by autosomal recessive inheritance in the remainder. Genetic heterogeneity exists even within the dominant and recessive forms. An X-linked form has been reported in fewer than 20 families. Linkage studies have mapped the abnormal gene to the long arm of the X chromosome (Cambi et al, 1995).

Autosomal Dominant Inheritance

Children with autosomal dominant spastic paraplegia (ADSP) usually have pure spastic paraplegia without prominent disturbances of other neurological systems. Even among these "pure" ADSPs, genetic heterogeneity exists. At least four loci have been identified: 2p, 8q23-24, 14q, and 15q13-15 (Figlewitz and Bird, 1999). Families with "complicated" ADSP (mental retardation, ataxia, and extraocular abnormalities) do not show linkage to any of these loci (Meierkord et al, 1997).

CLINICAL FEATURES. The age at onset ranges from 1 to 68 years, with the mean at 29 years. Early and late onset occur among members of the same family. Motor milestones are normal in affected infants except for toe walking. Their condition is frequently misdiagnosed as cerebral palsy, especially if the affected parent is asymptomatic or has only a mildly stiff gait. Increased tone is more prominent than weakness. Tone increases slowly for 10 years and then stabilizes. At this point, the child may have minimal stiffness of gait or be unable to stand or walk.

Tendon reflexes are usually increased in the legs and arms, and ankle clonus may be present. Occasionally, tendon reflexes at the ankle are diminished or absent. This may be caused by an associated axonal neuropathy. Increased reflexes are usually the only sign of involvement of the arms. Vibratory and position sense are diminished in half of patients. One third have urinary symptoms, usually in the form of frequency and urgency, and one third have a pes cavus deformity.

DIAGNOSIS. Familial spastic paraplegia is difficult to diagnose in the absence of a family history of the defect. It should be suspected in any child with very slowly progressive spastic paraplegia. Laboratory studies are not helpful except to exclude other conditions such as spinal cord compression, adrenoleukodystrophy, and argininemia.

MANAGEMENT. No treatment is available.

Autosomal Recessive Inheritance

Autosomal recessive inheritance of hereditary spastic paraplegia is characterized by involvement of other neurological systems. The associated features vary from family to family, suggesting genetic heterogeneity. One form has been linked to chromosome 8p12-q13.

CLINICAL FEATURES. Spastic paraplegia may begin during infancy but can be delayed until the teens. Involvement of other neurological systems follows. The common associated features, alone or in combination, include cerebellar dysfunction, pseudobulbar palsy, sensory neuropathy, and *pes cavus*.

Children with sensory neuropathy lose the once hyperactive tendon reflexes in the legs. Some have delayed development and never achieve bladder control. When sensory loss is progressive, the symptoms resemble those of familial sensory neuropathies described in Chapter 9. The outcome varies from mild disability to wheelchair confinement.

DIAGNOSIS. The onset of paraplegia is in infancy. In the absence of a family history, the course of disease suggests cerebral palsy until the progressive nature of the spasticity is recognized. Sensory neuropathy with mutilation of digits may lead to the erroneous diagnosis of syringomyelia. Laboratory tests are useful only to exclude other diagnoses. Argininemia, a treatable cause of autosomal recessive progressive spastic paraplegia, should be considered (Prasad et al, 1997).

MANAGEMENT. No treatment is available for the underlying defect, but supportive care for the sensory neuropathy is needed (see Chapter 9).

Infections

Primary myelitis from acquired immune deficiency syndrome (AIDS) is uncommon in children and is not discussed in this section.

Diskitis (Disk Space Infection)

Disk space infection is a relatively uncommon disorder of childhood in which one disk space is infected secondary to subacute osteomyelitis of the adjacent vertebral bodies. The cause is bacterial infection. *Staphylococcus aureus* is the organism most often grown on culture of disk material removed by needle biopsy and is probably the major cause. The same organism is rarely isolated from cultures of the blood, however, because the infection is subacute, cultures are rarely positive, and biopsy is not indicated.

CLINICAL FEATURES. The initial feature is either difficulty walking or back pain. Difficulty walking occurs almost exclusively in children less than 3 years of age. The typical child has a low-grade or no fever, is observed to be limping, and may refuse to stand or walk. This symptom complex evolves over 24 to 48 hours. Affected children prefer to lie on their sides rather than to rest supine, resist being brought to standing, and then seem uncomfortable and walk with a shuffling gait. Examination shows loss of lumbar lordosis and absolute resistance to flexion of the spine. The hips or back are sometimes tender.

Pain as an initial feature occurs more often after 3 years of age. The pain may be abdominal or vertebral. When abdominal, the pain gradually increases in intensity and may radiate from the epigastrium to the umbilicus or pelvis. Abdominal pain in association with low-grade fever and an elevated peripheral white blood cell count invariably suggests the possibility of appendicitis or other intra-abdominal disease. Fortunately, abdominal pain is the least common presenting feature.

Back pain is the most common complaint. Older children may indicate a specific area of pain and tenderness. Younger children may have only an abnormal posture intended to splint the painful area. Back pain usually leads to prompt diagnosis because attention is immediately directed to the spine. Examination reveals loss of lumbar lordosis and decreased movement of the spine, especially flexion.

DIAGNOSIS. Disk space infection should be considered in all children who have a sudden back pain or refuse to walk and in whom neurological findings are normal. Strength, tone, and tendon reflexes in the legs are normal. Radiographs of the spine reveal narrowing of the affected intervertebral space, most often in the lumbar region but sometimes as high as the C5 to C6 positions. The inflammation within the disk is best demonstrated by MRI, which shows osteomyelitis of the surrounding vertebrae as well as of the disk space (Figure 12-2).

MANAGEMENT. Antibiotics are effective in treating the infection. Antistaphylococcal antibiotics should be begun intravenously as soon as the diagnosis is confirmed. These may be switched to the oral route within 2 to 5 days and continued on an outpatient basis. Immobilization is not necessary because the children are nearly asymptomatic when discharged from hospital.

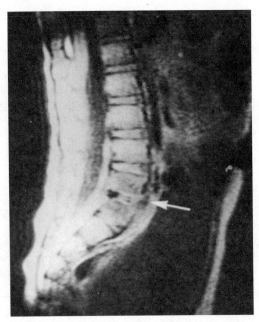

Figure 12-2. Diskitis. MRI reveals collapse of the disk space (*arrow*) and demineralization of the adjoining vertebral bodies.

Herpes Zoster Myelitis

Immunosuppressed individuals may experience reactivation of the varicella-zoster virus that had been latent in sensory ganglia following primary chickenpox infection.

CLINICAL FEATURES. The spinal cord becomes involved within 3 weeks after a truncal rash appears. The myelopathy usually progresses for 3 weeks, but progression may last as long as 6 months in people with AIDS. Cord involvement is bilateral in 80% of cases.

DIAGNOSIS. Diagnosis depends on recognition of the characteristic herpetic rash at the dermatomal level of the myelitis. Unfortunately, the myelitis sometimes precedes the onset of rash. The spine should be imaged to exclude other causes. The cerebrospinal fluid shows a pleocytosis and protein elevation that is greatest at the time of maximal neurological deficit.

MANAGEMENT. Corticosteroids and acyclovir are recommended for treatment, although their benefit is uncertain.

Tuberculous Osteomyelitis

Vertebral infection is caused by hematogenous dissemination. Any level of the vertebral column may be affected. The infection usually begins in one vertebral body and then spreads to adjacent vertebrae and the surrounding soft tissue. Fewer than 20% of patients with tuberculous osteomyelitis have symptoms of spinal cord dysfunction. The pathophysiological mechanisms include epidural abscess, arteritis, and vertebral collapse. In addition, tuberculous granuloma of the spine may occur in the absence of vertebral disease.

CLINICAL FEATURES. Tuberculosis of the vertebrae and spine is primarily a disease of children and young adults. Young children with vertebral osteomyelitis not extending to the spinal cord may refuse to walk because of pain, and their symptoms may mimic paraplegia. The prominent features are fever, anorexia, and back pain. In children less than 10 years of age, infection is generally diffuse, affecting several vertebrae and adjacent tissues. Older children tend to have localized infection, but with a higher incidence of spinal cord compression. The symptoms and signs of spinal cord compression from tuberculosis are similar to those described for epidural abscess, except that progression is slower.

DIAGNOSIS. The cerebrospinal fluid is usually under pressure and shows a pleocytosis with polymorphonuclear leukocytes predominating early in the course and lymphocytes predominating in the later stages. The total cell count rarely exceeds 500 cells/mm³. Protein concentrations are elevated, and glucose concentrations are depressed. Acid-fast organisms can be seen on a stained smear and can be isolated on cultures of the cerebrospinal fluid.

Early stages of vertebral osteomyelitis can be shown by a technetium bone scan or plain radiographs. MRI is needed to search for a contiguous abscess. As the disease progresses, radiographs reveal collapse of adjacent vertebrae and gibbus formation.

MANAGEMENT. Tuberculous osteomyelitis and meningitis should be treated in a similar fashion. The recommended drug combinations are oral isoniazid, intramuscular streptomycin, and oral rifampin. Streptomycin and rifampin are continued for 8 weeks following clinical improvement, and isoniazid is continued for 2 years (Dutt and Stead, 1997).

Lupus Myelopathy

Transverse myelopathy is a rare complication of systemic lupus erythematosus. The usual features are back pain, rapidly progressive paraplegia, and bowel and bladder dysfunction. Sensory loss is not a constant feature. The protein con-

centration of the cerebrospinal fluid is elevated. Recovery is poor and mortality is high.

Metabolic Disorders

Adrenomyeloneuropathy

Adrenomyeloneuropathy (AMN) is the second most common phenotype of adrenoleukodystrophy, an X-linked disorder caused by impaired ability to oxidize very-long-chain fatty acids (see Chapter 5).

CLINICAL FEATURES. Paraparesis begins after age 20 and slowly progresses throughout adult life. Intellect is not usually impaired, and prolonged survival is the rule (van Geel et al, 1997). Most patients develop Addison's disease, which predates the paraparesis almost half of the time. A sensory neuropathy may be associated. Approximately 20% of female heterozygotes develop AMN.

DIAGNOSIS. The disease is often misdiagnosed as multiple sclerosis, especially in female heterozygotes. The demonstration of increased plasma concentrations of very-long-chain fatty acids is essential for diagnosis.

Argininemia

Argininemia is a urea cycle disorder transmitted as an autosomal recessive trait. It is caused by deficiency of the enzyme arginase (see Figure 1-2). The gene locus is assigned to chromosome 6q23.

CLINICAL FEATURES. Motor and cognitive development slows in early childhood and then regresses. Most children develop a progressive spastic paraplegia or quadriplegia. Other features may include recurrent vomiting and seizures (Prasad et al, 1997).

DIAGNOSIS. The serum concentration of arginine is always elevated, and 90% of children have elevated blood concentrations of ammonia. Arginase is absent from red blood cells.

MANAGEMENT. Dietary protein restriction may slow the progression of the disorder and sometimes cause improvement.

Krabbe Disease

The early infantile form of Krabbe disease (globoid leukodystrophy) causes psychomotor regression (see Chapter 5) and a peripheral neuropathy (see Chapter 7). The disorder is due to mutations of the gene encoding glycosylceramidase (GALC) at chromosome 14q31.

A late-onset form of the disease, with onset from childhood to adolescence, may present as a pure spastic paraplegia. All forms show a deficiency of galactosylceramide β-galactosidase (Percy, 1997). Allogeneic hematopoietic stem cell transplantation shows promise in preventing, and even reversing, the neurological abnormalities (Krivit et al, 1998).

Neonatal Cord Infarction

Infarction of the spinal cord is a hazard in newborns undergoing umbilical artery catheterization. The artery of Adamkiewicz arises from the aorta at the level of T10 to T12 and is the major segmental artery to the thoracolumbar spinal cord. Embolization of the artery may occur if the catheter tip is placed between levels T8 and T11. The result is acute and sometimes irreversible paraplegia. A similar syndrome can occur in premature or small-for-date newborns who have not been catheterized. The mechanism is not established but may be caused by hypotension.

Transverse Myelitis

Transverse myelitis is an acute demyelinating disorder of the spinal cord that evolves in hours or days. It may occur alone or in combination with demyelination in other portions of the nervous system. The association of transverse myelitis and optic neuritis is called *Devic disease;* acute demyelination throughout the neuraxis is called *diffuse encephalomyelitis.* These terms are descriptive and do not suggest an underlying cause.

Multiple sclerosis is usually suspected in adults with transverse myelitis, although only 20% eventually have other demyelinating lesions. Multiple sclerosis is uncommon in childhood, and the initial feature is more likely to be cerebellar or extraocular dysfunction than myelitis (see Chapter 10).

Transverse myelitis, and especially encephalomyelitis, in children is frequently attributed to a preceding viral infection or immunization. No evidence supports such a notion. School-age children average four to six "viral" episodes annually. Therefore, half of children with any illness may give a history of a viral infection within the preceding 30 days. Similarly, despite several case reports, a cause-and-effect relationship has not been established between licensed vaccines and demyelinating disorders of the central nervous system.

CLINICAL FEATURES. Mean age at onset is 9 years. Symptoms progress rapidly, and maximal deficit is attained within 2 days. The level of myelitis is usually thoracic and demarcated by the sensory loss. Asymmetric leg weakness is common. The bladder fills and does not empty voluntarily. Tendon reflexes may be increased or reduced. Recovery begins after 6 days but may be incomplete. Fifty percent of patients make a full recovery, 10% have no recovery, and 40% recover incompletely. Most resume walking, but many continue to have sensory disturbances.

Several children have a *relapsing myelitis* in which attacks of acute myelitis recur over months or years. None develop multiple sclerosis or more disseminated disease. Recovery after each attack may be complete.

DIAGNOSIS. MRI of the spine is needed to exclude acute cord compression, and it sometimes shows swelling at the level of myelitis. Cranial MRI is indicated to exclude more widespread disease. Vision should be checked daily because of the possibility of Devic disease.

MANAGEMENT. Corticosteroids are generally used despite the absence of controlled studies. High-dose intravenous therapy followed by tapering doses of prednisone is recommended.

Devic Disease (Neuromyelitis Optica)

I believe that Devic disease is a distinct disorder that occurs mainly in children and is not part of the spectrum of multiple sclerosis. Many authorities in the field do not share this view. No cause can be determined in most children with Devic disease.

A temporal association between pulmonary tuberculosis and Devic disease is seen in adolescents and adults. In these cases, the neurological disease appears to be an immune reaction to tuberculosis and not caused by antituberculous therapy.

CLINICAL FEATURES. A history of anorexia or a flu-like syndrome a few days or a week before the first neurological symptoms is common. The anorexia may be part of the acute demyelinating illness rather than a viral infection. Myelitis precedes optic neuritis in 13% of patients and follows it in 76%; myelitis and neuritis occur simultaneously in 10%. Optic neuritis and transverse myelitis generally occur within 1 week of each other. The child remains irritable while the neurological symptoms are evolving.

Bilateral optic neuritis occurs in 80% of patients (see Chapter 16). Both eyes may be affected at onset, or one eye may become affected before the other. Loss of vision is acute and accompanied by pain. Blindness is often complete within hours. The initial ophthalmoscopic examination may have normal results but more often shows swelling of the disk. The pupils are dilated, and the response to light is sluggish.

Myelitis is heralded by back pain and discomfort in the legs. The legs become weak, and the patient has difficulty standing and walking. Paraplegia becomes complete; it is first flaccid and then becomes spastic. Tendon reflexes may be diminished at first but later become exaggerated and are associated with extensor plantar responses. The bladder is spastic, and the patient has overflow incontinence. In some patients, a sensory level may be detected, but more often the sensory deficit is patchy and difficult to delineate in an irritable child.

The course is variable. Some patients develop an encephalomyelitis (see following section on Diffuse Encephalomyelitis), some have permanent paraplegia, and most recover but not always completely.

DIAGNOSIS. MRI of the spine is needed to exclude spinal cord compression syndrome, and MRI of the head is indicated to look for other demyelinating lesions (Figure 12-3). The cerebrospinal fluid in children with Devic disease is usually abnormal. The protein content is mildly to moderately increased, and a mixed pleocytosis of neutrophils and mononuclear cells is present.

MANAGEMENT. A course of corticosteroids is usually suggested for children with Devic disease. Although the value of corticosteroids is not established, most physicians believe they are beneficial. The regimen is the same as for diffuse encephalomyelitis. Bladder care with intermittent catheterization is imperative, as are measures to prevent bed sores and infection. The family and the child often need psychological counseling.

Diffuse Encephalomyelitis

Diffuse encephalomyelitis is discussed in the section on Devic syndrome and in Chapter 2. The major clinical difference from Devic disease is that the cerebral hemispheres are affected as well as the spinal cord. Cerebral demyelination may precede, follow, or occur concurrently with the myelitis.

CLINICAL FEATURES. In addition to the myelitis, an encephalopathy characterized by decreased consciousness, irritability, and spastic quadriplegia occurs. If the brainstem is affected, dysphagia, fever, cranial nerve palsies, and irregular respiration are present.

DIAGNOSIS. The full extent of demyelination can be appreciated only with MRI. Multiple white matter lesions that become confluent are noted in the cerebral hemispheres (see Figure 2-2), cerebellum, and brainstem. Adrenoleukodystrophy must be excluded by measuring very-long-chain fatty acids.

MANAGEMENT. Most authorities agree that corticosteroids should be administered. Prednisone, 2 mg/kg/day (not to exceed 100 mg), or its equivalent in a parenteral form is the initial dose, which is then tapered over a 4-week period, depending on the response. The benefit of such a course of therapy is not established, and some patients become corticosteroid dependent and have a relapse when prednisone is discontinued. Such children require long-term alternate-day therapy.

Trauma

Spinal cord injuries are relatively rare, especially before adolescence. The major cause is motor vehicle accidents, followed by sports-related injuries. The injuries affect the cervical spinal cord in 65% of cases before 15 years of age and in 71% of cases before 9 years of age. Fifteen percent of patients have injuries at multiple levels.

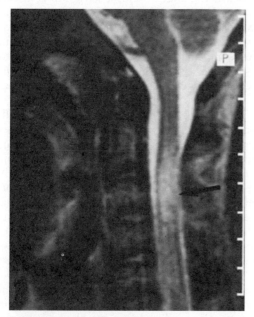

Figure 12-3. Demyelination of the spinal cord in an adolescent girl with multiple sclerosis.

Neurological function that is intact immediately after the injury remains intact afterward. Even those with incomplete function are likely to recover completely. Evidence of complete transection on initial examination indicates that paralysis is permanent.

Spinal Cord Concussion

A direct blow on the back may produce a transitory disturbance in spinal cord function. The dysfunction is caused by edema (spinal shock); the spinal cord is intact.

CLINICAL FEATURES. Most injuries occur at the level of the cervical cord or the thoracolumbar juncture. The major clinical features are flaccid paraplegia or quadriplegia, a sensory level at the site of injury, loss of tendon reflexes, and urinary retention. Recovery begins within a few hours and is complete within a week.

DIAGNOSIS. At the onset of weakness, a spinal cord compression syndrome such as epidural hematoma cannot be excluded, and an imaging study of the spine is necessary.

MANAGEMENT. Children with spinal cord concussion should be treated with methylprednisolone, as outlined in the section on fracture dislocation and spinal cord transection.

Compressed Vertebral Body Fractures

CLINICAL FEATURES. Compression fractures of the thoracolumbar region occur when a child jumps or falls from a height greater than 10 feet and lands in a standing or sitting position. The spinal cord itself is not transected, but spinal cord concussion may cause paraplegia. Back pain at the fracture site is immediate and intense. Nerve roots are compressed, causing pain that radiates into the groin and legs.

DIAGNOSIS. Thoracolumbar radiographs reveal the fracture, but when paraplegia is present, a spinal cord imaging study is usually performed as well, and the results prove to be normal.

MANAGEMENT. Immobilization relieves the back pain and promotes healing of the fracture.

Fracture Dislocation and Spinal Cord Transection

Transection of the spinal cord from fracture dislocation of the vertebral column injury is usually caused by a motor vehicle accident. A forceful flexion of the spine fractures the articular facets and allows the vertebral body to move forward or laterally, with consequent contusion or transection of the spinal cord. The common sites of traumatic transection are the levels C1 to C2, C5 to C7, and T12 to L2.

CLINICAL FEATURES. Neurological deficits at and below the level of spinal cord contusion or transection are immediate and profound. Many children with fracture dislocations sustained head injuries at the time of trauma and are unconscious.

Immediately after the injury, the child has flaccid weakness of the limbs below the level of the lesion associated with loss of tendon and cutaneous reflexes (spinal shock). In high cervical spinal cord lesions, the knee and ankle tendon reflexes, anal reflex, and plantar response may be elicited during the initial period of spinal shock. Spinal shock lasts for approximately 1 week in infants and young children and up to 6 weeks in adolescents.

First, the superficial reflexes return, then the plantar response becomes one of extension, and finally massive withdrawal reflexes (mass reflex) appear. The mass reflex is triggered by trivial stimulation of the foot or leg, usually in a specific zone unique to the patient. The response at first is dorsiflexion of the foot, flexion at the knees, and flexion and adduction at the thighs. Later, there are also contraction of the abdomen, sweating, piloerection, and emptying of the bladder and bowel. During this time of heightened reflex activity the tendon reflexes return and become exaggerated.

Below the level of injury, sensation is lost to a variable degree, depending on the completeness of the transection. When the injury is incomplete, sensation begins to return within weeks and may continue to improve for up to 2 years. Patients with partial or complete transections may complain of pain and tingling below the level of injury.

In addition to the development of a small, spastic bladder, autonomic dysfunction includes constipation, lack of sweating, orthostatic hypotension, and disturbed temperature regulation.

DIAGNOSIS. Radiographs of the vertebrae readily identify fracture dislocations. Imaging of the spinal cord produces further information on the presence of compressive hematomas and the structural integrity of the spinal cord (Figure 12-4). The presence of a complete block on myelography indicates a poor prognosis for return of function.

MANAGEMENT. The immediate treatment of fracture dislocation is to reduce the dislocation and prevent further damage to the cord by the use of corticosteroids, surgery, and immobiliza-

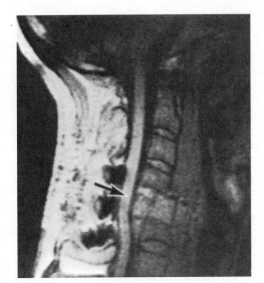

Figure 12-4. Fracture dislocation. C4 is dislocated on C5, causing compression (*arrow*) of the cord.

tion. An intravenous infusion of methylprednisolone, 30 mg/kg within the first 8 hours after injury followed by 4 mg/kg/hr for 23 hours, significantly reduces neurological morbidity. A discussion of the long-term management of spinal cord injuries is beyond the scope of this text. This management is best accomplished at specialized centers.

Spinal Epidural Hematoma

Spinal epidural hematoma usually results from direct vertebral trauma and is especially common in children with an underlying bleeding tendency. The hematoma causes symptoms by progressive compression of the cord and is manifested like any other extradural mass lesion. Diagnosis is usually based on MRI. Treatment is surgical evacuation.

Tumors of the Spinal Cord

Ewing's sarcoma accounts for nearly 20% of cases of spinal cord compression in children over 5 years of age, while neuroblastoma is the most common cause in younger children. Astrocytoma and ependymoma are the main primary tumors. Motor deficits, usually paraplegia, are an early feature in 86% of spinal cord tumors and back pain in 63%.

Astrocytoma

The problem of differentiating cystic astrocytoma of the spinal cord from syringomyelia is discussed in Chapter 9 (see section on Syringomyelia).

CLINICAL FEATURES. Astrocytomas are usually long and may extend from the lower brainstem to the conus medullaris. The initial features of multiple-segment spinal astrocytomas may be seen in the arms or legs. One syndrome is characterized primarily by weakness of one arm. Pain in the neck may be associated, but bowel and bladder function are normal. Examination shows mild spastic weakness of the legs. The solid portion of the tumor is in the neck, and its caudal extension is cystic.

A second syndrome is characterized by progressive spastic paraplegia, sometimes associated with thoracic pain. Scoliosis may be present. In these patients, the solid portion of the tumor is in the thoracic or lumbar region. When solid tumor extends into the conus medullaris, tendon reflexes in the legs may be diminished or absent and bowel and bladder function are impaired.

Intra-axial tumors of the cervicomedullary junction are often low-grade and have an indolent course. They may cause cranial nerve dysfunction or spinal cord compression. Cranial nerve dysfunction is manifested by difficulty in swallowing and nasal speech (see Chapter 17).

DIAGNOSIS. MRI is the definitive diagnostic procedure. It allows visualization of both the solid and cystic portions of the tumor (Figure 12-5).

MANAGEMENT. Evaluating proposed treatment options is difficult because the natural history of the tumor is one of slow progression. The 5-year survival rate with low-grade astrocytoma is greater than 90%. Complete resection should be attempted using microsurgical technique. The solid portion is removed and the cystic portion is aspirated. MRI should be repeated 1, 6, and 12 months after surgery. The benefits of radiation therapy, either after resection or at the time of recurrence, are not established.

Ependymoma

Ependymomas are composed primarily of ependymal cells and arise from the lining of the ventricular system or central canal. They are more often intracranial than intraspinal in children. When intraspinal, they tend to be located in the lumbar region or in the cauda equina but may occur anywhere along the neuraxis.

CLINICAL FEATURES. Clinical features vary with the location of the tumor. The initial feature may be scoliosis, pain in the legs or back, paresthesia, or weakness in one or both legs. Diagno-

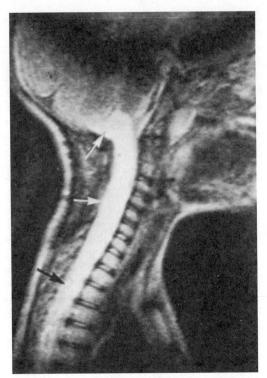

Figure 12-5. Astrocytoma of the cervical cord. The tumor demonstrates an intense signal (*arrows*) on T$_2$-weighted images.

sis may be delayed for years when scoliosis is the only sign. Eventually, all children have difficulty walking, and this is the symptom that usually leads to appropriate diagnostic testing.

Stiff neck and cervical pain that is worse at night are the early features of cervical ependymomas. Tumors of the cauda equina may sometimes rupture and produce meningismus, fever, and pleocytosis mimicking bacterial meningitis. Spastic paraplegia is the usual finding on examination. Cervical tumors cause weakness of one arm as well. Tumors of the cauda equina produce flaccid weakness and atrophy of leg muscles associated with loss of tendon reflexes.

DIAGNOSIS. MRI is the primary modality for imaging tumors of the spinal cord. Lumbar puncture is rarely indicated but shows an elevated protein content in the cerebrospinal fluid.

MANAGEMENT. Microsurgical techniques make possible the complete removal of intramedullary ependymoma. The role of postoperative local radiation therapy in treating benign tumors is uncertain. Malignant ependymomas of the spinal cord are unusual in children but require total neuraxis irradiation when present.

Neuroblastoma

Neuroblastoma is the most common extracranial solid tumor of infancy and childhood. It produces neurological dysfunction by direct invasion, by metastasis, and by distant "humoral" effects (see Chapter 10). Half of cases occur before 2 years of age and 60% occur before 1 year. Neuroblastoma is derived from cells of the sympathetic chain and cranial ganglia. Tumors in a paraspinal location may extend through a neural foramen and compress the spinal cord.

CLINICAL FEATURES. Paraplegia is the initial manifestation of neuroblastoma extending into the epidural space from a paravertebral origin. Because most affected children are infants, the first symptom is usually refusal to stand or walk. Mild weakness may progress to complete paraplegia within hours or days. Examination generally reveals a flaccid paraplegia, a distended bladder, and exaggerated tendon reflexes in the legs. Sensation may be difficult to test.

DIAGNOSIS. Radiographs of the chest usually show the extravertebral portion of the tumor, and the extent of spinal compression is delineated with MRI.

MANAGEMENT. In children with acute spinal cord compression, some relief can be provided by high-dose corticosteroids before surgical extirpation and radiation therapy. The survival rate in infants with neuroblastoma confined to a single organ is greater than 60%.

Cerebral Paraplegia and Quadriplegia

Almost all progressive disorders of the brain that result in quadriplegia also have dementia as an initial or prominent feature (see Chapter 5). Pure paraplegia of cerebral origin is unusual. At the very least, the patient has impairment of fine finger movements and increased tendon reflex activity in the arms. Pure paraplegia should always direct attention to the spinal cord.

Cerebral Palsy

Cerebral palsy (CP) is a chronic motor disability of cerebral origin, appearing early in life, and not caused by a progressive disease. The prevalence of moderately severe cases is approximately 2 per 1,000 live births; the prevalence of cerebral palsy has increased among very small premature infants, as more have survived (Hagberg et al, 1996). Life expectancy is reduced in children with CP who are immobile, profoundly retarded, or require special feeding (Strauss et al, 1998). Otherwise, children with CP may live well into adult life.

Many slowly progressive disorders are mistakenly diagnosed as CP (Table 12-2). Perinatal asphyxia is a known cause of CP but accounts for only a minority of cases. Most cases are caused by prenatal factors that are difficult to identify with precision in an individual patient.

CP is not always a permanent condition. Many infants with only mild motor impairments improve and achieve normal motor function in childhood. Unfortunately, up to 25% of such children will be retarded or will have some behavioral or cognitive disturbance.

Traditionally, the cerebral palsies have been classified by the pattern of motor impairment. The spastic types are paraplegia or diplegia, quadriplegia, and hemiplegia (see Chapter 11). The hypotonic types are ataxic (see Chapter 10) and athetoid (see Chapter 14).

Spastic Diplegia (Paraplegia)

Diplegia means that all four limbs are affected but that the legs are affected more severely than the arms. The motor impairment in the arms may be limited to increased responses of tendon reflexes; such children are classified as paraplegic. Spastic diplegia is usually caused by periventricular leukomalacia in children born prematurely. Cystic lesions in the white matter are often unilateral or at least asymmetric, causing a hemiplegia superimposed on spastic diplegia.

CLINICAL FEATURES. Many children with spastic diplegia have normal tone, or even hypotonia, during the first 4 months. The onset of spasticity in the legs is insidious and slowly progressive during the first year. Four-point creeping is impossible because of leg extension. Either rolling or crawling on the floor with the belly on the ground is used instead to achieve movement.

Sitting up alone is delayed or never achieved. From the supine position, the infant pulls to a standing rather than a sitting position. Sitting is later made possible by bending forward at the waist, to compensate for the lack of flexion at the hip and knee, and placing one hand on the floor for balance. Most children with spastic diplegia stand on their toes, with flexion at the knees and an increased lumbar lordosis. Walking is difficult because of the stiffness in the legs and can be accomplished only by throwing the body forward or from side to side to transfer weight.

Examination shows spasticity of the legs and less spasticity of the arms. The tendon reflexes are exaggerated in all limbs. Reflex sensitivity and responsiveness are increased; percussion at the knee causes a crossed adductor response. Ankle clonus and an extensor plantar response are usually present. When the infant is suspended vertically, strong contractions of the adductor muscles cause the legs to cross at the thigh (*scissoring*).

Subluxation or dislocation of the hips is relatively common in children with severe spasticity; this is caused in part by the constant adduction of the thighs and also by insufficient development of the hip joint resulting from delayed standing or inability to stand.

DIAGNOSIS. Spastic diplegia is a clinical diagnosis. Abnormalities in the deep white matter secondary to periventricular leukomalacia are easily identified by MRI, but children with a known history of perinatal distress secondary to prematurity do not require follow-up imaging studies. It is important not to mistake CP for a progressive disease of the brain or cervical portion of the spine. Features that suggest a progressive disease are a family history of CP, deterioration of mental function, loss of motor skills previously obtained, atrophy of muscles, and sensory loss.

MANAGEMENT. There are probably as many methods to manage spastic diplegia and quadriplegia as there are children with CP. In general,

---

Table 12-2
Slowly Progressive Disorders Sometimes Misdiagnosed as Cerebral Palsy

Condition	Chapter
Polyneuropathy	
GM$_1$ gangliosidosis type II	5
Hereditary motor and sensory neuropathies	7
Infantile neuroaxonal dystrophy	5
Metachromatic leukodystrophy	5
Ataxia	
Abetalipoproteinemia	10
Ataxia-telangiectasia	10
Friedreich ataxia	10
Spasticity-Chorea	
Familial spastic paraplegia	12
Glutaric aciduria type I	14
Lesch-Nyhan syndrome	5
Niemann-Pick disease type C	5
Pelizaeus-Merzbacher disease	5
Rett syndrome	5

a multidisciplinary approach, including infant stimulation, physical therapy, and occupational therapy, is used to help the child achieve an adequate functional status. Controlled clinical trials are rarely accomplished, and one such trial concluded that physical therapy offered no short-term advantage. Most drugs to relieve spasticity have marginal benefit and often cause unacceptable sedation. Motor function may be improved without sedation by using levodopa (Brunstrom et al, 2000).

Injections of botulinum toxin and selective posterior rhizotomy are useful procedures for the treatment of spasticity. Botulinum toxin should be tried first. The best results of selective posterior rhizotomy are obtained in children younger than 8 years. Surgery is also useful to relieve contractures but should be carefully planned so that it is performed only once. A program of physical therapy that maintains the desired range of motion must be started postoperatively.

Spastic Quadriplegia

All limbs are affected, the legs often more severely than the arms. If the arms are worse than the legs, the condition is sometimes called *double hemiplegia*. Most spastic quadriplegia is caused by intrauterine disease, usually malformations. Hypoxic-ischemic encephalopathy of the term newborn accounts for a minority of cases.

CLINICAL FEATURES. Developmental delay is profound, and the infant is quickly identified as neurologically abnormal. Failure to meet motor milestones, abnormal posturing of the head and limbs, and seizures are the common reasons for neurological evaluation.

In severely affected children, the supine posture is characteristic. The head and neck are retracted, the arms are flexed at the elbows with the hands clenched, and the legs are held in extension. Infantile reflexes (Moro and tonic-neck) are obligatory and stereotyped and persist after 6 months of age. Microcephaly is frequently an associated feature.

Because both hemispheres are damaged, supranuclear bulbar palsy (dysphagia and dysarthria) is common. Disturbances in vision and ocular motility are frequently associated features, and seizures occur in 50% of affected children.

DIAGNOSIS. Diagnosis is based on clinical findings. Laboratory studies are useful when the underlying cause is not obvious or the possibility of a genetically transmitted defect exists. MRI of the brain is especially useful to show malformations.

MANAGEMENT. Treatment is the same as described in the section on spastic diplegia (paraplegia).

References

Bindal AK, Dunsker SB, Tew JM Jr. Chiari I malformation: Classification and management. *Neurosurgery* 1995; 37:1069–1074.

Brunstrom JE, Bastian AJ, Wong M, et al. Motor benefit from levodopa in spastic quadraplegic cerebral palsy. *Ann Neurol* 2000;47:662–665.

Cambi F, Tartaglino L, Lublin F, et al. X-linked pure familial spastic paraparesis: Characterization of a large kindred with magnetic resonance imaging studies. *Arch Neurol* 1995;52:665–669.

Cornette L, Verpoorten C, Lagae L, et al. Tethered cord syndrome in occult spinal dysraphism. Timing and outcome of surgical release. *Neurology* 1998;50:1761–1765.

Crockard HA, Stevens JM. Craniovertebral junction anomalies in inherited disorders: Part of the syndrome or caused by the disorder? *Eur J Pediatr* 1995;154:504–512.

Dutt AK, Stead W. Tuberculosis. *Dis Mon* 1997;43:247–276.

Figlewitz DA, Bird TD. "Pure" hereditary spastic paraplegias: The story becomes more complicated. *Neurology* 1999;53:5–7.

Hagberg B, Hagberg G, Olow I, et al. The changing panorama of cerebral palsy in Sweden. VII. Prevalence and origin in the birth year period 1987-90. *Acta Paediatr* 1996;85:954–960.

Krivit W, Shapiro EG, Peters C, et al. Hematopoietic stem-cell transplantation in globoid-cell leukodystrophy. *N Engl J Med* 1998;338:1119–1126.

Meierkord H, Nürrnberg P, Mainz A, et al. "Complicated" autosomal dominant familial spastic paraplegia is genetically distinct from "pure" forms. *Arch Neurol* 1997;54:379–384.

Percy AK. Krabbe continuum or clinical conundrum? *Neurology* 1997;49:1203–1204.

Prasad AN, Breen JC, Ampola MG, et al. Argininemia: A treatable genetic cause of progressive spastic diplegia simulating cerebral palsy: Reports and literature review. *J Child Neurol* 1997;12:301–309.

Strauss DJ, Shavelle RM, Anderson TW. Life expectancy of children with cerebral palsy. *Pediatr Neurol* 1998;18:143–149.

Tulipan N, Hernanz-Schulman M, Bruner JP. Reduced hindbrain herniation after intrauterine myelomeningocele repair: A report of four cases. *Pediatr Neurosurg* 1998;29:274–278.

van Geel BM, Assies J, Wanders RJA, et al. X linked adrenoleukodystrophy: Clinical presentation, diagnosis, and therapy. *J Neurol Neurosurg Psychiatry* 1997;63:4–14.

Chapter 13
Monoplegia

FLACCID WEAKNESS OF one limb is usually caused by abnormalities of the spine or of the proximal portion of nerves. Many conditions that cause paraplegia or quadriplegia begin as monoplegia. Therefore the differential diagnosis of spinal paraplegia provided in Table 12-1 must also be consulted for monoplegia. In addition, several cerebral disorders that cause hemiplegia may begin as a monoplegia, so that tables in Chapter 11 should be consulted as well.

Approach to Monoplegia

Refusal to use a limb may be caused by either pain or weakness. Most painful limbs are caused by injuries. Other causes are arthritis, infection, and tumor. A trivial pull on an infant's arm may dislocate the radial head and cause an apparent monoplegia. Pain and weakness together is a feature of plexitis.

The differential diagnosis of acute monoplegia is summarized in Table 13-1. Plexopathies and neuropathies are the leading causes of pure monoplegia. Stroke often affects one limb more than another, usually the arm more than the leg. The presentation may suggest monoplegia, but careful examination often reveals increased tendon reflexes and an extensor plantar response in the seemingly unaffected leg. Any suggestion of hemiplegia rather than monoplegia, or increased tendon reflexes in the paretic limb, should focus attention on the brain and cervical cord as the pathological site.

Chronic progressive brachial monoplegia is uncommon. When it occurs, syringomyelia and tumors of the cervical cord or brachial plexus should be suspected. Chronic progressive weakness of one leg suggests a tumor of the spinal

Table **13-1**
**Differential Diagnosis
of Acute Monoplegia**

Complicated Migraine (see Chapter 11)

Dislocation of the Radial Head

Hemiparetic Seizures (see Chapter 11)

Monomelic Spinal Muscular Atrophy

Plexopathy and Neuropathy
Acute neuritis
  Asthmatic plexitis
  Idiopathic plexitis
  Osteomyelitis plexitis
  Poliomyelitis (see Chapter 7)
  Tetanus toxoid plexitis
Hereditary
  Hereditary brachial neuritis
  Hereditary neuropathy with liability to pressure palsy
Injury
  Lacerations
  Pressure injuries
  Traction injuries

Stroke (see Table 11-2)

cord or a neurofibroma of the lumbar plexus. A monomelic form of spinal muscular atrophy, affecting only one leg or one arm, should be considered when progressive weakness is unaccompanied by sensory loss.

Spinal Muscular Atrophies

A monomelic form of spinal muscular atrophy was first reported from Asia but is probably equally common among Europeans. The terms *benign focal amyotrophy* and *monomelic amyotrophy* are used to describe the entity. Trauma

273

and immobilization of the limb may precede the onset of atrophy by several months (Paradiso, 1997). A cause-and-effect relationship is not established.

Familial forms are transmitted by autosomal recessive inheritance, and a mutation in the superoxide dismutase 1 gene was identified in two brothers (Robberecht et al, 1997). In one set of male identical twins, both developed atrophy of first one hand and then the other.

CLINICAL FEATURES. Onset is usually in the second or third decade and has a male preponderance. The initial features are usually weakness and atrophy in one limb, the arm in 75% and the leg in 25%. Tendon reflexes in the involved limb are hypoactive or absent. Sensation is normal. The weakness and atrophy affect only one limb in half of cases and spread to the contralateral limb in the remainder. Tremor of one or both hands is often associated with the wasting. The appearance of fasciculations heralds weakness and wasting. Progression is slow, and spontaneous arrest within 5 years is the rule. However, another limb may become affected after a gap of 15 years.

DIAGNOSIS. Electromyographic (EMG) studies of all limbs are essential to show the extent of involvement. Motor conduction is normal. Magnetic resonance imaging (MRI) of the spine and plexus is needed to exclude a tumor.

MANAGEMENT. Physical therapy, occupational therapy, splinting, and bracing are the main treatment options.

Plexopathies

Acute Idiopathic Plexitis

Acute plexitis is a demyelinating disorder of the brachial or lumbar plexus thought to be immune mediated. Brachial plexitis is far more common than lumbar plexitis.

Brachial Plexitis

Brachial plexitis (brachial neuritis, neuralgic amyotrophy) occurs from infancy to adult life. Prior immunization with tetanus toxoid is recorded in 10% to 20% of childhood and adult cases and in almost all infants (Hamati-Haddad and Fenichel, 1997). The site of immunization does not correlate with the limb involved.

CLINICAL FEATURES. The onset of symptoms is usually explosive. Pain, the initial feature in 95% of patients, is frequently localized to the shoulder but may be more diffuse or limited to the lower arm. It is severe, may awaken the patient, and is described as sharp, stabbing, throbbing, or aching. The duration of pain, which is frequently constant, varies from several hours to 3 weeks. As the pain subsides, weakness appears. Weakness is in the distribution of the upper plexus alone in half of patients and the entire plexus in most of the rest. Lower plexitis alone is unusual. Although the initial pain abates, paresthesias may accompany the weakness.

Two thirds of people report improved strength during the month after onset. Upper plexus palsies improve faster than do lower plexus palsies. Among all patients, one third recover within 1 year, three quarters by 2 years, and 90% by 3 years. After 3 years, further improvement may occur but permanent residua should be expected. Recurrences are unusual and less severe than the initial episode.

DIAGNOSIS. Pain and weakness in one arm are also symptoms of spinal cord compression, and an imaging study of the spinal cord is often needed. However, when the onset is characteristic of brachial plexus neuritis, the diagnosis can be established by the clinical features and diagnostic tests can be deferred.

The cerebrospinal fluid is usually normal. A slight lymphocytosis and mild elevation in protein content are sometimes noted. EMG and nerve conduction studies are helpful in showing the extent of plexopathy. Electrical evidence of bilateral involvement may be present in patients with unilateral symptoms.

MANAGEMENT. Corticosteroids have not been shown to affect the outcome. Range of motion exercises are recommended.

Lumbar Plexitis

Lumbar plexitis occurs at all ages and is similar to brachial plexitis, except that the leg is affected instead of the arm. The mechanism is probably the same as in brachial plexitis.

CLINICAL FEATURES. Fever is often the first symptom and is followed, after 3 to 8 days, by pain in one or both legs. The pain has an abrupt onset and may occur in a femoral or sciatic distribution. Sciatica, when present, suggests disk disease. Young children refuse to stand or walk, and older children begin to limp.

Weakness may develop concurrently with pain or may be delayed for as long as 3 weeks. The onset of weakness is insidious and often difficult to date, but usually it begins 8 days after the onset of pain. Weakness progresses for a week and then stabilizes. Tendon reflexes are absent in the affected leg but are present in other limbs.

Recovery is characterized first by abatement of pain and then by increasing strength. The average time from onset of pain to maximal recovery is 18 weeks, with a range of 8 weeks to several years. Functional recovery is almost universal, but mild weakness may persist.

DIAGNOSIS. The sudden onset of pain and weakness in one leg suggests spinal cord or disk disease. MRI of the spine is a means of excluding other disorders; the results are invariably normal in lumbar plexitis. The cerebrospinal fluid is normal except for a mild elevation of the protein concentration. EMG performed 3 weeks after onset shows patchy denervation.

MANAGEMENT. Corticosteroids do not affect the outcome. Range of motion exercises are recommended.

Osteomyelitis-Neuritis

Apparent limb weakness caused by pain is a well-recognized phenomenon. However, a true brachial neuritis may occur in response to osteomyelitis of the shoulder. The mechanism is thought to be ischemic nerve damage caused by vasculitis.

CLINICAL FEATURES. Osteomyelitis-neuritis occurs predominantly during infancy. The initial feature is a flaccid arm without pain or tenderness. Body temperature may be normal at first but soon becomes elevated. Pain develops on movement of the shoulder, and tenderness to palpation follows. No swelling is present. The biceps and triceps reflexes may be depressed or absent.

DIAGNOSIS. Osteomyelitis of the proximal humerus should be suspected when brachial plexitis develops during infancy. Radiographs of the humerus become abnormal at the end of the first week, when they show destruction of the lateral margin of the humerus, but a focal area of uptake in the proximal humerus, the scapula, or both is seen shortly after onset using radioisotope bone scan. After 3 weeks EMG shows patchy denervation in the muscles innervated by the upper plexus. These results support the idea that this is a true plexitis and not just a painful limb.

The organism can be identified in an aspirate from the shoulder joint or by blood cultures. Group B *Streptococcus* is often isolated in specimens from young infants, and other species of bacteria are found in older children.

MANAGEMENT. Intravenous antibiotics, usually penicillin, must be administered for 3 to 4 weeks. Recovery of arm strength may be incomplete.

Asthmatic Amyotrophy (Hopkins Syndrome)

Sudden flaccid paralysis of one or more limbs, resembling poliomyelitis, may occur during recovery from an asthmatic attack. All affected children had been immunized against poliomyelitis. The probable cause of the syndrome is an infection by a neurotropic virus other than poliovirus. Adenovirus, echovirus, and coxsackievirus have been isolated from stool, throat, or cerebrospinal fluid in some cases.

CLINICAL FEATURES. Age at onset is from 1 to 11 years, and the male-to-female ratio is 7:4. The interval between the asthmatic attack and the paralysis is 1 to 11 days, with an average of 5 days. Monoplegia occurs in 90%, with the arm involved twice as often as the leg. The other 10% have hemiplegia or diplegia. Meningeal irritation is not present. Sensation is intact, but the paralyzed limb is painful in half of cases. Recovery is incomplete, and all affected children have some degree of permanent paralysis.

DIAGNOSIS. Asthmatic amyotrophy is primarily a clinical diagnosis based on the sequence of events. It must be distinguished from paralytic poliomyelitis and idiopathic brachial neuritis. The distinction from paralytic poliomyelitis is based on finding normal cerebrospinal fluid in asthmatic amyotrophy. A few white blood cells may be present in the cerebrospinal fluid but never to the extent encountered in poliomyelitis, and the protein concentration is normal. EMG during the acute phase shows active denervation of the paralyzed limb, but the pattern of denervation does not follow the radicular distribution expected in a brachial neuritis.

MANAGEMENT. Treatment is directed to the symptoms and includes analgesics for pain and physical therapy.

Hereditary Brachial Plexopathy

Focal familial recurrent neuropathy has two major phenotypes: hereditary brachial plexopathy (also called *hereditary neuralgic amyotrophy*) and hereditary neuropathy with liability to pressure palsies (see section on Mononeuropathies later in this chapter). The phenotypes can be confused because isolated nerve palsies may occur in hereditary brachial plexopathy, and brachial plexopathy occurs in patients with hereditary neuropathy with a liability to pressure palsies. Both disorders are transmitted by autosomal dominant inheritance, but the underlying mutations are at different sites on chromosome 17. The gene for hereditary brachial plexopathy maps to chromosome 17q25 (Stögbauer et al, 2000).

CLINICAL FEATURES. Hereditary brachial plexopathy may be difficult to distinguish from idiopathic brachial plexitis in the absence of a family history or a patient's history of similar episodes. Events that may trigger an attack in genetically predisposed individuals include infection, emotional stress, strenuous use of the affected limb, and childbirth. Immunization has not been implicated.

The initial attack usually occurs during the second or third decade but may appear in childhood. When brachial plexus palsy is present at birth, it is usually misinterpreted as traumatic even when the family history is known. Weakness resolves completely, only to recur later in childhood.

Attacks are characterized by severe arm pain that may be exacerbated by movement. Weakness follows in days to weeks; it is usually maximal within a few days and always by 1 month. The entire plexus may be involved, but most often the upper trunk is affected alone or most severely. Examination shows proximal arm weakness. Distal weakness may be present as well. Tendon reflexes cannot be elicited from affected muscles. Weakness persists for weeks to months, during which time atrophy and fasciculations are observed. Pain, which is frequently the only sensory finding, subsides after the first week.

Recovery begins weeks to months after maximal weakness is attained. Return of function is usually complete, although some residual weakness may persist after repeated attacks. The frequency of attacks is variable; several attacks may occur within a single year, but the usual pattern is two or three attacks per decade.

Occasional children have an episode of lumbar plexopathy, which is characterized by pain in the thigh and by proximal weakness. Brachial and lumbar plexopathies are never concurrent, although bilateral brachial plexopathy is a relatively common event. Isolated cranial nerve palsies are reported in families with hereditary brachial plexopathy. The vagus nerve is most often affected, causing hoarseness and difficulty in swallowing. Transitory facial palsies and unilateral hearing loss are reported as well.

DIAGNOSIS. The family history, early age at onset, unique triggering events, recurrences, and involvement of other nerves differentiate hereditary brachial plexopathy from idiopathic brachial neuritis. EMG shows a diffuse axonopathy in the affected arm and some evidence of denervation in the asymptomatic arm. Asymptomatic legs are electrically normal.

MANAGEMENT. Corticosteroid use is not beneficial. Analgesics may be needed at the onset of an attack. Range of motion exercises are recommended.

Neonatal Brachial Neuropathy

The incidence of neonatal brachial plexus birth injuries is estimated at 1/1,000 livebirths. It seems likely that the incidence has increased in recent years because of the societal and financial pressures to avoid cesarean section. Obstetrical brachial plexus palsies are caused by excessive traction. The upper plexus is injured when the head is suddenly pulled away from the arm. This occurs in the vertex position when the head is forcefully pulled to deliver the aftercoming shoulder or when the head and neck are forced downward by normal contractions while the shoulder is caught in the pelvis. Injuries in the breech position occur when the arm is pulled downward to free the aftercoming head or when the head is rotated to occipitoanterior, but the shoulder is fixed. Complete (upper and lower) plexus injuries occur during vertex deliveries when traction is exerted on a prolapsed arm and in breech deliveries when the trunk is pulled downward but an aftercoming arm is fixed.

CLINICAL FEATURES. Most neonatal brachial plexus injuries occur in large full-term newborns of primiparous mothers, especially when the fetus is malpositioned and the delivery is long and difficult. Although brachial plexus injuries are traditionally divided into those involving the upper roots (named for Erb and Duchenne) and those involving the lower roots (named for Klumpke), solitary lower root injuries are unusual (Eng et al, 1996). Only the C5 through C7 cervical roots are affected in 88% and the complete plexus in 12%. Bilateral, but not necessarily symmetric, involvement occurs in 8% of cases.

Because the upper plexus (C5 to C7) is almost always involved, the posture of the arm is typical and reflects weakness of the proximal muscles. The arm is abducted and internally rotated at the shoulder and is extended and pronated at the elbow, so that the partially flexed fingers face backward. Extension of the wrist is lost and the fingers are fisted. The biceps and triceps reflexes are absent. Injuries that extend higher than the C4 segment result in ipsilateral diaphragmatic paralysis.

Newborns with complete brachial plexus palsies have flaccid, dry limbs with neither proximal nor distal movement. A Horner syndrome is sometimes associated. Sensory loss to pinprick is present with partial or complete palsies but may not conform to the segmental pattern of weakness.

DIAGNOSIS. Brachial plexus palsy is easily recognized by the typical posture of the arm and by failure of movement when the Moro reflex is tested. Because the injury often takes place during a long and difficult delivery, asphyxia may be present as well. In such cases, focal arm weakness may be missed because of generalized hypotonia. Approximately 10% of newborns with brachial plexus injuries have facial nerve palsy and fractures of the clavicle or humerus.

MANAGEMENT. The spontaneous recovery rate is approximately 70%. One goal of therapy is to prevent the development of contractures. This is accomplished by range of motion exercises; splinting or other forms of immobilization should be avoided. Significant recovery occurs throughout the first year, but infants who show no improvement in strength at the end of 6 months are unlikely to show functional improvement later. Surgical reconstruction of the plexus (nerve grafts, neuroma excision, etc.) is a consideration in infants with no evidence of spontaneous recovery at 6 months. However, the benefit of reconstructive surgery is not established.

Postnatal Injuries

Brachial Plexus

Traction and pressure injuries of the brachial plexus are relatively common because of its superficial position. Motor vehicle and sports accidents account for the majority of severe injuries. However, mild injuries also occur in the following situations: (1) when an adult suddenly yanks a child's arm, either protectively or to force movement; (2) by a blow to the shoulder, such as in a football scrimmage or from the recoil of a rifle; (3) because of prolonged wearing of a heavy backpack; (4) when the arm is kept hyper-

extended during surgery; and (5) by pressure in the axilla from poorly positioned crutches.

CLINICAL FEATURES. Mild injuries do not affect all portions of the plexus equally. Diffuse weakness is uncommon. Pain may be an important initial feature, and sensory loss is uncommon. Recovery begins within days or weeks and is complete. Atrophy does not occur.

More severe injuries are usually associated with fractures of the clavicle and scapula and dislocation of the humerus. The upper plexus is generally affected more severely than is the lower plexus, but complete paralysis may be present at the onset. Sensory loss is less marked than weakness, and the two may not correspond in distribution. Pain is common, not only from the plexopathy but also from the bone and soft tissue injuries. The most painful injuries are those associated with root avulsion.

Tendon reflexes are absent, and atrophy develops in denervated muscle. Recovery progresses from proximal to distal and can be plotted by Tinel's sign: tingling in the distal part of a limb caused by tapping over the regenerating segment of a nerve. Complete reinnervation, when it occurs, may take several months or years. The completeness of recovery depends on the severity and nature of the injury. Pressure and traction injuries in which anatomical integrity is not disturbed recover best, whereas injuries that tear the nerve or avulse the root do not recover at all.

DIAGNOSIS. EMG is useful in identifying the pattern of nerve injury and in providing information on the prognosis. Even with mild traction injuries, the amplitude of motor and sensory action potentials is attenuated and motor and sensory conduction are slowed.

MANAGEMENT. Mild injuries do not require treatment other than range of motion exercises. For more severe traction injuries, resting the limb for the first month is usually necessary. During that time, analgesia is needed for pain and the muscles can be stimulated electrically, away from the site of injury, to maintain tone. Range of motion exercises should be started after the pain subsides.

Fractures and dislocations causing pressure on the brachial plexus must be corrected promptly. Where nerves have been lacerated, anatomical integrity must be restored surgically.

Lumbar Plexus

The lumbar plexus, surrounded by the pelvis and the very heavy muscles of the proximal leg, is much less likely to be injured than is the brachial plexus.

CLINICAL FEATURES. Lumbar plexus injuries are almost always associated with fracture dislocation of the pelvis. Motor vehicle accidents or falls from a considerable height are required to produce sufficient force to fracture the pelvis. Therefore the patient usually has multiple injuries, and the lumbar plexus injury may not be identified early. Lumbar plexus injuries produce a patchy weakness that is difficult to differentiate from mononeuritis multiplex.

DIAGNOSIS. EMG is very helpful in making the distinction between plexus injuries and nerve injuries.

MANAGEMENT. Fracture-dislocations must be treated to relieve pressure on the plexus. As with brachial plexus injuries, the completeness of recovery depends on the anatomical integrity of the nerves.

Plexus Tumors

Plexus tumors in childhood are rare. The most common primary tumor is the plexiform neurofibroma (Figure 13-1). These can be either in the brachial or the lumbar plexus. They grow very slowly and cause progressive but selected weakness over several years. Secondary tumors of the brachial plexus are the neuroblastoma and primitive neuroectodermal tumors arising in the chest.

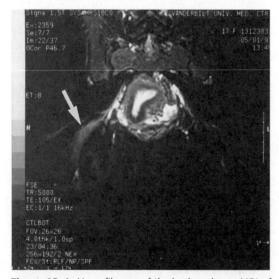

Figure 13-1. Neurofibroma of the lumbar plexus. MRI of the plexus using a subtraction technique shows enlargement of the sciatic nerve (*arrow*).

Plexus tumors are easily visualized on MRI when fat subtraction techniques are used.

Mononeuropathies

Radial Neuropathy

The radial nerve is most often injured in the spinal groove of the humerus, just below the takeoff of the motor branch to the triceps muscle. Injury may occur with fractures of the humerus or by external pressure. Such pressure usually results when a sleeping or sedated patient is in a position that compresses the nerve between the humerus and a hard surface, such as an operating room table or chair.

Isolated radial nerve injuries may occur in newborns with a history of failure of progression of labor. These may result from prolonged radial nerve compression (Hayman et al, 1999).

CLINICAL FEATURES. Injuries to the radial nerve within the spiral groove are characterized by wrist drop and finger drop. The brachioradialis muscle may be weak and its tendon reflex lost. Sensory disturbances are restricted to the back of the hand near the base of the thumb. With the wrist dropped, a fist is mechanically difficult to make but the finger flexors are not weak.

DIAGNOSIS. Electrophysiological studies are useful for locating the site of injury and assessing the anatomical integrity of the nerve and the prognosis for recovery.

MANAGEMENT. Pressure injuries recover completely in 6 to 8 weeks. During that time, a splint is useful for placing the wrist in extension so that the patient can flex the fingers.

Ulnar Neuropathy

The most common site of ulnar injury is the elbow. This type of injury can result from external pressure, recurrent dislocation of the nerve from its groove, and fracture of the distal humerus.

CLINICAL FEATURES. Paresthesias are experienced on the ulnar side of the hand, the little finger, and the ring finger. Tapping the ulnar groove increases the discomfort. Hand strength is lost, and the intrinsic muscles become wasted. Sensation over the little finger and the adjacent side of the ring finger is diminished or absent.

DIAGNOSIS. The injury's precise localization along the course of the nerve is readily determined by electrophysiological techniques.

MANAGEMENT. Minor pressure injuries do not require treatment, and recovery is complete within a few weeks. Surgical repair is often needed for injuries to the elbow that cause fracture or nerve dislocation.

Median Neuropathy

Nontraumatic median neuropathies are caused by compression of the nerve in the carpal tunnel, and traumatic injuries occur at the elbow. In children, a storage disease such as mucolipidosis may cause nerve compression in the carpal tunnel, but idiopathic cases occur as well. Fracture at the elbow is the usual cause of traumatic median neuropathy.

CLINICAL FEATURES. The most common features are numbness and pain in the hand. Nontraumatic median neuropathy is often bilateral. Weakness and atrophy are more likely to occur in traumatic injuries of the nerve than in carpal tunnel entrapment.

DIAGNOSIS. EMG is very useful to localize the lesion, especially when surgical decompression is an option.

MANAGEMENT. Surgical decompression may be beneficial for both nontraumatic and traumatic injuries.

Peroneal Neuropathy

The peroneal nerve lies in a superficial position adjacent to the fibula and is readily compressed against the bone by external force. This most often occurs in children who have undergone significant weight loss or trauma to the nerve. EMG evidence of a prenatal peroneal palsy, presumably caused by pressure, was documented in one newborn (Jones et al, 1996).

CLINICAL FEATURES. The prominent feature is an acute, painless foot drop. Both dorsiflexion and eversion of the foot are weak. Sensation is usually intact, but sometimes there is numbness over the lower lateral leg and dorsum of the foot. When only the deep branch of the peroneal nerve is involved, sensory loss is restricted to a small triangle between the first two toes. Complete or significant spontaneous recovery is the rule except when the palsy was caused by considerable trauma.

DIAGNOSIS. Electrodiagnosis is useful to discriminate peroneal nerve lesions from disturbances of the fifth lumbar root.

MANAGEMENT. A foot drop brace is a useful aid to walking until recovery is complete.

Hereditary Neuropathy with Liability to Pressure Palsy

Hereditary neuropathy with liability to pressure palsy (also called *tomaculous neuropathy*) is characterized by the development of a mononeuropathy following trivial trauma. In some cases, the brachial plexus is affected. The disorder is transmitted as an autosomal dominant trait, and most families have a deletion in chromosome 17p11.2 (Tyson et al, 1996).

CLINICAL FEATURES. The first episode usually occurs during the second or third decade. Typical precipitating factors include sleeping on a limb, body contact in sports, constrictive clothing, or positioning during surgery. Individuals quickly learn to avoid activities that provoke episodes. Superficial nerves (radial, ulnar, median, peroneal) are the ones most commonly affected. The resulting mononeuropathy is painless and affects both motor and sensory fibers. Tendon reflexes are lost. Recovery is complete within days to weeks.

DIAGNOSIS. Except for the family history, the first episode might suggest ordinary pressure palsy, although the trivial nature of the trauma should alert the physician to the underlying neuropathy. The diagnosis should be considered in children with repeated neuropathies or multifocal neuropathies even in the absence of a family history.

The diagnosis is established by molecular genetic testing. Electrophysiological studies show slow conduction time, not only in the affected limb but also in all limbs. Generalized slowing of conduction can be shown in other family members between attacks.

MANAGEMENT. No treatment is available for the underlying neuropathy. The lifestyle may need to be altered to avoid pressure palsies. Acute episodes should be treated with physical therapy. Some patients eventually develop a generalized motor and sensory neuropathy.

References

Eng GD, Binder H, Getson P, et al. Obstetrical brachial plexus palsy (OBPP) outcome with conservative management. *Muscle Nerve* 1996;19:884–891.

Hamati-Haddad A, Fenichel GM. Brachial neuritis following routine childhood immunization for diphtheria, tetanus, and pertussis (DTP): Report of two cases and review of the literature. *Pediatrics* 1997;99:602–603.

Hayman M, Roland EH, Hill A. Newborn radial nerve palsy: Report of four cases and review of published reports. *Pediatr Neurol* 1999;21:648–651.

Jones HR Jr, Herbison GJ, Jacobs SR, et al. Intrauterine onset of a mononeuropathy: Peroneal neuropathy in a newborn with electromyographic findings at age one day compatible with prenatal onset. *Muscle Nerve* 1996;19: 88–91.

Paradiso G. Monomelic amyotrophy following trauma and immobilization in children. *Muscle Nerve* 1997;20: 425–430.

Robberecht W, Aguirre T, Van Den Bosch L, et al. Familial juvenile focal amyotrophy of the upper extremity (Hirayama disease). *Arch Neurol* 1997;54:46–50.

Stögbauer F, Young P, Kuhlenbaumer G, et al. Hereditary recurrent focal neuropathies. Clinical and molecular features. *Neurology* 2000;54:546–551.

Tyson J, Malcom S, Thomas PK, et al. Deletions of chromosome 17p11.2 in multifocal neuropathy. *Ann Neurol* 1996;39:180–186.

Chapter 14
Movement Disorders

INVOLUNTARY MOVEMENTS ARE usually associated with abnormalities of the basal ganglia and their connections and occur in several different neurological disorders. Abnormal movements can be the main or initial features of disease, or they can occur as a late manifestation. The former type is discussed in this chapter, and the latter is discussed in other chapters.

Approach to the Patient

Movement disorders cannot be adequately described; they must be seen. If abnormal movements are not present at the time of examination, the parents should be instructed to videotape the movements at home. Some relatively common movements are recognizable by description, but the rich variety of abnormal movements and postures that may occur defies classification. The most experienced observer will at times mistake one movement for another or will have difficulty conceptualizing the nature of an abnormal movement.

Many abnormal movements are paroxysmal or at least intermittent. Movement, startle, emotional upset, or sleep induces some movements. The physician should ask what makes the movement worse and if it is action-induced. Children should be asked to perform the action during the examination. Paroxysmal movements raise the question of epilepsy. Indeed, many neurological disorders of childhood are characterized by the concurrent presence of seizures and involuntary movements. All cases of nocturnal paroxysmal dystonia are now recognized to be frontal lobe seizures (see Chapter 1). The clinical and conceptual distinction between spinal myoclonus and spinal seizures remains a gray area. The

following guidelines are useful to distinguish involuntary movements from seizures: (1) involuntary movements, with the exception of spinal myoclonus, abate or disappear during sleep and seizures persist or may worsen; (2) involuntary movements usually have a more stereotyped appearance and, with the exception of acute drug reactions, are more persistent than seizures; (3) seizures are often characterized by loss of consciousness or awareness, and involuntary movements are not; and (4) seizures are usually accompanied by epileptiform activity on electroencephalography (EEG), and involuntary movements are not.

Involuntary contractions of a muscle that do not move a joint may be fasciculations, focal seizures, or myoclonus. Low-amplitude jerking movements that move a joint or muscles may be focal seizures, chorea, myoclonus, tics, or hemifacial spasm. High-amplitude jerking movements that move a limb or limbs may be seizures, ballismus, or myoclonus. Slow, writhing movements and abnormal posturing may be due to athetosis, dystonia, continuous motor unit activity (see Chapter 8), or seizures. Rhythmic movements may be caused by tremors, seizures, or myoclonus.

Chorea and Athetosis

Chorea is a rapid movement affecting any part of the body that is often incorporated into a voluntary movement to hide it. The movements are repetitive but neither rhythmic nor stereotyped, and they migrate from side to side and limb to limb. Because the involuntary movement flows into a voluntary movement, it gives the appearance of constant movement (*restlessness*).

Restlessness is also caused by *akathisia,* an inward compulsion to move (discussed later). Depending on the condition, chorea may be unilateral or bilateral and may affect the face and trunk as well as the limbs. *An observer cannot precisely describe chorea because it has no fixed form.*

Chorea is more readily observed when separated from the superimposed voluntary movement that follows. This is achieved by asking the child to raise both hands upward beside the head with the palms facing each other. Low-amplitude jerking movements occur that turns the arm into pronation. When the child is asked to grip the examiner's fingers lightly, the grip alternately tightens and loosens, as if the patient is "milking" the examiner's hands. Hypotonia is common in many conditions causing chorea. Tendon reflexes may be normoreactive, but at times a choreic movement occurs during the patellar response, producing an extra kick.

Athetosis is a slow, writhing movement of the limbs that may occur alone but is often associated with chorea (*choreoathetosis*). Athetosis without chorea is almost always due to perinatal brain injury. Kernicterus was once a major cause of chorea but is now a rare event. Perinatal asphyxia is now the predominant etiology. Many children with athetosis have atonic cerebral palsy, and others have spastic diplegia.

Ballismus is a high-amplitude, violent flinging of a limb from the shoulder or pelvis. It is considered an extreme form of chorea. In adults it may occur in limbs contralateral to a vascular lesion in the subthalamic nucleus; in children it is almost always associated with chorea and is seen in Sydenham chorea and lupus erythematosus.

Tardive dyskinesia is a complex syndrome characterized by buccolingual masticatory movements that include tongue protrusion, lip smacking, puckering, and chewing. It is decidedly uncommon in children. Psychotropic drugs are the usual cause of tardive dyskinesia. It may be considered a subtype of chorea, or at least a related disorder, and is sometimes associated with choreic movements of the limbs. Most children who are thought to have developed tardive dyskinesia usually turn out to have motor tics.

The differential diagnosis of chorea and choreoathetosis is summarized in Tables 14-1 and 14-2. Chorea is a cardinal feature of the conditions listed in Table 14-1. Nevertheless, many are detailed elsewhere in the text because concurrent features are more prominent. Although abnormal movements are the only manifestation, familial paroxysmal choreoathetosis is described in Chapter 1 because it is more likely to be confused with epilepsy than with other causes of chorea.

Table 14-2 contains a partial list of conditions in which chorea and choreoathetosis may occur, but in which they are either late features or at least not prominent early in the course. Movement disorders are a relatively common feature of several cerebral degenerative disorders. In contrast, chorea may be misinterpreted as seizures when it develops during an acute illness such as bacterial meningitis, metabolic encephalopathies, or encephalitis. At times the movement disorder is due to the underlying brain disorder and at times to drugs used in treatment.

Cardiopulmonary Bypass Surgery

Severe choreoathetosis is seen in 1% to 10% of children with congenital heart disease following cardiopulmonary bypass surgery and profound hypothermia. Deep hypothermia and circulatory arrest are not essential factors in the pathophysiology but are often associated. The mechanism of basal ganglia injury is unknown.

Table 14-1
Differential Diagnosis of Chorea as an Initial or Prominent Symptom

Cardiopulmonary Bypass Surgery

Genetic Disorders
Abetalipoproteinemia (see Chapter 10)
Ataxia-telangiectasia (see Chapter 10)
Benign familial chorea
Fahr disease
Familial paroxysmal choreoathetosis (see Chapter 1)
Glutaric aciduria
Hepatolenticular degeneration (Wilson disease)
Huntington disease (see Chapter 5)
Lesch-Nyhan syndrome (see Chapter 5)
Machado-Joseph disease (see Chapter 5)
Neuroacanthocytosis

Drug-Induced Movement Disorders
Anticonvulsants
Antiemetics
Oral contraceptives
Psychotropic agents
Stimulants
Theophylline

Systemic Conditions
Hyperthyroidism
Lupus erythematosus
Pregnancy (chorea gravidarum)
Sydenham (rheumatic) chorea

Tumors of Cerebral Hemisphere (see Chapter 4)

CLINICAL FEATURES. Most affected children are more than 1 year of age and have cyanotic heart disease with systemic to pulmonary collaterals. Choreoathetosis begins within 2 weeks postoperatively and may be associated with oral-facial dyskinesias, hypotonia, affective changes, and pseudobulbar signs. Some children have only mild chorea that resolves spontaneously within 2 months. Others have severe exhausting chorea, unresponsive to treatment, that results in either death or severe neurological morbidity. Some cognitive disturbance is expected in all survivors.

DIAGNOSIS. The diagnosis is based on the clinical features alone. Magnetic resonance imaging (MRI) results are normal during the acute illness.

MANAGEMENT. Sedation is needed to prevent exhaustion in severely affected children. The choreoathetosis is refractory to drug therapy.

Drug-Induced Chorea

Choreiform movements and akathisia or dystonic posturing may occur as effects of drugs, especially dopamine antagonists (Janavs and Aminoff, 1998). Chorea and akathisia are more likely to be dose-related effects, whereas dystonia is usually an idiosyncratic reaction (see section on Dystonia later in this chapter). Phenytoin and ethosuximide may induce chorea as a toxic or idiosyncratic manifestation. Oral contraceptives are associated with chorea. The mechanism is unknown. Phenothiazines and haloperidol are associated with idiosyncratic dystonic reactions and tardive dyskinesia, and stimulant drugs (dextroamphetamine and methylphenidate) are associated with chorea, akathisia, and tic (see section on Tic and Tourette Syndrome later in this chapter).

Tardive Dyskinesia

The term *tardive dyskinesia* denotes drug-induced choreiform movements. These movements are often limited to the lingual facial and buccal muscles and appear late ("tardive") in the course of drug therapy. Drug-induced buccolingual dyskinesia is unusual in children.

Tardive dyskinesias are most often associated with drugs used to modify behavior (neuroleptics), such as phenothiazines or haloperidol, and antiemetics, such as metoclopramide and prochlorperazine; they also occur in children with asthma treated with theophylline. The incidence of tardive dyskinesia in children taking neuroleptic drugs is estimated at 1%. I suspect that such children were taking large dosages to treat major behavioral disorders.

CLINICAL FEATURES. Tardive dyskinesia is a complex of stereotyped movements. It usually affects the mouth and face, resembles chewing, and includes tongue protrusion and lip smacking; the trunk may be involved in rocking movements and the fingers in alternating flexion and extension resembling piano playing. Limb chorea, dystonia, myoclonus, tics, and facial grimacing may be associated features. These movements are exacerbated by stress and relieved by sleep.

Symptoms appear months to years after the start of therapy and are not related to changes in dosage. In children the movements usually cease when the drug is discontinued, but they may remain unchanged in adults.

DIAGNOSIS. Drug-induced dyskinesia should be suspected in any child who shows abnormal movements of the face or limbs while taking neuroleptic drugs. It is important to distinguish tardive dyskinesia from facial tics in children with Tourette syndrome and from facial mannerisms in children with schizophrenia.

MANAGEMENT. All neuroleptic drugs should be discontinued as quickly as possible after symptoms of dyskinesia develop. This may not be possible when drugs are needed to treat psychosis. In such circumstances the movements sometimes respond to diazepam.

Emergent Withdrawal Syndrome

Chorea and myoclonus may appear for the first time after neuroleptic drugs are abruptly discontinued or greatly reduced in dosage. Lingual-facial-buccal dyskinesia may be present as well. The symptoms are self-limited and cease in weeks to months.

Genetic Disorders

Cerebellar ataxia is often the initial feature of abetalipoproteinemia and ataxia-telangiectasia. Chorea may occur in both conditions, but only in ataxia-telangiectasia does chorea occur without ataxia. Huntington disease is an important cause of chorea and dystonia and is described in most texts as a movement disorder. However, because declining school performance is the usual initial feature of Huntington disease in children, it is discussed in Chapter 5.

Benign Familial (Hereditary) Chorea

Benign familial chorea is a rare disorder transmitted by autosomal dominant inheritance. Benign familial chorea and familial paroxysmal choreoathetosis (see Chapter 1) may be genetically related disorders.

CLINICAL FEATURES. The onset of chorea is usually in early childhood, often when the child is beginning to walk. Motor development is sometimes delayed. Other possible features are intention tremor, dysarthria, hypotonia, and athetosis. Intelligence is normal. Most children have only chorea, which becomes less pronounced by adolescence. Adults may be asymptomatic or may have mild hypotonia and ataxia.

DIAGNOSIS. Benign familial chorea may be difficult to distinguish from other causes of chorea in children, especially familial paroxysmal chorea. A family history of the disorder is critical to diagnosis but can be overlooked because of incomplete expression in parents. Chorea is con-

tinuous and not episodic or paroxysmal. Neuroimaging studies and EEG results are normal.
MANAGEMENT. Chlorpromazine or haloperidol is beneficial in some individuals.

Fahr Disease

The combination of encephalopathy and progressive calcification of the basal ganglia is called Fahr disease. It is also termed *idiopathic basal ganglia calcification* (IBGC). Calcification of the basal ganglia occurs with infectious, metabolic, and genetic disorders. IBGC disease is usually inherited as an autosomal dominant trait. It is uncertain whether the central nervous system calcification is a metastatic deposition or a primary disorder of neuronal calcium metabolism (Geschwind et al, 1999).

CLINICAL FEATURES. Onset may be in childhood, but the usual age is after 30 years. The core clinical features of IBGC are dysarthria, extrapyramidal signs, and ataxia. The expression of IBGC varies within a family.

DIAGNOSIS. Plain radiographs of the skull show bilateral calcifications in the region of the basal ganglia that are localized more precisely by CT. The most common area of calcification is the globus pallidus. However, additional areas of involvement may include the putamen, caudate, dentate, thalamus, and cerebral white matter. Parathyroid function must be assessed in every child with basal ganglia calcification to exclude the possibility of either hyperparathyroidism or pseudohypoparathyroidism.

MANAGEMENT. Specific treatment is not available. Symptoms may respond to drug therapy.

Neuroacanthocytosis (Choreoacanthocytosis)

Familial and nonfamilial cases of a progressive neurological disorder are described in which the main features are chorea and acanthocytosis with normal lipoprotein levels. The acanthocyte is an abnormal erythrocyte that has thorny projections from the cell surface. Acanthocytosis occurs in at least three neurological syndromes: McLeod syndrome (see Chapter 8), neuroacanthocytosis, and abetalipoproteinemia (see Chapter 10). The clinical features in severe cases of McLeod syndrome may be similar to those of neuroacanthocytosis.

CLINICAL FEATURES. Onset is usually in adult life but may occur as early as the first decade. The most consistent neurological findings are impairment of frontal lobe function and psychiatric symptoms. (Kartsounis and Hardie, 1996). Tics, oromandibular dyskinesia and dystonia, and self-mutilation of the lips may be associated features. Phenotypic variability is considerable and may include axonal neuropathy, loss of tendon reflexes, dementia, seizures, and neurosis. **DIAGNOSIS.** The association of acanthocytes or echinocytes (cells with rounded projections) and neurological disease in the absence of lipoprotein abnormality is required for diagnosis. McLeod syndrome is excluded by testing for the Kell antigen.

MANAGEMENT. Only the symptoms can be treated. Death occurs 10 to 20 years after onset.

Paroxysmal Choreoathetosis

Paroxysmal choreoathetosis occurs in children who are otherwise normal and in children with an obvious underlying static encephalopathy. The normal children have a genetic disease, *familial paroxysmal choreoathetosis* (see Chapter 1), and the abnormal children may have one of several nongenetic disorders.

Acquired paroxysmal choreoathetosis occurs most often in children with cerebral palsy. Either hemiplegia or diplegia may be present, and the involuntary movements affect only the paretic limbs. The onset of the movement disorder often begins 10 or more years after the acute encephalopathy. In one child, paroxysmal choreoathetosis precipitated by sound and light was attributed to an arteriovenous malformation of the parietal lobe.

Systemic Disorders

Hyperthyroidism

The ocular manifestations of thyrotoxicosis are discussed in Chapter 15. Tremor is the most common associated movement disorder. Chorea is unusual, but when present it may affect the face, limbs, and trunk. The movements cease when the child becomes euthyroid.

Lupus Erythematosus

CLINICAL FEATURES. Lupus-associated chorea is uncommon but may be the initial feature of the disease, beginning 7 years before to 3 years after the appearance of systemic features. It is indistinguishable from Sydenham chorea in appearance. Average duration is 12 weeks, but one fourth of patients have recurrences. Additional neurological features of lupus (ataxia, psycho-sis, and seizures) are common in children who have chorea but occur only after the appearance of systemic symptoms. Therefore, chorea may be a solitary manifestation of disease.

DIAGNOSIS. The diagnosis is clear in children with known lupus erythematosus. When chorea is the initial feature of lupus, it must be differentiated from Sydenham chorea. The erythrocyte sedimentation rate may be elevated in both conditions and is not a distinguishing feature. The presence of elevated concentrations of antinuclear antibodies is critical to diagnosis.

MANAGEMENT. Children with neurological manifestations of lupus erythematosus should be treated with high doses of corticosteroids. The overall outcome is poor.

Pregnancy (Chorea Gravidarum)

Chorea of any cause beginning in pregnancy is chorea gravidarum. Rheumatic heart disease was once the most frequent cause but it is now the antiphospholipid antibody syndrome, with or without systemic lupus erythematosus.

CLINICAL FEATURES. The onset of chorea is usually during the second to fifth month of pregnancy but may begin postpartum. Cognitive change may accompany the chorea. Symptoms usually resolve spontaneously within weeks to months.

DIAGNOSIS. Women who develop chorea during pregnancy should be studied for the rheumatic fever, antiphospholipid antibody syndrome, and systemic lupus erythematosus.

MANAGEMENT. This is a self-limited condition, and drugs should be used cautiously so as not to harm the fetus. Haloperidol and corticosteroids are useful.

Sydenham (Rheumatic) Chorea

Sydenham chorea is the most common cause of acquired chorea in children. It is a cardinal feature of rheumatic fever and is sufficient alone to make the diagnosis. It occurs primarily in populations with untreated streptococcal infections. One hypothesis is that when genetically predisposed children are exposed to group A β-hemolytic streptococcus infection, antibodies mistakenly attack cells in the basal ganglia and cause inflammation.

CLINICAL FEATURES. The onset is frequently insidious, and diagnosis is often delayed. Chorea, hypotonia, dysarthria, and emotional lability are cardinal features. Difficulty in school may bring the child to medical attention. Chorea causes the child to be restless, and discipline by the teacher results in emotional excess. Obsessive-compulsive behavior may be present. The behavioral change is often thought to be a sign of mental illness.

Examination reveals a fidgeting child with migratory chorea of limbs and face. The limbs of only one side may be affected initially, but the chorea eventually becomes generalized in most patients. Efforts to conceal chorea with voluntary movement only add to the appearance of restlessness.

Gradual improvement occurs over several months. Most patients recover completely. Rheumatic valvular heart disease develops in one third of untreated patients.

DIAGNOSIS. The diagnosis is established by the clinical features and cannot be confirmed by laboratory tests. The differential diagnosis is mainly between Sydenham chorea, lupus-associated chorea, and drug-induced chorea. Blood should be examined for lupus antinuclear antibodies and for thyroid function. The onset of Sydenham chorea is usually 4 months after the provocative streptococcal infection, and by that time the antistreptolysin O titer is back to normal or only slightly increased.

During the time of illness, T_2-weighted MRI images may show increased signal intensity in the putamen and globus pallidus that resolves when the child has recovered (Traill et al, 1995).

MANAGEMENT. Pimozide usually controls the acute neurological symptoms without producing sedation. If pimozide does not relieve the symptoms, benzodiazepines, phenothiazines, or haloperidol should be tried. All children with Sydenham chorea must be treated as if they had acute rheumatic fever: penicillin in high doses for 10 days to eradicate active streptococcal infection and prophylactic penicillin therapy until age 21.

Dystonia

Dystonia is characterized by sustained muscle contractions. The overall appearance is not of an involuntary movement but rather of an abnormal posture. The muscle contractions can affect the limbs, trunk, or face (grimacing). Involvement may be of a single body part (*focal dystonia*), two or more contiguous body parts (*segmental dystonia*), the arm and leg on one side of the body (*hemidystonia*), or one or both legs and the contiguous trunk and any other body part (*generalized dystonia*).

Table 14-3
Differential Diagnosis of Abnormal Posturing

Dystonia
Hysteria
Muscular dystrophy
Myotonia
Neuromyotonia
Rigidity
Spasticity
Stiffman syndrome

The differential diagnosis of abnormal posturing is summarized in Table 14-3. Continuous motor unit activity (see Chapter 8) may be difficult to distinguish from dystonia by clinical inspection alone, especially when only one or two limbs are affected. The two disorders are differentiated by electromyography, which is recommended in many cases.

Persistent focal dystonias are relatively common in adults but are unusual in children except when drug induced. Most dystonias in children that begin focally eventually become generalized. Children with focal, stereotyped movements of the eyelids, face, or neck are much more likely to have a tic than focal dystonia. Childhood forms of focal dystonia are listed in Table 14-4.

Generalized dystonia usually begins in one limb. The patient has difficulty performing an act rather than a movement, so that the foot becomes dystonic when walking forward but may not be dystonic when sitting, standing, or running.

Focal Dystonias

Blepharospasm

Blepharospasm is an involuntary spasmodic closure of the eyes. The differential diagnosis for children is summarized in Table 14-5. Essential blepharospasm, an incapacitating condition, is a disorder of middle or late adult life and never begins in childhood. Tics account for almost all cases of involuntary eye closure in children. Eye fluttering occurs during absence seizures (see Chapter 1) but is not confused with dystonia. Focal dystonia involving eye closure in children is almost always drug induced.

Blepharospasm and orofacial dystonia in adults may be helped by treatment with baclofen, clonazepam, trihexyphenidyl, tetrabenazine

Table 14-4
Differential Diagnosis of Dystonia in Childhood

Focal Dystonia
Blepharospasm
Drug-induced dystonia
Generalized dystonia beginning as focal dystonia
Torticollis
Writer's cramp

Generalized Genetic Dystonias
Ataxia with episodic dystonia (see Chapter 10)
Ceroid lipofuscinosis (see Chapter 5)
Dopa-responsive dystonia
Familial paroxysmal choreoathetosis (see Chapter 1)
Glutaric acidemia type I
Hallervorden-Spatz disease
Hepatolenticular degeneration (Wilson disease)
Huntington disease (see Chapter 5)
Idiopathic torsion dystonia
Infantile bilateral striatal necrosis
Leber disease (see Chapter 16)
Machado-Joseph disease (see Chapter 10)
Mitochondrial disorders (see Chapters 5, 8, and 11)
Transient paroxysmal dystonia of infancy (see Chapter 1)

Generalized Symptomatic Dystonias
Perinatal cerebral injury (see Chapter 1)
Postinfectious
Poststroke
Posttraumatic
Toxin-induced
Tumor-induced

Hemidystonia
Alternating hemiplegia (see Chapter 11)
Antiphospholipid syndrome (see Chapter 11)
Basal ganglia tumors
Neuronal storage disorders

with lithium, and injections of botulinum A toxin.

Drug-Induced Dystonia

Acute Reactions

Focal or generalized dystonia may occur as an acute idiosyncratic reaction following a first dose of phenothiazine or haloperidol. Possible reactions include trismus, opisthotonos, torticollis, and oculogyric crisis. Difficulty with swallowing and speaking may occur. Metoclopramide, a nonphenothiazine antiemetic that blocks postsynaptic dopamine receptors, may produce acute and delayed (tardive) dystonia. The acute reactions are usually self-limited or respond to treatment with benztropine, but they may be prolonged and resistant to therapy.

Table 14-5
Differential Diagnosis of Blepharospasm in Childhood

Continuous motor unit activity
Drug-induced
Encephalitis
Hemifacial spasm
Hepatolenticular degeneration (Wilson disease)
Huntington disease
Hysteria
Myokymia
Myotonia
Schwartz-Jampel syndrome
Seizures

Tardive Dystonia

The onset of dystonia is usually 3 to 11 days after treatment with neuroleptic drugs is initiated. The dystonia is usually generalized in children but may be focal in adults.

Spontaneous remissions are unusual. Tetrabenazine is helpful in most patients, and anticholinergics offer relief in others.

Torticollis

The differential diagnoses of torticollis and head tilt are summarized in Table 14-6. The first step in diagnosis is to distinguish fixed from nonfixed torticollis. In fixed torticollis the neck cannot be readily moved back to the neutral position. This may be caused by a structural disturbance of the cervical vertebrae or may occur because movement causes pain and is therefore resisted.

Evidence of concurrent dystonia in the face or limbs indicates the need for further evaluation

Table 14-6
Differential Diagnosis of Torticollis and Head Tilt

Benign paroxysmal torticollis
Cervical cord syringomyelia (see Chapter 12)
Cervical cord tumors (see Chapter 12)
Cervicomedullary malformations (see Chapters 10 and 18)
Diplopia (see Chapter 15)
Dystonia
Familial paroxysmal choreoathetosis (see Chapter 1)
Juvenile rheumatoid arthritis
Posterior fossa tumors (see Chapter 10)
Sandifer syndrome
Spasmus nutans (see Chapter 15)
Sternocleidomastoid injuries
Tic and Tourette syndrome

directed at underlying causes of dystonia. When torticollis is associated with corticospinal tract signs (hyperactive tendon reflexes, ankle clonus, or extensor plantar responses) a cervical spinal cord disturbance should be suspected and cervical MRI is indicated. Symptoms of increased intracranial pressure indicate a posterior fossa tumor with early herniation. When torticollis is the only abnormal feature, the underlying causes are focal dystonia, injury to the neck muscles, and juvenile rheumatoid arthritis.

Nonfixed torticollis that occurs in attacks suggests benign paroxysmal torticollis or familial paroxysmal choreoathetosis. The combination of head tilt and nystagmus in infants is termed *spasmus nutans* (see Chapter 15). Tic can cause head turning but is so spasmodic that it should not be confused with torticollis.

Benign Paroxysmal Torticollis

The cause of benign paroxysmal torticollis is not fully understood. It is believed to be a migraine variant closely related to benign paroxysmal vertigo (see Chapter 10) in some infants but not in others.

CLINICAL FEATURES. Onset is always in the first year and is characterized by episodes in which the head is tilted to one side (not always the same side) and may be slightly rotated. The child may resist efforts to return the head to a neutral position, but this can be overcome. Some children have no other symptoms, whereas others have pallor, irritability, malaise, and vomiting. Most attacks last for 1 to 3 days, end spontaneously, and tend to recur three to six times a year. Children who are old enough to stand and walk become ataxic during attacks.

With time the attacks may evolve into episodes characteristic of benign paroxysmal vertigo or classic migraine, or may simply cease without further symptoms. The disorder has been described in siblings, but more often the family history is only of migraine.

DIAGNOSIS. The disorder should be suspected in any infant with attacks of torticollis that remit spontaneously. A family history of migraine should be sought. Familial paroxysmal choreoathetosis and familial paroxysmal dystonia do not begin during early infancy. *Sandifer syndrome,* intermittent torticollis associated with hiatal hernia, is an alternative consideration.

MANAGEMENT. No treatment is available or needed for the acute attacks.

Writer's Cramp

Writer's cramp is a focal dystonia that may occur only when writing, when performing other specific manual tasks such as typing or playing the piano (*occupational cramp*), or with nonspecific use of the hands. The cramp is more often isolated but may be associated with other focal dystonias, such as torticollis, or with generalized dystonia.

CLINICAL FEATURES. Onset is almost always after 20 years of age but may be in the second decade. Initial features are any of the following: aching in the hand when writing, loss of handwriting neatness or speed, and difficulty in holding writing implements. All three symptoms are eventually present. Dystonic postures occur when the patient attempts to write. The hand and arm lift from the paper, and the fingers may flex or extend. Writing with the affected hand becomes impossible and the patient learns to write with the nondominant hand, which may also become dystonic.

Symptoms are at first intermittent and are especially severe when others observe the writing. Later the cramp occurs with each attempt at writing. Some patients have lifelong difficulty with using the dominant hand for writing and may have difficulty with other manual tasks as well. Others experience remissions and exacerbations. Progression to generalized dystonia is rare.

DIAGNOSIS. Unfortunately, most people with writer's or occupational cramp are thought to have psychiatric illness despite the lack of associated psychopathological features. Early diagnosis can save considerable expense and concern. Isolated focal dystonia must be distinguished from generalized dystonia with focal onset. The family history should be explored thoroughly, and repeated examinations are needed to determine the presence of dystonia in other body parts.

MANAGEMENT. The same medications used to treat generalized dystonia should be used in patients with focal dystonia (see section on Idiopathic Torsion Dystonia later in this chapter).

Generalized Genetic Dystonias

The autosomal dominant dystonias have been classified into a numeric system using the code DYT. Three are important entities in childhood.

Dopa-Responsive Dystonia

Dopa-responsive dystonia (DYT5) is also called *the dystonia-parkinsonism syndrome, dystonia with diurnal variation,* and *Segawa disease.* Dopa-responsive dystonia may be inherited as either an autosomal dominant or autosomal recessive trait. The dominant form is due to mutations in the gene for GTP cyclohydrolase 1, the cofactor for tyrosine hydroxylase, and the recessive form is due to mutations in the tyrosine hydroxylase gene. Most reported cases of "juvenile parkinsonism" are probably variants of dopa-responsive dystonia (Nygaard and Wooten, 1998).

CLINICAL FEATURES. Marked variation in expressivity occurs even between affected members of the same kindred. (Steinberger et al, 1998). Age at onset is usually between 4 and 8 years but may be as early as infancy. Early-onset cases are often misdiagnosed as cerebral palsy. The initial feature is nearly always a gait disturbance caused by leg dystonia. Flexion at the hip and knee and plantar flexion of the foot cause toe walking. Both flexor and extensor posturing of the arms develop, and finally parkinsonian features appear: cogwheel rigidity, mask-like facies, and bradykinesia. The disease reaches a plateau in adolescence. Postural or intention tremor occurs in almost half of patients, but typical parkinsonian tremor is unusual.

Diurnal fluctuation in symptoms occurs in more than half of patients. Symptoms are considerably improved on awakening and become worse later in the day. Movement and exercise exacerbate dystonia in some patients, and other disorders with exercise-induced dystonia as the main or only clinical features may be expressions of the same genetic error.

DIAGNOSIS. Dopa-responsive dystonia may be difficult to differentiate from other genetic disorders with dystonia because of phenotypic variation among family members (see also section on Rapid-Onset Dystonia-Parkinsonism later in this chapter). Diagnosis by mutation analysis is available. Important clues to diagnosis are features of parkinsonism without other neurological signs, diurnal variation in severity of symptoms, exacerbation of symptoms with exercise, and response to levodopa.

MANAGEMENT. A small dose of levodopa usually provides immediate and complete relief in most patients, even when treatment is initiated long after symptoms begin. No other dystonia responds so well. Carbidopa-levodopa should be started at the lowest possible dose and slowly increased until a response is established. Long-term therapy is beneficial and required; symptoms return when the drug is discontinued. Trihexyphenidyl, in doses lower than ordinarily needed to treat idiopathic torsion dystonia, and bromocriptine are also effective.

Glutaric Acidemia Type I

Glutaric acidemia type I is a rare inborn error in the catabolism of lysine, hydroxylysine, and tryptophan. It is transmitted by autosomal recessive inheritance and is caused by deficiency of glutaryl-coenzyme-A dehydrogenase (Superti-Furga and Hoffmann, 1997).

CLINICAL FEATURES. Megalencephaly is usually present at birth. Neurological findings may be otherwise normal. Two patterns have been described in affected infants. The initial feature in two thirds of infants is an acute encephalopathy characterized by somnolence, irritability, and excessive sweating. Seizures sometimes occur. The prognosis in such cases is poor. Afterward, development regresses and progressive choreoathetosis and dystonia occur. The other pattern is more insidious and the prognosis is better. Affected infants are at first hypotonic and later have mild developmental delay and dyskinesias. Many of these cases are often misdiagnosed as cerebral palsy (see Chapter 12).

DIAGNOSIS. Metabolic acidosis may be present. Abnormal amounts of glutaric, 3-hydroxyglutaric, 3-hydroxybutyric, and acetoacetic acids are found in the urine. The diagnosis is established by showing the enzyme deficiency in cultured fibroblasts. Prenatal diagnosis is available. CT often shows diffuse attenuation of cerebral white matter and cerebral atrophy, most marked in the frontal and temporal lobes.

MANAGEMENT. Disease progression may be slowed in patients with little or no neurological disease by oral carnitine supplementation together with the immediate administration of fluids, glucose, electrolytes, and antipyretics during febrile illnesses.

Hallervorden-Spatz Disease

Hallervorden-Spatz disease encompasses several disorders with the triad of pallidal iron deposition, axonal spheroids, and gliosis (Halliday 1995). Most cases are transmitted by autosomal recessive inheritance.

CLINICAL FEATURES. The disorder becomes symptomatic between 2 and 10 years of age in more than half of patients but may appear as late as the third decade. The initial feature is progressive rigidity, first in the foot, causing an equinovarus deformity, and then in the hand. Other features are choreoathetosis, rigidity, and dysarthria. Retinitis pigmentosa and seizures each occur in 20% to 25% of cases. Mental deterioration and spasticity follow, with progression to spastic immobility and death within 5 to 10 years.

DIAGNOSIS. Antemortem diagnosis is based primarily on the clinical presentation and is difficult to establish in the absence of a family history of the disorder. T_2-weighted MRI shows low-intensity signal images from the globus pallidus with a central area of increased signal intensity, known as *the eye-of-the-tiger* sign. Postmortem examination shows degeneration of the pallidum and substantia nigra with deposition of iron-containing material.

MANAGEMENT. Agents that chelate iron have not proved effective. Only symptomatic treatment is available.

Hepatolenticular Degeneration (Wilson Disease)

Hepatolenticular degeneration is transmitted by autosomal recessive inheritance. The defective gene site is chromosome 13q14-q21, and the abnormal gene product is the main copper transporter moving copper from the hepatocyte into the bile. Tissue damage occurs after excessive copper accumulation in the liver, brain, and cornea.

CLINICAL FEATURES. Wilson disease can present with hepatic, neurological, or psychiatric disturbances, alone or in combination. The age at onset ranges from 3 to over 50 years (Cox and Roberts, 1999). Hepatic failure is the prominent clinical feature in children less than 10 years of age, usually without neurological symptoms or signs. Neurological manifestations with only minimal symptoms of liver disease are more likely when the onset of symptoms is in the second decade. A single symptom, such as a disturbance of gait or speech, is often the initial feature and may remain unchanged for years. Eventually the initial symptoms worsen and new features develop (dysarthria, dystonia, dysdiadochokinesia, rigidity, gait and postural abnormalities, tremor, and drooling). Dystonia of bulbar muscles is responsible for three prominent features of the disease: dysarthria, a fixed pseudosmile (risus sardonicus), and a high-pitched whining noise on inspiration.

Psychiatric disturbances precede the neurological abnormalities in 20% of cases. They range from behavioral disturbances to paranoid psychoses. Dementia is not an early feature of the disease.

The Kayser-Fleischer ring, a yellow-brown granular deposit at the limbus of the cornea, is a certain indicator of the disease. It is caused by copper deposition in the Descemet membrane and is present in almost all patients with neurological manifestations, although it may be absent in children with liver disease alone.

DIAGNOSIS. Hepatolenticular degeneration should be considered in any child with dysarthria and dystonia. The further association of chronic liver disease increases the probability of hepatolenticular degeneration. The diagnosis is established by showing an increased copper content by liver biopsy or by the demonstration of a Kayser-Fleischer ring by slit-lamp examination. Ninety-six percent of patients will have a serum ceruloplasmin concentration of less than 20 mg/dl, corresponding to less than 56 g/dl of ceruloplasmin copper. Mutation analysis is available for early diagnosis in siblings at risk.

MANAGEMENT. Treatment is lifelong. Copper chelating agents (e.g., penicillamine or trientine) that increase urinary excretion of copper are the primary treatment for Wilson disease. The dose of *d*-penicillamine is 250 mg four times a day for children more than 10 years of age and half as much for younger children. Penicillamine must always be given on an empty stomach together with a daily dose of 25 mg pyridoxine. Twenty-four-hour urine copper excretion is used to confirm chelation, and urinary copper values should run 5–10 times normal. Improvement is slow, and neurological improvement frequently takes several months. Worsening may occur during the first months of therapy, but this should not be a cause for alarm. When treatment is started early, the results are quite satisfactory, without excess morbidity and mortality.

Oral administration of zinc may be used after initial decoppering with a chelating agent. Antioxidants, such as vitamin E, may be used along with a chelator or zinc to prevent tissue damage, particularly to the liver. Liver transplantation is reserved for patients who fail to respond or cannot tolerate medical therapy. Siblings of patients with Wilson disease should be carefully screened for disease and treated as early as possible.

Idiopathic Torsion Dystonia

Early-onset idiopathic torsion dystonia (DYT1) (*dystonia musculorum deformans*) is transmitted by autosomal dominant inheritance with reduced penetrance (30% to 40%) and variable expression. The gene locus is chromosome 9q34

(Warner and Jarman, 1998). The frequency of idiopathic torsion dystonia in Ashkenazi Jews is 5 to 10 times greater than in other groups. Nonfamilial cases probably represent autosomal dominant inheritance with incomplete penetrance.

CLINICAL FEATURES. Age at onset has a bimodal distribution; for early onset the mode is 9 years, and for late onset the mode is 45 years. The early-onset cases are more genetically homogeneous.

The limbs are usually affected before the trunk. The initial features may be in the arms, legs, or larynx. Early leg involvement is more common in children than in adults. Despite the focal features at onset, dystonia always becomes generalized in children, affecting the limbs and trunk. Spontaneous stabilization is the rule, but remission is unusual. The eventual outcome varies from complete disability to functional independence.

Other clinical features include dysarthria, orofacial movements, dysphagia, postural tremor, and blepharospasm. Mental deterioration does not occur, but as a group, patients with familial disease have a lower IQ than those with sporadic cases.

DIAGNOSIS. The clinical features of dystonic movements and postures, normal perinatal history, no exposure to drugs, no evidence of intellectual or corticospinal deterioration, and no demonstrable biochemical disorder suggest the diagnosis. Diagnosis is confirmed by genetic-based testing.

MANAGEMENT. Medical management is often ineffective. The best results are obtained with high-dose anticholinergic therapy (trihexyphenidyl, 30mg/day). While children tend to tolerate higher doses than do adults; confusion and memory impairment may limit usefulness. Other drugs that may be of value include baclofen, carbamazepine, and benzodiazepines. All juvenile-onset dystonic patients deserve a trial of L-dopa. Botulinum toxin may be used for selected focal problems. Surgical procedures are rarely useful and are associated with severe complications.

Infantile Bilateral Striatal Necrosis

Bilateral striatal necrosis occurs in several genetic disorders that share pathological features of bilateral, symmetric, spongy degeneration of the corpus striatum with variable degeneration of the globus pallidus. These disorders may appear in infancy or early childhood.

CLINICAL FEATURES. Three clinical syndromes are associated with infantile bilateral striatal necrosis. One is characterized by an insidious onset during infancy or childhood and with a long clinical course that includes dystonia, cognitive impairment, seizures, and death. Most of these cases are probably mitochondrial disorders; a point mutation in the mitochondrial ATPase 6 gene was shown in one child (Meirleir et al, 1995). A clinical and pathological overlap exists between progressive infantile bilateral striatal necrosis, subacute necrotizing encephalomyelopathy (see Chapter 5), and Leber's hereditary optic neuropathy (see Chapter 16).

A second syndrome begins as an acute encephalopathy, usually following a febrile illness with nausea and vomiting. The major features are dystonia and tremor. The severity of symptoms may fluctuate at the time of intercurrent illness. Some children recover spontaneously; others are permanently impaired.

The third syndrome occurs in Arab kinships but may have a wider distribution (Ozand et al, 1998). The etiology may be defective transport of biotin across the blood-brain barrier. The syndrome is probably transmitted by autosomal recessive inheritance. Onset is usually between age 3 and 5 years. The first symptoms are confusion, dysarthria, and dysphagia. These progress to cranial nerve palsies, cogwheel rigidity, dystonia, and quadriparesis.

DIAGNOSIS. The diagnosis is suggested by showing static or progressive striatal necrosis on serial MRI examinations.

MANAGEMENT. All features of biotin-responsive striatal necrosis clear after administration of biotin, 5 to 10 mg/kg/day, but reappear within 1 month after biotin is discontinued. Biotin should be tried in all children with evidence of bilateral striatal necrosis.

Rapid-Onset Dystonia-Parkinsonism

Rapid-onset dystonia-parkinsonism (DYT12) is a separate autosomal dominant form of dystonia characterized by an unusually rapid evolution of signs and symptoms (Brashear et al, 1996). The abnormal gene maps to chromosome 9q13.

CLINICAL FEATURES. The disorder is characterized by the acute (hours) or subacute (days to weeks) development of generalized dystonia and parkinsonism that responds poorly to treatment with levodopa. Age at onset is 14 to 45 years.

DIAGNOSIS. Diagnosis depends on the clinical features. The phenotypic variability is sufficient to hide the disease in family members.

MANAGEMENT. A trial of levodopa is reasonable in any child with new-onset dystonia even though it is not effective in idiopathic torsion dystonia. If dopa fails, then trihexyphenidyl is the drug of choice and is usually effective. High dosages are required, usually 30 mg/day in three divided doses. Dosages as high as 80 mg/day are sometimes necessary. Such high dosages can be tolerated in children if built up slowly but are rarely tolerated by adults. The response cannot be predicted from measurement of plasma concentrations.

If trihexyphenidyl is not effective, baclofen should be added. The initial dosage is 5 to 10 mg/day, increased 10 mg weekly until benefit is attained or adverse reactions occur. Diazepam is an alternative to baclofen and should also be added at low dosages and slowly increased as tolerated. If a patient does not respond to this combination, tetrabenazine or some combination of carbamazepine, benztropine, pimozide, or bromocriptine can be tried.

Symptomatic Generalized Dystonia

An underlying tumor, an active encephalopathy, or prior brain damage can cause dystonia.

CLINICAL FEATURES. The onset of dystonia may be at the time of an acute encephalopathy, after the acute phase is over, or several years later when the encephalopathy is thought to be static. Delayed-onset chorea and dystonia in children with perinatal disturbances such as asphyxia or kernicterus usually begin by 2 to 3 years of age but may be delayed for 17 years. After involuntary movements appear, they tend to become progressively more severe, but intellectual decline is not an associated feature. Delayed-onset dystonia is usually generalized.

Hemidystonia most often occurs after stroke or head injury but may be a symptom of neuronal storage diseases or tumors of the basal ganglia, alternating hemiplegia, and the antiphospholipid antibody syndrome (see Chapter 11). The dystonic limbs are contralateral to the damaged basal ganglia.

DIAGNOSIS. Children with a known cause for the development of dystonia or chorea do not require extensive studies. The new symptoms are discouraging for patients and families, who have adjusted to a fixed neurological deficit. They may be assured that this is not evidence of new degeneration in the brain, but only the appearance of new symptoms from old lesions. This sequence is most likely when injury is perinatal and brain maturation is required to manifest involuntary movements.

The appearance of hemidystonia, even when the predisposing event is known, necessitates MRI to look for localized changes that may require treatment, such as an expanding cyst. The possibility of tumor must be considered in children who had been neurologically intact before hemidystonia appeared.

MANAGEMENT. The drugs used to treat symptomatic dystonia are no different from those used for genetic dystonia, but the results may not be as favorable. Botulinum toxin may be useful when specific muscle contractions are causing severe disability.

Hemifacial Spasm

Hemifacial spasm is characterized by involuntary, irregular contraction of the muscles innervated by one facial nerve. It is very rare in children. The spasms may develop because of aberrant regeneration following facial nerve injury, as a result of posterior fossa tumor, or without apparent cause.

CLINICAL FEATURES. Spasms are embarrassing and disturbing but not painful. The orbicularis oculi muscles are affected first and most commonly, causing forced closure of the eye. As facial muscles on one side become affected, the mouth is pulled to one side. Spasms may occur several times a minute, especially during times of stress. The subsequent course depends on the underlying cause.

DIAGNOSIS. Hemifacial spasm in children may be mistaken for a focal seizure. The stereotyped appearance of the spasm and a concurrent normal EEG are distinguishing features. Posterior fossa tumor must be suspected in every child with hemifacial spasm. MRI is indicated unless symptoms can be explained by a known history of facial nerve injury.

MANAGEMENT. Some patients respond to treatment with carbamazepine at anticonvulsant doses (see Chapter 1), but most do not respond to medical therapy. Injection of botulinum toxin into the muscles in spasm is the treatment of choice. Surgical procedures to relieve pressure on the facial nerve from adjacent vessels are of questionable value.

Mirror Movements

Mirror movements are defined as involuntary movements of one side of the body, usually the hands, which occur as mirror reversals of an intended movement on the other side of the body. They are normal during infancy and tend to disappear before 10 years of age, coincident with myelination of the corpus callosum. Persistence of mirror movements may be a familial trait caused by ipsilateral and contralateral organization of the corticospinal pathways. Obligatory mirror movements are abnormal even in infants and suggest a congenital abnormality at the cervicomedullary junction.

Myoclonus

The term *myoclonus* encompasses several involuntary movements characterized by rapid muscle jerks. They are less frequent and severe during sleep but may not disappear. Myoclonus may be rhythmic or nonrhythmic; focal, multifocal, or generalized; or spontaneous or activated by movement (action myoclonus) or sensory stimulation (reflex myoclonus).

Nonepileptic myoclonus must be distinguished from tic, chorea, tremor, and seizures. Tics are usually more complex and stereotyped movements than myoclonus and can be briefly suppressed by voluntary effort; myoclonus cannot be suppressed. Chorea is more random than myoclonus and tends to be incorporated into voluntary movement; myoclonus is never part of a larger movement. Rhythmic myoclonus and tremor look alike and are distinguished with certainty only by special studies. Tremor is a continuous to-and-fro movement, whereas rhythmic myoclonus has a pause between movements.

An etiological classification of myoclonus is summarized in Table 14-7. *Physiological myoclonus* occurs in normal people when falling asleep, during sleep (nocturnal myoclonus), when waking up, and during times of anxiety. Nocturnal myoclonus is a rhythmic jerking of the legs during sleep that is common in children. It should be distinguished from the *restless legs syndrome*, a genetic disorder probably transmitted by autosomal dominant inheritance (Montplaisir et al, 1997). The syndrome is characterized by leg discomfort at rest that is relieved by movement. It is often attributed to "growing pains." Periodic limb movements mainly occur during sleep but also during wakefulness.

Epileptic myoclonus is associated with epileptiform activity on the EEG (see Chapter 1). *Symptomatic myoclonus* may be caused by drugs, may follow a cerebral injury, or may be

Table 14-7
Etiological Classification of Myoclonus

Physiological
Anxiety-induced
Exercise-induced
Sleep jerks and nocturnal myoclonus

Essential

Epileptic (see Chapter 1)

Symptomatic
Post-central nervous system injury
    Hypoxia (see Chapter 2)
    Trauma (see Chapter 2)
    Stroke (see Chapter 11)
Basal ganglia degenerations
    Idiopathic torsion dystonia
    Hallervorden-Spatz disease
    Hepatolenticular degeneration (Wilson disease)
    Huntington disease (see Chapter 5)
Drug-induced
    Carbamazepine
    Levodopa
    Tricyclic antidepressants
Lysosomal storage diseases (see Chapter 5)
Metabolic encephalopathies (see Chapter 2)
    Dialysis syndromes
    Disorders of osmolality
    Hepatic failure
    Renal failure
Myoclonic encephalopathy (see Chapter 10)
    Idiopathic
    Neuroblastoma
Spinal cord tumor (see Chapter 12)
Spinocerebellar degenerations (see Chapter 10)
Toxic encephalopathies (see Chapter 2)
Viral encephalitis

part of a generalized progressive encephalopathy.

Essential Myoclonus

Essential myoclonus is a chronic condition of focal, segmental, or generalized jerking that is aggravated by action or stress. Affected people are otherwise normal. Occurrence is usually sporadic, but when it is familial, transmission is by autosomal dominant inheritance.

CLINICAL FEATURES. Onset is in the first or second decade. Males and females are affected equally. The movements are predominantly in the face, trunk, and proximal muscles. They are usually generalized but may be restricted to one side of the body. No other neurological disturbances develop, and life expectancy is not affected. Essential tremor may be present in the same family.

DIAGNOSIS. The clinical features and family history establish the diagnosis. Careful neurological examination, EEG, and brain imaging are needed to exclude symptomatic and epileptic myoclonus. Even then, a period of observation and repeat laboratory investigations may be necessary to eliminate other causes.

MANAGEMENT. Mild essential myoclonus does not require treatment. When intervention is needed, clonazepam is the drug of choice. Carbamazepine, tetrabenazine, and valproate have been found useful in symptomatic myoclonus and may be beneficial in generalized myoclonus as well.

Symptomatic Myoclonus

Myoclonus is often a symptom of an underlying neurological disease. It tends to be generalized when caused by diffuse, progressive encephalopathies (such as lysosomal storage diseases) and segmental when there is a focal lesion of the brainstem or spinal cord. Multifocal myoclonus may occur as a non–dose-dependent side effect of carbamazepine therapy in children.

Posthypoxic Myoclonus (Lance-Adams Syndrome)

Posthypoxic myoclonus is a form of action myoclonus in patients who have suffered an episode of hypoxia. It does not follow hypoxic-ischemic encephalopathy of the newborn. Single or repetitive myoclonic jerks occur when voluntary movement is attempted. Facial and pharyngeal muscles may be affected, interfering with speech and swallowing. Cerebellar disturbances are usually associated findings.

Myoclonus usually begins during recovery from anoxic encephalopathy and once started never remits. It may respond to valproate, 5-hydroxytryptophan, or clonazepam.

Segmental (Focal) Myoclonus

Segmental myoclonus is an involuntary contraction of contiguous muscles innervated by the brainstem or spinal cord. It may be rhythmic or nonrhythmic. Rhythmic segmental myoclonus looks like a focal seizure. The underlying causes in children are limited mainly to demyelinating diseases and intrinsic tumors. Cystic astrocytoma of the spinal cord is the major cause of spinal myoclonus and may be the initial feature (see Chapter 12).

Palatal myoclonus is the most common segmental myoclonus of brainstem origin. It is a unilateral or bilateral rhythmic contraction of the palate (80 to 180/min) that usually persists during sleep. It may be associated with rhythmic contractions of the eyes, larynx, neck, diaphragm, trunk, and limbs. Lesions in the central tegmental tract or the dentato-olivary pathways cause palatal myoclonus. The median interval between the precipitating cause and the onset of palatal myoclonus is 10 to 11 months. Clonazepam and tetrabenazine are the most useful drugs in the treatment of segmental myoclonus.

Stereotypies

Stereotypies are repeated, purposeless movements that may be simple or complex. Simple sterotypies are foot or finger tapping and hair curling. Complex stereotypies range from shuddering attacks to sequential movements of the head, arms, and body. They appear intentional. A family history of similar movements can sometimes be elicited.

The main differential diagnosis is with seizures and complex tics. Seizures are never as stereotyped. Complex tics are more difficult to differentiate. Stereotypies differ from tics in that suppression of the movement does not cause tension, and other features of the Tourette syndrome are not present. Stereotypies tend to disappear as the child ages. Treatment is neither needed nor effective. The movements are best ignored.

Tic and Tourette Syndrome

Tics or *habit spasms* are complex, stereotyped movements (motor tic) or utterances (verbal tic) that are sudden, brief, and purposeless. They may be confused with chorea but can be readily distinguished by their stereotyped appearance. A tic can be accurately described and reproduced by an observer (e.g., "he blinks his eyes"); chorea cannot. Tics can be suppressed for short periods of time, with some discomfort, and are never incorporated into a voluntary movement. Chorea is harder to suppress and is usually elaborated into a voluntary movement. Tic and chorea are both exacerbated by stress and disappear during sleep.

Tourette syndrome is any combination of verbal and motor tics. It should not be considered a separate disease, but rather part of a phenotypic spectrum that includes simple motor tic, attention deficit disorder, and obsessive-compulsive behavior (Sadovnick and Kurlan, 1997). The syndrome is transmitted as a highly penetrant, autosomal dominant trait in which tics and attention deficit disorder are more commonly expressed in males and obsessive-compulsive behavior in females. Bilineal transmission is common and may correlate with the severity of disease. The abnormal gene locus is not known.

In addition to the strong evidence for a genetic basis for Tourette syndrome, environmental factors also play a role. Stimulants are known to provoke tics in predisposed children, and streptococcal infection may cause the sudden onset of severe tic or obsessive-compulsive disorder (Singer et al, 1998). The term PANDAS (pediatric autoimmune neuropsychiatric disorders associated with streptococcal infection) is used to acknowledge the association between streptococcal infection and the acute exacerbation of chorea or tic.

CLINICAL FEATURES. Affected children are not mentally disturbed before symptoms begin. Although the frequency of behavioral disturbances is increased in children with Tourette syndrome, the movement disorder and the behavioral disturbances should each be considered an expression of the same underlying genetic defect; one does not cause the other.

Onset is anytime from 2 to 15 years of age, with the mean between 6 and 7 years. The most severe period of tic severity is between 8 and 12 years of age, and half of children are tic-free by age 18 years (Leckman et al, 1998). Neck muscles are often affected first, causing a head movement in which the child appears to be tossing hair back from the face. New motor tics develop either in place of, or in addition to, existing tics. They usually affect the head, eyes, or face. Common tics include eye blinking, grimacing, lip smacking, and shrugging of one or both shoulders.

The initial verbal tics are usually a clearing of the throat, a snorting or sniffing noise, and a cough-like noise. Many children who make sniffing or coughing noises will undergo an extensive evaluation for allergy and are found to be allergic to something (isn't everyone?). Desensitization is then the next unsuccessful intervention. Grunting and hissing are other verbal tics. Uttering profanities (coprolalia) is rare in children. When it does occur, the profanity is quickly suppressed and replaced by barking or coughing noises.

Symptoms wax and wane spontaneously and in response to stress and excitement. Tics usually become less frequent when children are out of school. While half of children outgrow their tics, some have lifelong difficulty and others have prolonged remissions with recurrence in middle age or later.

Half of children with tics have an attention deficit disorder, and a third have an obsessive-compulsive disorder. Attention deficit disorder is characterized by hyperactivity, short attention span, restlessness, poor concentration, and impaired impulse control. This syndrome is often treated with methylphenidate, a drug that has the potential to accentuate tics in genetically predisposed children.

Obsessive-compulsive behavior is characterized by ritualistic actions and thoughts, which may include touching things repeatedly, placing objects in a certain place, washing and rewashing hands, obsessive thoughts about sex or violence, and counting objects. A history of obsessive-compulsive behavior in family members, especially mothers, can be elicited with the following questions: Do you routinely go back and check the door and lights after you leave the house? Do you have routines in the way that you clean the house or fold clothes that must be followed every time? The diagnosis of obsessive-compulsive behavior is assured if the mother responds that these habits are driving her family crazy.

DIAGNOSIS. The clinical features establish the diagnosis. Laboratory tests are not helpful and need not be done in obvious cases. EEG, MRI, and psychological test results are normal.

Tics do not ordinarily occur in degenerative diseases of the nervous system or as an adverse reaction to drugs. Drug-induced tics should be considered the potentiation of Tourette syndrome in a genetically predisposed child. Carbamazepine and lamotrigine (Lombroso, 1999), as well as amphetamine and methylphenidate, may trigger the symptoms. Withdrawal of the potentiating drug does not always stop the tics.

MANAGEMENT. Most children with tics and Tourette syndrome do not require drug treatment. The decision to prescribe medication depends on whether the tics bother the child. Drugs should not be used if the tics bother the parents but do not disturb the child's life. The parents must be told that tics are not a sign of progressive neurological or mental illness, are made worse by stress, and will diminish in frequency if ignored. Caffeine ingestion may exacerbate tics and should be reduced or removed from the diet (Davis and Osorio, 1998).

Drug treatment is difficult to evaluate because the disorder's natural history is one of exacerbation and remission. The most useful drugs to control tic are pimozide, fluphenazine, and haloperidol. I prefer pimozide, then fluphenazine, on the basis of a lower incidence of adverse effects. The dosage of pimozide is initially 1 mg/day and is increased 1 mg each week as needed. The maintenance dosage is usually 2–4 mg/day and never exceeds 10 mg/day. Fluphenazine is started at 1 mg/day and increased 1 mg each week. The usual maintenance dosage is 2–6 mg/day, and should not exceed 10 mg. Haloperidol is started as a single dose of 0.5 mg at night and is slowly increased 0.5 mg each week until tics are reasonably controlled or adverse reactions are noted. The usual maintenance dosage is 1–3 mg/day in two divided doses. The major toxic effects of all three drugs are sedation, irritability, and depression of appetite. Dystonia and akathisia are idiosyncratic reactions. Many neurologists recommend clonidine because it is also useful for attention deficit disorder, but it is not as effective for tics.

Any of these drugs may lose their efficacy after prolonged use, but effectiveness may return after an interval of withholding the drug. Interrupted therapy with one drug or alternating between two drugs is reasonable.

Obsessive-compulsive disorder (OCD), when it occurs as part of the Tourette phenotype, is best treated with serotonin reuptake inhibitors such as fluoxetine or sertraline. A modest dose of either may be effective not only for the OCD but also for the tics, either alone or in conjunction with pimozide.

Tremor

Tremor is an involuntary oscillating movement with a fixed frequency. The product of tremor frequency and amplitude is constant; because frequency decreases with age, amplitude increases. Shuddering, cerebellar ataxia or dysmetria, and asterixis are not tremors because they lack rhythm. Myoclonus may be rhythmic but is interrupted between oscillations.

All people have a low-amplitude *physiological tremor* inherent in movement that is not ordinarily observed without a measuring device. Physiological tremor may be enhanced to a clinically detectable level by situations (anxiety, excitement, exercise, fatigue, stress) and drugs (adrenergic agonists, nicotine, prednisone, thyroid hormone, xanthines). Hyperthyroidism is routinely associated with enhanced physiological tremor.

Parkinsonism is a common cause of pathological tremors in adults, but it does not occur in children except when drug induced or as part of a complex degenerative disorder. Typical parkinsonian tremor is seldom present in these situations. Essential (familial) tremor is the major cause of tremor in children.

Essential (Familial) Tremor

Essential (familial) tremor is a monosymptomatic condition transmitted as an autosomal dominant trait. Two different gene loci are identified. One maps to chromosome 3q13 (Gulcher et al, 1997) and the other to chromosome 2p. (Higgins et al, 1998). Penetrance is eventually complete, but the age at onset may be delayed until 65 years. The form associated with the 2p gene locus shows generational anticipation, and an expanded trinucleotide sequence is suspected. Childhood-onset essential tremor is not associated with other neurological disturbances.

CLINICAL FEATURES. Essential tremor occurs only in a limb being used. The head, face, and neck are sometimes affected. Neck tremor gives the appearance of torticollis. The frequency of essential tremor is typically between 4 and 8 Hz. Childhood-onset tremor usually appears in the second decade but can begin as early as 2 years of age. Essential tremor may impair function, especially schoolwork, and therefore disturbs the patient. In young children, the tremor has the appearance of restlessness or clumsiness. Later, its nature as an action tremor is appreciated.

Tremor is enhanced by greater precision of movement and therefore appears first and most prominently in the hands. It is further enhanced by anxiety, concentrated effort to stop the tremor, and fatigue. In such cases, the worsening of tremor may be due to enhanced physiological tremor rather than enhanced essential tremor. The distinction is important in considering treatment options. Essential tremor is generally lifelong.

DIAGNOSIS. Essential tremor in children is often mistaken for cerebellar dysfunction because it occurs with action (intention). The two are easily differentiated because essential tremor is rhythmic and not dysmetric (does not become worse at the endpoint) and because it is not associated with other signs of cerebellar dysfunction.

The distinction between essential tremor and enhanced physiological tremor may be more difficult because the two are often concurrent. Enhanced physiological tremor is always circumstantial, whereas essential tremor remains even when the patient is alone and relaxed.

MANAGEMENT. Not all people with essential tremor require treatment. Medication should be reserved for situations in which tremor impairs function. Propranolol, 1 to 2 mg/kg/day, or primidone, 2 to 10 mg/kg/day, is effective to control tremor in 70% of cases. Propranolol has fewer side effects and should be the first drug chosen.

Essential tremor is also relieved by alcohol ingestion. This treatment should be discouraged, as the incidence of alcoholism may be increased in adults with essential tremor.

Paroxysmal Dystonic Head Tremor

CLINICAL FEATURES. Paroxysmal dystonic head tremor is an uncommon nonfamilial syndrome of unknown cause. The major feature is attacks of horizontal head tremor (frequency 5 to 8 Hz), as if the person were saying "no." Onset occurs in adolescence, and two reported patients as well as three adolescents in my own practice were male. The attacks vary from 1 to 30 minutes, are not provoked by any single stimulus, and cannot be suppressed. A head tilt predates the onset of tremor by 5 to 10 years. The attacks are lifelong but do not progress to other neurological symptoms. Results of the examination are otherwise normal.

DIAGNOSIS. Imaging studies of the brain show no abnormalities. In an infant, the combination of head nodding and head tilt would be diagnosed as spasmus nutans even in the absence of nystagmus (see Chapter 15), and perhaps the underlying mechanism is similar.

MANAGEMENT. Daily use of clonazepam reduces the frequency and severity of attacks, but the head tilt may persist.

References

Brashear A, Farlow MR, Butler IJ, et al. Variable phenotype of rapid-onset dystonia-parkinsonism. *Mov Disord* 1996;11:151–156.

Cox DW, Roberts EA. (Updated 14 October 1999) Wilson Disease. In: GeneClinics: Medical Genetics Knowledge Base [database online]. University of Washington, Seattle. Available at http://www.geneclinics.org. Accessed November 1999.

Davis RE, Osorio I. Childhood caffeine tic syndrome. *Pediatrics* 1998;101:e4.

Geschwind DH, Loginov M, Stern JM. Identification of a locus on chromosome 14q for idiopathic basal ganglia calcification (Fahr disease). *Am J Hum Genet* 1999; 65:764–772.

Gulcher JR, Jonsson P, Kong A, et al. Mapping of a familial essential tremor gene, FET1, to chromosome 3q13. *Nature Genet* 1997;17:84–87.

Halliday W. The nosology of Hallervorden-Spatz disease. *J Neurol Sci* 1995;134:84–91.

Higgins JJ, Loveless JM, Jankovic J, et al. Evidence that a gene for essential tremor maps to chromosome 2p in four families. *Mov Disord* 1998;13:972–977.

Janavs JL, Aminoff MJ. Dystonia and chorea in acquired systemic disorders. *J Neurol Neurosurg Psychiatry* 1998;65:436–444.

Kartsounis LD, Hardie RJ. The pattern of cognitive impairments in neuroacanthocytosis: A frontosubcortical dementia. *Arch Neurol* 1996;53:77–80.

Leckman JF, Zhang H, Vitale A, et al. Course of tic severity in Tourette syndrome: The first two decades. *Pediatrics* 1998;102:14–19.

Lombroso C. Lamotrigine-induced tourettism. *Neurology* 1999;52:1191–1194.

Meirleir LD, Seneca S, Lissens W, et al. Bilateral striatal necrosis with a novel point mutation in the mitochondrial ATPase gene. *Pediatr Neurol* 1995;13:242–246.

Montplaisir J, Boucher S, Poirer G, et al. Clinical, polysomnographic, and genetic characteristics of restless legs syndrome: A study of 133 patients diagnosed with new standard criteria. *Mov Disord* 1997;12:61–65.

Nygaard TG, Wooten GF. Dopa-responsive dystonia: Some pieces of the puzzle are still missing. *Neurology* 1998; 50:853–855.

Ozand PT, Gascon GG, Al Essa M, et al. Biotin-responsive basal ganglia disease: A novel entity. *Brain* 1998; 121:1267–1279.

Sadovnick D, Kurlan R. The increasingly complex genetics of Tourette's syndrome. *Neurology* 1997;48:801–802.

Singer HS, Giuliano MSN, Hansen BH, et al. Antibodies against human putamen in children with Tourette syndrome. *Neurology* 1998;50:1618–1624.

Steinberger D, Weber Y, Korinthenberg R, et al. High penetrance and pronounced variation in expressivity of GCH1 mutations in five families with dopa-responsive dystonia. *Ann Neurol* 1998;43:634–639.

Superti-Furga A, Hoffman GF. Glutaric aciduria type 1 (glutaryl-CoA-dehydrogenase deficiency): Advances and unanswered questions. Report from an international meeting. *Eur J Pediatr* 1997;156:821–828.

Traill Z, Pike M, Byrne J. Sydenham's chorea: A case showing reversible striatal abnormalities on CT and MRI. *Dev Med Child Neurol* 1995;37:270–273.

Warner TT, Jarman P. The molecular genetics of the dystonias. *J Neurol Neurosurg Psychiatry* 1998;64:427–429.

Chapter 15
Disorders of Ocular Motility

THE MAINTENANCE OF binocular vision by conjugate movement of the eyes is perhaps the most delicate feat of muscular coordination achieved by the nervous system. Disorders of the visual sensory system, ocular muscles, ocular motor nerves, neuromuscular transmission, or gaze centers of the central nervous system may disturb ocular motility. This chapter deals with nonparalytic strabismus, paralytic strabismus (ophthalmoplegia), gaze palsies, ptosis, and nystagmus. Visual disorders and disorders of the pupil are discussed in Chapter 16.

Nonparalytic Strabismus

Strabismus (squint), or abnormal ocular alignment, affects 3% to 4% of preschool children. Many individuals have a latent tendency for ocular misalignment, *heterophoria*, which becomes apparent only under stress or fatigue. During periods of misalignment the child may have diplopia or headache. Constant ocular misalignment is called *heterotropia*. Children with heterotropia suppress the image from one eye to avoid diplopia. If only one eye is used for fixation, visual acuity may be permanently lost in the other (developmental amblyopia).

In nonparalytic strabismus the amount of deviation in different directions of gaze is relatively constant (comitant). Each eye moves through a normal range when tested separately (ductions), but the eyes are disconjugate when used together (versions). Many children with chronic brain damage syndromes, such as malformations or perinatal asphyxia, have faulty fusion or faulty control of conjugate gaze mechanisms (nonparalytic strabismus). In neurologically normal children, the most common cause of nonparalytic

strabismus is either a genetic influence or an intraocular disorder. Ocular alignment in the newborn is usually poor, with transitory shifts of alignment from convergence to divergence. Constant ocular alignment usually begins after 3 months of age. Approximately 2% of newborns exhibit tonic downward deviation of the eyes during the waking state. The eyes assume a normal position during sleep and are able to move upward reflexively.

Esotropia

Esotropia is an inward deviation (convergence) of the eyes. Early-onset or infantile esotropia is noted before 1 year of age, and accommodative esotropia is usually noted between 2 and 3 years but may be delayed until adolescence.

CLINICAL FEATURES. Children with infantile esotropia often alternate fixation between eyes and may cross-fixate, that is, look to the left with the right eye and to the right with the left eye. The misalignment is sufficient to be noticed by family members. Some children fixate almost entirely with one eye and are at risk for permanent loss of visual acuity, *amblyopia*, in the other.

Accommodative esotropia occurs when accommodation is used to correct hyperopia. Accommodation causes the blurred hyperopic image to be more sharply focused. Because accommodation is accompanied by convergence, the eyes turn inward. Some children with accommodative esotropia cross-fixate so that both eyes are used alternatively. However, if one eye is more hyperopic than the other, the better eye may be used exclusively for fixation, and the unused eye has a considerable potential for amblyopia.

DIAGNOSIS. An ophthalmologist should examine the eyes to determine whether hyperopia is present.

MANAGEMENT. Hyperopic errors should be corrected with eyeglasses. Early-onset esotropia in which only one eye is used for fixation is treated with alternate patching of the eyes. Early corrective surgery is required for persistent esotropia.

Exotropia

Exotropia is an outward divergence of the eyes. It may be intermittent or constant.

CLINICAL FEATURES. Intermittent exotropia is a relatively common condition that begins before 4 years of age. It is most often evident when the child is fatigued and fixating on a far object or in bright sunlight. The natural history of the condition is unknown. Constant exotropia may be congenital but can also be caused by poor vision in the outward-turning eye.

DIAGNOSIS. The eyes must be examined for intraocular disease.

MANAGEMENT. In children with intermittent exotropia, the decision to perform corrective surgery depends on the frequency and degree of the abnormality. When exotropia is constant, treatment depends on the underlying cause of visual loss.

Ophthalmoplegia

Paralytic strabismus can be caused by disorders of the ocular motor nerves, the ocular muscles, or neuromuscular transmission. The muscles, the nerves, and their functions are summarized in Table 15-1. The eye appears to deviate in a direction opposite to the field of action of the paralyzed ocular muscle, and diplopia is experienced. Strabismus and separation of images are made worse when the child gazes in the direction of action of the paralyzed muscle.

Congenital Ophthalmoplegia

Ophthalmoplegia in the newborn is often missed because eye movements are infrequently tested. It is common for strabismus to remain unnoticed for several months and then to be discounted as transitory esotropia. Therefore, congenital ophthalmoplegia should be considered even when there is no history of ophthalmoplegia at birth.

Oculomotor Nerve Palsy

CLINICAL FEATURES. Congenital oculomotor nerve palsy usually is unilateral and complete. Pupillary reflex paralysis is variable. Other cranial nerve palsies, especially abducens, may be associated. The palsy often is not recognized at birth. Most palsies are idiopathic, but some are familial or caused by orbital trauma (Holmes et al, 1999). The affected eye is exotropic and usually amblyopic. Aberrant regeneration may be evidenced by lid retraction on attempted adduction or downward gaze.

DIAGNOSIS. Magnetic resonance imaging (MRI) is indicated to exclude the possibility of an intracranial mass compressing the nerve. Exophthalmos suggests an orbital tumor. A dilated pupil excludes the diagnosis of myasthenia gravis, but an edrophonium chloride (Tensilon) test is indicated if the pupil is normal (see later section on Myasthenia Gravis).

MANAGEMENT. Extraocular muscle surgery may improve the cosmetic appearance but rarely improves ocular motility or visual function.

Trochlear Nerve Palsy

CLINICAL FEATURES. Congenital superior oblique palsy is unilateral in 94% of cases. Birth trauma is often suspected but is rarely established. Most congenital cases are idiopathic. The head is tilted away from the paralyzed side to keep the eyes in alignment and avoid diplopia. The major ocular features are noncomitant hypertropia, greatest in the nasal field of the involved eye; underaction of the paretic superior oblique muscle and overaction of the inferior oblique muscle; and increased hypertropia when the head is tilted to the paralyzed side (positive *Bielschowsky test*).

Table 15-1
The Extraocular Muscles

Ocular Muscles	Innervation	Functions
Lateral rectus	Abducens	Abduction
Medial rectus	Oculomotor	Adduction
Superior rectus	Oculomotor	Elevation, intorsion, adduction
Inferior rectus	Oculomotor	Depression, extorsion, adduction
Inferior oblique	Oculomotor	Extorsion, elevation, abduction
Superior oblique	Trochlear	Intorsion, depression, abduction

DIAGNOSIS. Head tilt, or *torticollis* (see Chapter 14), is not a constant feature. Once a superior oblique palsy is confirmed by examination, important etiological considerations other than congenital ones include trauma, myasthenia gravis, and brainstem glioma.

MANAGEMENT. Most patients require surgery. Several procedures are available to restore the balance between the superior and inferior oblique muscles.

Abducens Nerve Palsy

CLINICAL FEATURES. Congenital abducens nerve palsy may be unilateral or bilateral and is sometimes associated with other cranial nerve palsies. Lateral movement of the affected eye(s) is limited partially or completely. Most infants use cross-fixation and thereby retain vision in both eyes. In the few reported cases of congenital palsy with pathological correlation, the abducens nerve is absent and its nucleus is hypoplastic.

Möbius syndrome is the association of congenital facial diplegia and bilateral abducens nerve palsies (see Chapter 17). *Duane syndrome* is aplasia of one or both nuclei of the abducens nerve with innervation of the atrophic lateral rectus by fibers of the oculomotor nerve. It is characterized by lateral rectus palsy, some limitation of adduction, and narrowing of the palpebral fissure because of globe retraction on attempted adduction. Other ocular, ear, and systemic malformations may be associated.

DIAGNOSIS. MRI is indicated to exclude the possibility of an intracranial mass lesion. Hearing should be tested.

MANAGEMENT. Surgical procedures may be useful to correct head turn and to provide binocular vision, but they do not restore ocular motility.

Brown Syndrome

Brown syndrome consists of mechanical limitation of elevation in adduction as a result of congenital shortening of the superior oblique muscle or tendon. Only one eye may be involved.

CLINICAL FEATURES. Elevation is limited in adduction but is relatively normal in abduction. Passive elevation (forced duction) is also restricted. Other features include widening of the palpebral fissure on adduction and backward head tilt.

DIAGNOSIS. Brown syndrome must be differentiated from acquired shortening of the superior oblique muscle caused by juvenile rheumatoid arthritis, trauma, and inflammatory processes affecting the top of the orbit (see section on Orbital Inflammatory Disease later in this chapter).

MANAGEMENT. Surgical procedures that extend the superior oblique muscle can be useful in congenital cases.

Congenital Fibrosis of the Extraocular Muscles

Congenital fibrosis of the extraocular muscles (CFEOM) is inherited as an autosomal dominant trait and maps to chromosome 12 (Engle et al, 1997).

CLINICAL FEATURES. Affected children have congenital bilateral ptosis and restrictive ophthalmoplegia, with their eyes partially or completely fixed in a downward position. CFEOM is a relatively static disorder that is phenotypically homogeneous when completely penetrant. Some children have mild delay in achieving milestones during infancy, and some have a mild facial diplegia. The head is tilted back to allow vision, and diplopia is not associated despite the severe misalignment of the eyes.

DIAGNOSIS. The diagnosis is based on the clinical findings and the family history. Laboratory studies are useful only to exclude other possibilities.

MANAGEMENT. Treatment is directed at improving vision by correcting ptosis.

Congenital Myasthenia Gravis

Several clinical syndromes of myasthenia gravis occur in the newborn (see Chapter 6). Congenital myasthenia gravis is the only one with ophthalmoplegia as the primary clinical feature. It is probably transmitted by autosomal recessive inheritance and may be caused by several underlying defects, including abnormal acetylcholine resynthesis or immobilization, reduced endplate acetylcholinesterase, and impaired function of the acetylcholine receptor (Engel et al, 1999).

CLINICAL FEATURES. Although these disorders are transmitted by autosomal recessive inheritance, a male-to-female bias of 2:1 exists. Symmetric ptosis and ophthalmoplegia are noted at birth or shortly thereafter. Mild facial weakness may be present but is not severe enough to impair feeding. If partial at birth, the ophthalmoplegia becomes complete during infancy or childhood. Generalized weakness sometimes develops.

DIAGNOSIS. The diagnosis should be suspected in any newborn with bilateral ptosis or limitation of eye movement. Intramuscular injection of edrophonium chloride produces a transitory improvement in ocular motility. Repetitive nerve stimulation of the limbs at a frequency of 3 Hz may evoke a decremental response that is reversible with edrophonium chloride. This suggests that the underlying defect, although producing symptoms only in the eyes, is already generalized at birth.

MANAGEMENT. No evidence of an immunopathy exists, and immunosuppressive therapy is not indicated. Thymectomy and corticosteroids are ineffective. Anticholinesterases may decrease facial paralysis but have little or no effect on ophthalmoplegia. The weakness in some children responds to 3,4-diaminopyridine (DAP), an agent that releases acetylcholine (Anlar et al, 1996). This drug is not commercially available in the United States but can be obtained on a compassionate use basis for individual patients from Jacobus Pharmaceutical Company, Princeton, New Jersey.

Congenital Ptosis

CLINICAL FEATURES. Congenital drooping of one or both lids is relatively common, and the drooping is unilateral in 70%. The cause is unknown, but the condition rarely occurs in other family members. Congenital ptosis is often unnoticed until early childhood or even adult life and then is thought to be an "acquired" ptosis. Miosis is sometimes an associated feature and suggests the possibility of a Horner syndrome, except that the pupil responds normally to pharmacological agents. Some patients have a synkinesis between the oculomotor and trigeminal nerves; jaw movements produce opening of the eye (*Marcus-Gunn phenomenon*).

DIAGNOSIS. The differential diagnosis of ptosis is listed in Table 15-2. Distinguishing congenital ptosis from acquired ptosis is essential. This is best accomplished by examining baby pictures. If miosis is present, the eye must be tested with pharmacological agents to determine whether sympathetic hypersensitivity is present. Concurrent paralysis of extraocular motility is evidence against congenital ptosis.

MANAGEMENT. Early corrective surgery is useful in elevating the lid to improve the appearance or when ptosis impairs vision.

Acute Unilateral Ophthalmoplegia

The causes of acquired ophthalmoplegia are summarized in Table 15-3. Many of the conditions are discussed in other chapters.

Table 15-2
Causes of Ptosis

Congenital
Congenital fibrosis of extraocular muscles
Horner syndrome
Myasthenia
Oculomotor nerve palsy

Acquired
Horner syndrome
Lid inflammation
Mitochondrial myopathies (see Chapter 8)
Myasthenia gravis
Oculomotor nerve palsy
Oculopharyngeal dystrophy (see Chapter 17)
Ophthalmoplegic migraine
Orbital cellulitis
Trauma

Acute ophthalmoplegia is defined as reaching maximum intensity within 1 week of onset. It may be partial or complete (Table 15-4). Generalized increased intracranial pressure is always an important consideration in patients with unilateral or bilateral abducens palsy (see Chapter 4).

Aneurysm

Arterial aneurysms are discussed fully in Chapter 4, because the important clinical feature in children is hemorrhage rather than nerve compression. This section deals only with possible ophthalmoplegic features.

CLINICAL FEATURES. Aneurysms at the junction of the internal carotid and posterior communicating arteries are an important cause of unilateral oculomotor palsy in adults but are a rare cause in children. The palsy is attributed to compression of the nerve by expansion of the aneurysm. Intense pain in and around the eye is frequently experienced at the time of hemorrhage. Because the parasympathetic fibers are at the periphery of the nerve, mydriasis is an almost constant feature of ophthalmoplegia caused by aneurysms of the posterior communicating artery. However, pupillary involvement may develop several days after onset of an incomplete ophthalmoplegia. A normal pupil with complete ophthalmoplegia effectively excludes the possibility of aneurysm.

The superior branch of the oculomotor nerve is sometimes affected earlier and more severely than the inferior branch. Ptosis may precede the development of other signs by hours or days.

DIAGNOSIS. Contrast-enhanced MRI and magnetic resonance angiography (MRA) identify most aneurysms.

Table 15-3
Causes of Acquired Ophthalmoplegia

Brainstem
Brainstem encephalitis (see Chapter 10)
Intoxication
Multiple sclerosis (see Chapter 10)
Subacute necrotizing encephalopathy (see Chapter 10)
Tumor
   Brainstem glioma
   Craniopharyngioma (see Chapter 16)
   Leukemia
   Lymphoma
   Metastases
   Pineal region tumors
Vascular
   Arteriovenous malformation
   Hemorrhage
   Infarction
   Migraine
   Vasculitis

Nerve
Familial recurrent cranial neuropathies (see Chapter 17)
Increased intracranial pressure (see Chapter 4)
Infectious
   Diphtheria
   Gradenigo syndrome
   Meningitis (see Chapter 4)
   Orbital cellulitis
Inflammatory
   Sarcoid
   Tolosa-Hunt syndrome
Postinfectious
   Idiopathic (postviral)
   Miller Fisher syndrome (see Chapter 10)
   Polyradiculoneuropathy (see Chapter 7)
Trauma
   Head
   Orbital
Tumor
   Cavernous sinus hemangioma
   Orbital tumors
   Sellar and parasellar tumors (see Chapter 16)
   Sphenoid sinus tumors
Vascular
   Aneurysm
   Carotid-cavernous fistula
   Cavernous sinus thrombosis
   Migraine

Neuromuscular Transmission
Botulism (see Chapter 7)
Myasthenia gravis
Tic paralysis

Myopathies
Fiber-type disproportion myopathies (see Chapter 6)
Kearns-Sayres syndrome
Mitochondrial myopathies (see Chapter 8)
Oculopharyngeal dystrophy (see Chapter 17)
Orbital inflammatory disease
Thyroid disease
Vitamin E deficiency

MANAGEMENT. Surgical clipping is the treatment of choice whenever technically feasible. Oculomotor function often returns to normal after the aneurysm is clipped.

Brainstem Glioma

CLINICAL FEATURES. Symptoms begin between 2 and 13 years of age, with a peak between ages 5 and 8. The period from onset of symptoms to diagnosis is less than 6 months. Cranial nerve palsies, usually abducens and facial, are the initial features in most cases. Later, contralateral hemiplegia and ataxia, dysphagia, and hoarseness develop. Hemiplegia at onset is associated with a more rapid course. With time, cranial nerve and corticospinal tract involvement may become bilateral. Increased intracranial pressure is not an early feature, but vomiting may be caused by direct irritation of the brainstem emetic center. Intractable hiccough, facial spasm, personality change, and headache are early symptoms in occasional patients.

Brainstem gliomas carry the worst prognosis of any childhood tumor. The course is one of steady progression, with median survival times of 9 to 12 months.

DIAGNOSIS. MRI delineates the tumor well and differentiates tumor from inflammatory and vascular disorders (Figure 15-1).

Table 15-4
Causes of Acute
Unilateral Ophthalmoplegia

Aneurysm*†
Brain tumors
   Brainstem glioma
   Parasellar tumors (see Chapter 16)
   Tumors of pineal region (see Chapter 4)
Brainstem stroke*
Cavernous sinus fistula
Cavernous sinus thrombosis
Gradenigo syndrome
Idiopathic cranial nerve palsy*
Increased intracranial pressure (see Chapter 4)
Multiple sclerosis* (see Chapter 10)
Myasthenia gravis*
Ophthalmoplegic migraine*†
Orbital inflammatory disease*†
Orbital tumor†
Recurrent familial* (see Chapter 17)
Tolosa-Hunt syndrome*†
Trauma
   Head
   Orbital

* May be recurrent.
† May be associated with pain.

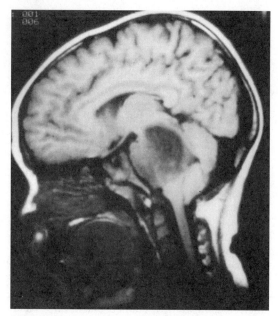

Figure 15-1. Brainstem glioma. MRI shows a large lesion infiltrating the brainstem.

MANAGEMENT. Radiation therapy is the treatment of choice. Several chemotherapeutic programs are undergoing experimental trials, but none is established as beneficial.

Brainstem Stroke

The causes of stroke in children are summarized in Table 11-2. Small brainstem hemorrhages resulting from emboli, leukemia, or blood dyscrasias have the potential to cause isolated ocular motor palsies, but this is not the rule. Other cranial nerves are also involved, and hemiparesis, ataxia, and decreased consciousness are often associated features.

Carotid-Cavernous Sinus Fistula

CLINICAL FEATURES. Arteriovenous communications between the carotid artery and the cavernous sinus may be congenital but are usually caused by trauma. The injury may be closed or penetrating. The carotid artery or one of its branches ruptures into the cavernous sinus, increasing pressure in the venous system. The results are a pulsating proptosis, redness and swelling of the conjunctiva, increased intraocular pressure, and ophthalmoplegia. A bruit, heard over the eye, is reduced in volume by compression of the ipsilateral carotid artery.

DIAGNOSIS. Carotid arteriography reveals rapid cavernous sinus filling, poor filling of the distal intracranial branches, and engorgement of and retrograde flow within venous drainage pathways.

MANAGEMENT. Transarterial balloon embolization of the affected cavernous sinus is the mainstay of treatment.

Cavernous Sinus Thrombosis

Cavernous sinus thrombosis may produce either unilateral or bilateral ophthalmoplegia. It is almost always caused by anterograde spread of infection from the mouth, face, nose, or paraspinal sinuses.

CLINICAL FEATURES. The development of fever, malaise, and frontal headache following dental infection is the typical history. Proptosis, orbital congestion, ptosis, external ophthalmoplegia, pupillary paralysis, and blindness may follow the initial symptoms. The infection begins in one cavernous sinus and spreads to the other. If untreated, it may extend to the meninges. Even with vigorous antibiotic treatment the mortality rate is 15%.

DIAGNOSIS. The ocular signs may suggest orbital cellulitis or orbital pseudotumor. The cerebrospinal fluid is normal early in the course. A mixed leukocytosis develops, and the protein concentration is moderately elevated even in the absence of meningitis. Once the meninges are involved, the pressure becomes elevated, the leukocytosis increases, and the glucose concentration falls.

Cranial CT may show clouding of infected paranasal sinuses. MRA shows decreased or absent flow in the cavernous portion of the carotid artery.

MANAGEMENT. The infection must be vigorously treated with intravenous antibiotics as if the child had meningitis. Surgical drainage of infected paranasal sinuses is sometimes necessary.

Gradenigo Syndrome

CLINICAL FEATURES. The abducens nerve lies adjacent to the medial aspect of the petrous bone before entering the cavernous sinus. Infections of the middle ear sometimes extend to the petrous bone and cause thrombophlebitis of the inferior petrosal sinus. The infection involves not only the abducens nerve but also the facial nerve and the trigeminal ganglion. The resulting syndrome is characterized by ipsilateral paralysis of abduction, facial palsy, and facial pain.

DIAGNOSIS. The combination of unilateral abducens and facial palsy can also be seen after closed head injuries. The diagnosis of Gradenigo syndrome requires the demonstration of middle-ear infection. Radiographs of the mastoid bone and lumbar puncture are indicated in all patients in whom the syndrome is suspected.

MANAGEMENT. Antibiotic therapy must be initiated early to prevent permanent nerve damage.

Idiopathic Cranial Nerve Palsy

CLINICAL FEATURES. The sudden onset of a single cranial neuropathy without apparent cause is frequently attributed to a prior viral infection. The pathophysiology is thought to be immune-mediated. However, a cause-and-effect relationship between viral infection and ocular motor palsies is not established.

The abducens nerve is more commonly affected than either the oculomotor or the trochlear nerve. Bilateral involvement is unusual. The complaints are of painless diplopia and paralytic strabismus. Girls are affected more often than are boys and the left eye more often than the right. Full motility is restored within 6 months, but shorter-duration recurrences occur in half of children.

DIAGNOSIS. Other causes of isolated nerve palsy must be excluded. Examination of the cerebrospinal fluid and MRI of the head and orbit are warranted in every child over the age of 15 years to exclude tumor and infection. Tumors in and around the orbit are sometimes difficult to demonstrate, and if ophthalmoplegia persists, a repeat MRI may be necessary. Younger children can be watched to see if the nerve palsy recovers spontaneously. Myasthenia gravis is always a consideration, and an edrophonium chloride test should be performed even though myasthenia gravis is less likely when there is a fixed single nerve deficit.

MANAGEMENT. Corticosteroids are not recommended. In children less than 9 years of age, intermittent patching of the normal eye may be necessary if the affected eye is not used for fixation.

Myasthenia Gravis

Some neonatal forms of myasthenia are discussed in Chapter 6; congenital myasthenia is included in the section "Congenital Ophthalmoplegia" earlier in this chapter, and limb-girdle myasthenia is discussed in Chapter 7. This section describes the immune-mediated form of myasthenia that is encountered from late infancy through adult life. Two clinical forms are recognized: *ocular myasthenia,* in which the eye muscles are primarily or exclusively affected but facial and limb muscles may also be mildly involved, and *generalized myasthenia,* in which weakness of bulbar and limb muscles is moderate to severe. The term *juvenile myasthenia* is sometimes used to denote immune-mediated myasthenia gravis in children, but because the disease is similar in children and adults the term should be discarded.

CLINICAL FEATURES. The initial symptoms do not appear until after 6 months of age; 75% of children first have symptoms after age 10. Prepubertal onset is associated with a male bias, only ocular symptoms, and seronegativity for acetylcholine receptor antibodies, whereas postpubertal onset is associated with a strong female bias, generalized myasthenia, and seropositivity. In general, boys have less severe disease than girls.

The initial features of both the ocular and the generalized form are usually ptosis, diplopia, or both. Myasthenia is the most common cause of unilateral or bilateral acquired ptosis. Pupillary function is normal. Between 40% and 50% of patients have weakness of other bulbar or limb muscles at the time of onset. Ocular motor weakness is generally not constant initially, and the specific muscles affected may change from examination to examination. Usually both eyes are affected, but one more than the other.

Children with ocular myasthenia may have mild facial weakness and easy fatigability of the limbs. However, they do not have respiratory distress or difficulty speaking or swallowing. The subsequent courses of ocular myasthenia may be characterized by steady progression to complete ophthalmoplegia or by relapses and remissions. The relapses are of varying severity and last for weeks to years. At least 20% of patients have permanent remissions. Prepubertal onset is more commonly associated with spontaneous remission than postpubertal onset.

Children with generalized myasthenia have generalized weakness within 1 year of the initial ocular symptoms. Dysarthria, dysphagia, difficulty chewing, and limb muscle fatigability are observed. Spontaneous remissions are unusual. Respiratory insufficiency (*myasthenic crisis*) occurs in a third of untreated children.

Children with generalized myasthenia, but not those with ocular myasthenia, have a higher than expected incidence of other autoimmune disorders, especially thyroiditis and collagen vascular diseases. Thymoma is present in 15% of adults with generalized myasthenia but occurs in less than 5% of children.

DIAGNOSIS. The edrophonium chloride test has been used as a standard of diagnosis for both the ocular and generalized forms of myasthenia gravis, but it has limitations. Edrophonium chloride is a short-acting anticholinesterase that is administered intravenously at a dose of 0.15 mg/kg. Before the test is initiated, an endpoint for the study must be determined. The best endpoint is the resolution of ptosis or the restoration of ocular motility, and test results are difficult to evaluate in their absence. Ptosis generally responds better to edrophonium chloride than does ocular motor paralysis.

Some patients with myasthenia are supersensitive to edrophonium chloride. Fasciculations and respiratory arrest may develop when a full dose is administered. For this reason, a test dose of one-tenth the full dose is injected first. Unfortunately, respiratory embarrassment sometimes develops in response to the test dose, and a hand ventilator should be readily available before any drug is given. Atropine is an effective antidote to the muscarinic side effects of edrophonium chloride but does not counteract the nicotinic effects on the motor endplate that result in paralysis of the skeletal muscles.

After the test dose is given, the remainder should be injected one third at a time (approximately 0.05 mg/kg), allowing up to 1 minute after each injection to test the response. Interpretation may be difficult. The judgment of improved strength is always subjective and may be influenced by examiner bias. The test becomes more objective when combined with electrophysiological studies. *I rarely use the edrophonium test for diagnosis and rely more on the clinical features, the serum antibody concentrations, and electrophysiological studies.*

Repetitive nerve stimulation study findings are abnormal in 66% of children when proximal nerves are stimulated but in only 33% when distal nerves are studied. Abnormal repetitive nerve study findings are unusual in children with ocular myasthenia but are the rule in children with generalized myasthenia. Patients with mild myasthenia show a decremental response at low rates of stimulation (2 to 5/sec) but not at high rates (50/sec). In severe myasthenia a decremental response is recorded at both low and high rates of stimulation.

The clinical features of myasthenia gravis are attributed to the presence of antibodies against the acetylcholine receptor. Elevated concentra-

tions of the antibody, greater than 10 nmol/L, are detected in the sera of 90% of patients with generalized myasthenia. Patients with ocular myasthenia may be seronegative or have low antibody concentrations. Early-onset, seronegative cases of immune-mediated ocular myasthenia are difficult to distinguish from genetic myasthenia. The distinction is important because one responds to immunotherapy and the other does not.

MANAGEMENT. The treatment selected depends on whether the child has ocular or generalized myasthenia. Children with ocular myasthenia have a reasonable hope of spontaneous remission, but those with generalized disease do not. Anticholinesterase therapy is the treatment of choice for ocular myasthenia. The initial dose of neostigmine is 0.5 mg/kg every 4 hours in children younger than 5 years of age and 0.25 mg/kg in older children, not to exceed 15 mg in any child. The equivalent dose of pyridostigmine is four times greater. After treatment is initiated, the dose is slowly increased as tolerated. Diarrhea and gastrointestinal cramps are the usual limiting factors. Edrophonium chloride should not be administered to determine whether the child would benefit from higher oral doses of anticholinesterases. It is not an accurate guide and may cause cholinergic crisis in children with generalized myasthenia.

Ocular myasthenia is difficult to treat. The response to anticholinesterase is often transitory, and the addition of corticosteroids is usually without benefit. The efficacy of any drug regimen in ocular myasthenia is difficult to assess because of the fluctuating course of the disease.

The place of thymectomy in the management of myasthenia is not established. Experience indicates that most children will be in remission within 3 years if thymectomy is performed early in the course of disease. However, the same result can be obtained with corticosteroids, and prior thymectomy does not reduce the need for long-term corticosteroid treatment.

Corticosteroids should be started at a dose of 1.5 mg/kg, not to exceed 100 mg/day. High-dose corticosteroids may make the patient weaker at first. After 5 days of daily treatment, an alternate-day regimen is used for the remainder of the month. The prednisone dose is then tapered by 10% each month until a dose is reached that keeps the patient symptom free. The usual maintenance dose is 10–20 mg every other day. I have been unsuccessful in eventually stopping prednisone. Anticholinesterase medication need not be given concurrently with corticosteroids but may be used if the patient weakens on the alternate days that corticosteroids are not taken.

The clinical characteristics and response to treatment of individuals with generalized myasthenia who are seronegative do not differ from the characteristics and response of those who are seropositive, except that seronegative patients are unlikely to show thymic abnormalities and are unlikely to benefit from thymectomy. Plasmapheresis, intravenous immunoglobulin, and high-dose intravenous corticosteroids are useful for acute intervention in patients who have respiratory insufficiency.

Ophthalmoplegic Migraine

The mechanism of ophthalmoplegia in migraine is not established. Although migraine is hereditary, the tendency for ophthalmoplegia is not.
CLINICAL FEATURES. Transitory ocular motor palsy, lasting sometimes as long as 4 weeks, may occur as part of a migraine attack in children and adults. The palsy affects the oculomotor nerve alone in 83% of cases and all three nerves in the remainder. Ptosis usually precedes ophthalmoplegia. Partial or complete pupillary involvement is present in 60%. The average age at onset is 15 years, but the onset may be as early as infancy. In infants, recurrent painless ophthalmoplegia or ptosis may be the only feature of the migraine attack. In older children, ophthalmoplegia usually occurs during the headache phase and is ipsilateral to the headache.
DIAGNOSIS. The diagnosis is obvious when ophthalmoplegia occurs during a typical migraine attack in a child previously known to have migraine. Diagnostic uncertainty is greatest when an infant has transitory strabismus or ptosis as an isolated sign. In such cases, a family history of migraine is essential for diagnosis. Even so, most infants with a first episode of ophthalmoplegia should be studied with MRI of the head and orbit to exclude other causes. A reversible enhancement and thickening of the cisternal segment of the oculomotor nerve is seen on contrast-enhanced MRI (Mark et al, 1998).
MANAGEMENT. Children with ophthalmoplegic migraine should be managed in the same manner as other children with migraine (see Chapter 3).

Orbital Inflammatory Disease

The term *orbital inflammatory disease* encompasses a group of nonspecific inflammatory conditions involving the orbit. Some experts include the Tolosa-Hunt syndrome as part of the spectrum. Inflammation may be diffuse or localized to specific tissues within the orbit (*orbital myositis*).
CLINICAL FEATURES. The disorder is unusual before age 20 years but may occur as early as 3 months of age. Males and females are affected equally. Acute and chronic forms are described.

The main features are pain, ophthalmoplegia, proptosis, and lid edema evolving over several days or weeks. One eye or both eyes may be involved. Ocular motility is disturbed in part by the proptosis but mainly by myositis. Some patients have only myositis, whereas others have inflammation in other orbital structures. Vision is initially preserved, but loss of vision is a threat if the condition remains untreated.
DIAGNOSIS. The development of unilateral pain and proptosis in a child should suggest an orbital tumor. Bilateral proptosis suggests thyroid myopathy. MRI shows a soft tissue mass without sinus involvement or bone erosion. This radiographic appearance may also be seen with orbital involvement by lymphoma or leukemia. The extraocular muscles may appear enlarged.
MANAGEMENT. Orbital inflammatory disease has a self-limited course but must be treated to prevent vision loss or permanent ophthalmoplegia. Prednisone, 1 mg/kg/day, should be administered for at least 1 month and then tapered. If the disorder recurs during the tapering, the full dose should be reinitiated.

Orbital Tumors

CLINICAL FEATURES. The initial feature of intraorbital tumors is proptosis, ophthalmoplegia, or ptosis. When the globe is displaced forward, the palpebral fissure is widened and it may not be possible to close the eye fully. As a consequence, the exposed portion of the eye becomes dry and erythematous and may suffer exposure keratitis. The direction of displacement of the globe is the best clue to the tumor's position. Ophthalmoplegia may occur because the globe is displaced forward, causing direct pressure on one or more ocular muscles.
DIAGNOSIS. The differential diagnosis of proptosis in children includes infection and inflammation, hemorrhage and other vascular disorders, orbital tumors, hyperthyroidism and other metabolic disorders, developmental anomalies, and Hand-Schüller-Christian disease and related disorders; some are idiopathic. The most common orbital tumors are dermoid

cyst, hemangioma, metastatic neuroblastoma, optic glioma, and rhabdomyosarcoma.

MANAGEMENT. Treatment varies with the tumor type. Surgical resection is indicated for many.

Tolosa-Hunt Syndrome

Tolosa-Hunt syndrome is a painful ophthalmoplegia attributed to an idiopathic granulomatous disease of the cavernous sinus or superior orbital fissure. No other structures are involved.

CLINICAL FEATURES. The pain is described as steady and penetrating, involving the entire hemicranium but centered around or behind the eye. It may precede the ophthalmoplegia by several days, may occur concurrently, or may appear later. The oculomotor nerve is ordinarily involved first and more severely than the two others, but all three ocular motor nerves, as well as the first and second divisions of the trigeminal nerve and the ocular sympathetic system, may be affected. Vision may be diminished; the pupil is usually small and may be reactive or nonreactive. Symptoms last for days or months. Spontaneous remissions occur, but partial neurological deficits may persist.

DIAGNOSIS. Tolosa-Hunt syndrome is easily confused with ophthalmoplegic migraine. The main features that distinguish the two entities are that patients with ophthalmoplegic migraine also have migraine without ophthalmoplegia, have family histories of migraine, and do not have trigeminal nerve involvement.

Tolosa-Hunt syndrome differs from orbital inflammatory disease by the absence of proptosis and the presence of trigeminal nerve involvement. Other diseases of the cavernous sinus, such as tumor or thrombosis, may resemble the Tolosa-Hunt syndrome.

The erythrocyte sedimentation rate is elevated in most patients. MRI shows alterations in the shape and signal of the cavernous sinus that are almost diagnostic.

MANAGEMENT. Prednisone, 1 mg/kg/day, is both diagnostic and therapeutic. If pain subsides within 2 days of initial administration, the diagnosis is likely but not certain. Other lesions in the cavernous sinus or orbit may also respond to corticosteroids. Ophthalmoplegia may subside but can take several days or weeks to clear completely. If prednisone fails to relieve the pain, the diagnosis of Tolosa-Hunt syndrome can be excluded and another cause must be identified.

Trauma

Trauma accounts for 40% of isolated acquired ocular motor nerve palsies and 55% of multiple nerve palsies in children. Hemorrhage and edema into the nerves or muscles may occur from closed head injuries even in the absence of direct orbital injury. When orbital fracture is present, the nerves and muscles may be lacerated, avulsed, or trapped by bone fragments.

CLINICAL FEATURES. Superior oblique palsy, caused by trochlear nerve damage, is a relatively common consequence of closed head injuries. Usually the trauma is severe, often causing loss of consciousness, but it may be mild. The palsy is more often unilateral than bilateral. Patients with unilateral superior oblique palsy have a marked hypertropia in the primary position and a compensatory head tilt to preserve fusion; 65% of cases resolve spontaneously. When bilateral involvement is present, the hypertropia is milder and alternates between the two eyes; spontaneous recovery occurs in only 25% of cases.

Transitory lateral rectus palsy is rare in newborns and has been attributed to birth trauma. The palsy is unilateral and clears completely within 6 weeks.

DIAGNOSIS. Direct injuries to the orbit with associated hemorrhage and swelling do not pose a diagnostic dilemma. CT of the head with orbital views shows the extent of fracture so that the need for surgical intervention can be determined. CT may also show a lateral midbrain hemorrhage as the cause of trochlear nerve palsy.

A greater problem of diagnosis is caused by a delay between the time of injury and the onset of ophthalmoplegia. The possible mechanisms of delayed ophthalmoplegia following trauma to the head include progressive local edema in the orbit; progressive brainstem edema; progressive increased intracranial pressure; development of meningitis, mastoiditis, or petrous osteomyelitis; venous sinus or carotid artery thrombosis; and carotid cavernous fistula.

MANAGEMENT. Local trauma and fracture of the orbit may require surgical repair. Permanent paralysis of ocular motor nerves following head injury is sometimes improved by surgery directed at rebalancing the extraocular muscles. Botulinum toxin is used for bilateral sixth nerve palsies.

Acute Bilateral Ophthalmoplegia

Many of the conditions that cause acute unilateral ophthalmoplegia (see Table 15-4) may also cause acute bilateral ophthalmoplegia. The con-

Table 15-5
Causes of Acute Bilateral Ophthalmoplegia

Basilar meningitis (see Chapter 4)
Brainstem encephalitis (see Chapter 10)
Carotid-cavernous fistula
Cavernous sinus thrombosis
Diphtheria
Intoxication
Miller Fisher syndrome (see Chapter 10)
Myasthenia gravis
Polyradiculoneuropathy (see Chapter 7)
Subacute necrotizing encephalomyelopathy (see Chapter 5)
Tick paralysis (see Chapter 7)

ditions listed in Table 15-5 often have a high incidence of bilateral involvement. Thyrotoxicosis is discussed with the chronic conditions because progression of ophthalmoplegia usually occurs over a period greater than 1 week.

Botulism

Several strains of the bacterium *Clostridium botulinum* elaborate a toxin that disturbs neuromuscular transmission. The infantile form of botulism causes ptosis but not ophthalmoplegia and is discussed in Chapter 6. This section deals with cases of later onset.

CLINICAL FEATURES. Botulism is most often caused by ingestion of toxin in home-canned food. This is most likely when canning is done at high altitudes, where the boiling temperature is too low to destroy spores. Because *C. botulinum* spores are ubiquitous in soil, infection may also follow burns and wounds. Blurred vision, diplopia, dizziness, dysarthria, and dysphagia begin 12 to 36 hours after ingestion of toxin. The pupillary response is usually normal. The early symptoms are followed by an ascending paralysis that suggests the Guillain-Barré syndrome and may lead to death from respiratory paralysis. Patients remain conscious and alert throughout. Most patients make a complete recovery within 2 to 3 months, but those with severe involvement may not return to normal for a year.

DIAGNOSIS. Botulism is distinguished from the Guillain-Barré syndrome by the presence of ophthalmoplegia and the EMG findings. The motor and sensory nerve conduction velocities are normal, evoked muscle action potentials are usually reduced in amplitude, and a decremental response is not ordinarily present at low rates of stimulation, although facilitation may be present at high rates of stimulation. The diagnosis is established by showing the organism or the toxin in food, stool, or a wound.

MANAGEMENT. The administration of antitoxin, 20,000 to 40,000 units two or three times a day, is recommended. The stomach and intestines should be emptied. 3,4-Diaminopyridine is effective in some patients and should be used for those with potential respiratory failure. Mechanical respiratory support must be made available as soon as the diagnosis is suspected.

Intoxications

CLINICAL FEATURES. Anticonvulsants, tricyclic antidepressants, and many other psychoactive drugs selectively impair ocular motility at toxic blood concentrations. The overdose may be accidental or intentional. A child is found unconscious and brought to the emergency department. The state of consciousness varies from obtundation to stupor, but the eyes cannot be made to move either by rapidly rotating the head laterally or with ice water irrigation of the ears. Complete ophthalmoplegia may be expected in a comatose child if brainstem function is otherwise impaired (see Chapter 2), but if it occurs in a noncomatose child with otherwise intact brainstem function, ingestion of a drug that selectively impairs ocular motility should be suspected.

DIAGNOSIS. The family should be questioned about drugs available in the household, and the blood and urine should be screened for toxic substances.

MANAGEMENT. Specific treatment depends on the drug ingested; in most cases, supportive care is sufficient.

Chronic Bilateral Ophthalmoplegia

The conditions responsible for bilateral ophthalmoplegia developing over a period longer than 1 week are listed in Table 15-6. Most are discussed in previous sections of this chapter or in other chapters.

Graves Ophthalmopathy

The association of ophthalmopathy with hyperthyroidism is not causal. The two conditions are associated autoimmune diseases. One hypothesis suggests the presence of a cross-reacting antigen in thyroid and orbital tissues. Myasthenia gravis may be associated as well.

Table 15-6
Causes of Chronic
Bilateral Ophthalmoplegia

Brainstem glioma
Chronic meningitis (see Chapter 4)
Chronic orbital inflammation
Graves ophthalmopathy
Kearns-Sayre syndrome
Myasthenia gravis
    Congenital
    Juvenile
Myopathies
    Fiber-type disproportion myopathy (see Chapter 6)
    Mitochondrial myopathies (see Chapter 8)
    Myotubular myopathy (see Chapter 6)
    Oculopharyngeal muscular dystrophy (see Chapter 17)
Subacute necrotizing encephalomyelopathy (see Chapter 5)
Thyroid disease
Vitamin E deficiency

CLINICAL FEATURES. Disorders of ocular motility are present in most patients with hyperthyroidism and may precede systemic features of nervousness, heat intolerance, diaphoresis, weight loss, tachycardia, tremulousness, and weakness. The main orbital pathology is a myopathy of the extraocular muscles. They become inflamed, swollen with interstitial edema, and finally fibrotic. If the two eyes are affected equally, the patient may not complain of diplopia despite considerable limitation of ocular motility. Staring or lid retraction (*Dalrymple sign*) occurs in more than 50% of cases, lid lag on downward gaze (*von Graefe sign*) in 30% to 50%, and proptosis (exophthalmos) in almost 90%. Severe exophthalmos is due to edema and infiltration of all orbital structures.

DIAGNOSIS. Thyroid disease should be considered in any child with evolving ophthalmoplegia. CT of the orbit shows enlargement of the extraocular muscles. Thyroid function tests are often normal, but a thyroid-releasing hormone stimulation test and a measure of the concentration of thyroid-stimulating immunoglobulin may confirm the diagnosis.

MANAGEMENT. Meticulous control of hyperthyroidism provides the best relief of the ophthalmopathy but is not necessarily curative. Hypothyroidism must be avoided. If the exophthalmos progresses, even after the patient is euthyroid, corticosteroids may prevent further proptosis, but surgical decompression is indicated if optic nerve compression persists.

Kearns-Sayre Syndrome

Kearns-Sayre syndrome is caused by deletions of mitochondrial DNA. Variability in the clinical syndrome reflects variability in the size of the deletion and the specific respiratory complex affected (see Chapter 8). Most cases are sporadic.

CLINICAL FEATURES. The invariable features of the disease are onset before 20 years of age, progressive external ophthalmoplegia, and pigmentary degeneration of the retina. At least one of three other features must also be present for diagnosis: heart block, cerebrospinal fluid protein level above 100 mg/dl, or cerebellar dysfunction.

DIAGNOSIS. Diagnosis is based on the major clinical criteria. Electrocardiographic monitoring for cardiac arrhythmia and examination of the cerebrospinal fluid are essential.

MANAGEMENT. Treatment with vitamins or co-enzyme Q, depending on the specific respiratory complex defect, may be beneficial in some patients. A cardiac pacemaker may be lifesaving.

Gaze Palsies

This section deals with supranuclear palsies. The examiner must show that the eyes move normally in response to brainstem gaze center reflexes (doll's head maneuver, caloric testing, and Bell's phenomenon) to verify supranuclear palsy. The differential diagnosis of gaze palsies is listed in Table 15-7.

Apraxia of Horizontal Gaze

Ocular motor apraxia is a deficiency in voluntary, horizontal, lateral, fast eye movements (saccades) with retention of slow pursuit movements. Jerking movements of the head are used to bring the eyes to a desired position. The rapid phase of optokinetic nystagmus is absent.

Congenital Ocular Motor Apraxia

CLINICAL FEATURES. Although ocular motor apraxia is present at birth, it is usually not detected until late infancy. Visual impairment may be suspected because of failure of fixation. Overshooting head thrusts, often accompanied by blinking of the eyes, are used for refixation. When the head is held immobile, the child makes no effort to initiate horizontal eye movements.

Many children with ocular motor apraxia have other signs of cerebral abnormality, such as psychomotor retardation, learning disabilities, and clumsiness. When hypotonia is present, the child may have difficulty making the head movements needed for refixation. Agenesis of the corpus callosum and agenesis of the cerebellar ver-

Table 15-7
Gaze Palsies

Apraxia of Horizontal Gaze
Ataxia-telangiectasia (see Chapter 10)
Ataxia-ocular motor apraxia (see Chapter 10)
Brainstem glioma
Congenital ocular motor apraxia
Huntington's disease (see Chapter 5)

Internuclear Ophthalmoplegia
Brainstem stroke
Brainstem tumor
Exotropia (pseudo-internuclear ophthalmoplegia [INO])
Multiple sclerosis
Myasthenia gravis (pseudo-INO)
Toxic-metabolic

Vertical Gaze Palsy
Aqueductal stenosis (see Chapter 18)
Congenital vertical ocular motor apraxia
Gaucher's disease (see Chapter 5)
Hydrocephalus (see Chapters 4 and 18)
Miller Fisher syndrome (see Chapter 10)
Niemann-Pick's disease, type C (see Chapter 5)
Tumor (see Chapter 4)
    Midbrain
    Pineal region
    Third ventricle

Horizontal Gaze Palsy
Adversive seizures (see Chapter 1)
Brainstem tumors
Destructive lesions of the frontal lobe (see Chapter 11)
Familial horizontal gaze palsy

Convergence Paralysis
Head trauma
Idiopathic
Multiple sclerosis (see Chapter 10)
Pineal region tumors (see Chapter 4)

mis are concurrent conditions in some children. The association does not indicate that the malformations are responsible for ocular motor apraxia.

DIAGNOSIS. The possibility of ocular motor apraxia must be considered in any infant referred for evaluation of visual impairment. Once the presence of apraxia is established, MRI is indicated to search for other cerebral malformations, and tests for ataxia-telangiectasia (see Chapter 10) and lysosomal storage diseases (see Chapter 5) should be performed.

MANAGEMENT. Management depends on the underlying condition.

Internuclear Ophthalmoplegia

The medial longitudinal fasciculus (MLF) contains fibers that connect the abducens nucleus to the contralateral oculomotor nucleus for the purpose of performing horizontal conjugate lateral gaze. Unilateral lesions in the MLF disconnect the two nuclei, so that when the patient attempts lateral gaze, the adducting eye ipsilateral to the abnormal MLF is unable to move medially but the abducting eye is able to move laterally. Nystagmus (actually *overshoot dysmetria*) is often present in the abducting eye. This symptom complex, which may be unilateral or bilateral, is called *internuclear ophthalmoplegia* (INO). Unilateral INO is usually caused by vascular occlusive disease and bilateral INO by demyelinating disease or toxic-metabolic causes.

Patients with myasthenia gravis sometimes have ocular motility dysfunction that resembles an INO except that nystagmus is usually lacking. The disorder is referred to as *pseudo-INO* because the MLF is intact. Pseudo-INO can also be caused by exotropia. When the normal eye is fixating in full abduction, there is no visual stimulus to bring the paretic eye into full adduction. Nystagmus is not present in the abducting eye.

The combination of an INO in one direction of lateral gaze and complete gaze palsy in the other is called a *one-and-a-half syndrome*. The underlying pathology is a unilateral lesion in the dorsal pontine tegmentum that affects the pontine lateral gaze center and the adjacent MLF. It is usually caused by multiple sclerosis but may be caused by brainstem glioma, infraction, or myasthenia gravis.

Toxic-Metabolic Disorders

CLINICAL FEATURES. Toxic doses of several drugs may produce the clinical syndrome of INO. The patient is usually found comatose and may have complete ophthalmoplegia that evolves into a bilateral INO, or a bilateral INO may be present at onset. The drugs reported to produce INO include amitriptyline, barbiturates, carbamazepine, doxepin, phenothiazine, and phenytoin. INO may also occur during hepatic coma.

DIAGNOSIS. Drug intoxications are always a consideration in children with decreased consciousness who were previously well. The presence of INO following drug ingestion suggests the possibility of anticonvulsant or psychotropic drug ingestion.

MANAGEMENT. The INO resolves as the blood concentration of the drug falls.

Vertical Gaze Palsy

Children with supranuclear vertical gaze palsies are unable to look upward or downward fully, but they retain reflex eye movements such as the Bell phenomenon. Disorders of upward gaze in children are generally due to damage to the dorsal midbrain and are almost always caused by tumors in the pineal region. The usual features are impaired upward and downward gaze, eyelid retraction, and occasional disturbances in horizontal movement, convergence, and skew deviation. Mydriasis with light-near dissociation is an early feature of extrinsic compression of the dorsal midbrain. Isolated paralysis of upward gaze may be the initial feature of the Miller Fisher syndrome and of vitamin B_1 deficiency.

Bilateral lesions in the midbrain reticular formation cause isolated disturbances of downward gaze. They are rare in children but may occur in neurovisceral lipid storage disease.

Congenital Vertical Ocular Motor Apraxia

CLINICAL FEATURES. Congenital vertical ocular motor apraxia is a rare syndrome similar to congenital horizontal ocular motor aparxia, except for the direction of gaze palsy. At rest the eyes are fixed in either an upward or a downward position, with little random movement. Head flexion or extension is used initially to fixate in the vertical plane; later, the child learns to use head thrusts. The Bell phenomenon is present. DIAGNOSIS. Vertical gaze palsy suggests intracranial tumor, and MRI must be performed. However, gaze palsies present from birth without the later development of other neurological signs usually indicate a nonprogressive process. Bilateral restriction of upward eye movement resulting from muscle fibrosis must also be considered. However, in children with ocular motor apraxia, the eyes can move upward reflexively or by forced ductions; in children with muscle fibrosis, the eyes will not move upward by any means.

Horizontal Gaze Palsy

Inability to look to one side is generally caused by a lesion in the contralateral frontal or ipsilateral pontine gaze center. Immediately after frontal lobe lesions develop, the eyes are tonically deviated toward the side of the lesion and contralateral hemiplegia is often present. The eyes can be made to move horizontally by stimulation of the brainstem gaze center with ice water caloric techniques. In contrast, an irritative frontal lobe lesion, such as one causing an epileptic seizure, generally causes the eyes to deviate in a direction opposite to the side with the seizure

focus. Movements of the head and eyes during a seizure are called *adversive seizures* (see Chapter 1). The initial direction of eye movement reliably predicts a contralateral focus, especially if the movement is forced and sustained in a unilateral direction. Later movements that are mild and unsustained are not predictive.

Convergence Paralysis

Convergence paralysis, inability to adduct the eyes to focus on a near object in the absence of medial rectus palsies, can be caused by a pineal region tumor; in such cases, however, other signs of midbrain compression are usually present. Convergence paralysis is sometimes factitious or due to lack of motivation or attention. This can be identified by the absence of pupillary constriction when convergence is attempted.

Convergence insufficiency is frequently encountered after closed head injuries. The head injury need not be severe. Diplopia, headache, or eyestrain during reading or other close work is reported. Convergence insufficiency also occurs in the absence of prior head injury. The onset often follows a change in study time or intensity, poor lighting in the workplace, or the use of new contact lenses or eyeglasses. Treatment consists of convergence exercises.

Nystagmus

Nystagmus is an involuntary, rhythmic oscillation of the eyes in which at least one phase is slow. With *pendular nystagmus,* the movements in each direction are slow. The oscillations of congenital pendular nystagmus are in the horizontal plane even on vertical gaze. On lateral gaze the oscillations may change to jerk nystagmus.

Movements of unequal speed characterize *jerk nystagmus.* An initial slow component in one direction is followed by a fast component with saccadic velocity in the other direction. Oscillation may be horizontal or vertical. The direction of jerk nystagmus is named for the fast (saccadic) component. Nystagmus intensity increases in the horizontal plane when gaze is in the direction of the fast phase.

Table 15-8 describes other eye movements that cannot be classified as nystagmus but that have diagnostic significance. *Opsoclonus* consists of conjugate, rapid, chaotic movements in all directions of gaze, often referred to as "dancing eyes." It occurs in infants with neuroblas-

Table 15-8
Abnormal Eye Movements

Movement	Appearance	Pathology
Nystagmus	Rhythmic oscillation	Variable
Opsoclonus	Nonrhythmic, chaotic conjugate movements	Neuroblastoma
Ocular flutter	Intermittent bursts of rapid horizontal oscillations during fixation	Cerebellar/brainstem disease
Ocular dysmetria	Overshooting, undershooting, or oscillation on refixation	Cerebellar disease
Ocular bobbing	Intermittent, rapid downward movement	Pontine lesions
Periodic alternating gaze	Cyclic conjugate lateral eye deviations, alternating from side to side	Posterior fossa

toma (see Chapter 10). *Ocular flutter* is a brief burst of conjugate horizontal saccadic eye movements that interrupt fixation. It occurs in the recovery phase of opsoclonus or in association with cerebellar disease. *Ocular dysmetria* is either an overshoot or undershoot of the eyes during refixation or an oscillation before the eyes come to rest on a new fixation target. *Ocular bobbing* is not downbeat nystagmus, but is a sudden downward movement of both eyes with a slow drift back to midposition. It is most often seen in comatose patients with pontine dysfunction. Congenital and acquired nystagmus are discussed separately because their differential diagnoses are different (Table 15-9).

Physiological Nystagmus

A high-frequency (1 to 3 Hz), low-amplitude oscillation of the eyes occurs normally when lateral gaze is sustained to the point of fatigue. A jerk nystagmus, present at the endpoint of lateral gaze, is also normal. A few beats are usual, but even sustained nystagmus occurring at the endpoint should be considered normal unless it is associated with other signs of neurological dysfunction or is distinctly asymmetric.

Congenital Nystagmus

Although congenital nystagmus is present at birth, it may not be noticed until infancy or childhood and then is misdiagnosed as acquired nystagmus. One reason that it may not be noticed is that the *null point,* the angle of ocular movement at which the nystagmus is minimal, may be very wide. Often the nystagmus is observed but is mistaken for normal movement.

The cause of congenital nystagmus is thought to be a defect in the gaze-holding mechanism. In the past, it was thought that loss of visual

acuity before the age of 2 years, regardless of cause, could produce nystagmus and that the nystagmus could be reversed by correction of the visual disturbance. It is now generally accepted that the visual defect is not causal, but associated, and intensifies the underlying defect in neural control.

Congenital nystagmus is sometimes inherited. The pattern of inheritance may be autosomal recessive, autosomal dominant, or X linked.

Table 15-9
Differential Diagnosis of Nystagmus

Physiological

Congenital
Associated with blindness
Familial
Idiopathic

Spasmus Nutans
Idiopathic
Tumors of optic nerve and chiasm (see Chapter 16)

Acquired Nystagmus
Pendular
   Brainstem infarction
   Multiple sclerosis (see Chapter 10)
   Oculopalatal syndrome
      Brainstem infarction
      Spinocerebellar degeneration
Jerk
   Horizontal
      Drug induced
      Ictal nystagmus
      Vestibular nystagmus
   Vertical
      Downbeat
      Upbeat
Dissociated
   Divergence
   Monocular
   See-saw

CLINICAL FEATURES. Congenital nystagmus is almost always horizontal in plane but may be either pendular or jerk in character. It is generally diminished by convergence and increased by fixation. Because a null zone exists where nystagmus is minimal, the head may be held to one side, or tilted, or both to improve vision. Periodic head turning may accompany periodic alternating nystagmus.

Two forms of head oscillation are associated with congenital nystagmus. One is involuntary and does not improve vision. The other, also seen in spasmus nutans, is opposite in direction to the nystagmus but not phase locked and improves vision. Many children have impaired vision from the nystagmus in the absence of a primary disturbance in visual acuity.

DIAGNOSIS. Determination that the nystagmus was present at birth is important but not always possible. The eyes must be carefully examined for abnormalities in the sensory system that may be accentuating nystagmus. If the neurological findings are otherwise normal, MRI is unnecessary.

MANAGEMENT. Nystagmus may be reduced by correcting a visual defect, particularly with contact lenses rather than eyeglasses, and by the use of prisms or surgery to move the eyes into the null zone without the head's turning.

Spasmus Nutans

Spasmus nutans is difficult to classify as either a congenital or an acquired nystagmus. It is probably never present at birth; the onset is early in infancy. Nystagmus, head nodding, and abnormal head positioning are the clinical features of spasmus nutans.

CLINICAL FEATURES. Onset typically occurs between 6 and 12 months of age. Nystagmus is characteristically binocular (but may be monocular), has high frequency and low amplitude, is often dysconjugate, and can be horizontal, vertical, or torsional in direction. The head is held in a tilted position and titubates in a manner that resembles nodding. Head tilt and movement may be more prominent than nystagmus, and torticollis is often the first complaint (see Chapter 14). The syndrome usually lasts for 1 to 2 years, sometimes as long as 5 years, and then resolves spontaneously.

DIAGNOSIS. Spasmus nutans is ordinarily a transitory, benign disorder of unknown cause. On rare occasions, the syndrome may be mimicked by a glioma of the anterior visual pathways or by subacute necrotizing encephalopathy (see

Chapter 10). Tumor should be considered if the nystagmus is monocular, the optic nerve is pale, or the onset is after 1 year of age. Imaging of the head and orbit is not needed in typical cases (Arnoldi and Tychsen, 1995).

MANAGEMENT. Treatment is not needed.

Acquired Nystagmus

Pendular Nystagmus

Pendular nystagmus may be either congenital or acquired. In adults, the usual causes of acquired pendular nystagmus are brainstem infarction and multiple sclerosis. In children, pendular nystagmus in the absence of other neurological signs is either congenital or the first sign of spasmus nutans. However, the development of optic atrophy in a child with pendular nystagmus indicates a glioma of the anterior visual pathway.

Vertical pendular nystagmus is unusual and sometimes occurs in association with rhythmic vertical oscillations of the palate (*palatal myoclonus or tremor*). This syndrome of oculopalatal oscillation is encountered in some spinocerebellar degenerations and ischemic disorders of the deep cerebellar nuclei and central tegmental tract.

Jerk Nystagmus

Drug-Induced Nystagmus

CLINICAL FEATURES. Many psychoactive drugs, including tranquilizers, antidepressants, anticonvulsants, and alcohol, produce nystagmus at high therapeutic or toxic blood concentrations. The nystagmus is horizontal or horizontal-rotary and is augmented by lateral gaze. Vertical nystagmus may be present on upward but rarely on downward gaze. Phenytoin and carbamazepine occasionally produce primary-position downbeat nystagmus as well.

DIAGNOSIS. Drug overdose should be suspected in patients with nystagmus and decreased consciousness. A drug screen and measurement of drug blood concentrations are indicated.

MANAGEMENT. Nystagmus resolves when the blood concentration of the drug falls.

Ictal Nystagmus

CLINICAL FEATURES. Nystagmus as a seizure manifestation is binocular. It can be jerk, pendular, or rotary, and it may occur alone or in association with other ictal manifestations. Pupillary oscillations synchronous with the nystagmus may be observed. As a rule, concurrent epileptiform discharges are focal, contralateral to the fast phase of nystagmus, and frontal, parietooccipital, or occipital. However, individual cases of nystagmus accompanying generalized 3-Hz spike-wave discharges, ipsilateral focal discharges, and periodic lateralized epileptiform discharges are reported.

DIAGNOSIS. Other seizure manifestations that identify the nature of the nystagmus are usually present. The electroencephalogram (EEG) confirms the diagnosis by the presence of epileptiform activity concurrent with nystagmus.

MANAGEMENT. Ictal nystagmus responds to anticonvulsant drug therapy (see Chapter 1).

Vestibular Nystagmus

Vestibular nystagmus occurs with disorders of the labyrinth, vestibular nerve, vestibular nuclei of the brainstem, or vestibulocerebellum.

CLINICAL FEATURES. Labyrinthine disease (especially labyrinthitis) is usually associated with severe vertigo, nausea, and vomiting (see Chapter 17). Deafness or tinnitus is often present as well. Movement of the head enhances the nystagmus and is more critical to the mechanism of nystagmus than the position obtained. Nystagmus is usually horizontal and torsional, with an initial linear slow phase followed by a rapid return. It is worse when gaze is in the direction of the fast phase. Fixation reduces nystagmus and vertigo.

Vertigo and nausea are mild when nystagmus is of central origin. Nystagmus is constantly present and is not affected by head position. It may be horizontal or vertical and is not affected by fixation. Other neurological disturbances referable to the brainstem or cerebellum are frequently associated features.

DIAGNOSIS. Vestibular nystagmus is readily identified by observation and is identical to the nystagmus provoked by caloric stimulation or rotation. Labyrinthine disorders in children are almost always infectious, sometimes viral, and sometimes a result of otitis media. Central causes of vestibular nystagmus include spinocerebellar degeneration, brainstem glioma or infarction, subacute necrotizing encephalomyelitis, periodic ataxias, and demyelinating disorders.

MANAGEMENT. Several different classes of drugs appreciably reduce the vertigo and nausea associated with labyrinthine disease. Diazepam is especially effective. Other useful drugs include scopolamine, antihistamines, and tranquilizers.

Downbeat Nystagmus

CLINICAL FEATURES. In primary position the eyes drift slowly upward and then spontaneously beat downward. The intensity of the nystagmus is usually greatest when the eyes are directed slightly downward and laterally. Downbeat nystagmus should be distinguished from *downward-beating nystagmus,* in which the nystagmus is present only on downward gaze. Downward-beating nystagmus is usually caused by toxic doses of anticonvulsant and sedative drugs, whereas downbeat nystagmus indicates a structural abnormality of the brainstem, especially the cervicomedullary junction or cerebellum. Patient complaints include dizziness, oscillopsia, blurred vision, and difficulty reading. Approximately one third of patients are asymptomatic. Cerebellar ataxia is present in about half of patients and usually is the only associated neurological sign.

DIAGNOSIS. Cerebellar degenerations, both congenital and acquired, are the most common identifiable cause. The Chiari malformation must be considered as well. Metabolic disturbances include phenytoin toxicity and hypomagnesemia resulting from either dietary depletion or the use of lithium salts.

A congenital hereditary downbeat nystagmus in a mother and son was noted in the boy at birth. By infancy he needed to keep his chin down to look at people. He had no other neurological abnormalities, but the nystagmus caused difficulty in learning to read. His mother had a subclinical downbeat nystagmus evident only in oblique downward gaze.

MANAGEMENT. Oscillopsia and acuity can be improved in some individuals by the use of clonazepam. A single test dose of 1 mg can be tried to determine whether long-term therapy will be useful. Trihexyphenidyl may prove effective when clonazepam fails. Prisms that increase convergence may also be useful.

Upbeat Nystagmus

CLINICAL FEATURES. In primary position the eyes drift slowly downward and then spontaneously beat upward. Upward gaze accentuates the nystagmus. A large- and a small-amplitude type are described. Large-amplitude nystagmus increases in intensity during upward gaze and indicates a lesion in the anterior vermis of the cerebellum or an abnormality in the anterior visual pathway. Anterior visual pathway abnormalities include Leber congenital amaurosis, bilateral optic nerve hypoplasia, and congenital cataract (see Chapter 16). Small-amplitude nystagmus decreases in intensity during upward gaze and, when present, suggests an intrinsic lesion of the medulla.

DIAGNOSIS. Upbeat nystagmus is usually an acquired disorder caused by vascular lesions or tumors of the brainstem or cerebellar vermis. Therefore, cranial MRI is indicated in every child with a normal anterior visual pathway. Upbeat nystagmus also occurs with impairment of smooth pursuit movements in dominantly inherited cerebellar vermian atrophy.

MANAGEMENT. No specific treatment is available.

Dissociated Nystagmus

Divergence Nystagmus

Divergence nystagmus is a rare condition in which both eyes beat outward simultaneously. The mechanism is poorly understood, but the condition suggests an abnormality in the posterior fossa and may be seen with spinocerebellar degenerations.

Monocular Nystagmus

Monocular nystagmus may be congenital or acquired. The most important diagnostic considerations in children are spasmus nutans and chiasmal tumors. Although no clinical feature consistently differentiates the two groups, optic nerve abnormalities, especially optic hypoplasia, are sometimes found in children with tumors but not in those with spasmus nutans.

A coarse pendular vertical nystagmus may develop in an amblyopic eye years after the visual loss. The nystagmus is noted in the blind eye when distance fixation is attempted with the sighted eye and is inhibited by convergence.

See-Saw Nystagmus

See-saw nystagmus is the result of two different oscillations. One is a pendular vertical oscillation. The other is a torsional movement in which one eye rises and intorts while the other falls and extorts. It may be congenital or acquired. The congenital form is sometimes associated with absence of the chiasm and a horizontal pendular nystagmus. Acquired cases are usually due to tumors of the sellar and parasellar regions and are associated with bitemporal hemianopia.

References

Anlar B, Varli K, Ozdimir E, et al. 3, 4-Diaminopyridine in childhood myasthenia: Double-blind, placebo-controlled trial. *J Child Neurol* 1996; 11:458–461.

Arnoldi KA, Tychsen L. Prevalence of intracranial lesions in children initially diagnosed with disconjugate nystagmus (spasmus nutans). *J Pediatr Ophthalmol Strabismus* 1995;32:296–301.

Engel AG, Ohno K, Sine SM. Congenital myasthenic syndromes. *Arch Neurol* 1999;56:163–167.

Engle EC, Goumnerov BC, McKeown CA, et al. Oculomotor nerve and muscle abnormalities in congenital fibrosis of the extraocular muscles. *Ann Neurol* 1997;41:314–327.

Holmes JM, Mutyala S, Maus T, et al. Pediatric third, fourth, and sixth nerve palsies: A population-based survey. *Am J Ophthalmol* 1999;127:388–392.

Mark AS, Casselman J, Brown D, et al. Ophthalmoplegic migraine: Reversible enhancement and thickening of the cisternal segment of the oculomotor nerve on contrast-enhanced MR images. *AJNR* 1998;19:1887–1891.

Waltz K, Lavin PJM. Accommodative insufficiency. In: Margo CE, Hamed RN, eds. *Diagnostic Problems in Clinical Ophthalmology*. WB Saunders: Philadelphia; 1993;862–866.

Chapter 16
Disorders of the Visual System

BOTH CONGENITAL AND acquired visual impairments in children are often associated with neurological disorders. The most common causes are refractive errors, congenital cataracts, and genetic disorders. Two conditions that are increasing in frequency are retrolental fibroplasia as a consequence of improved survival of premature babies and retinal hemorrhage caused by child abuse.

Assessment of Visual Acuity

The assessment of visual acuity in preverbal children relies mainly on assessing fixation and following and on observing the way an infant or young child interacts with the environment.

Clinical Assessment

The pupillary light reflex is an excellent test of the functional integrity of the afferent and efferent pathways and is reliably present after 31 weeks' gestation. A blink response to light develops at about the same time, and the lid may remain closed for as long as light is present (the *dazzle reflex*). The blink response to threat may not be present until 5 months of age. These responses are integrated in the brainstem and do not provide information on the cognitive (cortical) aspects of vision.

Fixation and following are the principal means to assess visual function in newborns and infants. The human face, at a distance of approximately 30 cm, is the best target for fixation. After fixation is obtained, the examiner slowly moves from side to side to test the *following response*.

Visually directed grasping is present in normal children by 3 months of age but is difficult to test before 6 months of age. Absence of visually directed grasping may indicate a motor rather than a visual disturbance.

Visual fields can be evaluated in infants and young children by eliciting a refixation reflex when a stimulus is moved in the peripheral field.

Clues to visual impairment are structural abnormalities (e.g., microphthalmia, cloudy cornea), an absent or asymmetric pupillary response to light, dysconjugate gaze, nystagmus, and failure to fixate or follow.

Visual Evoked Response

The visual evoked response to strobe light is an excellent technique for showing the anatomical integrity of subcortical visual pathways without patient cooperation. A positive "cortical" wave with a peak latency of 300 ms is first demonstrated at 30 weeks' gestation. The latency linearly declines at a rate of 10 ms each week throughout the last 10 weeks of gestation. In the newborn, the morphology of the visual evoked response is variable during wakefulness and active sleep and is best studied just after the child goes to sleep. By 3 months of age, the morphology and latency of the visual evoked response are mature.

Congenital Blindness

Cortical blindness is the most common cause of congenital blindness among children referred to a neurologist. The causes are numerous and include prenatal and perinatal disturbances. Optic nerve hypoplasia, with or without other ocular

Table 16-1
Corneal Clouding in Childhood

Cerebrohepatorenal syndrome (Zellweger syndrome)
Congenital syphilis
Fabry disease (ceramide trihexosidosis)
Familial high-density lipoprotein deficiency (Tangier island disease)
Fetal alcohol syndrome
Infantile GM_1 gangliosidosis
Juvenile metachromatic dystrophy
Marinesco-Sjögren disease
Mucolipidosis
Mucopolysaccharidoses
Multiple sulfatase deficiency
Pelizaeus-Merzbacher disease

malformations, is second in frequency, followed by congenital cataracts and corneal opacities. Corneal abnormalities usually do not cause visual loss unless clouding is extensive. Such extensive clouding may occur in the mucopolysaccharidoses and Fabry disease. Table 16-1 lists those conditions in which corneal clouding is present during childhood.

Congenital Cataract

For the purpose of this discussion, congenital cataract includes cataracts discovered within the first 3 months. The differential diagnosis is listed in Table 16-2.

Table 16-2
Lens Abnormalities in Childhood

Congenital Cataract
Chromosomal aberrations
  Trisomy 13
  Trisomy 18
  Trisomy 21*
  Turner syndrome*
Drug exposure during pregnancy
  Chlorpromazine
  Corticosteroids
  Sulfonamides
Galactokinase deficiency
Galactose-1-phosphate uridyltransferase deficiency
Galactosemia
Genetic
  Autosomal dominant inheritance
    Hereditary spherocytosis*
    Incontinentia pigmenti*
    Marshall syndrome*
    Myotonic dystrophy*
    Schafer syndrome*
    Without other anomalies
  Autosomal recessive inheritance
    Congenital ichthyosis*
    Congenital stippled epiphyses (Conradi disease)
    Marinesco-Sjögren syndrome*
    Siemens syndrome*
    Smith-Lemli-Opitz syndrome
  X-linked inheritance (oculocerebrorenal syndrome)*
    Idiopathic
    Intrauterine infection*
    Mumps
    Rubella
    Syphilis
  Maternal factors
    Diabetes
    Malnutrition
    Radiation
    Prematurity

Syndromes of uncertain etiology
  Hallerman-Streiff syndrome
  Pseudo-Turner syndrome*
  With oxycephaly
  With polydactyly

Acquired Cataract
Drug induced
  Corticosteroids
  Long-acting miotics
Genetic
  Autosomal dominant inheritance (Alport syndrome)
  Autosomal recessive inheritance
    Cockayne disease
    Hepatolenticular degeneration (Wilson disease)
    Rothmund-Thompson syndrome
    Werner syndrome
  X-linked inheritance (pseudo-pseudohypoparathyroidism)
Chromosomal (Prader-Willi syndrome)
Metabolic
  Cretinism
  Hypocalcemia
  Hypoparathyroidism
  Juvenile diabetes
  Pseudohypoparathyroidism
Trauma
Varicella (postnatal)

Dislocated Lens
Crouzon syndrome
Ehlers-Danlos syndrome
Homocystinuria
Hyperlysinemia
Marfan syndrome
Sturge-Weber syndrome
Sulfite oxidase deficiency

* Cataracts may not be noted until infancy or childhood.

In previous studies, approximately one third of congenital cataracts were attributed to intrauterine infection. That percentage has declined with prevention of rubella embryopathy by immunization. Genetic and chromosomal disorders account for at least one third, and the cause cannot be determined in half of the cases. When cataract is the only hereditary abnormality, genetic transmission is usually by autosomal dominant inheritance; when hereditary cataracts are associated with other features composing a syndrome, the mode of genetic transmission varies. In many hereditary syndromes, cataracts can be either congenital or delayed in appearance until infancy, childhood, or even adulthood. Several of these syndromes are associated with dermatoses: *incontinentia pigmenti* (irregular skin pigmentation), *Marshall syndrome* (anhidrotic ectodermal dysplasia), *Schafer syndrome* (follicular hyperkeratosis), *congenital ichthyosis,* and *Siemens syndrome* (cutaneousatrophy).

Congenital cataracts occur in approximately 10% of children with trisomy 13 and trisomy 18 and in most children with trisomy 21. Cataracts develop by puberty in up to 40% of children with Turner syndrome. The association of congenital cataract and lactic acidosis or cardiomyopathy indicates a mitochondrial disorder.

CLINICAL FEATURES. Small cataracts do not impair vision and may be difficult to detect by direct ophthalmoscopy. Large cataracts appear as a white mass in the pupil and, if left in place, quickly lead to loss of visual acuity. The initial size of a cataract does not predict its course; congenital cataracts may remain stationary or increase in density but never improve spontaneously. Other congenital ocular abnormalities, aniridia, coloboma, and microphthalmos occur in 40% to 50% of newborns with congenital cataracts.

DIAGNOSIS. Large cataracts are obvious on inspection. Smaller cataracts distort the normal red reflex when the direct ophthalmoscope is held at arm's length distance from the eye and a +12 to +20 lens is used.

Genetic disorders and maternal drug exposure should be considered when cataracts are the only abnormality. Intrauterine disturbances, such as maternal illness and fetal infection, are usually associated with growth retardation and other malformations. Chromosome analysis should be performed for all children with dysmorphic features. Galactosemia is suspected in children with hepatomegaly and milk intolerance (see Chapter 5), but cataracts may be present even before the development of systemic features.

MANAGEMENT. Early recognition and removal of cataracts before age 3 months is important to prevent developmental amblyopia. Urgent referral to a pediatric ophthalmologist is warranted.

Congenital Optic Nerve Hypoplasia

Optic nerve hypoplasia is a developmental defect in the number of optic nerve fibers and may result from excessive regression of retinal ganglion cell axons. Hypoplasia may be bilateral or unilateral and varies in severity. It may occur as an isolated defect and cause astigmatism or it may be associated with intracranial anomalies. The most common association is with midline defects of the septum pellucidum and hypothalamus (*septo-optic dysplasia*). Septo-optic dysplasia is familial in some cases and probably transmitted as an autosomal recessive trait (chromosome 3p21).

CLINICAL FEATURES. When hypoplasia is severe, the child is blind and attention is drawn to the eyes at birth because of strabismus and nystagmus. Ophthalmoscopic examination reveals a small, pale nerve head (Figure 16-1). A pigmented area surrounded by a yellowish mottled halo is sometimes present at the edge of the disk margin, giving the appearance of a double ring.

The degree of hypothalamic-pituitary involvement varies. Possible symptoms include neonatal hypoglycemia and seizures, recurrent

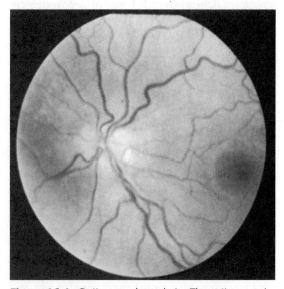

Figure 16-1. Optic nerve hypoplasia. The optic nerve is small and pale, but the vessels are of normal size.

hypoglycemia in childhood, growth retardation, diabetes insipidus, and sexual infantilism. Some combination of mental retardation, cerebral palsy, and epilepsy is often present and indicates malformations in other portions of the brain.

DIAGNOSIS. Cranial magnetic resonance imaging (MRI) and an assessment of endocrine status should be performed on all infants with ophthalmoscopic evidence of optic nerve hypoplasia. The common findings on MRI are cavum septum pellucidum, hypoplasia of the cerebellum, aplasia of the corpus callosum, aplasia of the fornix, and an empty sella (Willnow et al, 1996). Endocrine studies should include assays of growth hormone, antidiuretic hormone, and the integrity of hypothalamic-pituitary control of the thyroid, adrenal, and gonadal systems. Infants with hypoglycemia usually have growth hormone deficiency.

MANAGEMENT. No treatment is available for optic hypoplasia, but endocrine abnormalities respond to replacement therapy. Children with corticotrophin deficiency may experience sudden death (Brodsky et al, 1997).

Congenital Coloboma

Congenital coloboma is a defect in embryogenesis that may affect only the disk or may include the retina, iris, ciliary body, and choroid. Colobomas isolated to the nerve head appear as deep excavations. They may be unilateral or bilateral. The causes of congenital coloboma are genetic (monogenic and chromosomal) and intrauterine disease (toxic and infectious). Retinochoroidal colobomas are glistening white or yellow defects inferior or inferonasal to the disk. The margins are distinct and surrounded by pigment. *Morning glory disk,* a form of coloboma, is an enlarged dysplastic disk with a white excavated center surrounded by an elevated annulus of pigmentary change. Retinal vessels enter and leave at the margin of the disk, giving the appearance of a morning glory flower.

Leber Congenital Amaurosis

Leber congenital amaurosis (LCA), a group of autosomal recessive retinal dystrophies, is the most common genetic causes of congenital visual impairment. Mutations on chromosomes 17, 1, and 19 cause a similar clinical syndrome.

CLINICAL FEATURES. Blindness is present at birth or shortly thereafter and may be associated with pendular nystagmus, upbeat nystagmus, and photophobia. Ophthalmoscopy of the retina shows no abnormality in infancy and early childhood, but with time, progressive retinal stippling and pallor of the disk appear. Mental retardation and other neurological disturbances may be associated.

DIAGNOSIS. The disease is seldom diagnosed in infancy because the retina appears normal. Electroretinography is the primary method for detecting the widespread retinal degeneration. Neuroimaging shows cerebellar atrophy in children who are mentally slow (Casteels et al, 1996). Other disorders that may be mistaken for LCA are peroxisomal disorders and several varieties of infantile-onset progressive retinal degeneration.

MANAGEMENT. The retinopathy is not reversible.

Acute Monocular or Binocular Blindness

The differential diagnoses of acute and progressive blindness show a considerable overlap. Although older children recognize sudden visual loss, slowly progressive ocular disturbances may produce an asymptomatic decline until vision is severely disturbed. When finally noticed, the child's loss of visual acuity seems to be recent. Slowly progressive visual disturbances are often noted first by a teacher or parent rather than by the child. Table 16-3 lists conditions in which visual acuity is normal and then suddenly lost. Table 16-4 lists disorders in which the underlying pathological process is progressive; in most of these conditions the patient quickly perceives the visual loss. Therefore, both tables should be consulted in the differential diagnosis of acute blindness. The duration of a transitory monocular visual loss suggests the underlying cause: seconds indicate disk swelling, minutes indicate emboli, hours indicate migraine, and days indicate optic neuropathy, most commonly optic neuritis.

Cortical Blindness

Cortical blindness in children may be permanent or transitory, depending on the cause. Transitory cortical blindness in childhood can be caused by migraine (see Chapter 3), mild head trauma, brief episodes of hypoglycemia or hypotension, mitochondrial disorders, and benign occipital epilepsy (see Chapter 1). Acute and sometimes permanent blindness may occur following anoxia; as a result of massive infarction of, or hemorrhage into, the visual cortex; and when

Table 16-3
Causes of Acute Loss of Vision

Carotid Dissection (see Chapter 11)

Cortical Blindness
Anoxic encephalopathy (see Chapter 2)
Benign occipital epilepsy (see Chapter 1)
Hydrocephalus
Hypoglycemia
Hypertension (malignant or accelerated)
Hyperviscosity
Hypotension
Migraine (see Chapter 3)
Occipital metastatic disease
Posttraumatic transient cerebral blindness
Systemic lupus erythematosus
Toxic (cyclosporine, etc.)
Trauma

Hysteria

Optic Neuropathy
Demyelinating
    Idiopathic optic neuritis
    Multiple sclerosis (see Chapter 10)
    Neuromyelitis optica (see Chapter 12)
Ischemic
Toxic
Traumatic

Pituitary Apoplexy

Pseudotumor Cerebri (see Chapter 4)

Retinal Disease
Central retinal artery occlusion
Migraine
Trauma

---

multifocal metastatic tumors or abscesses are located in the occipital lobes.

The main feature of cortical blindness is loss of vision with preservation of the pupillary light reflex. Fundoscopic examination is normal.

Hypoglycemia

Repeated episodes of acute cortical blindness may occur at the time of mild hypoglycemia in children with glycogen storage diseases and following insulin overdose in diabetic children.
CLINICAL FEATURES. Sudden blindness is associated with clinical evidence of hypoglycemia (sweating and confusion). Ophthalmoscopic and neurological findings are normal. Recovery is complete in 2 to 3 hours.
DIAGNOSIS. During an episode of cortical blindness caused by hypoglycemia, electroencephalography (EEG) shows high-voltage slowing over both occipital lobes. Afterward the EEG returns to normal.

MANAGEMENT. Glucose can be given during the attack, but treatment may not be needed.

Transitory Posttraumatic Cerebral Blindness

CLINICAL FEATURES. Transitory posttraumatic cerebral blindness is a benign syndrome that most often occurs in children with a history of migraine or epilepsy. The spectrum of visual disturbance is broad, but a juvenile and an adolescent pattern have been delineated. In children younger than 8 years, the precipitating trauma is usually associated with either a brief loss of consciousness or a report that the child was "stunned." Blindness is noted almost immediately on recovery of consciousness and lasts for an hour or less. During the episode, the child may be lethargic and irritable but is usually coherent. Recovery is complete, and the child may not recall the event.

In older children, a syndrome of blindness, confusion, and agitation begins several minutes

---

Table 16-4
Causes of Progressive Loss of Vision

Compressive Optic Neuropathies
Aneurysm (see Chapters 4 and 15)
Arteriovenous malformations (see Chapters 4, 10, and 11)
Craniopharyngioma
Hypothalamic and optic tumors
Pituitary adenoma
Pseudotumor cerebri (see Chapter 4)

Disorders of the Lens (see Table 16-3)
Cataract
Dislocation of the lens

Hereditary Optic Atrophy
Leber hereditary optic neuropathy
Wolfram syndrome

Intraocular Tumors

Tapetoretinal Degenerations
Abnormal carbohydrate metabolism
    Mucopolysaccharidosis (see Chapter 5)
    Primary hyperoxaluria
Abnormal lipid metabolism
    Abetalipoproteinemia (see Chapter 10)
    Hypobetalipoproteinemia (see Chapter 10)
    Multiple sulfatase deficiency (see Chapter 5)
    Neuronal ceroid lipofuscinosis (see Chapter 5)
    Niemann-Pick disease (see Chapter 5)
    Refsum disease (see Chapter 7)
Other syndromes of unknown etiology
    Bardet-Biedl syndrome
    Cockayne syndrome
    Laurence-Moon syndrome
    Refsum disease (see Chapter 7)
    Usher syndrome (see Chapter 17)

or hours after trivial head trauma. Consciousness is not lost. All symptoms resolve after several hours, and the child has complete amnesia for the event. These episodes share many features with acute confusional migraine and are probably a variant of that disorder (see Chapter 2).

DIAGNOSIS. Children with any neurological abnormality following head trauma invariably have a head computed tomography (CT), but this is probably unnecessary if the blindness has cleared. Those with persistent blindness require MRI to exclude injury to the occipital lobes. Occipital intermittent rhythmic delta on EEG suggests migraine as the underlying cause. Recognition of the syndrome can avoid the trouble and expense of other studies. The family history should be scrutinized for the possibility of migraine or epilepsy. The rapid and complete resolution of all symptoms confirms the diagnosis.

MANAGEMENT. Treatment is not needed if the symptoms resolve spontaneously.

Hysterical Blindness

A claim of complete binocular blindness is easily identified as spurious. A pupillary response to light indicates that the anterior pathway is intact and only cerebral blindness is a possibility. Visual function can be assessed by using a full-field optokinetic stimulus tape or by moving a large mirror in front of the patient to stimulate matching eye movements. When monocular blindness is claimed, the same tests can be performed with a patch covering the normal eye.

Spurious claims of partial visual impairment are more difficult to challenge. Helpful tests include observing visual behavior, failure of acuity to improve linearly with increasing test size, inappropriate ability to detect small test objects on a tangent screen, and constricted (tunnel) visual fields to confrontation.

Optic Neuropathies

Demyelinating Optic Neuropathy

Demyelination of the optic nerve (optic neuritis) may occur as an isolated finding affecting one or both eyes, or it may be associated with demyelination in other portions of the nervous system. *Neuromyelitis optica* (Devic syndrome), the syndrome combining optic neuritis and transverse myelitis, is discussed in Chapter 12 and multiple sclerosis in Chapter 10. MRI is a useful technique for surveying the central nervous system for demyelinating lesions (see Figure 10-3). The incidence of later multiple sclerosis among children with optic neuritis is 15% or less if the child has no evidence of more diffuse involvement when brought to medical attention. The incidence is almost 100% when diffuse involvement is present or when optic neuritis recurs within 1 year. Unilateral optic neuritis has a higher incidence of later multiple sclerosis than does bilateral optic neuritis.

CLINICAL FEATURES. Monocular involvement is the rule in adults, but binocular involvement occurs in more than half of children. Binocular involvement may be concurrent or sequential, sometimes occurring over a period of weeks. The initial feature in some children is pain in the eye, but for most it is blurred vision, progressing within hours or days to partial or complete blindness. Visual acuity is reduced to less than 20/200 in almost all patients within 1 week. A history of a preceding "viral" infection or immunization is often presented, but a cause-and-effect relationship between optic neuritis and these events is not established.

Results of ophthalmoscopic examination may be normal at the onset of symptoms if neuritis is primarily retrobulbar. However, most children have papillitis rather than retrobulbar neuritis, and the nerve head is swollen and hemorrhagic, resembling papilledema. The two conditions are readily distinguished because optic neuritis is characterized by early and severe visual loss with afferent pupillary defect and papilledema is not.

Neuroretinitis is the association of swelling of the optic nerve head with macular edema or a macular star. Ophthalmoscopic examination shows disk swelling, peripapillary retinal detachment, and a macular star (Figure 16-2). Neuroretinitis suggests the possibility of conditions other than idiopathic optic neuritis.

In the absence of myelitis, the prognosis in children with bilateral optic neuritis is good. Complete recovery occurs in 90% of those affected.

DIAGNOSIS. Optic neuritis must be considered when monocular or binocular blindness develops suddenly in a child. The diagnosis is often established by ophthalmoscopic or slit-lamp examination. Further confirmation can be accomplished by testing the visual evoked response. MRI of the orbit often reveals swelling and demyelination of the optic nerve. Examination of the cerebrospinal fluid is unnecessary. Such examination sometimes shows a leukocytosis and an increased concentration of protein but does

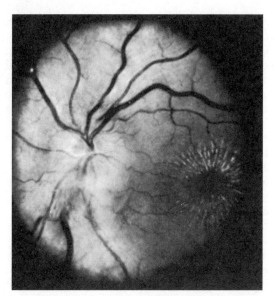

Figure 16-2. Neuroretinitis. The optic disk is swollen with peripapillary nerve fiber layer opacification. Exudates surround the macula in a star pattern. (Courtesy of Patrick Lavin, MD)

not provide information about the etiology or prognosis.

MANAGEMENT. Intravenous methylprednisolone, 250 mg every 6 hours for 3 days, followed by oral prednisone, 1 mg/kg/day for 14 days, speeds the recovery of visual loss and, in adults, may reduce the rate of development of multiple sclerosis over a 2-year period. Oral corticosteroids should not be used alone.

Ischemic Optic Neuropathy

Infarction of the anterior portion of the optic nerve is rare in children and is usually associated with systemic vascular disease or hypotension. **CLINICAL FEATURES.** Ischemic optic neuropathy usually occurs as a sudden segmental loss of vision in one eye, but slow or stepwise progression over several days is possible. Recurrent episodes are unusual except with migraine and some idiopathic cases. **DIAGNOSIS.** Altitudinal visual field defects are present in 70% to 80% of patients. Color vision loss is roughly equivalent in severity to visual acuity loss, whereas in demyelinating optic neuritis, color vision is affected more than visual acuity. Ophthalmoscopic examination reveals diffuse or partial swelling of the optic disk. When swelling is diffuse, it gives the appearance of papilledema and flame-shaped hemorrhages may be present adjacent to the disk margin.

After acute swelling subsides, optic atrophy follows.
MANAGEMENT. Treatment depends on the underlying disorder causing ischemia.

Leber Hereditary Optic Neuropathy

This condition is described in the section on Hereditary Optic Neuropathy.

Toxic-Nutritional Optic Neuropathies

Drugs, toxins, and nutritional deficiencies alone or in combination may cause an acute or progressive optic neuropathy. These factors may cause optic neuropathy by inducing mitochondrial changes, perhaps in susceptible populations with mitochondrial DNA (mtDNA) mutations.
CLINICAL FEATURES. Implicated drugs include barbiturates, antibiotics (chloramphenicol, isoniazid, streptomycin, sulfonamides), chemotherapeutic agents, chlorpropamide, digitalis, ergot, halogenated hydroxyquinolines, penicillamine, and quinine. Nutritional deficiencies that may cause such optic neuropathies include folic acid vitamins B_1, B_2, B_6, and B_{12}.

Symptoms vary with the specific drug, but progressive loss of central vision is typical. In some cases, visual loss is rapid and develops as acute binocular blindness that may be asymmetric at onset, suggesting monocular involvement. Many of the drugs produce optic neuropathy by interfering with the action of folic acid or vitamin B_{12} and thereby causing a nutritional deficiency.
DIAGNOSIS. Drug toxicity should be suspected whenever central and paracentral scotomas develop during the course of drug treatment. Optic nerve hyperemia with small paracentral hemorrhages may be an early feature. Later the disk becomes pale.
MANAGEMENT. Drug-induced optic neuropathy is dose related. Dosage reduction may be satisfactory in some cases, especially if concurrent treatment with folic acid or vitamin B_{12} reverses the process. Some drugs must be discontinued completely.

Traumatic Optic Neuropathies

Trauma to the head may cause an indirect optic neuropathy in one or both eyes. The nerve is tethered along its course and therefore subject to shearing forces when the skull suddenly accelerates or decelerates. Possible consequences include acute swelling, hemorrhage, or tear. This is particularly common in children who sustain bicycle injuries when not wearing a helmet.

CLINICAL FEATURES. Loss of vision is usually immediate. Delayed visual loss caused by a hematoma or edema may respond to corticosteroids and has a better prognosis. Traumatic optic neuropathy is readily distinguished from cortical blindness because the pupillary response is diminished or absent. The prognosis for recovery is best if there is a brief delay between the time of injury and the onset of blindness.

DIAGNOSIS. The loss of vision and pupillary light response immediately following a head injury should suggest the diagnosis. Peripapillary hemorrhages may be seen by ophthalmoscopic examination.

MANAGEMENT. Corticosteroids and surgical decompression of the nerve are suggested.

Pituitary Apoplexy

Pituitary apoplexy is a rare, life-threatening condition caused by hemorrhagic infarction of the pituitary gland.

CLINICAL FEATURES. Pituitary infarction occurs most often when there is a preexisting pituitary tumor but may also occur in the absence of tumor. Several different clinical features are possible, depending on which structures are affected by the swollen gland. These include any of the following, alone or in combination: monocular or binocular blindness, visual field defects, ophthalmoplegia, chemical meningitis, cerebrospinal fluid rhinorrhea, and shock from hypopituitarism. Leakage of blood and necrotic material into the subarachnoid space causes chemical meningitis associated with headache, meningismus, and loss of consciousness.

DIAGNOSIS. MRI of the head with views of the pituitary gland establishes the diagnosis. Endocrine testing may show a deficiency of all pituitary hormones.

MANAGEMENT. Patients deteriorate rapidly and may die within a few days if corticosteroids are not administered promptly. Other hormones must also be replaced but are not lifesaving. In patients who continue to do poorly, as evidenced by loss of consciousness, hypothalamic instability, or loss of vision, require urgent surgical decompression of the expanding pituitary mass.

Retinal Disease

Central Retinal Artery Occlusion

Migraine and coagulopathies are the main predisposing disorders among children with retinal artery obstruction. Others are sickle cell disease, cardiac disorders, vasculitis, and pregnancy. Congenital heart disease is the usual preexisting condition causing emboli to the central retinal artery in young people. Mitral valve prolapse is a potential cause but is more likely to produce transitory cerebral ischemia than monocular blindness.

CLINICAL FEATURES. Most affected children have an abrupt loss of monocular vision of variable intensity without premonitory symptoms. Some describe spots, a shadow, or a descending veil before the loss of vision. Bilateral retinal artery occlusion is uncommon in children.

DIAGNOSIS. The diagnosis of retinal artery obstruction is usually based on the clinical history and ophthalmoscopic examination. The posterior pole of the retina becomes opacified except in the foveal region, where a cherry-red spot is seen. The peripheral retina appears normal. Visual field examination and fluorescein angiography help confirm the diagnosis in some cases. Once the diagnosis is established, the underlying causes must be found. Evaluation should include auscultation of the heart, radiographs of the chest, echocardiography in selected cases, complete blood cell count with sedimentation rate, cholesterol and triglyceride screening, coagulation studies, hemoglobin electrophoresis, and lupus anticoagulant and antiphospholipid antibodies.

MANAGEMENT. Acute treatment requires immediate ophthalmological consultation. The management of idiopathic occlusion of the retinal artery in adults is controversial, with some authorities recommending the use of corticosteroids. In children, giant cell arteritis is not a consideration and corticosteroids are not indicated. Visual acuity is more likely to improve when the obstruction is in a branch artery rather than in the central retinal artery.

Retinal Migraine

CLINICAL FEATURES. Visual symptoms are relatively common during an attack of classic migraine (see Chapter 3). The typical scintillating scotomas, or "fortification spectra," are field defects caused by altered neuronal function in the occipital cortex. The affected field is contralateral to the headache.

Transitory monocular blindness is an unusual feature of migraine. Careful questioning is needed to differentiate a field defect from a monocular defect. Migraine is the main cause of transitory monocular blindness in children. The visual loss is sudden in most cases, may be partial or complete, and often precedes and is ipsilateral to the headache. Recurrences are usually in the same eye, and attacks may occur without headache.

Typical patients have a long history of migraine with aura in which both field defects and monocular blindness are experienced separately or together. The visual aberrations are often described as a mosaic or jigsaw pattern of scotomas that clear within minutes. Permanent monocular blindness is unusual and occurs mainly in adolescent and adult women. Many patients with persistent blindness have other risk factors for vascular disease, such as the use of oral contraceptives or vasculitis.

DIAGNOSIS. The diagnosis can be considered when there is a history of migraine with aura. Ophthalmoscopic findings may be normal initially and then include retinal edema with scattered hemorrhages. Several patterns of retinal vaso-occlusive disease may be observed by fluorescein angiography: branch retinal artery, central retinal artery, central retinal vein, and cilioretinal artery.

MANAGEMENT. Children who have retinal ischemia during migraine attacks should be treated with agents that prevent further episodes. Verapamil is the most effective drug against retinal migraine.

Retinal Trauma

Direct blunt injury to the orbit causes visual impairment by retinal contusion, tear, or detachment. All three are characterized by a diminished pupillary response. Contusion is associated with retinal edema. Although visual loss is immediate, the retina appears normal for the first few hours and only later becomes white and opaque. The severity of visual loss varies, but complete recovery is the rule.

Retinal tear is often associated with vitreous hemorrhage. Visual loss is usually immediate and easily diagnosed by its ophthalmoscopic appearance. Recovery is spontaneous unless there is detachment, for which cryotherapy is required.

Progressive Loss of Vision

Compressive Optic Neuropathy

Compression of one or both optic nerves often occurs in the region of the chiasm. Visual loss may be confined to one eye or to a visual field. In children with tumors in and around the diencephalon, the most constant feature is growth failure. This may not be recognized until other symptoms develop.

Craniopharyngioma

CLINICAL FEATURES. The initial features of craniopharyngioma in children are growth retardation, visual disturbances, endocrinopathies, and failure of sexual maturation. Field defects are frequently asymmetric or unilateral. Bitemporal hemianopsia is present in 50% of children, with craniopharyngioma and homonymous hemianopsia in 10% to 20%. Visual acuity is always diminished in one or both eyes.

Approximately 25% of children have hydrocephalus that causes headache and papilledema. Hypothalamic involvement may produce diabetes insipidus or the *hypodipsia-hyponatremia syndrome,* characterized by lethargy, confusion, and hypotension. Other features depend on the direction of tumor growth. Anterior extension may compress the olfactory tract, causing anosmia, whereas lateral extension may compress the third and fifth nerves.

DIAGNOSIS. MRI readily visualizes craniopharyngiomas.

MANAGEMENT. Surgical resection is the initial treatment, but the recurrence rate is 50%, and radiotherapy is then initiated. The 5- and 10-year survival rates after postoperative radiotherapy are 84% and 72% for children. Radiation improves visual field defects and visual acuity without causing optic atrophy. The treatment causes endocrine disturbances and intellectual impairment. Hormone replacement therapy is needed.

Optic Pathway and Diencephalic Gliomas

Optic pathway gliomas are pilocytic astrocytomas. They are difficult to distinguish by histological criteria from tumors arising in the thalamus and hypothalamus. Optic gliomas represent 3% to 5% of childhood brain tumors. More than 50% of children with optic gliomas have neurofibromatosis type 1 (NF1). Precocious puberty is a common initial feature in children with NF1. The rate of tumor growth is slower in children with NF1 than when NF1 is not present.

CLINICAL FEATURES. Initial symptoms depend on the location, but hypothalamic tumors eventually affect the optic chiasm and optic chiasm tumors affect the hypothalamus. In children younger than 3 years, tumors of the hypothalamus may produce the *diencephalic syndrome,* characterized by marked loss of subcutaneous fat and total body weight with maintenance or acceleration of long bone growth. Despite the appearance of cachexia, the infant is mentally alert and does not seem as sick as the appearance suggests. Pendular nystagmus is usually associated. The precise endocrine mechanism of the diencephalic syndrome has never been clarified. Hamartomas of the tuber cinereum, optic pathway gliomas that compress the hypothalamus, and craniopharyngiomas are also associated with the diencephalic syndrome. Precocious puberty, rather than the diencephalic syndrome, can be the initial feature of hypothalamic tumors in infants and children.

Slowly progressive loss of vision is the initial feature in children with optic gliomas (Listernick et al, 1997). Monocular visual loss suggests optic nerve involvement but also may occur with tumors of the chiasm. Binocular involvement suggests involvement of the optic chiasm or tract. Visual field deficits vary. Tumors in or near the orbit may produce proptosis, optic disk swelling in which blurring of the disk resembles papilledema, and central loss of vision. Ophthalmoplegia is unusual.

Increased intracranial pressure suggests extension of tumor from the chiasm to the hypothalamus. When this is the initial feature, the site of tumor origin is difficult to determine.

DIAGNOSIS. MRI of the hypothalamus identifies gliomas as high-density signals on T_2-weighted studies. MRI permits visualization of the hypothalamus in several different planes and identification of brainstem extension of tumor (Figure 16-3).

MRI with enhancement identifies optic pathway gliomas as an enlarged tubular appearance of the nerve and chiasm. In evaluating children with optic gliomas, the entire visual pathway must be visualized, because many tumors involve the chiasm and retrochiasmal pathways. MRI screening for optic pathway gliomas in asymptomatic children with NF1 does not affect the outcome (Listernick et al, 1997).

MANAGEMENT. Stereotaxic-guided biopsy of hypothalamic tumors may cause more damage than diagnostic information, and imaging criteria are often used to develop a therapeutic plan. Tumors located in the floor of the fourth ventricle, lateral recesses, cerebellar pontine angle, or cervical medullary junction may be surgically accessible and have a more benign course. Radiotherapy provides 5-year survival rates of 20% to 30%.

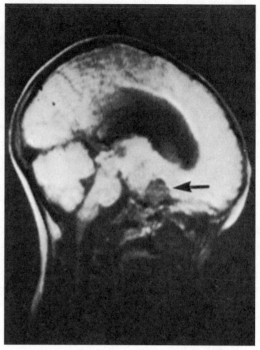

Figure 16-3. Optic nerve glioma identified by MRI (*arrow*).

Optic pathway gliomas are slow-growing tumors, and those associated with NF1 rarely progress after the time of diagnosis. The decision to biopsy or remove a tumor from a sighted eye is recommended only when the tumor is believed to be malignant and likely to cause blindness or death.

Pituitary Adenoma

Pituitary adenomas represent only 1% to 2% of intracranial tumors of childhood. Visual field defects may be unilateral temporal, bitemporal, or occasionally homonymous. Optic atrophy is present in 10% to 20% of cases.

CLINICAL FEATURES. The onset of symptoms is usually during adolescence. The presenting features relate to the hormone secreted by the tumor. Approximately one third of adenomas secrete prolactin, one third are nonfunctioning, and many of the rest secrete growth hormone or adrenocorticotropic hormone (ACTH) (Thapar et al, 1995). Amenorrhea is usually the first symptom in girls with prolactin-secreting tumors. Galactorrhea may also be present. In boys, the initial features are growth retardation, delayed puberty, and headache.

Gigantism results when concentrations of growth hormone are increased before the epiphyses close. After closure, growth hormone causes acromegaly. Increased concentrations of ACTH cause Cushing's syndrome.

DIAGNOSIS. Visualization of the tumor and identification of its extrasellar extent are best accomplished by MRI. Measurement of hormone production is useful in distinguishing the tumor type.

MANAGEMENT. Surgical resection is the preferred treatment for tumors that compress the optic pathways. Small tumors are often treated medically.

Hereditary Optic Neuropathy

Hereditary optic neuropathies may affect only the visual system, or the visual system and central nervous system, or multiple systems. The underlying abnormality may lie in the nuclear or the mitochondrial DNA. These disorders can cause acute, subacute, or chronic decline in visual acuity. The two conditions discussed below are selected because optic neuropathy is not the only feature.

Leber Hereditary Optic Neuropathy

Leber hereditary optic neuropathy (LHON) is a multisystem mitochondrial disease caused by one or more mutations of the mtDNA. All mutations are missense mutations in complexes I, III, and IV of the respiratory chain (Riordan-Eva et al, 1995). Intrafamily phenotypic variability may be caused by the ratio of mutant to normal mtDNA within an individual, but interfamily variability is probably caused by alternative mutations.

CLINICAL FEATURES. Less than half of patients have a family history of similar disease. The characteristic early symptom is rapid loss of vision in young, otherwise healthy men. Onset is usually between 18 and 23 years, but children younger than 10 years of age may be affected. Age at onset may vary by several decades within a kindred.

The initial complaint is usually painless blurred central vision in one eye, described as fogging of vision or central fading of color. The other eye ordinarily shares the symptoms within days or weeks but may remain unimpaired for several years. Examination of the visual fields reveals first central and then cecocentral scotomas.

The characteristic changes in the ocular fundus include circumpapillary telangiectatic microangiopathy, swelling of the nerve fiber layer around the disk, and absence of peripapillary staining on fluorescein angiography. However, some patients never have these characteristic features even at the time of acute visual loss. Telangiectatic microangiopathy may be observed in presymptomatic maternal family members. As the patient's symptoms develop, the nerve fiber layer becomes swollen; retinal vessels on and around the disk become dilated, tortuous, and telangiectatic; and hemorrhages appear in the nerve fiber layer. Atrophy first appears in the papillomacular bundle and then involves the rest of the retina. The vascular bed involutes, leaving a pale retina and optic atrophy.

Visual impairment is permanent in patients with the most common mtDNA mutation causing LHON. Visual improvement can occur with some of the other mutations, but only 10% regain full vision. Childhood-onset cases have the greatest chance of regaining vision. Neurological impairment is an associated feature in some families. Associated disturbances include dystonia, spastic paraplegia, and ataxia. Some family members may have neurological impairment without optic atrophy, and some have optic atrophy without neurological impairment.

DIAGNOSIS. LHON should be suspected in every kindred with optic neuropathy or with progressive neurological impairment in which transmission is restricted to the maternal line. The optic fundus changes, especially the microangiopathy, are the basis for diagnosis in the context of a compatible family history. Fluorescein angiography shows the development and involution of the telangiectatic microangiopathy and is useful in the diagnosis before symptoms occur.

MANAGEMENT. Treatment is rehabilitative.

Wolfram Syndrome

Wolfram syndrome is the combination of diabetes insipidus and mellitus with optic atrophy and bilateral neurosensory hearing loss (DID-MOAD). A mutation in a gene in the 4p16 region predisposes to multiple mitochondrial DNA deletions in families with Wolfram syndrome (Barrientos et al, 1996).

CLINICAL FEATURES. The onset of diabetes is usually in the first decade. Insulin therapy is required soon after diagnosis. Visual loss progresses rapidly in the second decade but does not lead to complete blindness. Diabetes is not thought to cause optic atrophy. It is more likely that all clinical features result from a progressive neurodegenerative process. The sensorineural hearing loss affects high frequencies first and progresses slowly, rarely leading to severe hearing loss. Features reported in some patients include anosmia, autonomic dysfunction, ptosis, external ophthalmoplegia, tremor, ataxia, nystagmus, seizures, central diabetes insipidus, and endocrinopathies. Psychiatric illness occurs in most cases of Wolfram syndrome, and heterozygous carriers have a predisposition for psychiatric disorders.

DIAGNOSIS. Diagnosis depends on the combination of the preceding list of clinical features. mtDNA analysis confirms the clinical suspicion.

MANAGEMENT. Each of the clinical features is treated symptomatically.

Intraocular Tumors

Although retro-orbital tumors generally cause strabismus and proptosis, intraocular tumors always diminish visual acuity. Retinoblastoma is the most common malignant intraocular tumor. Its prompt recognition can be lifesaving.

The typical features of intraocular tumor in a young child are an abnormal appearance of the eye, loss of vision, and strabismus. Monocular blindness is usually unrecognized by parents. Older children may complain of visual blurring and floaters. Ocular pain is uncommon.

Leukokoria, a white pupillary reflex, is the initial feature in most children with retinoblastoma. This is first noted in bright sunlight or in a flash photograph; the pupil does not constrict and has a white color. Strabismus occurs when visual acuity is impaired. The sighted eye is used for fixation, and the other remains deviated outward in all directions of gaze.

Most children with intraocular tumors are referred directly to an ophthalmologist. A neurologist may be the primary consulting physician when the tumor is part of a larger syndrome that includes mental retardation. Such syndromes include retinoblastoma associated with deletion of the long arm of chromosome 13, retinal astrocytoma associated with tuberous sclerosis, choroidal hemangioma associated with Sturge-Weber disease, and optic nerve glioma in children with neurofibromatosis.

Tapetoretinal Degenerations

Most tapetoretinal degenerations are hereditary and due to inborn errors of lipid or carbohydrate metabolism. These disorders also cause dementia, peripheral neuropathy, and ataxia as initial features and are discussed in several chapters. The conditions discussed here are less common,

but other neurological features are not prominent initial complaints.

Bardet-Biedel and Laurence-Moon Syndromes

The Bardet-Biedel syndrome is characterized by mental retardation, pigmentary retinopathy, polydactyly, obesity, and hypogenitalism. The abnormal gene in Bardet-Biedel syndrome maps to chromosome 16q21. The Laurence-Moon syndrome is a distinct disorder with mental retardation, pigmentary retinopathy, hypogenitalism, and spastic paraplegia without polydactyly and obesity. The genetic abnormality is unknown.

CLINICAL FEATURES. Pigmentary retinopathy usually is manifested in the second decade. It may be characterized by salt-and-pepper retinopathy, macular pigmentation, or macular degeneration. In some patients, the retina appears normal, but the electroretinogram always shows abnormalities. Heterozygotes have an increased frequency of obesity, hypertension, diabetes mellitus, and renal disease.

DIAGNOSIS. Diagnosis depends on recognition of the clinical constellation of symptoms and signs.

MANAGEMENT. Treatment is symptomatic.

Cockayne Syndrome

Cockayne syndrome, like xeroderma pigmentosum (see Chapter 5), is a disorder of DNA repair (Broughton et al, 1995). It is believed to be transmitted by autosomal recessive inheritance, with a male-to-female bias of 3:1.

CLINICAL FEATURES. Primary pigmentary degeneration of the retina occurs during infancy. Affected children appear cachectic, and a disproportionate dwarfism develops in which the limbs are large compared with the trunk. The characteristic facies includes lack of subcutaneous fat with prominence of facial bones, enophthalmos, a beak-like nose, and large ears. Mental deficiency and microcephaly are constant features. Neurological signs may include cerebellar ataxia, involuntary movements, spasticity, peripheral neuropathy, sensorineural hearing loss, and ocular motor apraxia. Disproportionately long limbs with large hands and feet and flexion contractures of joints are usual skeletal features.

DIAGNOSIS. The constellation of clinical signs suggests the diagnosis. Hyperbetaglobulinemia, hyperinsulinemia, and hyperlipoproteinemia are present in some cases.

TREATMENT. Treatment is directed at symptoms, but ultraviolet light exposure must be avoided.

Disorders of the Pupil

When the person is awake, the size of the pupil is constantly changing in response to light and autonomic input. This pupillary unrest is called *hippus*. An isolated disturbance of pupillary size is not evidence of intracranial disease.

Aniridia

Hypoplasia of the iris may occur as a solitary abnormality or may be associated with mental retardation, genitourinary abnormalities, and Wilms tumor. About two thirds of cases are genetic and transmitted as an autosomal dominant trait. One third of sporadic cases are associated with Wilms tumor. In some cases, the short arm of chromosome 11 is abnormal.

Argyll Robertson Pupil

Argyll Robertson pupil is associated with tertiary syphilis and is almost never seen in children. Both pupils are irregularly shaped and miotic. Iris atrophy may be present. The pupils respond poorly to light, but the response to near fixation is present.

Essential Anisocoria

Between 20% and 30% of healthy people have an observable difference in the size of their pupils. Like congenital ptosis, it may go unnoticed until late childhood or adult life and then it is thought to be a new finding. The difference is constant at all levels of illumination but may be greater in darkness. The absence of other pupillary dysfunction or disturbed ocular motility suggests essential anisocoria, but old photographs are invaluable to confirm the diagnosis.

Fixed, Dilated Pupil

CLINICAL FEATURES. A fixed, dilated pupil is an ominous sign in unconscious patients because it suggests transtentorial herniation (see Chapter 4). However, a dilated pupil that does not respond to light or accommodation in a child who is otherwise well and has no evidence of ocular motor dysfunction can result only from the application of a pharmacological agent or from a ruptured sphincter. The application may be accidental, as when a drug or chemical is inadvertently wiped from the hand to the eye. Many cosmetics contain chemicals that can induce mydriasis. A careful history must be obtained.

Factitious application of mydriatics is a relatively common attention-seeking device, and convincing parents that the problem is self-inflicted may be difficult. Occasionally, a parent is the responsible party.

DIAGNOSIS. Pilocarpine 1% should be instilled in both eyes using the normal eye as a control. Parasympathetic denervation produces prompt constriction. A slow or incomplete response indicates pharmacological dilation.

MANAGEMENT. Most pharmacological agents are long-acting, and their effects are not rapidly reversed.

Horner Syndrome

Horner syndrome is characterized by sympathetic denervation; it may be congenital or acquired. When acquired, it may occur at birth as part of a brachial plexus injury, during infancy from neuroblastoma, or in childhood from tumors or injuries affecting the superior cervical ganglion or the carotid artery.

CLINICAL FEATURES. Unilateral Horner syndrome consists of the following ipsilateral features: mild to moderate ptosis (ptosis of the lower lid in one third); miosis, which is best appreciated in dim light so that the normal pupil dilates; anhidrosis of the face, heterochromia, and apparent enophthalmos when the syndrome is congenital.

DIAGNOSIS. Horner syndrome may be caused by disruption of the sympathetic system anywhere from the hypothalamus to the eye. Brainstem disturbances from stroke are common in adults, but peripheral lesions are more common in children. Topical instillation of 1% hydroxyamphetamine usually produces pupillary dilation after 30 minutes when postganglionic denervation is present. However, false-negative results can occur during the first week after injury (Donahue et al, 1996). Ten percent cocaine solution produces little or no dilatation, regardless of the site of abnormality.

MANAGEMENT. Treatment depends on the underlying cause.

Tonic Pupil Syndrome (Adie Syndrome)

CLINICAL FEATURES. Tonic pupil syndrome is caused by a defect in the orbital ciliary ganglion.

The onset usually occurs after childhood but has been reported as early as 5 years. Women are affected more often than men.

The defect is usually monocular and is manifested as anisocoria or photophobia. The abnormal pupil is slightly larger in bright light but changes little, if at all, with alteration in illumination. In a dark room the normal pupil dilates and then is larger than the tonic pupil. With attempted accommodation, which may also be affected, the pupil constricts slowly and incompletely and redilates slowly afterward. Binocular tonic pupils are seen in children with dysautonomia and are also seen in association with diminished tendon reflexes (*Holmes-Adie syndrome*). DIAGNOSIS. The tonic pupil is supersensitive to parasympathomimetic agents; constriction is achieved with 0.125% pilocarpine.
MANAGEMENT. The condition is benign and seldom needs treatment.

References

Barrientos A, Volpini V, Casademont J, et al. A nuclear defect in the 4p16 region predisposes to multiple mitochondrial DNA deletions in families with Wolfram syndrome. *J Clin Invest* 1996;97:1570–1576.

Brodsky MC, Conte FA, Taylor D, et al. Sudden death in septo-optic dysplasia: Report of 5 cases. *Arch Ophthalmol* 1997;115:66–70.

Broughton BC, Thompson AF, Harcourt SA, et al. Molecular and cellular analysis of the DNA repair defect in a patient in xeroderma pigmentosum complementation group D who has the clinical features of xeroderma pigmentosum and Cockayne syndrome. *Am J Hum Genet* 1995;56:167–174.

Casteels I, Spileers W, Demaerel Ph, et al. Leber congenital amaurosis—Differential diagnosis, ophthalmological and neuroradiological report of 18 patients. *Neuropediatrics* 1996;27:189–193.

Donahue SP, Lavin PJM, Digre K. False-negative hydroxyamphetamine (Paredrine) test in acute Horner's syndrome. *Am J Ophthalmol* 1996;122:900–901.

Listernick R, Louis DN, Packer RJ, et al. Optic pathway gliomas in children with neurofibromatosis 1: Consensus statement from the NF1 optic pathway glioma task force. *Ann Neurol* 1997;41:143–149.

Riordan-Eva P, Sanders MD, Govan GG, et al. The clinical features of Leber's hereditary optic neuropathy defined by the presence of a pathogenic mitochondrial DNA mutation. *Brain* 1995;118:319–337.

Thapar K, Kovacs K, Muller PJ. Clinical-pathological correlations of pituitary tumors. *Clin Endocrinol Metab* 1995;9:243–270.

Willnow S, Kiess W, Butenandt O, et al. Endocrine disorders in septo-optic dysplasia (De Morsier syndrome): Evaluation and follow-up of 18 patients. *Eur J Pediatr* 1996;155:179–184.

Chapter 17
Lower Brainstem and Cranial Nerve Dysfunction

THIS CHAPTER CONSIDERS disorders causing dysfunction of the seventh through twelfth cranial nerves. Many such disorders also disturb ocular motility and are discussed in Chapter 15. The chapter assignment is based on the usual initial clinical feature. For example, myasthenia gravis is discussed in Chapter 15 because diplopia is a more common initial complaint than dysphagia.

An acute isolated cranial neuropathy, such as facial palsy, is usually a less ominous sign than multiple cranial neuropathies and is likely to have a self-limited course. However, an isolated cranial neuropathy may be the first sign of progressive cranial nerve dysfunction. Therefore conditions causing isolated and multiple cranial neuropathies are discussed together because they may not be separable at onset.

Facial Weakness and Dysphagia

Anatomical Considerations

Facial Movement

The motor nucleus of the facial nerve is a column of cells in the ventrolateral tegmentum of the pons. Nerve fibers leaving the nucleus take a circuitous path in the brainstem before emerging close to the pontomedullary junction, where they enter the internal auditory meatus with the acoustic nerve. Fibers for voluntary and reflexive facial movements separate rostral to the lower pons. After bending forward and downward around the inner ear, the facial nerve traverses the temporal bone in the facial canal and exits the skull at the stylomastoid foramen. Extracranially, the facial nerve passes into the

parotid gland, where it divides into several branches and is distributed to all muscles of facial expression except the levator palpebra superioris.

Sucking and Swallowing

The sucking reflex requires the integrity of the trigeminal, facial, and hypoglossal nerves. Stimulation of the lips produces coordinated movements of the face, jaw, and tongue. The automatic aspect of the reflex disappears after infancy but returns in bilateral disease of the cerebral hemispheres.

The afferent arc of the swallowing reflex is formed by fibers of the trigeminal and glossopharyngeal nerves that end in the nucleus solitarius. The motor roots of the trigeminal nerve, the glossopharyngeal and vagus fibers from the nucleus ambiguus, and the hypoglossal nerves form the efferent arc. A swallowing center that coordinates the reflex is located in the lower pons and upper medulla. A bolus of food stimulates the pharyngeal wall or back of the tongue, and food is moved into the esophagus by action of the tongue, palatine arches, soft palate, and pharynx.

Approach to Diagnosis

Weakness of facial muscles may be caused by supranuclear palsy (pseudobulbar palsy), intrinsic brainstem disease, or disorders of the motor unit: facial nerve, neuromuscular junction, and facial muscles (Tables 17–1 and 17–2). The differential diagnosis of dysphagia is similar (Table 17–3), except that isolated dysfunction of the nerves that enable swallowing is very uncommon.

Table 17-1
Causes of Congenital Facial Weakness

Aplasia of facial muscles
Birth injury
Congenital myotonic dystrophy (see Chapter 6)
Congenital bilateral perisylvian syndrome
Fiber-type disproportion myopathies (see Chapter 6)
Myasthenic syndromes
    Congenital myasthenia (see Chapter 15)
    Familial infantile myasthenia (see Chapter 6)
    Transitory neonatal myasthenia (see Chapter 6)

Table 17-2
Causes of Postnatal Facial Weakness

Autoimmune and Postinfectious
Bell's palsy
Idiopathic cranial polyneuropathy
Miller Fisher syndrome (see Chapter 10)
Myasthenia gravis (see Chapter 15)

Genetic
Juvenile progressive bulbar palsy (Fazio-Londe disease)
Muscular disorders
    Facioscapulohumeral syndrome (see Chapter 7)
    Facioscapulohumeral syndrome, infantile form
    Fiber-type disproportion myopathies (see Chapter 6)
    Myotonic dystrophy (see Chapter 7)
    Oculopharyngeal dystrophy
Myasthenic syndromes
    Congenital myasthenia (see Chapter 15)
    Familial infantile myasthenia (see Chapter 6)
Osteopetrosis (Albers-Schönberg disease)
Recurrent facial palsy
Melkersson syndrome

Hypertension

Infectious
Diphtheria
Herpes zoster oticus
Infectious mononucleosis
Lyme disease (see Chapter 2)
Otitis media
Sarcoidosis
Tuberculosis

Metabolic Disorders
Hyperparathyroidism
Hypothyroidism

Multiple Sclerosis (see Chapter 10)

Syringobulbia

Toxins

Trauma
Delayed
Immediate

Tumor
Glioma of brainstem (see Chapter 15)
Histiocytosis X
Leukemia
Meningeal carcinoma
Neurofibromatosis

Table 17-3
Neurological Causes of Dysphagia

Autoimmune/Postinfectious
Dermatomyositis (see Chapter 7)
Guillain-Barré syndrome (see Chapter 7)
Idiopathic cranial polyneuropathy
Myasthenia gravis (see Chapter 15)
Transitory neonatal myasthenia gravis (see Chapter 6)

Congenital or Perinatal
Aplasia of brainstem nuclei
Cerebral palsy (see Chapter 5)
Chiari malformation (see Chapter 10)
Congenital bilateral perisylvian syndrome
Syringobulbia

Genetic
Degenerative disorders (see Chapter 5)
Familial dysautonomia (see Chapter 6)
Familial infantile myasthenia (see Chapter 6)
Fiber-type disproportion myopathies (see Chapter 6)
Myotonic dystrophy (see Chapters 6 and 7)
Oculopharyngeal dystrophy

Glioma of Brainstem

Infectious
Botulism (see Chapters 6 and 7)
Diphtheria
Poliomyelitis (see Chapter 7)

Juvenile Progressive Bulbar Palsy

Pseudobulbar Palsy

Because the corticobulbar innervation of most cranial nerves is bilateral, pseudobulbar palsy occurs only when hemispheric disease is bilateral. Many children with pseudobulbar palsy have a progressive degenerative disorder of gray or white matter. Most of these disorders are discussed in Chapter 5 because dementia is usually the initial feature. Bilateral strokes, simultaneous or in sequence, causes pseudobulbar palsy in children; the usual causes are coagulation defects, leukemia, and trauma (see Chapter 11). Pseudobulbar palsy is a major feature of the *congenital bilateral perisylvian syndrome,* discussed in this chapter. Episodic pseudobulbar palsy (oral apraxia, dysarthria, and drooling) may indicate *the acquired epileptiform opercular syndrome* (see Chapter 1).

Pseudobulbar palsy is characterized by inability to use bulbar muscles in voluntary effort, whereas reflex movements initiated at a brainstem level are performed normally. Extraocular motility is unaffected. The child can reflexly suck, chew, and swallow but cannot coordinate these reflexes for eating; movement of a food bolus from the front of the mouth to the back has a volitional component. Emotionally derived facial expression occurs, but facial movements do not occur on command. Severe dysarthria is often present. Affected muscles do not show atrophy or fasciculations. The gag reflex and jaw jerk are usually exaggerated, and emotional volatility is often an associated feature.

Newborns with familial dysautonomia have difficulty feeding, despite normal sucking and swallowing, because they fail to coordinate the two reflexes (see Chapter 6). The differential diagnosis of feeding difficulty in an alert newborn is summarized in Table 6–8. Children with cerebral palsy often have a similar disturbance in the coordination of chewing and swallowing, and feeding is impaired.

Motor Unit Disorders

Disorders of the facial nuclei and nerves always cause ipsilateral facial weakness and atrophy, but associated features vary with the site of abnormality:

1. Motor nucleus: Hyperacusis is present, but taste, lacrimation, and salivation are normal.

2. Facial nerve between the pons and the internal auditory meatus: Taste is spared, but lacrimation and salivation are impaired and hyperacusis is present.

3. Geniculate ganglion: Taste, lacrimation, and salivation are impaired, and hyperacusis is present.

4. Facial nerve from the geniculate ganglion to the stapedius nerve: Taste and salivation are impaired and hyperacusis is present, but lacrimation is normal.

5. Facial nerve from the stapedius nerve to the chorda tympani: Taste and salivation are impaired, hyperacusis is not present, and lacrimation is normal.

6. Facial nerve below the exit of the chorda tympani nerve: Only facial weakness is present.

Disturbances of cranial nerve nuclei seldom occur in isolation; they are often associated with other features of brainstem dysfunction (bulbar palsy). Usually some combination of dysarthria, dysphagia, and diplopia is present. Examination may show strabismus, facial diplegia, loss of the gag reflex, atrophy of bulbar muscles, and fasciculations of the tongue.

The weakness of myasthenia gravis and facial myopathies is almost always bilateral, whereas brainstem disorders usually begin on one side but eventually cause bilateral impairment. Facial

---

Table 17-4
Causes of Recurrent Cranial Neuropathies/Palsies

Familial
  Isolated facial palsy
  Melkersson syndrome
Hypertensive facial palsy
Myasthenia gravis
Sporadic multiple cranial neuropathies
Toxins

---

nerve palsies are usually unilateral. The differential diagnosis of recurrent facial palsy or dysphagia is limited to disorders of the facial nerve and neuromuscular junction (Table 17–4).

Congenital Bilateral Perisylvian Syndrome

This is a migrational disorder that results in pachygyria of the sylvian and rolandic regions. Most cases are sporadic. Some familial cases are transmitted by X-linked inheritance; such cases are more severe in males than in females (Borgatti et al, 1999).

CLINICAL FEATURES. All affected children have a pseudobulbar palsy that causes failure of speech development and dysphagia. Mental retardation and seizures are present in approximately 85% of cases. The retardation varies from mild to severe, and the seizures, which begin between 4 and 12 years, may be atypical absence, atonic/tonic, partial, or generalized tonic-clonic.

DIAGNOSIS. Magnetic resonance imaging (MRI) shows bilateral perisylvian gyral malformations, pachygyria, and polymicrogyria (Figure 17-1). Postmortem studies have confirmed the MRI impression.

MANAGEMENT. The seizures are usually difficult to control, and corpus callosotomy has been useful in some cases with intractable drop attacks. Speech therapy does not overcome the speech disorder, and sign language should be taught to children of near-normal intelligence.

Congenital Facial Asymmetry

Most facial asymmetries observed at birth are caused by congenital aplasia of muscle and are not traumatic. Facial diplegia, whether complete or incomplete, suggests the Möbius syndrome or other congenital muscle aplasia. Complete unilateral palsies are likely to be traumatic in origin, whereas partial unilateral palsies may be

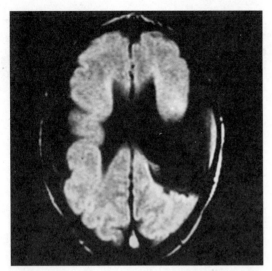

Figure 17-1. MRI of congenital bilateral perisylvian syndrome. This child has lissencephaly and schizencephaly. Bilateral disturbances in the perisylvian region caused a pseudobulbar palsy.

either traumatic or aplastic. The term *neonatal facial asymmetry* is probably more accurate than *facial nerve palsy* to denote partial or complete unilateral facial weakness in the newborn and emphasizes the difficulty in differentiating traumatic nerve palsies from congenital aplasias.

Aplasia of Facial Muscles

CLINICAL FEATURES. The Möbius syndrome is the best-known congenital aplasia of facial nerve nuclei and facial muscles. The site of pathology is usually the facial nerve nuclei and their internuclear connections (Jaradeh et al, 1996). Facial diplegia may occur alone, with bilateral abducens palsies, or with involvement of several cranial nerves. Congenital malformations elsewhere in the body—dextrocardia, talipes equinovarus, absent pectoral muscle, and limb deformities—may be associated features. The abnormal genes in one family with dominantly inherited Möbius syndrome were mapped to the long arm of chromosome 3.

Other developmental causes of unilateral facial palsy are Goldenhar's syndrome, the Poland anomoly, DiGeorge syndrome, osteopetrosis, and trisomy 13 and 18 (Shapiro et al, 1996). **DIAGNOSIS.** Congenital facial diplegia is by definition a Möbius syndrome. MRI of the brain is indicated in all such cases to determine whether other cerebral malformations are present. Causes other than primary malformation must be considered as well. Some cases are due to intrauterine toxins (e.g., thalidomide) or structural disturbances of the brainstem, such as vascular malformation of infarction.

Electromyography (EMG) can help determine the timing of injury. Denervation potentials are present only if the facial nuclei or nerves were injured 2 to 6 weeks before the study. Facial muscles that are aplastic as a result of Möbius syndrome or nerve injury occurring early in gestation do not show active denervation. **MANAGEMENT.** Surgical procedures that provide partial facial movement are being developed.

Depressor Anguli Oris Muscle Aplasia

CLINICAL FEATURES. Isolated unilateral weakness of the depressor anguli oris muscle (DAOM) is the most common cause of facial asymmetry at birth. One corner of the mouth fails to move downward when the child cries. All other facial movements are symmetric. The lower lip on the paralyzed side feels thinner to palpation, even at birth, suggesting antepartum hypoplasia.

DIAGNOSIS. Traumatic lesions of the facial nerve would not selectively injure nerve fibers to the DAOM and spare all other facial muscles. Electrodiagnostic studies aid in differentiating aplasia of the DAOM from traumatic injury. In aplasia the conduction velocity and latency of the facial nerve are normal. Fibrillations are not present at the site of the DAOM. Instead, motor unit potentials are absent or decreased in number.

MANAGEMENT. No treatment is available or needed. The DAOM is not a significant component of facial expression in older children and adults, and its absence is hardly noticed.

Birth Injury

Perinatal traumatic facial palsy is a disorder of large term newborns delivered vaginally after a prolonged labor. The palsy is more often caused by nerve compression against the sacrum during labor than by misapplication of forceps. Children with forceps injuries, an unusual event, have forceps marks on the cheeks. **CLINICAL FEATURES.** The clinical expression of complete unilateral facial palsy in the newborn can be subtle and may not be apparent immediately after birth. Failure of eye closure on the affected side is the first noticeable evidence of weakness. Only when the child cries does flaccid paralysis of all facial muscles become obvious. The eyeball rolls up behind the open lid, the nasolabial fold remains flat, and the corner of the mouth droops during crying. The normal side, which appears to pull and distort the face, may be thought to be paralyzed and the paralyzed side normal.

When paralysis of the facial nerve is partial, the orbicularis oculi is the muscle most frequently spared. In these injuries the compression site is usually over the parotid gland, with sparing of nerve fibers that course upward just after leaving the stylomastoid foramen.

DIAGNOSIS. Facial asymmetry is diagnosed by observation of the crying newborn. The facial skin must be carefully examined for laceration. Otoscopic examination is useful to establish the presence of hemotympanum. EMG does not alter the management of the palsy.

MANAGEMENT. Prospective studies regarding the natural outcome of perinatal facial nerve injuries are not available. Most authors are optimistic and indicate a high rate of spontaneous recovery. The optimism may be warranted, but it is based on anecdotal experience alone. In the absence of data on the long-term outcome, the efficacy of suggested therapeutic measures cannot be evaluated. Most newborns should not be subjected to surgical intervention unless the nerve is lacerated at delivery. In that event, the best response is to reconstitute the nerve if possible or at least to allow the proximal stump a clear pathway toward regeneration by debridement of the wound.

Congenital Dysphagia

Congenital dysphagia is usually associated with infantile hypotonia and is therefore discussed in Chapter 6. Because the neuroanatomical substrates of swallowing and breathing are contiguous, congenital dysphagia and dyspnea are often concurrent. Isolated aplasia of cranial nerve nuclei subserving swallowing has not been documented, but I have seen one infant in whom the clinical syndrome was consistent with isolated aplasia.

Autoimmune and Postinfectious Disorders

Most cases of acute unilateral facial neuritis (Bell's palsy) or bilateral facial neuritis are attributed to postinfectious demyelination of the nerve. A bilateral Bell's palsy is distinguished from the Guillain-Barré syndrome (acute inflammatory demyelinating polyneuropathy) mainly on the basis that in Bell's palsy the tendon reflexes are preserved in the limbs. The Guillain-Barré syndrome is discussed in Chapter 7.

Bell's Palsy

Bell's palsy is an acute idiopathic paralysis of the face caused by dysfunction of the facial nerve. The pathogenesis is believed to be viral (most often herpes simplex) but may also be postviral immune-mediated demyelination. The annual incidence is approximately 3/100,000 in the first decade, 10/100,000 in the second decade, and 25/100,000 in adults. Only 1% of cases have clinical evidence of bilateral involvement, but many have electrophysiological abnormalities on the unaffected side.

CLINICAL FEATURES. A history of viral infection, usually upper respiratory, is recorded in many cases, but the frequency is not significantly greater than expected by chance. The initial feature of neuritis is often pain or tingling in the ear canal ipsilateral to the subsequent facial palsy. Sensory symptoms, when present, are usually mild and do not demand medical attention.

The palsy has an explosive onset and becomes maximal within hours. It may be noticed first by either the child or the parents. The palsy affects all muscles on one side of the face. Half of the face sags, enlarging the palpebral fissure. Weakness of the levator palpebrae muscle prevents closure of the lid. Efforts to use muscles of expression cause the face to pull to the normal side. Eating and drinking become difficult, and the dribbling of liquids from the weak corner of the mouth causes embarrassment.

The most commonly affected portion of the nerve is within the temporal bone; taste, lacrimation, and salivation are impaired; and hyperacusis is present. However, examination of all facial nerve functions in small children is difficult, and precise localization is not critical to diagnosis or prognosis. The muscles remain weak for 2 to 4 weeks, and then strength returns spontaneously. The natural history of Bell's palsy in children has not been studied, but experience indicates that almost all patients recover completely.

DIAGNOSIS. Every child with acute unilateral facial weakness must be fully examined to determine whether the palsy is an isolated abnormality. Mild facial weakness on the other side or the absence of tendon reflexes in the limbs suggests the possibility of Guillain-Barré syndrome. Such children must be watched carefully for the development of progressive limb weakness.

Possible underlying causes (e.g., hypertension, infection, trauma) of facial nerve palsy should be excluded before the diagnosis of Bell's palsy is considered satisfactory. The ear ipsilateral to the facial palsy should be examined for herpetic lesions (see the later discussion of herpes zoster oticus). MRI shows contrast enhancement of the involved nerve (Sartoretti-Schefer et al, 1998), but *MRI is not indicated for every child with acute, isolated facial palsy*. A more reasonable approach is to watch the child and recommend an imaging study if other neurological disturbances develop or if the palsy does not begin to resolve within 1 month.

MANAGEMENT. If the blink reflex is absent, the cornea must be protected. The eye should be patched when the child is outside the home or at play, and artificial tears should be applied several times a day to keep the cornea moist.

The use of corticosteroids has been advocated in adults, but has no scientific basis in children because their prognosis for complete spontaneous recovery is excellent. The clinician who elects to use corticosteroid therapy must first exclude hypertension or infection as an underlying cause.

Idiopathic Cranial Polyneuropathy

As the name implies, idiopathic cranial neuropathy is of uncertain nosology. A postinfectious basis is presumed, and some consider it to be an abortive form of the Guillain-Barré syndrome.

CLINICAL FEATURES. Onset is usually in adults, and most childhood cases occur in adolescence. Similar cases had been described in infants, but because many subsequently developed limb weakness, infantile botulism was the more likely diagnosis (see Chapter 6).

Constant, aching facial pain usually precedes weakness by hours or days. The pain is often localized to the temple or frontal region but can be anywhere in the face. Weakness may develop within 1 day or may evolve over several weeks. Extraocular motility is usually affected. Facial and trigeminal nerve disturbances occur in half of cases, but lower cranial nerve involvement is uncommon. Occasional patients have transitory visual disturbances, ptosis, pupillary abnormalities, and tinnitus. Tendon reflexes in the limbs remain active. Recurrent idiopathic cranial neuropathies occur as sporadic cases in adults but are usually familial in children.

DIAGNOSIS. The differential diagnosis includes the Guillain-Barré syndrome, infant and childhood forms of botulism, brainstem glioma, juvenile progressive bulbar palsy, pontobulbar palsy with deafness, and the Tolosa-Hunt syndrome. Preservation of tendon reflexes in idiopathic cranial polyneuropathy is the major feature distinguishing it from the Guillain-Barré syndrome. Botulism can be separated clinically by its prominent autonomic dysfunction and limb weakness (see Chapters 6 and 7). Cranial nerve dysfunction in patients with brainstem glioma, juvenile progressive bulbar palsy, and pontobulbar palsy with deafness usually evolves over a longer period. The Tolosa-Hunt syndrome of painful ophthalmoplegia and idiopathic cranial polyneuropathy shares many features and may be a variant of the same disease process (see Chapter 15).

All laboratory findings are normal. MRI of the brainstem should be performed in all cases to exclude the possibility of a brainstem glioma. Examination of the cerebrospinal fluid occasionally reveals a mild elevation of protein concentration and a lymphocyte count of 5 or 6/mm^3.

MANAGEMENT. The disease is self-limited, and full recovery is expected 2 to 4 months after onset. Corticosteroids are used routinely and are believed to relieve facial pain and shorten the course. The relief of pain may be dramatic, but evidence documenting a shortened course is lacking.

Genetic Disorders

Facioscapulohumeral Syndrome

The facioscapulohumeral (FSH) syndrome (see Chapter 7) sometimes begins during infancy as facial diplegia (Brouwer et al, 1995). All forms of the disease are transmitted by autosomal dominant inheritance. The responsible gene maps to chromosome 4q35 in many, but not all, families.

CLINICAL FEATURES. The onset of infantile FSH is usually during infancy and no later than age 5. Facial diplegia, the first feature, is often misdiagnosed as congenital aplasia of facial muscles when the onset is in infancy. Later, nasal speech and sometimes ptosis develop. Progressive proximal weakness begins 1 to 2 years after onset, first affecting the shoulders and then the pelvis. Pseudohypertrophy of the calves may be present. Tendon reflexes are depressed and then absent in weak muscle. Progression of weakness is often rapid and unrelenting, leading to disability and death from respiratory insufficiency before age 20, but may also stabilize for long intervals and not cause severe disability until adult life.

Retinal telangiectasia and high-frequency hearing loss occur in about half of affected families (Padberg et al, 1995). Both conditions are progressive and may not be symptomatic in early childhood.

DIAGNOSIS. The diagnosis should be suspected in any child with progressive facial diplegia. A family history of FSH syndrome cannot always be obtained because the defect may be only minimally expressed in the affected parent. Molecular-based testing is reliable for diagnosis.

Myasthenia gravis and brainstem glioma must be considered in infants with progressive facial diplegia. The serum concentration of creatine kinase is helpful in differentiating these disorders. It is usually elevated in the infantile FSH syndrome and is normal in myasthenia gravis and brainstem glioma. Electrophysiological studies show brief, small-amplitude polyphasic potentials in weak muscles and a normal response to repetitive nerve stimulation.

MANAGEMENT. Treatment is supportive.

Oculopharyngeal Muscular Dystrophy

Oculopharyngeal muscular dystrophy is usually transmitted by autosomal dominant inheritance. It is most often described in families of French Canadian descent but is not restricted to any ethnic group. Most cases that are not clearly transmitted by autosomal dominant inheritance will prove to be mitochondrial myopathies (Schröder et al, 1995).

CLINICAL FEATURES. Onset is usually in the fourth decade but may be as early as adolescence. The initial features are ptosis and dysphagia, followed by proximal weakness in the legs and external ophthalmoplegia. Eventually all skeletal muscle is affected, but smooth muscle and cardiac muscle are spared.

Many patients with oculopharyngeal muscular dystrophy also have EMG or biopsy evidence of denervation in the limbs. The neurogenic features may be attributed to neuronopathy rather than neuropathy, suggesting that this disorder is actually a spinal (bulbar) muscular atrophy.

DIAGNOSIS. Myasthenia gravis must be excluded with an edrophonium chloride (Tensilon) test and a repetitive nerve stimulation study. The serum concentration of creatine kinase is normal, but EMG of affected muscles shows brief, small-amplitude polyphasic potentials, as well as prolonged polyphasic potentials and fibrillations. The presence of ragged-red fibers on histo-

logical examination of muscle indicates an underlying mitochondrial myopathy.

MANAGEMENT. Therapy is directed at the symptoms. Ptosis can be corrected by levator palpebral shortening, and constrictor or cricopharyngeal myotomy may help dysphagia.

Melkersson Syndrome

As many as 7% of facial palsies are recurrent. Autosomal dominant inheritance with variable expression is suspected in many cases. Some members of a kindred may have only recurrent facial nerve palsy, whereas others have recurrent neuropathies of the facial and ocular motor nerves. The Melkersson syndrome may be genetically distinct from other recurrent facial palsies with a gene locus at chromosome 9p11.

CLINICAL FEATURES. Melkersson syndrome is a rare disorder characterized by the triad of recurrent facial palsy, lingua plicata, and facial edema. Attacks of facial palsy usually begin in the second decade, but the deeply furrowed tongue is present from birth.

The first attack of facial weakness is indistinguishable from Bell's palsy except that it may be preceded by a migraine-like headache. Subsequent attacks are associated with facial edema, which is soft, painless, nonerythematous, and nonpruritic. The edema is most often asymmetric, involving only the upper lip on the paralyzed side, but it may affect the cheek and eyelid of one or both sides. Attacks of facial swelling may be precipitated by cold weather or emotional stress and are not coincident with attacks of facial palsy.

Lingua plicata is present in 30% to 50% of cases. Furrowing and deep grooving on the dorsal surface of the tongue are permanent from birth. This feature is transmitted by autosomal dominant inheritance and occurs as an isolated finding in some families.

DIAGNOSIS. Melkersson syndrome can be diagnosed when two features of the triad are present. It should be considered in any child with a personal or family history of recurrent facial palsy or recurrent facial edema. The presence of lingua plicata in any member of the kindred confirms the diagnosis.

MANAGEMENT. This disease has no established treatment. A short course of high-dose intravenous methylprednisolone was beneficial in one patient (Kesler et al, 1998).

Hypertension

Unilateral facial palsy may be a feature of malignant hypertension in children. The palsy is caused by swelling and hemorrhage into the facial canal.

CLINICAL FEATURES. The course of the facial paralysis is indistinguishable from that in Bell's palsy. The nerve is compressed in its proximal segment, impairing lacrimation, salivation, and taste. The onset coincides with a rise in blood pressure to greater than 120 mm Hg, and recovery begins when pressure is reduced. The duration of palsy varies from days to weeks. Recurrences are associated with repeated episodes of hypertension.

DIAGNOSIS. The occurrence of facial palsy in a child with known hypertension suggests that the hypertension is out of control.

MANAGEMENT. Control of hypertension is the only effective treatment.

Infection

The facial nerve is sometimes involved when bacterial infection spreads from the middle ear to the mastoid. External otitis may lead to facial nerve involvement by spread of infection from the tympanic membrane to the chorda tympani.

Diphtheria may cause single or multiple cranial neuropathies from a direct effect of its toxin. Facial palsy, dysarthria, and dysphagia are potential complications. Basilar meningitis, from tuberculosis or other bacterial infections, causes inflammation of cranial nerves as they leave the brain and enter the skull. Multiple and bilateral cranial nerve involvement is usually progressive.

Herpes Zoster Oticus (Ramsay Hunt Syndrome)

Herpes zoster oticus is caused by herpes zoster infection of the geniculate ganglion.

CLINICAL FEATURES. The initial feature is pain in and behind the ear. This pain is often more severe and persistent than that expected with Bell's palsy. Unilateral facial palsy, which cannot be distinguished from Bell's palsy by appearance, follows. However, examination of the ipsilateral ear, especially in the fossa of the helix and behind the lobule, shows a vesicular eruption characteristic of herpes zoster. Hearing loss is associated in 25% of cases.

DIAGNOSIS. The only historical feature distinguishing herpes zoster oticus from Bell's palsy is the severity of ear pain. Examination of the ear for vesicles is critical to the diagnosis.

MANAGEMENT. Herpes zoster infections are usually self-limited but painful. A combination of oral acyclovir, 800 mg, five times a day for 7 days, and oral prednisone, 1 mg/kg for 5 days

and then tapered, improves the outcome for facial nerve function in people 15 years and older (Murakami et al, 1997). Complete recovery occurs in 75% of those treated within 7 days of onset and in 30% treated after 7 days. The varicella vaccine may reduce the incidence of new cases and decrease the severity of symptoms (Hato et al, 2000).

Sarcoidosis

Cranial nerve dysfunction is the most common neurological complication of sarcoidosis. It is usually caused by basilar granulomatous meningitis, but the facial nerve may also be involved when parotitis is present.

CLINICAL FEATURES. Onset is usually in the third decade but may be as early as adolescence. Neurological complications occur in only 5% of patients with sarcoidosis but, when present, are often an early feature of the disease. Facial nerve palsy, unilateral or bilateral, is the single most common feature. Visual impairment or deafness is next in frequency. Single cranial neuropathies are present in 73% and multiple cranial neuropathies in 58%. Any cranial nerve except the accessory nerve may be involved. Systemic features of sarcoidosis occur in almost every case: intrathoracic involvement is present in 81% and ocular involvement in 50%. Uveoparotitis is an uncommon manifestation of sarcoidosis. The patient ordinarily comes to medical attention because of visual impairment and a painful eye. The mouth is dry and the parotid gland swollen. Facial nerve compression and palsy are present in 40% of cases.

DIAGNOSIS. Sarcoidosis should be considered in any patient with single or multiple cranial neuropathies. The suspicion is confirmed by documentation of multisystem disease. Radiographs of the chest either establish or are compatible with the diagnosis in almost all patients with neurological manifestations.

Increased serum concentrations of serum angiotensin-converting enzyme (ACE) are detected in approximately 75% of patients with active pulmonary disease, and patients with neurosarcoidosis may have elevated cerebrospinal fluid concentrations of ACE. Biopsy of lymph nodes or other affected tissues provides histological confirmation.

MANAGEMENT. Prednisone, 0.5 to 1 mg/kg/day, should be maintained until a clinical response is evident and then tapered at a slow enough rate to prevent relapse. The prognosis for neurological complications of sarcoidosis is good without treatment, but corticosteroids appear to hasten recovery.

Juvenile Progressive Bulbar Palsy

Juvenile progressive bulbar palsy, also known as *Fazio-Londe disease,* is a motor neuron disease limited to bulbar muscles. Most cases are sporadic; autosomal recessive inheritance is suspected, and a rare autosomal dominant subtype may also occur.

CLINICAL FEATURES. Two clinical patterns are described. Stridor is the initial feature in early-onset cases (ages 1 to 5 years). Progressive bulbar palsy follows, and respiratory compromise causes death within 2 years of onset. Respiratory symptoms are less common in later-onset cases (ages 6 to 20 years). The initial feature may be facial weakness, dysphagia, or dysarthria. Eventually, all the lower motor cranial nerve nuclei are affected, but the ocular motor nerve nuclei are spared. Fasciculations and atrophy of the arms are reported in some cases, but limb strength and tendon reflexes are usually spared despite severe bulbar palsy.

DIAGNOSIS. The major diagnostic considerations are myasthenia gravis and brainstem glioma. MRI of the brainstem is needed to exclude brainstem tumors, and EMG is useful to show active denervation of facial muscles, with sparing of the limbs and normal repetitive stimulation of nerves. Children with rapidly progressive motor neuron disease affecting the face and limbs should be considered to have a childhood form of amyotrophic lateral sclerosis.

MANAGEMENT. The disorder is often devastating. A previously normal child is no longer able to speak intelligibly or swallow. Feeding gastrostomy is soon required. The child needs considerable psychological support. Treatment is not available for the underlying disease.

Metabolic Disorders

Hyperparathyroidism

The most common neurological features of primary hyperparathyroidism are headache and confusion (see Chapter 2). Occasionally, hyperparathyroidism is associated with a syndrome that is similar to amyotrophic lateral sclerosis and includes ataxia and internuclear ophthalmoplegia. Dysarthria and dysphagia are prominent features.

Hypothyroidism

Cranial nerve abnormalities are unusual in hypothyroidism. Deafness is the most common feature, but acute facial nerve palsy resembling Bell's palsy also occurs.

Osteopetrosis (Albers-Schönberg Disease)

The term *osteopetrosis* encompasses at least three hereditary skeletal disorders of increased bone density. The most common form is transmitted by autosomal recessive inheritance (chromosome 11q). Its features are macrocephaly, progressive deafness and blindness, hepatosplenomegaly, and severe anemia beginning in fetal life or early infancy. The calvarium becomes thickened, and cranial nerves are compressed and compromised as they pass through the bone.

The main clinical features of the dominant form (1p) are fractures and osteomyelitis, especially of the mandible. Treatment with high-dose calcitrol is effective in reducing the sclerosis and preventing many neurological complications.

Syringobulbia

Syringobulbia is usually the medullary extension of a cervical syrinx (see Chapter 12) but may also originate in the medulla. The syrinx usually involves the nucleus ambiguus and the spinal tract and motor nucleus of the trigeminal nerve. Symptoms in order of frequency are headache, vertigo, dysarthria, facial paresthesias, dysphagia, diplopia, tinnitus, and palatal palsy.

Toxins

Most neurotoxins produce either diffuse encephalopathy or peripheral neuropathy. Only ethylene glycol, trichlorethylene, and chlorocresol exposure cause selective cranial nerve toxicity. Ethylene glycol is used as an antifreeze. Ingestion causes facial diplegia, hearing impairment, and dysphagia. Trichlorethylene intoxication can cause multiple cranial neuropathies but has a predilection for the trigeminal nerve and was previously used in the treatment of tic douloureux.

Chlorocresol, a compound used in the industrial production of heparin, was reported to cause recurrent unilateral facial palsy in an exposed worker. Inhalation of the compound caused tingling of one side of the face followed by weakness of the muscles. The neurological disturbance was brief, relieved by exposure to fresh air, and could be reproduced experimentally.

Trauma

Facial palsy following closed head injury is usually associated with bleeding from the ear and fracture of the petrous bone.

CLINICAL FEATURES. The onset of palsy may be immediate or may be delayed for as long as 3 weeks after injury. In most cases the interval is between 2 and 7 days. The mechanism of delay is unknown.

DIAGNOSIS. Electrophysiological studies are helpful in prognosis. If the nerve is intact but shows a conduction block, recovery usually begins within 5 days and is complete. Most patients with partial denervation recover full facial movement but have evidence of aberrant reinnervation. Full recovery is not expected when denervation is complete.

MANAGEMENT. The management of traumatic facial palsy is controversial. Some authors have recommended surgical decompression and corticosteroids, but no evidence supporting either mode of therapy is available.

Tumors

Tumors of the facial nerve are rare in children. The major neoplastic cause of facial palsy is brainstem glioma (see Chapter 15), followed by tumors that infiltrate the meninges, such as leukemia, meningeal carcinoma, and histiocytosis X. Acoustic neuromas are unusual in childhood and are limited to children with neurofibromatosis type 2. These neuromas cause hearing impairment before facial palsy and are discussed in the next section.

Hearing Impairment and Deafness

Anatomical Considerations

Sound is mechanically funneled through the external auditory canal to the tympanic membrane, causing it to vibrate. The vibrations are transmitted by ossicles to the oval window of the cochlea, the sensory organ of hearing. The air-filled space from the tympanic membrane to the cochlea is the middle ear. The membranous labyrinth within the osseous labyrinth is the principal structure of the inner ear. It contains the cochlea, the semicircular canals, and the vestibule. The semicircular canals and vestibule are the sensory organs of vestibular function. The cochlea consists of three fluid-filled canals wound into a snail-like configuration.

The organ of Corti is the transducer within the cochlea that converts mechanical to electrical energy. Impulses are transmitted in the auditory portion of the eighth nerve to the ipsilateral cochlear nuclei of the medulla. The cochlear nuclei on each side transmits information to both superior olivary nuclei, causing bilateral representation of hearing throughout the remainder of the central pathways. From the superior olivary nuclei, impulses are transmitted by the lateral lemniscus to the inferior colliculus. Further cross-connections occur in collicular synapses. Rostrally directed fibers from the inferior colliculi ascend to the medial geniculate and auditory cortex of the temporal lobe.

Symptoms of Auditory Dysfunction

The major symptoms of disturbance in the auditory pathways are hearing impairment, tinnitus, and hyperacusis. Hearing impairment is characterized in infants by failure to develop speech (see Chapter 5) and in older children by inattentiveness and poor school performance.

Fifty percent of infants use words with meaning by 12 months and join words into sentences by 24 months. Failure to accomplish these tasks by 21 months and 3 years, respectively, is always abnormal. A hearing loss of 25 to 30 dB is sufficient to interfere with normal acquisition of speech.

Hearing Impairment

Hearing impairment is classified as conductive, sensorineural (perceptive), or central.

Conductive hearing impairment is caused by disturbances in the external or middle ear. The mechanical vibrations that make up the sensory input of hearing are not faithfully delivered to the inner ear because the external canal is blocked or the tympanic membrane or ossicles are abnormal. The major defect in conductive hearing loss is sound amplification. Patients with conductive hearing impairment are better able to hear loud speech in a noisy background than soft speech in a quiet background. Tinnitus may be associated.

Sensorineural hearing impairment may be congenital or acquired and is caused by disturbances of the cochlea or auditory nerve. The frequency content of sound is improperly analyzed and transduced. High frequencies may be selectively lost. Individuals with sensorineural hearing impairment have difficulty discriminating speech when there is background noise.

Central hearing impairment results from disturbance of the cochlear nuclei or their projections to the cortex. Brainstem lesions usually cause bilateral hearing impairment. Cortical lesions lead to difficulty in processing information. Pure-tone audiometry is normal, but speech discrimination is impaired by background noise or competing messages.

Approximately one third of childhood deafness is genetic in origin, one third is acquired, and the remaining third is idiopathic. Many of the idiopathic cases are probably genetic as well (Das, 1996).

Tinnitus

Tinnitus is the illusion of noise in the ear. The noise is usually high-pitched and constant. In most cases tinnitus is caused by disturbances of the auditory nerve, but it may occur as a simple partial seizure originating from the primary auditory cortex. Sounds generated by the cardiovascular system (heartbeat and bruit) are sometimes audible, especially while a person is lying down, but should not be confused with tinnitus.

Hyperacusis

Hyperacusis is caused by failure of the stapedius muscle to dampen sound by its effect on the ossicles. This occurs when the chorda tympani branch of the facial nerve is damaged (see the discussion of Bell's palsy earlier in this chapter).

Approach to the Patient

Hearing assessment in the office is satisfactory for severe hearing impairment but is unsatisfactory for detecting loss of specific frequency bands. The speech and hearing handicap generated by a high-frequency hearing impairment should not be underestimated.

When testing an infant, the physician should stand behind the patient and provide interesting sounds to each ear. Bells, chimes, rattles, or a tuning fork are useful for that purpose. Dropping a large object and watching the infant and parents startle from the noise is not a test of hearing. Once the infant sees the source of the interesting sound or hears it several times, interest is lost. Therefore, different high- and low-frequency sounds should be used for each ear. The normal responses of the infant are to become alert and to attempt to localize the source of the sound.

Older children can be tested by observing their response to spoken words at different intensities and with tuning forks that provide pure tones of different frequencies. The *Rinne test* compares air conduction (conductive plus sensorineural hearing) with bone conduction (sensorineural hearing). A tuning fork is held against the mastoid process until the sound fades and is then held 1 inch from the ear. Normal children hear the vibration produced by air conduction twice as long as that produced by bone conduction. Impaired air conduction with normal bone conduction indicates a conductive hearing loss.

The *Weber test* compares bone conduction in the two ears. It is based on the principle that signals transmitted by bone conduction are localized to the better-hearing ear or the ear with the greater conductive deficit. A tuning fork is placed at the center of the forehead, and the patient is asked whether sound is perceived equally in both ears. A normal response is to hear the sound in the center of the head. If bone conduction is normal in both ears, sound is localized to the ear with impaired air conduction because the normal blocking response of air conduction is lacking. If a sensorineural hearing impairment is present in one ear, bone conduction is perceived in the good ear.

Otoscopic examination is imperative in every child with hearing problems or tinnitus. The cause may be seen through the speculum in the form of impacted wax, otitis media, perforated tympanic membrane, or cholesteatoma.

Hearing Tests

The usual battery of audiologic tests includes pure-tone air and bone conduction testing, and measures of speech threshold and word discrimination.

Pure-Tone Audiometry

Selected frequencies are presented by earphones (air conduction) or by a vibrator applied to the mastoid (bone conduction), and the subject is asked to determine the minimum level perceived for each frequency. Normal hearing levels are defined by an international standard. The test can be performed adequately only in children old enough to cooperate. With conductive hearing impairment, air conduction is abnormal and bone conduction is normal; with sensorineural hearing impairment, both are abnormal; and with central hearing impairment, both are normal.

Speech Tests

The *speech reception threshold* measures the intensity at which a subject can repeat 50% of presented words. The *speech discrimination test* measures the subject's ability to understand speech at normal conversational levels. Both tests are abnormal out of proportion to pure-tone loss with auditory nerve disease, abnormal in proportion to pure-tone loss with cochlear disease, and normal with conductive and central hearing loss.

Special Tests

Cochlear lesions may cause *diplacusis* and *recruitment*. Auditory nerve lesions produce *tone decay*. Diplacusis is a distortion of pure tones so that the subject perceives a mixture of tones. With recruitment the sensation of loudness increases at an abnormally rapid rate as the intensity of sound is increased. Tone decay is diminished perception of a suprathreshold tone with time.

Brainstem Auditory Evoked Response

The brainstem auditory evoked response (BAER) is used to test hearing and the integrity of the brainstem auditory pathways in infants and small children. No cooperation is required, and sedation improves the accuracy of results.

When each ear is stimulated with repetitive clicks and simultaneous recordings are made from an electrode over the ipsilateral mastoid referenced to the forehead, five waves are recorded. Wave I is generated by the acoustic nerve, wave II by the cochlear nerve, wave III by the superior olivary complex, wave IV by the lateral lemniscus, and wave V by the inferior colliculus.

The BAER first appears at a conceptional age of 26 to 27 weeks. The absolute latencies of waves I and V and the V-I interpeak interval decline progressively with advancing conceptional age. The latency of wave V bears an inverse relationship to the intensity of the stimulus and can be used to test hearing.

An initial test is performed with a stimulus intensity of 70 dB. If wave V is not produced, hearing is impaired and the test should be repeated at higher intensities until a response threshold is found. If wave V is present, the test is repeated at sequential reductions of 10 dB until the lowest intensity capable of producing wave V, the *hearing threshold*, is established.

Because the latency of wave V is proportional to the intensity of the stimulus, a latency-intensity curve can be drawn. In normal newborns, the latency of wave V will decrease by 0.24 to 0.44 ms for each 10 dB in sound intensity between 70 and 110 dB.

In children with conductive hearing impairment, the time required to transmit sound across the middle ear and activate the cochlea is prolonged and the total amount of sound energy is reduced. As a consequence, the latency of wave I is prolonged and the latency-intensity curve of wave V shifts to the right by an amount equivalent to the hearing impairment, without any alteration in the slope of the curve.

In children with sensorineural hearing impairment, the latency-intensity curve of wave V is shifted to the right because of the hearing impairment. In addition, the slope of the curve becomes steeper, exceeding 0.55 ms/dB.

Congenital Deafness

Congenital deafness is often missed in the newborn unless a deformity of the external ear is present or a family history of genetic hearing loss is obtained. Congenital ear malformations are present in approximately 2% of newborns with congenital deafness. Genetic factors account for about one third of all congenital deafness and half of profound deafness.

Aplasia of Inner Ear

Inner ear aplasia is always associated with auditory nerve abnormalities. The three main types are the *Michel defect*, complete absence of the otic capsule and eighth cranial nerve; the *Mondini defect*, incomplete development of the bony and membranous labyrinths and dysgenesis of the spiral ganglion; and the *Scheibe defect*, dysplasia of the membranous labyrinth and atrophy of the eighth nerve.

Chromosome Disorders

Hearing impairment is relatively uncommon in children with chromosomal disorders. Abnormalities of chromosome 18 are often associated with profound sensorineural hearing loss and malformations of the external ear.

Genetic Disorders

Several hundred genes are known to cause hereditary hearing loss and deafness. The hearing loss may be conductive, sensorineural, or mixed. Some are congenital and some develop later in childhood.

Infantile Refsum Disease

Infantile Refsum disease, like Zellweger syndrome, is a disorder of peroxisome biogenesis (see Chapter 6). It differs from later-onset Refsum disease (see Chapter 7), a single-enzyme peroxisomal disorder. The gene locus is on chromosome 7q21–q22. Autosomal recessive inheritance is suspected.

CLINICAL FEATURES. Features include early onset, mental retardation, minor facial dysmorphism, retinitis pigmentosa, sensorineural hearing deficit, hepatomegaly, osteoporosis, failure to thrive, and hypocholesterolemia.

DIAGNOSIS. The concentration of protein in the spinal fluid is elevated, and EEG may show epileptiform activity. Liver transaminase levels are elevated, as is the serum concentration of bile acids. An elevated plasma concentration of very-long-chain fatty acids is essential to the diagnosis.

MANAGEMENT. Treatment is directed at the symptoms.

Isolated Deafness

Isolated deafness in newborns and infants is usually genetic and may be transmitted by autosomal dominant, autosomal recessive, or X-linked inheritance. In many sporadic cases the hearing loss proves to be transmitted by autosomal recessive inheritance. The association of congenital deafness and external ear deformities is often caused by genetic disorders transmitted by autosomal dominant inheritance, but chromosomal disorders and fetal exposure to drugs and toxins must be considered as well. Maternal use of heparin during pregnancy produces an embryopathy characterized by skeletal deformities, flattening of the nose, cerebral dysgenesis, and deafness.

In the absence of external malformation, a sporadic case of deafness may not be suspected until the infant fails to develop speech. Intrauterine infection with cytomegalovirus is an important cause of congenital deafness (see Chapter 5). Nearly 1% of newborns in the United States are infected with cytomegalovirus, and sensorineural hearing loss develops in approximately 10%. Rubella embryopathy was once a significant cause of deafness, but it has been almost eliminated in the United States by mass immunization.

Pendred Syndrome

Pendred syndrome is a genetic defect in thyroxine synthesis transmitted by autosomal recessive inheritance and characterized by goiter and sensorineural hearing impairment.

CLINICAL FEATURES. Sensorineural hearing impairment is present at birth and is severe in 50% of cases. Milder hearing impairment may not be detected until the child is 2 years of age. Vestibular function may also be impaired.

A diffuse, nonnodular goiter becomes apparent during the first decade, often in infancy. No clinical signs of hypothyroidism are present. Growth and intelligence are usually normal.

DIAGNOSIS. The laboratory method for assessing iodide organification is the perchlorate discharge test. It is a measure of thyroidal radioactive iodine content following the administration of potassium perchlorate. A decline of 10% or more from baseline levels of thyroidal radioactive iodine is considered a positive result.

Thin-section high-resolution MRI in the axial and sagittal planes shows enlargement of the endolymphatic sac and duct in association with a large vestibular aqueduct (Phelps et al, 1998). Recognized mutations in the chromosomal locus 7q22–q31 can be detected in approximately 75% of cases.

MANAGEMENT. Goiter is best treated medically, not surgically. Exogenous hormone decreases production of thyroid-stimulating hormone, with subsequent reduction in goiter size. The hearing loss is irreversible.

Usher Syndrome

Usher syndrome is the most common type of autosomal recessive syndromic hearing loss. It is characterized by congenital deafness and retinitis pigmentosa.

CLINICAL FEATURES. Bilateral severe sensorineural deafness is present at birth. Slowly progressive loss of vision caused by retinitis pigmentosa begins during the second decade and leads to blindness in the fifth decade or later. Vestibular responses to caloric testing are absent, and mild ataxia may be present. Mental retardation is present in 25% of cases.

DIAGNOSIS. The combination of retinitis pigmentosa and hearing impairment is also present in other syndromes: *Alstrom syndrome*, obesity and diabetes mellitus; *Cockayne syndrome* (see

Chapter 16); *Laurence-Moon-Biedel syndrome,* mental deficiency, hypogonadism, obesity; and *Refsum disease* (see Chapter 7). Usher syndrome is the only one in which profound deafness is present at birth.

MANAGEMENT. Deafness is too profound to be corrected with hearing aids. Treatment is unavailable.

Waardenburg Syndrome

Waardenburg syndrome is the most common type of autosomal dominant syndromic hearing loss. It consists of sensorineural hearing loss and pigmentary abnormalities of the skin, hair (white forelock), and eyes (heterochromia iridis). Several clinical forms exist (Read and Newton, 1997). The gene map locus is chromosome 2q35.

CLINICAL FEATURES. Waardenburg syndrome is relatively easy to recognize because of its cutaneous features: a white forelock, eyes of different colors (usually different shades of blue), hypertelorism, and depigmented dermal patches. Hearing loss is not a constant feature. An additional feature is a wide bridge of the nose owing to lateral displacement of the inner canthus of each eye.

DIAGNOSIS. The family history and the cutaneous features establish the diagnosis. Five gene abnormalities have been identified that can be tested by DNA analysis.

MANAGEMENT. Treatment is unavailable.

Acquired Hearing Impairment

Drug-Induced Impairment

Antibiotics are the most commonly used class of drugs with potential ototoxicity in children. The incidence of toxic reactions is greatest with amikacin, furosemide, and vancomycin and only a little less with kanamycin and neomycin. Permanent damage is unusual with any of these drugs. The characteristic syndrome consists of tinnitus and high-frequency hearing impairment. Vancomycin produces hearing loss only when blood concentrations exceed 45 μg/ml.

By contrast, aminoglycosides may cause irreversible cochlear toxicity, which begins as tinnitus, progresses to vertigo and high-frequency hearing impairment, and finally impairs all frequencies. This is of special concern in sick preterm newborns given aminoglycosides for periods of 15 days or longer.

β-adrenoceptor blocking drugs are a rare cause of hearing impairment and tinnitus. Cessa-

tion of therapy reverses symptoms. Cisplatin, an anticancer drug, has ototoxic effects in 30% of recipients. Tinnitus is the major feature. The hearing impairment is at frequencies above those used for speech.

Salicylates tend to concentrate in the perilymph of the labyrinth and are ototoxic. Tinnitus and high-frequency hearing impairment result from long-term exposure to high doses.

Genetic Neurological Disorders

Several of the disorders listed in Table 17-5 are discussed in other chapters. Sensorineural hearing impairment occurs as part of several spinocerebellar degenerations, hereditary motor sensory neuropathies, and sensory autonomic neuropathies. It is a major feature of Refsum disease (hereditary motor sensory neuropathy type IV) and can be controlled by dietary measures to reduce serum concentrations of phytanic acid.

Pontobulbar Palsy with Deafness

Pontobulbar palsy with deafness is a rare hereditary motor neuron disorder. The mode of transmission is not established. It shares many clinical features with juvenile progressive bulbar palsy, and some cases may be variant expressions of the same genetic error.

CLINICAL FEATURES. Onset most often occurs during the second decade. Progressive sensorineural hearing loss is the initial symptom and may affect first one ear and then the other. Deafness is accompanied or quickly followed by facial weakness and dysphagia. Tongue atrophy occurs in most cases, but masseter and ocular motor palsies are uncommon.

Approximately half of patients have evidence of pyramidal tract dysfunction, such as extensor plantar responses, and half have atrophy and fasciculations of limb muscle. Loss of tendon reflexes is an early feature of most cases. Respiratory insufficiency is a common feature and a frequent cause of death.

DIAGNOSIS. The presence of deafness and areflexia distinguishes pontobulbar palsy from juvenile progressive bulbar palsy but can also suggest a hereditary motor sensory neuropathy if symptoms of bulbar palsy are delayed. The diagnosis depends on the clinical features and cannot be confirmed by laboratory tests. MRI of the brainstem should be performed to exclude the possibility of tumor.

Table 17-5
Hearing Impairment and Deafness

Congenital
Aplasia of inner ear
   Michel defect
   Mondini defect
   Scheibe defect
Chromosome disorders
   Trisomy 13
   Trisomy 18
   18q-syndrome
Genetic disorders
   Isolated deafness
   Pendred syndrome
   Usher syndrome
   Waardenburg syndrome
Intrauterine viral infection (see Chapter 5)
Maternal drug use

Drugs
Antibiotics
β-blockers
Chemotherapy

Genetic Neurological Disorders
Adhalin deficiency (see Chapter 7)
Facioscapulohumeral dystrophy (see Chapter 7)
Familial spastic paraplegia (see Chapter 12)
Hereditary motor sensory neuropathies (see Chapter 7)
Hereditary sensory autonomic neuropathies (see Chapter 9)
Infantile Refsum disease
Neurofibromatosis type 2 (see Acoustic Neuroma)
Pontobulbar palsy with deafness
Mitochondrial disorders (see Chapter 8)
Spinocerebellar degenerations (see Chapter 10)
Wolfram syndrome (see Chapter 16)
Xeroderma pigmentosum (see Chapter 5)

Infectious Diseases
Bacterial meningitis
Otitis media (see Vertigo)
Sarcoidosis (see Facial Weakness)
Viral encephalitis (see Chapter 2)
Viral exanthemas

Metabolic Disorders
Hypothyroidism
Mèniére disease (see Vertigo)

Skeletal Disorders
Apert acrocephalosyndactyly
Cleidocranial dysostosis
Craniofacial dysostosis (Crouzon disease)
Craniometaphyseal dysplasia (Pyle disease)
Klippel-Feil syndrome
Mandibulofacial dysostosis (Treacher Collins syndrome)
Osteogenesis imperfecta
Osteopetrosis (Albers-Schönberg disease)

Trauma (see Vertigo)

Tumor
Acoustic neuroma
Cholesteatoma (see Vertigo)

MANAGEMENT. A feeding gastrostomy is needed in most patients. Treatment is not available for the underlying disease.

Infectious Diseases

Otitis media is a common cause of reversible conductive hearing impairment in children, but only rarely does suppurative infection spread to the inner ear (see section on Vertigo later in this chapter). Hearing impairment is a relatively common symptom of viral encephalitis (see Chapter 2) and may be an early feature. Sudden hearing loss may also accompany childhood exanthemas (chickenpox, mumps, and measles), and in such cases virus can be isolated from the cochlear and auditory nerves.

The overall incidence of persistent unilateral or bilateral hearing loss in children with acute bacterial meningitis is 10%. The risk can be reduced by early treatment with dexamethasone (see Chapter 4). *Streptococcus pneumoniae* meningitis is also associated with a 20% incidence of persistent dizziness, gait ataxia, and other neurological deficits.

The site of disease is probably the inner ear or auditory nerve. Organisms may gain access to the inner ear from the subarachnoid space. Otitis media is the source of meningitis in many children and produces a transitory conductive hearing loss but does not cause a permanent sensorineural hearing loss. It is common in many centers to screen all children hospitalized for treatment of acute bacterial meningitis with BAER audiometry prior to discharge.

Metabolic Disorders

Mèniére disease is characterized by vertigo, tinnitus, and hearing impairment. Vertigo is often the presenting feature (see the later discussion of Vertigo). Tinnitus and decreased hearing are common features of hypothyroidism and are reversible by thyroid replacement therapy.

Skeletal Disorders

The combination of hearing impairment and skeletal deformities almost always indicates a genetic disease. Skeletal disorders may be limited, usually to the face and digits, or generalized. The partial list in Table 17-6 highlights the more common syndromes. Almost all are transmitted by autosomal dominant inheritance with variable expression. The exceptions are osteopetrosis, which is transmitted by autosomal

Table 17-6
Causes of Vertigo

Drugs and toxins
Epilepsy
  Complex partial seizures
  Simple partial seizures
Infections
  Otitis media
  Vestibular neuronitis
Mèniére disease
Migraine
  Basilar migraine (see Chapter 10)
  Benign paroxysmal vertigo (see Chapter 10)
Motion sickness
Multiple sclerosis (see Chapter 10)
Psychogenic
  Hyperventilation syndrome (see Chapter 1)
  Panic attacks
Trauma
  Migraine
  Posttraumatic neurosis
  Temporal bone fracture
  Vestibular concussion
  Whiplash injury

recessive inheritance; craniometaphyseal dysplasia, which has both a dominant and a recessive form; and the Klippel-Feil anomaly, for which the pattern of transmission is uncertain.

Trauma

Acute auditory and vestibular injuries occur with fractures of the petrous portion of the temporal bone. Vestibular function is more likely to be impaired than auditory function (see section on Vertigo later in this chapter).

Tumor

Acoustic neuroma and cholesteatoma are the tumors most likely to impair children's hearing. Other cerebellopontine angle tumors are extremely rare before the third or fourth decade. Cholesteatoma is discussed in the section on vertigo.

Acoustic Neuroma

Acoustic neuromas are more properly classified as schwannomas of the eighth nerve. Only 6% of acoustic neuromas come to medical attention in the second decade, and even fewer are seen in the first decade. Children with acoustic neuroma almost always have *neurofibromatosis type 2*

(NF2), a genetic disease distinct from neurofibromatosis type 1 (see Chapter 5). NF2 is transmitted by autosomal dominant inheritance, with the gene locus on chromosome 22. The phenotype is characterized by acoustic neuromas. Later, other cerebral tumors such as meningioma, glioma, schwannoma, and juvenile posterior subcapsular lenticular opacity may develop. Café au lait spots may be present on the skin but are fewer than five in number.

CLINICAL FEATURES. Deafness or tinnitus is the usual initial complaint. Approximately one third of patients have nonaudiological symptoms, such as facial numbness or paresthesia, vertigo, headache, and ataxia. Hearing impairment is present in almost every patient; ipsilateral diminished corneal reflex occurs in half; and ataxia, facial hypesthesia or weakness, and nystagmus are found in 30% to 40%. Large tumors cause obstructive hydrocephalus with symptoms of increased intracranial pressure and brainstem compression.

DIAGNOSIS. Molecular-based testing is available. The criteria for the clinical diagnosis of NF2 are bilateral vestibular schwannomas or a family history of NF2 in one or more first-degree relative(s) plus (1) unilateral vestibular schwannomas at age less than 30 years or (2) any two of the following: meningioma, glioma, schwannoma, or juvenile posterior subcapsular

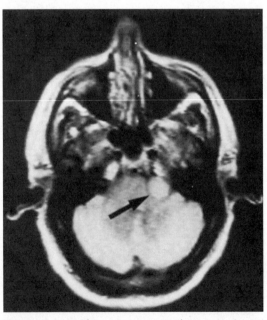

Figure 17-2. CT of acoustic neuroma. A large tumor (*arrow*) is pressing on and displacing the brainstem.

lenticular opacities/juvenile cortical cataract (Gutmann et al, 1997). Every child with progressive hearing impairment or tinnitus should be carefully examined for café au lait spots on the skin. The family history should be explored for acoustic neuroma or other neurological disturbance.

Abnormalities in pure-tone audiometry and in the BAER are present in almost every patient, but these tests are not needed for diagnosis. Gadolinium-enhanced MRI is the test of choice to visualize tumors in the cerebellopontine angle (Figure 17-2).

MANAGEMENT. Acoustic neuromas must be resected, either by surgery or by the photon (gamma ray) knife. Surgery often sacrifices residual hearing and sometimes causes a facial palsy. The superiority of the photon knife to standard surgery is not yet established.

Vertigo

Vertigo is the sensation of rotation or spinning. It is terrifying to small children. Balance is lost and posture is difficult to maintain, giving the appearance of ataxia (see Chapter 10). Nausea and nystagmus are often associated features. When nystagmus is present, the fast phase is in the same direction as the perceived rotation. Movement of the head exacerbates all symptoms.

Anatomical Considerations

The semicircular canals and the vestibule, within the labyrinth, are the sensory organs of the vestibular system. The stimulus for excitation of the semicircular canals is rotary motion of the head; for the vestibule it is gravity. Information from the sensory organs is transmitted by the vestibular portion of the eighth cranial nerve to the vestibular nuclei in the brainstem and the cerebellum. The vestibular nuclei have extensive connections with the cerebellum and medial longitudinal fasciculus. Cortical projections terminate in the superior temporal gyrus and frontal lobe.

Approach to Vertigo

History and Physical Examination

Children often complain of dizziness or lightheadedness but rarely complain of vertigo. Those who complain of dizziness or lighthead-

edness must be carefully questioned about the sensation of rotation. Whether the subject or the environment is perceived to rotate is irrelevant. The illusion of rotation separates vertigo from presyncope, ataxia, and other disturbances of balance and localizes the disturbance to the vestibular system. Vertigo implies dysfunction of the labyrinth or vestibular nerve (peripheral vertigo) or the brainstem or temporal lobe (central vertigo).

Important historical points to document include the course of vertigo (acute, recurrent, chronic), precipitating events (trauma, infection, position change), association of hearing impairment and tinnitus, drug exposure, cardiovascular disease, and family history of migraine.

Acute, episodic attacks of vertigo, not induced by motion, are most often caused by migraine or epilepsy, with migraine as the more common of the two. A single, prolonged attack of vertigo, especially when combined with nausea and vomiting, is usually due to infection of the labyrinth or vestibular nerve. Chronic vertigo often waxes and wanes and may seem intermittent rather than chronic. Both central and peripheral causes of vertigo must be considered (see Table 17-6), but the clinical and laboratory features readily distinguish central from peripheral vertigo (Table 17-7).

Special Tests

Caloric and audiometric testing is indicated for most children with chronic vertigo. Caloric testing is described in this section and audiometric testing in the section on hearing impairment. The Nylen-Hallpike test is useful to define position-induced vertigo.

Caloric Testing

The simplest method of caloric testing is to instill small quantities of cool water into the external auditory canal with a rubber-tipped syringe. The canal must first be inspected to determine whether there is clear passage to an intact tympanic membrane. A sufficient quantity of water is used, depending on the child's size, to keep the tympanic membrane cooled for 20 seconds. The eyes are then observed for nystagmus. A normal response is slow deviation of the eyes to the side stimulated, followed by a fast component to the opposite side. If stimulation with cool water fails to produce a response, the procedure is repeated with ice water. Absence of nystagmus indicates absence of peripheral vestibu-

---

Table **17-7**
Distinguishing Peripheral and Central Vertigo

Peripheral Vertigo
Clinical Features
Hearing loss, tinnitus, and otalgia may be associated features.
Past pointing and falling in the direction of unilateral disease occur.
Ataxia occurs with the eyes closed in bilateral disease.
Vestibular and positional nystagmus is present.

Laboratory Features
Caloric testing reveals vestibular paresis, directional preponderance, or both.
Pure-tone audiometry reveals sensorineural hearing loss.
Recruitment is present with end-organ disease and tone decay with nerve disease.

Central Vertigo
Clinical Features
Cerebellar and cranial nerve dysfunction are frequently associated.
Hearing is intact.
Loss of consciousness may be associated.

Laboratory Features
Pure-tone audiometry and speech discrimination are normal.
Comprehension of competing messages is impaired.
Caloric testing may reveal directional preponderance but not vestibular paresis.
Brainstem evoked response, EEG, CT, or MRI may be abnormal.

---

lar function. Partial dysfunction of one vestibular apparatus results in asymmetry of response (*directional preponderance*).

Electronystagmography

Electronystagmography is a technique that allows better quantification of caloric testing. A standard caloric stimulus is delivered into the ear, and the duration and velocity of nystagmus are recorded on paper by a machine designed for this purpose.

Nylan-Hallpike Test

In the Nylan-Hallpike test, the patient is tilted backward from the sitting position to the supine position so that the head hangs down below the level of the examining table. The head is then turned 45 degrees to the right, and the eyes are observed for position-induced nystagmus. Several minutes later, the maneuver is repeated twice, first with the head turned 45 degrees to the left and then tilted 45 degrees backward.

Causes of Vertigo

Drugs

Many drugs that disturb vestibular function also disturb auditory function. This section deals only with drugs affecting vestibular function more than auditory function. Toxic doses of anticonvulsants and neuroleptics produce ataxia, incoordination, and measurable disturbances of vestibular function, but patients do not ordinarily complain of vertigo.

Antibiotics are the main class of drugs with vestibular toxicity. Streptomycin, minocycline, and aminoglycosides have a high incidence of toxic reactions, and sulfonamides have a low incidence.

Streptomycin disturbs vestibular function but has little effect on hearing. A toxic milligram-per-kilogram dose has not been established because of variation in individual susceptibility. However, the vestibular toxicity of streptomycin is so predictable at high doses that the drug has been used to destroy vestibular function in patients with severe Mèniére disease. Dihydro-streptomycin affects auditory function and spares vestibular function. It is so ototoxic that its use has been abandoned.

Minocycline produces nausea, vomiting, dizziness, and ataxia at standard therapeutic doses. Symptoms begin 2 to 3 days after treatment is started and cease 2 days after it is stopped. Gentamicin and other aminoglycosides have an adverse effect on both vestibular and auditory function. Some disturbance is noted in 2% of patients treated with gentamicin. Vestibular dysfunction, either alone or in combination with auditory dysfunction, occurs in 84% of cases, whereas auditory dysfunction alone occurs in only 16%. Ototoxic effects develop when the total dose exceeds 17.5 mg/kg.

Epilepsy

Vertigo can be the only feature of a simple partial seizure or the initial feature of a complex partial seizure. From 10% to 20% of patients with complex partial seizures experience vertigo as an aura.

CLINICAL FEATURES. When vertigo is followed by a complex partial seizure, it is readily recognized as an aura. Diagnosis is more problematic when vertigo is the only feature of a simple partial seizure. The child ceases activity, becomes pale, appears frightened, and then recovers. Unsteadiness and nausea may be associated features.

DIAGNOSIS. Electroencephalography (EEG) is indicated in children with unexplained brief attacks of vertigo, especially when vestibular and auditory function are normal between attacks. Ambulatory EEG or 24-hour video monitoring may be needed to capture an attack if interictal EEG is normal.

MANAGEMENT. Management of simple and complex partial seizures is discussed in Chapter 2.

Infections

Bacterial Infection

Otitis media and meningitis are leading causes of vestibular and auditory impairment in children. Acute suppurative labyrinthitis resulting from extension of bacterial infection from the middle ear has become uncommon since the introduction of antibiotics. However, even without direct bacterial invasion, bacterial toxins may cause serous labyrinthitis.

Chronic otitic infections cause labyrinthine damage by the development of *cholesteatoma*. A cholesteatoma is a sac containing keratin, a silvery-white debris shed by squamous epithelial cells. Such cells are not normal constituents of the middle ear but gain access from the external canal when the eardrum is repeatedly perforated by infection. Cholesteatomas erode surrounding tissues, including bone, and produce a fistula between the perilymph and the middle ear.

CLINICAL FEATURES. Acute suppurative or serous labyrinthitis is characterized by the sudden onset of severe vertigo, nausea, vomiting, and unilateral hearing loss. Meningismus may also be present. Chronic otitis causes similar symptoms. Severe vertigo that is provoked by sneezing, coughing, or merely applying pressure on the external canal indicates fistula formation. Otoscopic examination reveals evidence of otitis media and tympanic membrane perforation and allows visualization of cholesteatoma.

DIAGNOSIS. When vestibular dysfunction develops in children with otitis media, radiographs or CT of the skull is needed to visualize erosion of bone or mastoiditis. The presence of meningismus or increased intracranial pressure (see Chapter 4) necessitates CT to exclude the possibility of abscess and then examination of cerebrospinal fluid to exclude meningitis.

MANAGEMENT. Vigorous antibiotic therapy and drainage of the infected area are required in every case. Myringotomy and mastoidectomy may be needed for drainage. Cholesteatomas are progressive and must be surgically excised.

Viral Infections

Viral infections may affect the labyrinth or vestibular nerve. The two are difficult to differentiate by clinical features, and the terms *vestibular neuritis* or *neuronitis* are used to describe acute peripheral vestibulopathies. Vestibular neuritis may be part of a systemic viral infection, such as mumps, measles, and infectious mononucleosis, or it may occur in epidemics without an identifiable viral agent, or as part of a postinfectious cranial polyneuritis. The incidence in children is low, accounting for less than 7% of all cases.

CLINICAL FEATURES. The main feature is the acute onset of vertigo. Any attempt to move the head is met with severe exacerbation of vertigo, nausea, and vomiting. Nystagmus is present on fixation and increased by head movement. The patient is unable to maintain posture and lies motionless in bed. Recovery begins during the first 48 hours. Spontaneous nausea diminishes, and nystagmus on fixation ceases. With each day, vertigo decreases in severity but positional nystagmus is still present. Recovery is usually complete within 3 weeks.

DIAGNOSIS. The diagnosis is usually established on the basis of clinical features alone. Brain imaging is unnecessary when acute-onset vertigo is an isolated symptom and begins improving within 48 hours (Hotson and Baloh, 1998).

MANAGEMENT. During the acute phase the child must be kept in bed and provided with vestibular sedation. Diazepam is very effective in dampening the labyrinth and relieving the symptoms. Transdermal scopolamine should not be used in children. As recovery progresses, activity is gradually increased and sedation reduced.

Mèniére Disease

Mèniére disease is believed to be an overaccumulation of endolymph resulting in rupture of the labyrinth. It is uncommon in children.

CLINICAL FEATURES. The clinical features of hearing impairment, tinnitus, and vertigo are attributed to rupture of the labyrinth. Hearing impairment fluctuates and may temporarily return to normal when the rupture heals. Tinnitus may be ignored, but vertigo demands attention and is often the complaint that brings the disorder to attention.

A typical attack consists of disabling vertigo and tinnitus lasting for 1 to 3 hours. The vertigo may be preceded by tinnitus, fullness in the ear, or increased loss of hearing. Tinnitus becomes worse during the attack. Pallor, sweating, nausea, and vomiting are often associated features. Afterward, the patient is tired and sleeps. Attacks occur at unpredictable intervals for years and then subside, leaving the patient with permanent hearing loss. Bilateral involvement is present in 20% of cases.

Nystagmus is present during an attack. At first the fast component is toward the abnormal ear (irritative); later, as the attack subsides, the fast component is away (paralytic). Between attacks the results of examination are normal, with the exception of unilateral hearing impairment.

DIAGNOSIS. Pure-tone audiometry shows threshold fluctuation. Speech discrimination is preserved, and recruitment is present on the abnormal side. Caloric stimulation demonstrates unilateral vestibular paresis or directional preponderance.

MANAGEMENT. The underlying disease cannot be reversed. Treatment is directed at management of the acute attack and attempts to increase the interval between attacks. The acute attack is treated with bed rest, sedation, and antiemetics. Maintenance therapy usually consists of a low-salt diet and diuretics; neither provides substantial benefit.

Migraine

Seventeen percent of migraineurs report vertigo at the time of an attack. Such individuals have no difficulty in recognizing vertigo as a symptom of migraine. Another 10% experience vertigo in the interval between attacks and may have difficulty relating vertigo to migraine.

Brief (minutes), recurrent episodes of vertigo in infants and small children are recognized as a migraine equivalent, despite the absence of headache, because the attacks later evolve into classic migraine. Affected children appear ataxic, and for this reason the disorder is discussed in Chapter 10 (see the section on Benign Paroxysmal Vertigo).

Motion Sickness

Motion sickness is induced by unfamiliar body accelerations or a mismatch in information provided to the brain by the visual and vestibular systems during acceleration of the body. It is inhibited when motion in the visual field is in opposition to actual body movement. Therefore, looking out the window when driving reduces motion sickness. Small children in the back seat, where the only visual input is the car interior, are at the greatest risk for motion sickness. A minivan may reduce the incidence of motion sickness by allowing children access to a window.

The prevalence of motion sickness depends on how violent the movement is and approaches 100% in the worst case. Twenty-five percent of a ship's passengers become sick during a 2- to 3-day Atlantic crossing, and 0.5% of commercial airline passengers are affected.

The first symptom is pallor, which is followed by nausea and vomiting. Because nausea usually precedes vomiting, there is time to prevent vomiting in some situations. Stopping the motion is the best way to abort an attack. Watching the environment move opposite the direction of body movement may inhibit early attacks. Individuals with known susceptibility to motion sickness should take an antihistamine, diazepam, or scopolamine before travel.

Trauma

Fifty percent of children complain of dizziness and headache during the first 3 days after a closed head injury, with or without loss of consciousness. One third have persistent vertigo without hearing loss. This group may be separated into patients with direct trauma to the labyrinth (*vestibular concussion*) and those in whom the vestibular apparatus is not injured. Children with posttraumatic neurosis complain of dizziness or giddiness but do not experience the illusion of rotation.

Vestibular Concussion

CLINICAL FEATURES. Vestibular concussion follows blows to the parieto-occipital or temporo-parietal region of the skull. Severe vertigo is present immediately after injury. The child is unsteady and sways toward the affected side. Symptoms persist for several days and then resolve completely, but specific movements of the head (*paroxysmal positional vertigo*) precipitate recurrent episodes of vertigo and nausea lasting for 5 to 10 seconds.

DIAGNOSIS. Radiography of the skull is indicated in all children with vertigo following head injury. Special attention should be paid to fractures through the petrous pyramid. Bleeding from the ear or a facial palsy should raise suspicion of such a skull fracture.

Positional nystagmus is induced by the Nylan-Hallpike technique when the injured ear is moved down. Caloric testing or electronystagmography shows a reduced response from the injured ear.

MANAGEMENT. Immediately after injury the patient should be treated with an antihistamine and diazepam until the acute phase is over. Individuals with paroxysmal positional vertigo are treated with *fatigue therapy*. The patient is tilted to a position that reproduces symptoms. The patient remains in that position until the vertigo subsides for at least 30 seconds and then sits up for 30 seconds. The procedure is repeated four times. This exercise is performed several times each day until the patient is no longer sensitive to positional change.

Whiplash Injury

Whiplash injuries are frequently associated with vestibular and auditory dysfunction. Symptoms are probably caused by basilar artery spasm.

CLINICAL FEATURES. Vertigo may be present immediately after injury and subsides within a few days. Brief attacks of vertigo and tinnitus, sometimes associated with headache or nausea, may develop months later in children who appear fully recovered from the injury. Many features of the attacks suggest basilar artery migraine (see Chapter 10) and probably represent a post-traumatic migraine.

DIAGNOSIS. During the acute phase, vertigo may be induced by the Nylan-Hallpike technique and unilateral dysfunction is documented by caloric testing. Vestibular function may also be abnormal in children who are experiencing basilar artery migraine, especially at the time of an attack. EEG often shows occipital intermittent rhythmic delta activity (see Figure 10-2).

MANAGEMENT. Treatment is symptomatic.

References

Borgatti R, Triulzi F, Zucca C, et al. Bilateral perisylvian polymicrogyria in three generations. *Neurology* 1999;52:1910–1913.

Brouwer OF, Padberg GW, Bakker E. Early onset facioscapulohumeral muscular dystrophy. *Muscle Nerve* 1995;2(suppl):S67–S72.

Das VK. Aetiology of bilateral sensorineural hearing impairment in children. *Arch Dis Child* 1996;74:8–12.

Gutmann D, Aylsworth A, Carley J, et al. The diagnostic evaluation and multidisciplinary management of neurofibromatosis 1 and neurofibromatosis 2. *JAMA* 1997;278:51–57.

Hato N, Kisaki H, Honda N, et al. Ramsay-Hunt syndrome in children. *Arch Neurol* 2000;48:254–256.

Hotson JR, Baloh RW. Acute vestibular syndrome. *N Engl J Med* 1998;333:680–686.

Jaradeh S, D'Cruz O, Howard JF, Jr, et al. Mobius syndrome: Electrophysiologic studies in seven cases. *Muscle Nerve* 1996;19:1148–1153.

Kesler A, Vainstein G, Gadoth N. Melkersson-Rosenthal syndrome treated with methylprednisolone. *Neurology* 1998;51:1440–1441.

Murakami S, Hato N, Horiuchi J, et al. Treatment of Ramsay Hunt syndrome with acyclovir-prednisone: Significance of early diagnosis and treatment. *Ann Neurol* 1997;41:353–357.

Padberg GW, Brouwer OF, de Keizer RJW, et al. On the significance of retinal vascular disease and hearing loss in facioscapulohumeral muscular dystrophy. *Muscle Nerve* 1995;2(suppl):S73–S80.

Phelps PD, Coffey RA, Trembath RC, et al. Radiological malformations of the ear in Pendred syndrome. *Clin Radiol* 1998;53:268–273.

Read AP, Newton VE, Waardenburg syndrome. *J Med Genet* 1997;34:656–665.

Sartoretti-Schefer S, Kollias S, Wichmann W, et al. T2-weighted three-dimensional fast spin-echo MR in inflammatory peripheral facial nerve palsy. *AJNR* 1998;19:491–495.

Schröder JM, Krabbe B, Weis J. Oculopharyngeal muscular dystrophy: Clinical and morphological follow-up study reveals mitochondrial alterations and unique nuclear inclusions in a severe autosomal recessive type. *Neuropathol Appl Neurobiol* 1995;21:68–73.

Shapiro NL, Cunningham MJ, Parikh SJ, et al. Congenital unilateral facial palsy. *Pediatrics* 1996;98:261–265.

Chapter 18
Disorders of Cranial Volume and Shape

THE VOLUME OF the three compartments that fill the skull (brain, cerebrospinal fluid, and blood) determines the size of the skull during infancy. Expansion of one compartment is at the expense of another so that intracranial volume and pressure remain constant (see Chapter 4). The extracerebral spaces (epidural, subdural, and subarachnoid) may expand with blood and significantly affect cranial volume. Less important factors contributing to head size are the thickness of the skull bones and the rate of their fusion.

The skull's shape is determined in part by its content, but external forces on the skull and the rate at which individual skull bones fuse are even more important factors. The recent move to have infants sleep supine instead of prone may be leading to a generation of children with flat occiputs (Hunt and Puczynski, 1996).

Measuring Head Size

Head circumference is determined by measuring the greatest occipitofrontal circumference. The accuracy of the measurement in estimating cranial volume is influenced by fluid in and beneath the scalp and by head shape. The scalp can be thickened from edema or blood following a prolonged and difficult delivery, and cephalohematoma may be present as well. Fluid that infiltrates from a scalp infusion can markedly increase head circumference.

A round head has a larger intracranial volume than an oval head of equal circumference. A head with a relatively large occipitofrontal diameter has a larger volume than a head with a relatively large biparietal diameter.

Head circumference measurements are most informative when plotted over time. The head

sizes of male and female infants are different, and head growth charts that provide median values for both sexes should not be used. The rate of head growth in premature infants is considerably faster than in full-term newborns (Figure 18-1). For this reason, head circumference must always be charted by conceptional age and not by postnatal age.

Macrocephaly

Macrocephaly means a large head, larger than two standard deviations from the normal distribution. Thus 2% of the "normal" population has macrocephaly. Investigation of such individuals may show an abnormality that has caused macrocephaly, but many are normal, often with a familial tendency for a large head. *When asked to evaluate a large head in an otherwise normal child, first ask the parents for their hat sizes.*

The causes of a large head include *hydrocephalus,* or an excessive volume of cerebrospinal fluid in the skull; *megalencephaly,* or enlargement of the brain; thickening of the skull; and hemorrhage into the subdural or epidural spaces. Hydrocephalus is traditionally *communicating* (nonobstructive) or *noncommunicating* (obstructive), depending on whether cerebrospinal fluid communicates between the ventricles and subarachnoid space (Table 18-1). Hydrocephalus is the main cause of macrocephaly at birth in which intracranial pressure is increased.

The causes of megalencephaly are anatomical and metabolic. The anatomical disorders are primary megalencephaly and neurocutaneous disorders (Table 18-2). Children with anatomical megalencephaly are often macrocephalic at birth but have normal intracranial pressure.

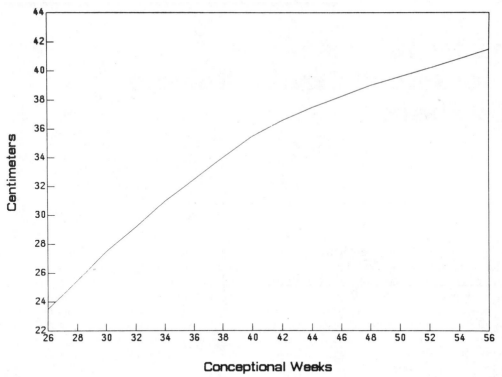

Figure 18-1. Normal growth of head circumference in boys. The rate of growth in premature infants is greater than in full-term infants.

Table 18-1
Causes of Hydrocephalus

Communicating
Achondroplasia
Basilar impression (see Chapter 10)
Benign enlargement of subarachnoid space
Choroid plexus papilloma (see Chapter 4)
Meningeal malignancy
Meningitis (see Chapter 4)
Posthemorrhagic (see Chapter 4)

Noncommunicating
Aqueductal stenosis
  Infectious
  X-linked
Chiari malformation (see Chapter 10)
Dandy-Walker malformation
Klippel-Feil syndrome
Mass lesions
  Abscess (see Chapter 4)
  Hematoma (see Chapter 1 and 2)
  Tumors and neurocutaneous disorders
  Vein of Galen malformation
  Walker-Warburg syndrome

Hydranencephaly
Holoprosencephaly
Massive hydrocephalus
Porencephaly

Table 18-2
Causes of Megalencephaly

Anatomical Megalencephaly
Genetic megalencephaly
Megalencephaly with achondroplasia
Megalencephaly with gigantism (Sotos syndrome)
Megalencephaly with a neurological abnormality
Neurocutaneous disorders
  Epidermal nevus syndrome
  Hypomelanosis of Ito
  Incontinentia pigmenti (see Chapter 1)
  Neurofibromatosis (see Chapter 5)
  Tuberous sclerosis (see Chapter 5)

Metabolic Megalencephaly
Alexander disease (see Chapter 5)
Canavan disease (see Chapter 5)
Galactosemia: transferase deficiency (see Chapter 5)
Gangliosidosis (see Chapter 5)
Globoid leukodystrophy (see Chapter 5)
Glutaric aciduria type I (see Chapter 14)
Leukoencephalopathy with swelling and cysts
Maple syrup urine disease (see Chapter 1)
Metachromatic leukodystrophy (see Chapter 5)
Mucopolysaccharidoses (see Chapter 5)

Table 18-3
Conditions with a Thickened Skull Causing Macrocephaly

Anemia
Cleidocranial dysostosis
Craniometaphyseal dysplasia of Pyle
Epiphyseal dysplasia
Hyperphosphatemia
Leontiasis ossea
Orodigitofacial dysostosis
Osteogenesis imperfecta
Osteopetrosis
Pyknodysostosis
Rickets
Russell dwarf

Children with metabolic megalencephaly are usually normocephalic at birth and develop megalencephaly from cerebral edema during the neonatal period.

Macrocephaly caused by increased thickness of the skull bones is not present at birth or in the newborn period but develops during infancy. The conditions associated with increased skull growth are summarized in Table 18-3 but are not discussed in the text. Intracranial hemorrhage in the newborn is discussed in Chapter 1, and intracranial hemorrhage in older children is discussed in Chapter 2.

Communicating Hydrocephalus

Communicating hydrocephalus is usually caused by impaired absorption of cerebrospinal fluid secondary to meningitis or subarachnoid hemorrhage. Meningeal malignancy, usually caused by leukemia or primary brain tumor, is a less common cause. The excessive production of cerebrospinal fluid by a choroid plexus papilloma rarely causes communicating hydrocephalus because the potential rate of cerebrospinal reabsorption far exceeds the productive capacity of the choroid plexus (see Chapter 4). Such tumors more commonly cause hydrocephalus by obstructing one or more ventricles.

Achondroplasia

Achondroplasia is a genetic disorder, transmitted as an autosomal dominant trait (4p16.3). Most cases are new mutations. It is the most frequent form of short-limbed dwarfism.

CLINICAL FEATURES. The main features are short stature caused by rhizomelic shortening of the limbs (the proximal portion of the limbs is shorter than the distal portion), frontal bossing and mid-face hypoplasia, lumbar lordosis, and limitation of elbow extension. The typical recessed facial appearance is caused by stunted formation of enchondral bone.

Affected newborns have true megalencephaly. Hydrocephalus, when it occurs, may be caused by increased intracranial pressure from stenosis of the sigmoid sinus at the level of the jugular foramina. Despite considerable, and sometimes alarming, enlargement of head circumference, achondroplastic dwarfs seldom show clinical evidence of increased intracranial pressure or progressive dementia. Respiratory disturbances are common. Dyspnea is sometimes caused by cervicomedullary compression. Other features of cervicomedullary compression are hyperreflexia, spasticity, and sensory disturbances of the limbs (Lachmann, 1997).

DIAGNOSIS. The diagnosis of achondroplasia is established by clinical examination. The mutation rate is high, and no other family member may be affected. Computed tomography (CT) shows a small posterior fossa and enlargement of the sphenoid sinuses. Basilar impression is sometimes present. Ventricular size varies from normal in newborns and young infants to moderate or severe dilatation in older children and adults.

MANAGEMENT. Ventricular size, after initial dilatation, usually remains stable and surgical diversion of cerebrospinal fluid is rarely needed. Decompressive surgery is required in children with evidence of progressive cervicomedullary compromise.

Benign Enlargement of Subarachnoid Space

Benign enlargement of the subarachnoid space is described under several names in the literature: *external hydrocephalus, extraventricular hydrocephalus, benign subdural effusions,* and *benign extracerebral fluid collections.* It is a relatively common cause of macrocephaly in infants, a fact not fully appreciated before the widespread use of CT to investigate large head size. A genetic cause of this condition is likely in some cases, with the infant's father often having a large head.

CLINICAL FEATURES. The condition occurs more commonly in males than females. A large head circumference is the only feature. An otherwise

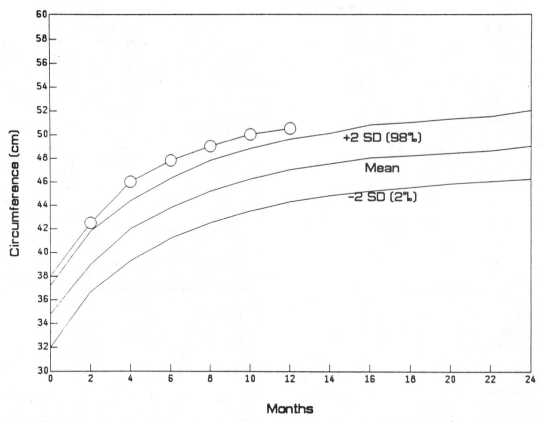

Figure 18-2. Benign enlargement of the subarachnoid space. Head circumference is already large at birth, grows to exceed the 98th percentile, and then parallels the curve.

normal infant is brought to medical attention because serial head circumference measurements show an enlarging head size. The circumference is usually above the 90th percentile at birth, grows to exceed the 98th percentile, and then parallels the normal curve (Figure 18-2). The anterior fontanelle is large but soft. Neurological findings and developmental status are normal.

DIAGNOSIS. Cranial CT shows an enlarged frontal subarachnoid space, widening of the sylvian fissures and other sulci, and normal or minimally enlarged ventricular size (Figure 18-3). Normal ventricular size distinguishes this condition from cerebral atrophy. In infants, the upper limit of normal size for the frontal subarachnoid space is 5.7 mm and for the sylvian fissure is 7.6 mm.

MANAGEMENT. Most affected infants develop normally and do not require ventricular shunts. Head circumference measurements should be plotted monthly for the next 6 months after diagnosis to be certain that growth is paralleling the normal curve. Repeat CT is not needed un-

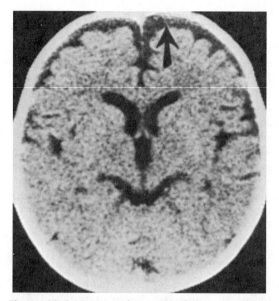

Figure 18-3. Benign enlargement of the subarachnoid space. CT reveals an enlarged frontal subarachnoid space (*arrow*), prominent sulci, and normal ventricular size.

less head growth deviates upward from the normal curve, neurological findings become abnormal, or development is delayed.

Meningeal Malignancy

Tumors that infiltrate the meninges and subarachnoid space impair the reabsorption of cerebrospinal fluid and cause communicating hydrocephalus. The primary site of tumor is usually established before its meningeal spread, but hydrocephalus may be the initial feature of diffuse meningeal gliomatosis.

CLINICAL FEATURES. Tumors that infiltrate the meninges are usually aggressive, causing a rapid progression of symptoms. Headache and vomiting are the initial features and are followed by lethargy and personality change. Meningismus and papilledema are common features and may suggest bacterial meningitis. Multifocal neurological disturbances may be present.

DIAGNOSIS. Magnetic resonance imaging (MRI) shows dilatation of the entire ventricular system but not of the subarachnoid space, which may appear obliterated except for a layer of enhancement. The pressure of the cerebrospinal fluid and its protein concentration are increased. The glucose concentration may be depressed or normal. Tumor cell identification in the cerebrospinal fluid is essential for early diagnosis and treatment, although it is rarely accomplished unless large volumes are examined. Meningeal biopsy is required for tissue diagnosis in many cases.

MANAGEMENT. A ventricular shunt is necessary to relieve symptoms of increased intracranial pressure. Radiation therapy and chemotherapy provide palliation and extend life in some cases, but the outcome is generally poor.

Noncommunicating Hydrocephalus

Complete obstruction of the egress of cerebrospinal fluid from the ventricles to the subarachnoid space causes increased pressure and dilation of all ventricles proximal to the obstruction. The incidence of congenital hydrocephalus is 0.4–0.8 per 1,000 liveborns and stillbirths. X-linked hydrocephalus accounts for 4% of all cases (Schrander-Stumpel and Fryns, 1998).

Noncommunicating hydrocephalus is the most common form of hydrocephalus in fetuses. Aqueductal stenosis is the usual cause of congenital hydrocephalus in the absence of other associated cerebral malformations. It becomes less common during infancy but increases in frequency again during childhood. Mass lesions are the most common cause of aqueductal obstruction during childhood. Children with congenital hydrocephalus who have seizures usually have other cerebral malformations. Such children have a higher incidence of mental retardation.

Congenital Aqueductal Stenosis

At birth, the mean length of the cerebral aqueduct is 12.8 mm and its smallest cross-sectional diameter is usually 0.5 mm. The small lumen of the cerebral aqueduct, in relation to its length, makes it especially vulnerable to internal compromise from infection and hemorrhage and to external compression by tumors and venous malformations. Congenital atresia or stenosis of the cerebral aqueduct can occur as a solitary malformation or can occur in families as an X-linked trait (Haverkamp et al, 1999).

CLINICAL FEATURES. Hydrocephalus is present at birth. Head circumference ranges from 40 to 50 cm and may cause cephalopelvic disproportion and poor progress of labor. The forehead is bowed, the scalp veins are dilated, the skull sutures are widely separated, and the fontanelles are large and tense. These signs are exaggerated when the child cries but are also present in the quiet state. The eyes are deviated downward so that the sclera shows above the iris (*setting-sun sign*), and abducens palsies may be present.

Adduction and flexion of the thumbs are seen in approximately 20% of newborns with X-linked aqueductal stenosis. The thumb position was thought to be an associated malformation but probably represents a nonspecific sign of corticospinal tract compression by the dilated lateral ventricles.

DIAGNOSIS. Antenatal diagnosis is accomplished by intrauterine sonography. However, the ventricles do not expand before 20 weeks, and sonograms performed earlier are misleading. When macrocephaly is present in the fetus, α-fetoprotein should be assayed in the amniotic fluid for the detection of neural tube defects (see Chapter 12) and chromosomal analysis should be performed. Information concerning the integrity of the fetal nervous system is needed to develop a management plan.

The postpartum diagnosis of aqueductal stenosis is readily accomplished with CT. The lateral and third ventricles are markedly enlarged, as is the cephalic end of the cerebral aqueduct. The remainder of the cerebral aqueduct and the fourth ventricle cannot be visualized (Figure 18-4).

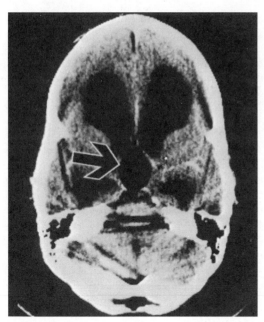

Figure 18-4. Aqueductal stenosis. CT demonstrates marked enlargement of the third ventricle (*arrow*) and the lateral ventricles.

MANAGEMENT. Congenital hydrocephalus caused by aqueductal stenosis is severe, does not respond to medical therapy directed at decreasing the volume of cerebrospinal fluid, and progresses to a stage that harms the brain. Diversion of the cerebrospinal fluid from the ventricular system to an extracranial site is the only effective method of management.

The management of fetal hydrocephalus depends on the presence of other malformations. Between 70% and 80% of patients have other abnormalities, usually spina bifida. Many pregnancies with an affected fetus are terminated voluntarily.

Ventriculoperitoneal shunt is generally considered the procedure of choice for newborns and small infants with aqueductal stenosis. It is easier to revise and better tolerated than ventriculoatrial shunt. Mechanical obstruction and infection are the most common complications of shunt placement in infancy (see Chapter 4).

The relief of hydrocephalus increases the potential for normal development, even when the cerebral mantle appears very thin preoperatively, but does not necessarily result in a normal child. The growth of intelligence is often uneven, with better development of verbal skills than of nonverbal skills. Associated anomalies may cause motor deficits and seizures.

Dandy-Walker Malformation

The Dandy-Walker malformation consists of partial or complete agenesis of the cerebellar vermis, cystic dilatation of the posterior fossa communicating with the fourth ventricle, and hydrocephalus. The hydrocephalus may not be present at birth and more often develops during childhood or even later. The size of the lateral ventricles does not correlate with the size of the cyst in the fourth ventricle. Other malformations are present in 68% of patients. The most common associated malformation is agenesis of the corpus callosum. Other malformations are heterotopia, abnormal gyrus formation, dysraphic states, aqueductal stenosis, and congenital tumors (Cavalcanti and Salomao, 1999).

CLINICAL FEATURES. The diagnosis is made at birth in only 25% of cases and by 1 year in 75%. Macrocephaly is the usual initial feature. Bulging of the skull, when present, is more prominent in the occipital than in the frontal region. The rapidity of head growth is considerably slower than with aqueductal stenosis. Compression of posterior fossa structures leads to neurological dysfunction, including apneic spells, nystagmus, truncal ataxia, cranial nerve palsies, and hyperreflexia in the legs.

DIAGNOSIS. CT or MRI is usually ordered because of macrocephaly or ataxia. Either study shows cystic dilatation of the posterior fossa and partial or complete agenesis of the cerebellar vermis (Figure 18-5). MRI is more useful

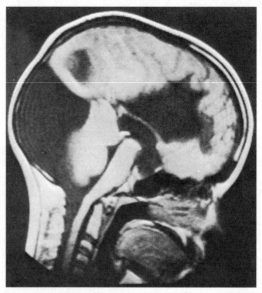

Figure 18-5. Dandy-Walker malformation. CT demonstrates cystic dilatation of the fourth ventricle and partial agenesis of the cerebellar vermis.

because it also identifies other cerebral abnormalities such as heterotopia. Incomplete vermian agenesis may be difficult to differentiate from an enlarged cisterna magna. The Dandy-Walker malformation is part of the spectrum of anomalies associated with trisomy 9 and with mutations on the X chromosome.

MANAGEMENT. Decompression of the cyst alone provides immediate relief of symptoms; however, hydrocephalus recurs and ventricular shunting is required in two thirds of affected children. Shunting of the lateral ventricle alone provides immediate relief of hydrocephalus but fails to relieve brainstem compression. The procedure of choice is a dural shunt of both the lateral ventricle and the posterior fossa cyst.

Even after successful shunt placement, many children have transitory episodes of lethargy, personality change, and vomiting. Shunt failure is suspected but cannot be substantiated. The mechanism of such episodes, which may prove fatal, is unknown.

Klippel-Feil Syndrome

Klippel-Feil syndrome is a malformation of the craniocervical skeleton that may be associated with the Chiari malformation and with basilar impression. Hydrocephalus is caused by obstruction of the egress of cerebrospinal fluid from the fourth ventricle to the subarachnoid space. There are clearly several entities in this general category. One or more may be recessive, one is dominant, and some may have no genetic basis. The malformation is classified into three types: I, extensive fusion of thoracic and upper cervical vertebrae; II, one or two interspace fusions with hemivertebrae and occipitoatlantal fusion; and III, cervical and lower thoracic or lumbar fusion. Type II is the most common form.

CLINICAL FEATURES. The essential features of the Klippel-Feil syndrome are a low posterior hairline, a short neck, and limitation of neck movement. Head asymmetry, facial asymmetry, scoliosis, and mirror movements of the hands are common. Unilateral or bilateral failure of downward migration of the scapula (Sprengel deformity) is present in 25% to 35% of patients. Malformations of the genitourinary system and deafness are associated features. The deafness may be of the sensorineural, conductive, or mixed type (McGaughran et al, 1998).

Hydrocephalus affects the fourth ventricle first and then the lateral ventricles. This results in symptoms of posterior fossa compression: ataxia, apnea, and cranial nerve dysfunction.

DIAGNOSIS. The characteristic fusion and malformations of vertebrae are seen on radiographs of the spine. MRI may show an associated Chiari malformation and dilatation of the ventricles.

MANAGEMENT. Children with unstable cervical vertebrae require cervical fusion to prevent myelopathy. Those with symptoms of obstructive hydrocephalus require a ventriculoperitoneal shunt to relieve pressure in the posterior fossa.

Congenital Brain Tumors

Congenital brain tumors and congenital brain malformations are both disorders of cellular proliferation. A noxious agent active during early embryogenesis might stimulate either or both abnormalities. The relative oncogenicity or teratogenicity depends on the virulence of the agent, the timing of the insult, the duration of exposure, and the genetic background and health of the fetus. The most common tumors of infancy are astrocytoma, medulloblastoma, teratoma, and choroid plexus papilloma.

CLINICAL FEATURES. Congenital tumors are more often supratentorial than infratentorial and more often in the midline than situated laterally. Newborns with hemispheric gliomas and teratomas may develop hydrocephalus in utero or in the first days or weeks postpartum. The point of obstruction is usually at the cerebral aqueduct (see Chapter 4). Choroid plexus papillomas are usually located in one lateral ventricle and usually become symptomatic during infancy rather than in the perinatal period. They produce hydrocephalus either by obstruction of the foramen of Monro or by excessive production of cerebrospinal fluid (see Chapter 4). Medulloblastomas are located in the posterior fossa and obstruct the fourth ventricle and cerebral aqueduct (see Chapter 10).

The clinical features of all congenital tumors are those of increasing intracranial pressure: enlarging head size, separation of the sutures, lethargy and irritability, difficult feeding, and vomiting. Seizures are unusual. Because of its posterior fossa location, medulloblastoma also produces nystagmus, downward deviation of the eyes, opisthotonus, and apnea.

DIAGNOSIS. CT or MRI, performed to investigate hydrocephalus, readily visualizes all congenital tumors. Some are identified by intrauterine sonography.

MANAGEMENT. Complete resection of congenital brain tumors is unusual, with the exception of choroid plexus papilloma. The management of individual tumors is discussed in Chapters 4 and 10.

Vein of Galen Malformation

Arteriovenous malformations of the cerebral circulation may become symptomatic during infancy and childhood (see Chapters 4 and 10), but the one associated with congenital hydrocephalus is the vein of Galen malformation. Vein of Galen vascular malformations are actually not aneurysms and do not involve the vein of Galen. Instead, the normal vein of Galen does not develop and the median prosencephalic vein of Markowsky persists, dilates, and drains to the superior sagittal sinus. Multiple arteriovenous fistulas are associated.

CLINICAL FEATURES. Eighty percent of newborns with vein of Galen malformations are male. The usual initial feature is either high-output cardiac failure or an enlarging head size. Hemorrhage almost never occurs early in the course. A cranial bruit is invariably present. Unexplained, persistent hypoglycemia has been noted in some children.

Large midline arteriovenous malformations produce a hemodynamic stress in the newborn because of the large quantities of blood shunted from the arterial to the venous system. The heart enlarges in an effort to keep up with the demands of the shunt, but high-output cardiac failure ensues. Affected newborns often come to the attention of a pediatric cardiologist first because congenital heart disease is suspected. The intracranial malformation is then diagnosed during cardiac catheterization.

When the hemodynamic stress is not severe and cardiac compensation is possible, symptoms are delayed until infancy or early childhood. In such a case, the initial feature of the malformation is obstructive hydrocephalus because it compresses the tegmentum and aqueduct. Symptoms usually begin before age 5 and always before age 10. The lateral ventricles enlarge, causing headache, lethargy, and vomiting. In infants, the head enlarges and the fontanelle feels full.

DIAGNOSIS. Vein of Galen malformations are readily visualized by contrast-enhanced CT (Figure 18-6) or MRI. The lateral and third ventricles are dilated behind the compressed cerebral aqueduct. Radiographs of the chest in newborns with high-output cardiac failure show an enlarged heart that has a normal shape.

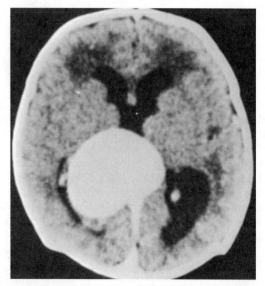

Figure 18-6. Vein of Galen malformation. The malformation is visible on contrast-enhanced CT as a large aneurysmal sac compressing the midbrain and producing obstructive hydrocephalus.

MANAGEMENT. The overall results of direct surgical approaches are poor; the mortality rate is high, as is neurological morbidity in survivors. Embolization has become the treatment of choice, but the long-term results are not established.

Walker-Warburg Syndrome

The Walker-Warburg syndrome is characterized by cerebral and ocular abnormalities. Hydrocephalus is a constant feature. The combination of the Walker-Warburg syndrome and congenital muscular dystrophy is called *cerebro-ocular dysplasia* (see Chapter 6). The abnormal gene locus has been mapped to chromosome 9q31. The risk of recurrence among siblings exceeds 50%, but the syndrome is not transmitted from one generation to the next, suggesting autosomal recessive inheritance.

CLINICAL FEATURES. Hydrocephalus is usually present at birth. It may be caused by aqueductal stenosis or the Dandy-Walker malformation. Most children with both a Dandy-Walker malformation and ocular abnormalities have the Walker-Warburg syndrome. Some children are born with microcephaly, yet have enlarged ventricles. Severe neurological abnormalities are caused by partial or total agyria (lissencephaly) resulting from failure of neuronal migration. The pattern of architectural abnormalities throughout the neuraxis suggests a disruption of cerebral maturation in the fourth conceptional month.

Several ocular abnormalities may be present, usually in combination: hypoplasia of the iris, abnormal anterior chamber, microphthalmos, cataracts, persistence of primary vitreous, optic disk coloboma, retinal detachment, retinal dysplasia, and hypoplasia of the optic nerve. In addition to having hydrocephalus and blindness, affected infants are hypotonic and have difficulty feeding. Seizures are uncommon. Most affected children die during the neonatal period or early infancy.

DIAGNOSIS. The diagnosis is based on the characteristic combination of cerebral and ocular abnormalities. Congenital infections may produce similar disturbances and must be excluded, but multisystem disease (visceromegaly and disturbed hematopiesis), an expected feature of most intrauterine infections, is lacking in the Warburg syndrome.

Cerebro-ocular abnormalities at birth are also encountered in septo-optic dysplasia (see Chapter 16) and the oculocerebrorenal syndrome (see Chapter 6), but hydrocephalus is not a component of either syndrome.

MANAGEMENT. Hydrocephalus can be managed by ventricular shunt, but the outcome is poor because of the concomitant severe cerebral malformations.

Hydranencephaly

The term *hydranencephaly* encompasses several conditions that result in the extensive replacement of brain by cerebrospinal fluid. Hydranencephaly may be caused by failure of normal brain development or from an intrauterine disorder that destroys the brain parenchyma. Progressive obstructive hydrocephalus may cause hydranencephaly if left untreated. Excessive pressure within the lateral ventricles destroys the midline structures and reduces the cerebral mantle to a thin membrane.

Head circumference at birth is large when hydranencephaly is caused by obstructive hydrocephalus, is small when the condition is caused by intrauterine diseases, and may be large or small with primary malformations.

Porencephaly

Porencephaly is a term used loosely in the literature. It was originally used to describe defects in the final stage of prosencephalization resulting in a hemispheric cyst that communicated with the subarachnoid space and the lateral ventricle. The term is now used broadly for any hemispheric cyst; most are caused by intrauterine or perinatal infarction or trauma. The injured immature brain loses neurons, glia, and supporting structures. A fluid-filled cyst in formed in the injured area and may not communicate with either the ventricular system or the subarachnoid space. Pressure within the cyst often becomes excessive, causing compression of adjacent structures and macrocrania.

Congenital Midline Porencephaly

Congenital midline porencephaly is a distinct malformation characterized by congenital hydrocephalus, alopecia or encephalocele in the parietal midline, and a midline defect in the posterior cerebral mantle. Midline porencephaly differs from holoprosencephaly, because the forebrain divides into two separate hemispheres. It may be caused by early hydrocephalus with upward outpouching and destruction of adjacent structures, including the corpus callosum, cerebral mantle, skull, and scalp. The syndromes of *giant interhemispheric cyst* and *dygenesis of the corpus callosum* are probably the same (Griebel et al, 1995).

CLINICAL FEATURES. The head is large in utero and may cause cephalopelvic disproportion at delivery. Possible defects in the parietal midline range from a small, round area of alopecia to an encephalocele. Affected children are severely retarded and blind. Most die during infancy or early childhood.

DIAGNOSIS. A large dorsal cyst that has destroyed the septum pellucidum and corpus callosum is seen on CT or MRI. The cyst communicates with enlarged lateral ventricles and extends through a skull defect to produce an encephalocele.

MANAGEMENT. Shunting the cyst may ease care by reducing the size of the head or encephalocele, but it does not prevent severe neurological impairment from the underlying cerebral malformation.

Anatomical Megalencephaly

Anatomical megalencephaly includes conditions in which the brain is enlarged because the number or size of cells increases. There is no evidence of metabolic disease or acute encephalopathy.

Benign Familial Macrocephaly

CLINICAL FEATURES. The term describes a familial condition in which neurological and mental function are normal but head circumference is larger than the 98th percentile. Autosomal dominant inheritance is suspected, but the genetic basis for nonsyndromic macrocephaly is probably multifactorial, with a polymorphic genetic basis (Arbour et al, 1996). Head circumference may not be large at birth but increases during infancy, usually to between 2 and 4 cm above the 98th percentile. Body size is normal, and no physical deformities are present.

DIAGNOSIS. The enlargement is indistinguishable by physical examination from benign enlargement of the subarachnoid space, but the two can be distinguished by CT. CT is normal in benign familial macrocephaly.

MANAGEMENT. Treatment is not required.

Megalencephaly with a Neurological Disorder

The term *megalencephaly with a neurological disorder* is used to encompass all disorders, other than neurocutaneous syndromes, in which the head is large and the child is neurologically abnormal.

CLINICAL FEATURES. Head circumference may be large at birth or may become large during infancy. It is generally 2 to 4 cm greater than the 98th percentile. Results of neurological tests are normal, but the children have learning disabilities, mental deficiency, or seizures. Neurological status remains stable.

DIAGNOSIS. The skin of the patient and other family members must be carefully examined to exclude the possibility of a neurocutaneous disorder. Ophthalmoscopic examination of family members should be carried out. Results of CT or MRI may be normal or may show mild dilatation of the ventricular system. Agenesis of the corpus callosum is the only abnormality found in some families with macrocrania and borderline intelligence.

MANAGEMENT. Seizures often respond to anticonvulsant drugs. Special education is usually required. Treatment is not available for the underlying disorder.

Megalencephaly with Gigantism

Megalencephaly with gigantism is also termed *cerebral gigantism* or *Sotos syndrome* (Opitz et al, 1998). It probably encompasses several disorders, most of them sporadic and some clearly genetic, transmitted by autosomal recessive or dominant inheritance. Chromosome studies are normal.

CLINICAL FEATURES. Affected children are in the 75th to 90th percentile at birth and grow at an excessive rate in height, weight, head circumference, and bone age up to the age of 3. Afterward, the rate of growth is normal. All children with the syndrome are large as adults, but they are not usually giants.

A prominent forehead, high-arched palate, and hypertelorism are present in almost every case. Several other dysmorphic features are reported in small numbers of patients. Many have mild learning problems that are less apparent as they become adults.

DIAGNOSIS. Cranial CT is usually normal except for mild ventricular widening. Extensive studies of endocrine function have failed to show a consistent abnormality other than glucose intolerance. Plasma somatomedin levels are elevated during the first year in some infants and fall below normal during early childhood.

MANAGEMENT. Girls may benefit from high doses of estrogens to curtail excessive growth, but treatment is not available for the underlying disorder.

Neurocutaneous Disorders

Seizures (see Table 1-8) and mental retardation (see Chapter 5) are the common features of most neurocutaneous disorders. The cutaneous features may be present at birth (incontinentia pigmenti) or during infancy (neurofibromatosis, tuberous sclerosis). Macrocrania is caused by either hydrocephalus or megalencephaly. Hemimegalencephaly, hemihypertrophy of the body, or hypertrophy of a single limb should always suggest the possibility of a neurocutaneous disorder.

Hypomelanosis of Ito

Hypomelanosis of Ito, also called *incontinentia pigmenti achromians,* does not represent a distinct entity but rather a symptom of many different states of mosaicism (Kuster et al, 1998). Most cases are sporadic, and several different chromosomal anomalies have been associated.

CLINICAL FEATURES. The cutaneous feature is a large, hypopigmented area that has a whorled or streaked appearance. It appears in the first year and is a negative image of the hyperpigmented lesions of incontinentia pigmenti (see Chapter 1). Other cutaneous features are café au lait spots, angiomatous nevi, heterochromia of the iris or hair, and other nevi. Seizures and mental retardation are the most common neurological abnormalities. IQ scores are below 70 in more than half of patients, but approximately 20% have IQ scores above 90. Approximately half of patients have seizures, usually with onset in the first year. Focal seizures are most common, although occasional patients have infantile spasms and Lennox-Gastaut syndrome. Spastic diplegia may also be present. These symptoms are caused by disturbances of neuronal migration. Megalencephaly occurs in approximately 25% of cases.

One third of patients have skeletal and eye anomalies, including limb hypertrophy or atrophy, facial hemiatrophy, poorly formed ears, dysplastic teeth, hypertelorism, strabismus, and corneal opacities.

DIAGNOSIS. The characteristic cutaneous lesions are critical to the diagnosis and should be sought in the parents and siblings as well as the child. Chromosome studies in the child and parents are indicated. MRI usually shows generalized cerebral or cerebellar hypoplasia, severe cortical neuronal migration anomalies, and hemimeganencephaly and lissencephaly. Hemimeganencephaly may be ipsilateral or contralateral to the cutaneous hypopigmentation.

MANAGEMENT. Treatment is directed at the symptoms.

Epidermal Nevus Syndrome

Epidermal nevus syndrome, also called the *linear nevus sebaceous syndrome,* refers to several disorders that have in common an epidermal nevus and neurological manifestations such as seizures or hemimeganencephaly (Dodge and Dobyns, 1995).

CLINICAL FEATURES. A unilateral linear nevus is present on the skin of the face or scalp. It may not be visible at birth but darkens during infancy and becomes verrucous. Hemihypertrophy of the face, head and limbs ipsilateral to the nevus may be present at birth or may develop during infancy.

The spectrum of neurological disability is considerable. Developmental delay and seizures are expected. The head may be enlarged generally or unilaterally. Focal neurological deficits, such as hemiplegia and hemianopia, contralateral to the nevus are relatively common. Eye abnormalities, such as microphthalmia and coloboma, occur in one third of children.

DIAGNOSIS. Diagnosis relies on recognition of the linear nevus. Electroencephalography (EEG) usually shows unilateral slowing and epileptiform discharges ipsilateral to the nevus. Hypsarrhythmia is seen on EEG when infantile spasms are the initial feature (see Chapter 1). Hemihypsarrhythmia may also occur.

Megalencephaly ipsilateral to the epidermal nevus is the most frequent finding on MRI. Several types of cerebal dysplasia may be associated, usally ipsilateral to the epidermal nevus. Focal pachygyria is the most common.

MANAGEMENT. Seizures may respond to standard anticonvulsant therapy (see Chapter 1), but treatment is not available for the underlying cerebral malformation.

Metabolic Megalencephaly

Several inborn errors of metabolism produce megalencephaly by storage of abnormal substances or by producing cerebral edema (Table 18-2). They are discussed elsewhere in the text because the initial features are usually developmental regression (see Chapter 5) or seizures (see Chapter 1). Two exceptions are glutaric aciduria type I (see Chapter 14) and *leukoencephalopathy with swelling and cysts.* Infants with glutaric aciduria type I are normal up to 3 years, except for macrocephaly, any then develop an acute encephalitic illness that resembles encephalitis.

Most infants with metabolic megalencephaly have a normal head circumference at birth. Head enlargement parallels neurological regression and clinical evidence of increased intracranial pressure. The ventricles are often small.

Leukoencephalopathy with Swelling and Cysts

The metabolic defect has not been established, but autosomal recessive inheritance is suspected because of an affected sibling pair and instances of parental consanguinity (van der Knaap et al, 1995).

CLINICAL FEATURES. The initial feature is abnormal head enlargement in a child whose development is either normal or only mildly delayed. A slowly progressive ataxia and spasticity develop, with intellectual functioning preserved for years after onset. The subsequent course is characterized by very slowly progressive ataxia and spasticity. Seizures and mild mental deterioration may occur late in the course.

DIAGNOSIS. MRI shows a severe leukoencephalopathy that suggests a demyelinating white matter disorder. The hemispheres appear swollen, with cyst-like spaces in the frontoparietal and anterior temporal areas. The occipital white matter is relatively spared.

MANAGEMENT. Treatment is directed at the symptoms.

Microcephaly

Microcephaly means a head circumference that is smaller than two standard deviations below the normal distribution. The standard for head circumference varies among different ethnic groups. A small head circumference indicates a small brain. Most full-term newborns whose head circumferences are smaller than two standard deviations, but who are neurologically normal, will have normal intelligence at age 7, but a head circumference smaller than three standard deviations usually indicates later mental retardation.

A small head circumference at birth establishes the antepartum timing of brain damage but does not distinguish primary from secondary microcephaly (Table 18-4). *Primary microcephaly* encompasses conditions in which the brain is small and never formed properly because of genetic or chromosomal abnormalities. *Secondary microcephaly* implies that the brain was forming normally but a disease process im-

paired further growth. Normal head circumference at birth, followed by failure of normal head growth, usually indicates a secondary microcephaly. Chromosomal disorders are an exception to that rule unless they cause defective prosencephalization or cellular migration.

Perinatal brain damage does not cause a recognizable decrease of head circumference until 3 to 6 months postpartum. Failure of normal brain growth removes the force keeping the cranial bones separated, and they fuse prematurely. A primary disorder of the skull (craniostenosis) may cause premature closure of the cranial sutures even though the brain is attempting to grow normally (Chumas et al, 1997). The distinction between the two is relatively simple: craniostenosis is always associated with an abnormal skull shape and heaping up of bone along the cranial sutures; failure of brain growth produces a relatively normal-shaped skull with some overlapping of skull bones.

Cranial MRI may be informative in distinguishing primary from secondary microcephaly. In most children with primary microcephaly, either MRI results are normal or a recognizable pattern of cerebral malformation is present. In those with secondary microcephaly, the brain image is usually abnormal, characterized by one or more of the following features: ventricular enlargement, cerebral atrophy, and porencephaly.

Primary Microcephaly

Many cerebral malformations are of uncertain cause and cannot be classified as primary or secondary. Morphogenetic errors, although lacking in the traditional stigmata of tissue injury, could result from exposure of the embryo to a noxious agent during the first weeks after conception. At this early stage, the delicate sequencing of neuronal development could be disorganized at a time when the brain is incapable of generating a cellular response.

Microcephaly Vera (Genetic)

Microcephaly vera is a term applied to genetic defects that decrease bulk growth of the brain. The defect is mainly transmitted as an autosomal recessive trait. Jackson et al (1998) identified a genetic locus, which they named MCPH1, for primary microcephaly, at chromosome 8pter-p22.

CLINICAL FEATURES. Children with the autosomal recessive form of microcephaly vera are usu-

---

Table 18-4
Conditions Causing Microcephaly

Primary Microcephaly
Microcephaly vera (genetic)
Chromosomal disorders
Defective neurolation
    Anencephaly
    Encephalocele
Defective prosencephalization
    Agenesis of the corpus callosum
    Holoprosencephaly (arhinencephaly)
Defective cellular migration

Secondary Microcephaly
Intrauterine disorders
    Infection
    Toxins
    Vascular
Perinatal brain injuries
    Hypoxic-ischemic encephalopathy
    Intracranial hemorrhage
    Meningitis and encephalitis
    Stroke
Postnatal systemic diseases
    Chronic cardiopulmonary disease
    Chronic renal disease
    Malnutrition

ally short and have a characteristic disproportion in size between the face and the skull. The forehead slants backward, and the reduced size of the skull causes the scalp to wrinkle in the occipital region. The chin is small, and the ears and nose are prominent. Mental retardation is moderate to severe, and other neurological abnormalities, such as spastic diplegia and seizures, may be present.

DIAGNOSIS. Results of brain imaging are normal.

MANAGEMENT. Treatment is directed at symptoms.

Chromosomal Disorders

Chromosomal disorders are not usually a cause of microcephaly at birth unless cerebral aplasia, such as holoprosencephaly, is part of the syndrome. Hypotonia and dysmorphism are the prominent features of chromosomal disorders in the newborn (see Chapter 5), and microcephaly becomes evident during infancy.

Defective Neurulation

At the end of the first week, a rostrocaudal axis appears on the dorsal aspect of the embryo. This axis is responsible for the subsequent induction of a neural plate, the anlage of the nervous system. The neural plate is converted into a closed neural tube during the third and fourth weeks. Defects in closure are called *dysraphic states*. The most rostral portion of the neural tube, the anterior neuropore, closes at about the 24th day.

Anencephaly

Anencephaly is the result of defective closure of the anterior neuropore, just as myelomeningocele is the result of defective closure of the posterior neuropore (see Chapter 12). The rate of each is declining. The cause of the malformations and the reason for their decline in prevalence are unknown.

CLINICAL FEATURES. Less than half of anencephalics are born alive, and those who are rarely survive the first month. The scalp is absent, and the skull is open from the vertex to the foramen magnum. The brain, appearing hemorrhagic and fibrotic, is exposed to view. It consists mainly of the hindbrain and parts of the diencephalon; the forebrain is completely lacking. The orbits are shallow, and the eyes protrude. The neck is held in retroflexion, and the proximal portions of the arms seem overgrown compared with the legs. The overall appearance of the anencephalic newborn is grotesque and described as "toad-like."

DIAGNOSIS. Following the birth of a child with a neural tube defect, the chance of anencephaly or myelomeningocele in subsequent pregnancies increases twofold to fivefold. After two affected children have been born, the chance of having another affected child doubles again. The prenatal diagnosis of dysraphic states is discussed in the section on myelomeningocele (see Chapter 12).

MANAGEMENT. No effort to prolong life should be attempted.

Encephalocele

An encephalocele is a protrusion of cortex and meninges, covered by skin, through a defect in the skull. Encephaloceles may occur in any location; however, most are midline-occipital, except in Asians, in whom the defects are usually midline-frontal.

CLINICAL FEATURES. The size of the encephalocele may range from a small protrusion to a cyst as big as the skull. When the protrusion is large, the skull is likely to be microcephalic. No conclusion can be drawn concerning the contents of the mass by its size, but an encephalocele with a sessile base is more likely to contain cerebral tissue than is one with a pedunculated base.

Encephaloceles rarely occur as a solitary cerebral malformation and are usually associated with abnormalities of the cerebral hemispheres, cerebellum, and midbrain.

DIAGNOSIS. Cranial MRI is reasonably accurate in defining the contents of the encephalocele. Despite its midline location, the protruded material is usually derived from one hemisphere that is smaller than the other and is displaced across the midline by the larger hemisphere.

MANAGEMENT. The desire to remove the encephalocele surgically should be tempered by its contents and the extent of associated anomalies. Occipital meningocele, in which the sac contains no neural tissue, should be surgically removed, and the outcome is often excellent. Children with protruded brain material and associated malformations usually die during infancy.

Defective Prosencephalization

The forebrain develops between 25 and 30 days' gestation from a midline vesicle that is generated from the closed anterior neuropore. Between 30 and 40 days' gestation, bilateral cerebral vesicles are formed by the cleavage and outpouching of the midline vesicle. The midline vesicle is the primordium of the third ventricle, and the bilateral cerebral vesicles are the primordia of the lateral ventricles.

Holoprosencephaly

A spectrum of malformations has been described as resulting from defective cleavage of the embryonic forebrain. The term *arhinencephaly* is often used to refer to the full spectrum of abnormalities, but *holoprosencephaly* is a more accurate term.

Total failure of cleavage produces a small brain with a midline vesicle covered by a horseshoe of limbic cortex. With less severe defects, the third ventricle and diencephalon differentiate, and the hemispheres are partially cleaved in the occipital lobe. The corpus callosum is hypoplastic or absent. The minimal defect (arhinencephaly) is the unilateral or bilateral absence of the olfactory bulbs and tracts associated with some degree of rhinic lobe aplasia. Hemispheric cleavage is complete, the ventricles are normal, and the corpus callosum is present in part or in total.

Holoprosencephaly may result from defects of several genes or their transcription products. An autosomal dominant form maps to the chromosome 7p36.2 locus, and a defect at the same locus results in sacral agenesis. Abnormalities of chromosome 13 account for most chromosomal abnormalities that cause holoprosencephaly (Brown et al, 1998).

CLINICAL FEATURES. Craniofacial dysplasia is almost always associated, and malformations in other organs are common. The facial deformities are primarily in the midline (cyclopia or ocular hypotelorism, flat nose, cleft lip, and cleft palate), and their severity is often predictive of the severity of the brain malformation. Associated malformations include congenital heart defects, clubbing of the hands or feet, polydactyly and syndactyly, hypoplasia of the genitourinary system, accessory spleen and liver, and malrotation of the intestine.

Most children with severe defects in cleavage of the forebrain are stillborn or die in the neonatal period. Microcephaly, hypotonia, apnea, and seizures are prominent features. Hypotonia is especially severe when the defect is associated with a chromosomal abnormality. Infants who survive have severe intellectual, motor, and sensory impairment. Children with only arhinencephaly may appear physically normal and may display minor disturbances in neurological function such as learning disabilities and seizures.

DIAGNOSIS. Holoprosencephaly should be suspected in every child with midline facial deformities, especially when malformations are present in other organs. MRI provides excellent visualization of the malformation.

MANAGEMENT. Considering the multiplicity of malformations, measures to extend life are inappropriate.

Agenesis of the Corpus Callosum

Anomalous development of the three telencephalic commissures (the corpus callosum and the anterior and hippocampal commissures) is an almost constant feature of defective prosencephalization. The prevalence of agenesis of the corpus callosum on CT is 2% to 3% in North America and 7% to 9% in Japan. Most cases are isolated malformations. Agenesis also occurs in association with other prosencephalic dysplasias and with some metabolic defects (see the section on Glycine Encephalopathy in Chapter 1) and as a solitary genetic defect. When only the corpus callosum is absent, the anterior and hippocampal commissures may be normal or enlarged. Callosal agenesis is part of the Aicardi syndrome (see Chapter 1), the *Andermann syndrome* (autosomal recessive callosal agenesis, mental deficiency, and peripheral neuropathy), and trisomies 8, 11, and 13.

CLINICAL FEATURES. Solitary agenesis of the corpus callosum is clinically inapparent except for subtle disturbances in the interhemispheric transfer of information, for which special testing is needed. Mental retardation or learning disabilities occur in most cases, and epilepsy usually indicates concurrent focal heterotopia.

DIAGNOSIS. Neuroimaging shows lateral displacement of the lateral ventricles and upward displacement of the third ventricle. Intraventricular pressure is normal.

MANAGEMENT. Treatment is directed at symptoms.

Defective Cellular Migration

When neurons that should form the superficial layers of the cerebral cortex are unable to pass through the already established deeper layers of neurons, the results are a simplification of the cortical convolutional pattern (*agyria*) and an abnormal accumulation of neurons in the white matter (*heterotopia*). Complete absence of gyri causes a smooth cerebral surface (*lissencephaly*), whereas incomplete gyral formation causes the existing convolutions to be reduced in number and enlarged (*pachygyria*).

Lissencephaly is divided into several types. Some affect only the cerebral cortex, some affect the cortex, cerebellum and brainstem, and others are combined with facial dysmorphism. The *Miller-Dieker syndrome* is characterized by microcephaly and a peculiar facies that includes micrognathia, high forehead, thin upper lip, short nose with anteverted nares, and low-set ears. A microdeletion at the 17p13.3 locus occurs in most patients with Miller-Dieker syndrome, and deletions on chromosome 17 are also shown in other lissencephaly syndromes (Dobyns, 1999). Lissencephaly is also transmitted as an X-linked dominant trait with two different phenotypes; classical lissencephaly is seen in males and bilateral periventricular nodular heterotopia (BPNH) in females (Dobyns et al, 1996).

CLINICAL FEATURES. Most children with lissencephaly are referred for evaluation of developmental delay or intractable myoclonic seizures. Many initially exhibit muscular hypotonia that later evolves into spasticity and opisthotonus. Microcephaly is not always present, but all children have mental retardation, epilepsy, and cerebral palsy. BPNH usually presents with sporadic or familial epilepsy and normal intelligence. Isolated heterotopia is an important cause of intractable epilepsy in an otherwise normal child (see Chapter 1).

DIAGNOSIS. The diagnosis is based on MRI abnormalities. A smooth cortical surface except for rudimentary sulci (agyria) may be limited to the parietal or frontal regions or encompass the whole brain. The sylvian fissure is broad and triangular, the interhemispheric fissure is widened, and nests of gray matter are present within the white matter. The ventricles may be enlarged and the corpus callosum absent. Genetic tests are available that detect the mutations on chromosomes 17 and X.

MANAGEMENT. Seizures are usually intractable but may be partially controlled by standard drugs for the management of infantile spasms or myoclonic seizures (see Chapter 1). Death often occurs during infancy, but long survival is possible.

Secondary Microcephaly

Intrauterine Disorders

Intrauterine infection is an established cause of microcephaly. Cytomegalovirus infection (see Chapter 5) can be manifest as microcephaly, without any features of systemic disease. Because maternal infection is asymptomatic, such cases are difficult to identify as being caused by cytomegalovirus disease. However, surveys of cytomegalovirus antibody demonstrate a higher rate of seropositive individuals among microcephalic than normocephalic children. This suggests that such cases do exist.

Efforts to identify environmental toxins that produce cerebral malformation have had only limited success. Drugs of abuse and several pharmaceutical agents have been implicated, but the evidence is rarely compelling. The only absolute conclusion that can be derived from an abundance of studies is that a negative impact occurs on fetuses of women whose lifestyle includes some combination of heavy alcohol or drug use, poor nutrition, and inadequate health care. This negative impact is usually expressed as intrauterine growth retardation, dysmorphic features, and microcephaly.

Aplasia of major cerebral vessels is a rare malformation of unknown cause. Brain tissue that should have been supplied by the aplastic vessels either never forms or is infarcted and replaced by calcified cystic cavities. The cavities are present at birth, and the CT appearance suggests an intrauterine infection except that the cysts conform to a vascular distribution.

Perinatal Brain Injuries

Perinatal brain injuries are an important cause of failure of brain growth during infancy when head circumference is normal at birth. The initial features of this group of disorders are neonatal encephalopathy and seizures (see Chapter 1). Children with microcephaly and mental retardation from perinatal brain injuries always have cerebral palsy and often have epilepsy. Microcephaly and mental retardation in the absence of motor impairment are always of prenatal origin.

Postnatal Systemic Disease

Infants who are chronically ill and malnourished fail to thrive. All growth is retarded, but head circumference is usually maintained better than length and weight. If body size is below the 3rd percentile, head circumference might be at the 5th or 10th percentile. If the systemic disturbance is not corrected, brain injury generally occurs, brain growth slows, and head circumference falls into the microcephalic range.

Abnormal Head Shape

Whereas the size of the skull is determined almost exclusively by its contents, the shape of the skull is the result of forces acting from within and without, and of the time of closure of the cranial sutures.

Intracranial Forces

The shape of the brain contributes to the shape of the skull by influencing the time of closure of cranial sutures. Temporal lobe agenesis results in a narrower calvarium, and cerebellar agenesis results in a small posterior fossa. Hydrocephalus produces characteristic changes in skull shape. Large lateral ventricles cause bowing of the forehead, and the Dandy-Walker malformation causes bowing of the occiput. In infants with subdural hematomas, bitemporal widening may be seen because of separation of the sagittal suture.

Extracranial Forces

Head shape may be influenced in utero by constricting forces, such as a bicornuate uterus or multiple fetuses. Physical constraint of the skull in utero may contribute to premature closure of a cranial suture, but perinatal and postnatal constraints do not. Molding of the skull is common during a prolonged vaginal delivery, but the closure of cranial sutures is unaffected. Molding does not influence eventual head shape.

In premature infants, *scaphocephaly* (Table 18-5) often develops because the poorly mineralized skull becomes flattened on one side and then the other as the child is turned back and forth. The shape of the skull becomes normal with maturity.

Table 18-5
Terms That Describe Head Shapes

Acrocephaly	High, tower-like head with vertical forehead
Brachycephaly	Broad head with recessed lower forehead
Oxycephaly	Pointed head
Plagiocephaly	Flattening of one side of head
Scaphocephaly (dolicocephaly)	Abnormally long, narrow head
Trigonocephaly	Triangular head with prominent vertical ridge in the midforehead

Table 18-6
Disorders Associated with Craniostenosis

Ataxia-telangiectasia
Familial hypophosphatemia
Hyperthyroidism
Idiopathic hypercalcemia
Mucopolysaccharidoses
Polycythemia vera
Rickets
  Renal rickets
  Vitamin D deficient
  Vitamin D resistant
Sickle cell disease
Thalassemia major

Plagiocephaly or occipital flattening is a frequent finding in hypotonic infants. This is caused by constantly lying in the same position. The hair over the flattened portion of skull is usually sparse from rubbing against the bed surface. A normal head shape is resumed if the infant's lying position can be changed.

Craniostenosis

Craniostenosis and *craniosynostosis* are terms used for premature closure of one or more cranial sutures; the result is always an abnormal skull shape. These terms should be applied only to infants in whom the sutures close while the brain is growing. Early closure of sutures in infants with microcephaly is not premature because the intracranial pressure required to keep sutures apart is lacking.

Most cases of craniostenosis are sporadic and of uncertain etiology. Autosomal dominant and recessive forms of single-suture closure occur. Autosomal dominant inheritance is more common than autosomal recessive inheritance but is also more easily identified as hereditary. Many sporadic cases could represent autosomal recessive inheritance.

Craniostenosis may be one feature of a larger recognized syndrome of chromosomal or genetic abnormality. Genetic disorders are often associated with syndactyly or polydactyly (see the section on Acrocephalosyndactyly later in this chapter), whereas chromosomal disorders are usually characterized by other limb malformations and growth retardation.

Craniostenosis is also reported in association with other disorders (Table 18-6). Some of these associations are coincidental, but a cause-and-effect relationship probably does exist with metabolic disorders of bone.

CLINICAL FEATURES. In nonsyndromic craniostenosis, the only clinical feature is an abnormal head shape. Normal bone growth is impaired in a plane perpendicular to the fused sutures but is able to occur in a parallel plane. Scaphocephaly is caused by premature fusion of the sagittal suture, brachycephaly by fusion of both coronal sutures, plagiocephaly by fusion of one coronal or one lambdoid suture, trigonocephaly by fusion of the metopic suture, and oxycephaly by fusion of all sutures.

When several sutures close prematurely, the growing brain is constricted and symptoms of increased intracranial pressure develop. Communicating and noncommunicating hydrocephalus occur more frequently in children with craniostenosis than in normal children. It is more likely that a common underlying factor causes both rather than one causing the other.

Two-suture craniostenosis is common. The sagittal suture is almost always involved, in combination with either the metopic or coronal suture (Chumas et al, 1997).

DIAGNOSIS. Visual inspection of the skull and palpation of the sutures are sufficient for diagnosis in most cases of one- or two-suture craniostenosis. Radiography of the skull shows a band of increased density at the site of the prematurely closed sutures. CT is indicated in all children with craniostenosis of multiple sutures and in children with craniostenosis of a single suture if hydrocephalus is suspected.

MANAGEMENT. The two indications for surgery to correct craniostenosis are to improve the appearance of the head and to relieve increased intracranial pressure. The cosmetic indication should be used sparingly and only to make severe deformities less noticeable.

Acrocephalosyndactyly

Acrocephalosyndactyly is characterized by the combination of craniostenosis and fusion of fingers and toes. Some degree of mental retardation is often present.

Apert syndrome is characterized by syndactyly and premature closure of the coronal suture resulting in brachycephaly. The gene abnormality, inherited as a dominant trait, is a mutation in the gene encoding fibroblast growth factor receptor-2 (10q26). The forehead is high and prominent, and the face is similar to but less severely deformed than the face in Crouzon disease. Agenesis of the corpus callosum and limbic

structures may be an associated feature. The IQ is greater than 70 in 50% of the children who have a skull decompression before 1 year of age versus only 7% in those operated on later in life (Reiner et al, 1996).

Carpenter syndrome differs from Apert syndrome because it is transmitted by autosomal recessive inheritance and the patient has polydactyly as well as syndactyly, premature closure of all sutures, obesity, and hypogonadism. Approximately 75% of patients are retarded secondary to cerebral malformations that are demonstrable on MRI.

Crouzon Disease (Craniofacial Dysostosis)

Crouzon disease is the combination of premature closure of any or all cranial sutures and maldevelopment of facial bones. The disorder is caused by mutations in the gene for fibroblast growth factor receptor-2 and is transmitted by autosomal dominant inheritance.

CLINICAL FEATURES. The facial deformity is present at birth and becomes worse during infancy. The skull is usually widened anteriorly as a result of premature closure of the coronal suture. The eyes are widely separated and prominent, but the lower face appears recessed because of maxillary hypoplasia and prognathism. Adding to the deformity are a beak-like nose and a large, protuberant tongue. Intracranial pressure is often increased because several cranial sutures are usually involved.

DIAGNOSIS. The typical facies and genetic pattern of inheritance are diagnostic. Cranial CT is indicated in every case to follow the progression of cerebral compression.

MANAGEMENT. A sequential neurosurgical and plastic surgical approach has been successful in opening the sutures to relieve intracranial pressure and in advancing the facial bones forward to improve the cosmetic appearance.

References

Arbour L, Watters GV, Hall JG, et al. Multifactorial inheritance of non-syndromic macrocephaly. *Clin Genet* 1996;50:57–62.

Brown SA, Warburton D, Brown LY, et al. Holoprosencephaly due to mutations in Zic2, a homologue of *Drosophila* odd-paired. *Nat Genet* 1998;20:180–183.

Cavalcanti DP, Salomao MA. Dandy-Walker malformation with postaxial polydactyly: Further evidence for autosomal recessive inheritance. *Am J Med Genet* 1999; 85:83–184.

Chumas PD, Cinalli G, Arnaud E, et al. Classification of previously unclassified cases of craniosynostosis. *J Neurosurg* 1997;86:177–181.

Dobyns WB. Lissencephaly and Subcortical Band Heterotopia (Agyria-Pachygyria-Band Spectrum): Overview. In: GeneClinics: Medical Genetic Knowledge Base. University of Washington, Seattle (http://www.geneclinics.org). accessed 4 October 1999.

Dobyns WB, Andermann E, Andermann F, et al. X-linked malformations of neuronal migration. *Neurology* 1996; 47:331–339.

Dodge NN, Dobyns WB. Agenesis of the corpus callosum and Dandy-Walker malformation associated with hemimegalencephaly in the sebaceous nevus syndrome. *Am J Med Genet* 1995;56:147–150.

Griebel ML, Williams JP, Russell SS, et al. Clinical and developmental findings in children with giant interhemispheric cysts and dysgenesis of the corpus callosum. *Pediatr Neurol* 1995;13:119–124.

Haverkamp F, Wolfle J, Aretz M, et al. Congenital hydrocephalus internus and aqueduct stenosis: Aetiology and implications for genetic counseling. *Eur J Pediatr* 1999;158:474–478.

Hunt CE, Puczynski MS. Does supine sleeping cause asymmetrical heads? *Pediatrics* 1996;98:127–129.

Jackson AP, McHale DP, Campbell DA, et al. Primary autosomal recessive microcephaly (MCPH1) maps to chromosome 8p22-pter. *Am J Hum Genet* 1998;63:541–546.

Kuster W, Ehrig T, Happle R. Hypomelanosis of Ito: No entity, but a cutaneous sign of mosaicism. In: Nordlund JJ, Boissy R, Hearing V, King R, Ortonne JP eds. *The Pigmentary System and Its Disorders*. New York: Oxford University Press, 1998:594–601.

Lachman RS. Neurologic abnormalities in the skeletal dysplasias: A clinical and radiological perspective. *Am J Med Genet* 1997;69:33–43.

McGaughran JM, Kuna P, Das V. Audiological abnormalities in the Klippel-Feil syndrome. *Arch Dis Child* 1998; 79:352–355.

Opitz JM, Weaver DW, Reynolds JF Jr. The syndromes of Sotos and Weaver: Reports and review. *Am J Med Genet* 1998;79:294–304.

Reiner D, Arnaud E, Cinalli G, et al. Prognosis for mental function in Apert's syndrome. *J Neurosurg* 1996; 85:66–72.

Schrander-Stumple C, Fryns J-P. Congenital hydrocephalus: Nosology and guidelines for clinical approach and genetic counseling. *Eur J Pediatr* 1998;157:355–362.

van der Knaap MS, Barth PG, Stroink H, et al. Leukoencephalopathy with swelling and a discrepantly mild clinical course in eight children. Ann Neurol 1995;37:324–334.

Index

Note: Pages in *italic* indicate illustrations; those followed by t refer to tables.